Third Edition

Critical Care

C E R T I F I C A T I O N
PREPARATION & REVIEW

Thomas Ahrens, RN, DNS, CCRN
Clinical Specialist in Critical Care
Barnes Hospital
St. Louis, Missouri

Donna Prentice, RN, MSN(R), CCRN, TNS
Clinical Specialist in Critical Care
Barnes Hospital
St. Louis, Missouri

APPLETON & LANGE
Norwalk, Connecticut

0-8385-1251-8

Copyright © 1993 by Appleton & Lange
Simon & Schuster Business and Professional Group
Previous editions © 1991, © 1984 by Appleton & Lange

93 94 95 96 97 / 10 9 8 7 6 5 4 3 2 1

Prentice Hall International (UK) Limited, *London*
Prentice Hall of Australia Pty. Limited, *Sydney*
Prentice Hall Canada, Inc., *Toronto*
Prentice Hall Hispanoamericana, S.A., *Mexico*
Prentice Hall of India Private Limited, *New Delhi*
Prentice Hall of Japan, Inc., *Tokyo*
Simon & Schuster Asia Pte. Ltd., *Singapore*
Editora Prentice Hall do Brasil Ltda., *Rio de Janeiro*
Prentice Hall, *Englewood Cliffs, New Jersey*

Library of Congress Cataloging-in-Publication Data

Ahrens, Thomas.
    Critical care, certification preparation & review. — Ed. 3/
Thomas Ahrens, Donna Prentice.
        p.   cm.
    Includes bibliographical references and index.
    ISBN 0-8385-1251-8
    1. Intensive care nursing. I. Prentice, Donna. II. Title.
III. Title: Critical care. IV. Title: Critical care, certification
preparation and review.
    [DNLM: 1. Critical Care—nurses' instruction.   WY 154 A287c 1993]
RT120.I5A392   1993
610.73′61—dc20   92-48534
DNLM/DLC   CIP
for Library of Congress

Contributors

Thomas S. Ahrens, RN, DNS, CCRN
Clinical Specialist—Critical Care
Barnes Hospital
St. Louis, Missouri

Donna Prentice, RN, MSN(R), CCRN, TNS
Clinical Specialist—Critical Care
Barnes Hospital
St. Louis, Missouri

Patricia A. Ahrens, RN
Staff/Charge Nurse—Emergency Department
St. Mary's Medical Center
St. Louis, Missouri

Pamela Becker-Weilitz, RN, MSN(R)
Clinical Specialist—Pulmonary
Specialist in Critical Care
Manager
Barnes Hospital
St. Louis, Missouri

Nelda K. Martin, RN, MSN, CCRN
Clinical Specialist—Cardiology
Barnes Hospital
St. Louis, Missouri

Lori Geisman, RN, MSN(R), CCRN
Clinical Specialist
Specialist in Critical Care
St. Louis, Missouri

Paula Goldberg, RN, MSN
Clinical Specialist—Oncology
Barnes Hospital
St. Louis, Missouri

Teresa Halloran, RN, MSN, CCRN
Head Nurse
St. Johns Medical Center
St. Louis, Missouri

Deborah Klein, RN, MSN, CCRN
Clinical Specialist—Critical Care
Metro Health Medical Center
Cleveland, Ohio

To Pat. You have been my teacher in matters that are really important. TSA

To Michael for his continued love and support and to Alex and Nicole, whose precious smiles make anything possible. DP

Reviewers

Captain Mary Ellen Frantz, RN, MSN, CCRN
Clinical Specialist—Critical Care
Scott Air Force Base, Illinois

Mitch Mahon, RN, BSN
Nurse Clinician
Barnes Hospital
St. Louis, Missouri

Lisa Meyer-Mayfield, RN, BSN
Barnes Hospital
St. Louis, Missouri

Shawn E. Ray, RN, BSN, CCRN
Head Nurse—Surgical ICU
Barnes Hospital
St. Louis, Missouri

Kim Tucker, RN, BSN, CCRN
Head Nurse—Medical ICU
Barnes Hospital
St. Louis, Missouri

First and Second Edition Contributors

Doris Wilmsmeyer Conn, RN, MN, OCN
Clinical Specialist
Barnes Hospital
St. Louis, Missouri

Lori Kohles Geisman, RN, MSN(R), CCRN
Nurse Clinician
Barnes Hospital
St. Louis, Missouri

Richard Abels Geisman, MD
Gastroenterologist
Member of the Boonslick Medical Group
St. Charles, Missouri

Dot Langfitt, RN, MSN
Columbia, South Carolina

Mary Ann Shea, JD, RN
Private Practice
St. Louis, Missouri

Susan Smith, RN, MSN, CCRN
Clinical Specialist
Emory University
Atlanta, Georgia

Contents

Preface xi

Acknowledgments xiii

PART I: CARDIOVASCULAR 1

Chapter 1
Cardiac Anatomy 3

Chapter 2
Cardiac Physiology 15

Chapter 3
The Normal ECG 23

Chapter 4
Sinus and Atrial Dysrhythmias 31

Chapter 5
AV Node and Ventricular
    Dysrhythmias 41

Chapter 6
Angina Pectoris and Myocardial
    Infarction 61

Chapter 7
Congestive Heart Failure,
    Pulmonary Edema, and
    Pericarditis 69

Chapter 8
Hemorrhagic (Hypovolemic) and
    Cardiogenic Shock 75

Chapter 9
Cardiac and Vascular Surgery 85

Bibliography 91

PART II: PULMONARY 93

Chapter 10
Pulmonary Anatomy 95

Chapter 11
Pulmonary Physiology 109

Chapter 12
Acute Respiratory Failure and
    Adult Respiratory Distress 127

Chapter 13
Chronic Obstructive Pulmonary
    Disease and Status Asthmaticus 135

Chapter 14
Pulmonary Embolism and
    Chest Trauma 141

Bibliography 152

PART III: NEUROLOGY 155

Chapter 15
Anatomy of the Nervous System 157

Chapter 16
Physiology of the Nervous System 175

Chapter 17
The Vertebrae and the Spinal Cord:
    Function and Dysfunction 181

Chapter 18
Acute Head Injuries and Craniotomies 191

Chapter 19
Meningitis, Guillain-Barré Syndrome,
    and Myasthenia Gravis 201

Chapter 20
Seizures, Status Epilepticus,
    Cerebrovascular Accidents 207

Chapter 21
Intracranial Pressure, Aneurysm,
    Coma, and Brain Herniation 213

Bibliography 228

PART IV: GASTROENTEROLOGY 229

Chapter 22
Anatomy and Physiology of the
Gastrointestinal System 231

Chapter 23
Gastrointestinal Hemorrhage and
Esophageal Varices 255

Chapter 24
Viral Hepatitis 261

Chapter 25
Cirrhosis, Hepatic Failure, and
Pancreatitis 265

Chapter 26
Intestinal Infarction, Obstruction,
and Perforation 271

Chapter 27
Gastrointestinal Surgery and
Treatment 275

Bibliography 283

PART V: RENAL 285

Chapter 28
Anatomy of the Renal System 287

Chapter 29
Physiology of the Renal System 293

Chapter 30
Renal Regulation of Electrolytes
and Electrolyte Imbalances 303

Chapter 31
Acute Renal Failure 313

Chapter 32
Dialysis 317

Bibliography 324

PART VI: ENDOCRINE 327

Chapter 33
Introduction to the Endocrine
System 329

Chapter 34
Anatomy, Physiology, and
Dysfunction of the Pituitary
Gland 335

Chapter 35
Anatomy, Physiology, and
Dysfunction of the Thyroid and
Parathyroid Glands 343

Chapter 36
Anatomy, Physiology, and
Dysfunction of the Adrenal
Glands 351

Chapter 37
Anatomy, Physiology, and
Dysfunction of the Pancreas 359

Bibliography 363

**PART VII: IMMUNOLOGY AND
HEMATOLOGY** 365

Chapter 38
Introduction to Immunology and
Hematology 367

Chapter 39
Blood and Component Therapy 383

Chapter 40
Normal Coagulation and Pathologic
Hematologic Conditions 387

Chapter 41
Disorders of the Immune System 399

Bibliography 409

**PART VIII: MULTISYSTEM PATIENT-
CARE PROBLEMS** 411

Chapter 42
Burns and Toxicology 413

Chapter 43
Sepsis and Multiple Organ
Dysfunction Syndrome 431

Bibliography 438

Index 441

Preface

The successful completion of the Critical Care Registered Nurse (CCRN) examination offered by the American Association of Critical Care Nurses (AACN) is both a personal and professional mark of achievement. Nurses who have passed the examination earn the right to list the prized CCRN credential after their name. CCRN certification carries the distinction of beginning excellence in the area of critical care nursing and marks the achievement of proficiency as defined by AACN in the area of critical care nursing.

The CCRN examination requires knowledge of eight conceptual areas as defined by the AACN Certification Corporation. These areas are cardiovascular, neurology, pulmonary, renal, gastroenterology, immunology, hematology, endocrine, and multisystem patient-care problems. Unfortunately, essential knowledge of these eight areas is not necessarily easy to acquire. Undergraduate education does not consistently teach critical care concepts, and clinical experience teaches practical content but not thorough learning in the eight conceptual areas necessary for the CCRN examination.

This text is an attempt to help any nurse interested in passing the CCRN examination attain that goal. The book is written with two purposes: to provide information that is likely to be seen on the CCRN examination and to provide information that is useful in clinical settings and valuable beyond the CCRN examination. The reason for the second purpose is less obvious but just as important as passing the test. For any nurse to retain enough information to pass the test, she or he must study intensely before the examination to learn material presented in the CCRN examination and use the information in practice. Application of the material presented in this text in the clinical setting will allow both better retention of content and improvement in patient care. The improved nursing practices that lead to improved patient care are actually what the certification examination is all about. This text attempts to help

realize the goal of improving your knowledge so you can both pass the CCRN examination and apply the material to practice settings. Ultimately, patient care will be improved through your increased knowledge.

To help you pass the test, content experts (who have passed the CCRN examination) in each of the major areas tested have reviewed the original text. Included in each chapter are Editor's Notes which highlight how important each section is likely to be for the CCRN examination. Some sections have been edited and updated and others completely redone in an attempt to maintain the currency of the text. The information is current and based on both recent research and standard practice. As a rule, the CCRN examination does not necessarily require an in-depth understanding of recent research.

One key point must be remembered when preparing in each content area. The areas in which you are weak will require extra preparation. Study these sections in the text closely. Content areas in which you believe you are strong can be tested by using the practice examination text written in conjunction with this text. If you can score 80 percent or better on the content areas in the practice examinations, you should be prepared in that content area. At that point, concentrate on content areas in which you may not be as strong.

REFERENCES IN THE TEXT

The references included in bibliography lists at the end of each section are intended to provide you with supplemental reading if points in the text are not clear. Because this text covers most of the content that will be addressed on the examination, you should not have to use outside readings to any great extent.

This text, however, like any general text, is not meant to contain a comprehensive review of any one topic. If you would like more material than is in this text, please consult the bibliography lists. Many questions from the examination may be derived from articles in *Heart & Lung, Focus on Critical Care, Critical Care Nurse,* and *American Journal of Critical Care.* Review articles from these journals first if you have questions about a particular topic. If an article is not listed for the area in which you have questions, you may need to refer to other general references. General texts that are listed, however, are intended as a source for background reading in the content area, and not for specific information.

STANDARDS FOR PASSING THE EXAMINATION

To pass the CCRN examination, you will have to achieve a minimum passing score of 130 on a scaled examination. This does not mean that you must get 130 out of 200 correct. It means you must score adequately in all areas. It is difficult to identify how well you must score on practice examinations (such as those written to supplement this text) to give some degree of confidence in passing the CCRN examination. Although there are no guarantees, if you can achieve a 70 to 80 percent success rate for each content area in the practice examination text, your chances of passing are good.

Different versions of the test exist, possibly with different levels of difficulty. The scaled examination, however, compensates for a more difficult examination by requiring fewer correct answers. In any event, the scaled score of 130 must be achieved.

Each content area is represented, but in differing percentages on the test. The percent each content area represents on the examination and the approximate numbers of questions in each examination are listed below:

Cardiovascular	39% of the test	78 questions
Pulmonary	22% of the test	44 questions
Multisystem Problems	10% of the test	20 questions
Neurology	8% of the test	16 questions
Gastroenterology	8% of the test	16 questions
Renal	5% of the test	10 questions
Immunology/ Hematology	4% of the test	8 questions
Endocrine	4% of the test	8 questions

You must attain a cumulative score high enough to reach 130. Doing well in cardiopulmonary, for example, will not be enough if you do poorly in neurology, renal, and gastroenterology. You should not have any areas of great weakness. Strong scores in one section can offset some weak areas but to a limited extent. You cannot rely on being strong in a few areas to pull you through the test.

Successful completion of the CCRN examination is an important step for your career. You can best prepare for taking the examination by noting the following tips.

TIPS ON TEST TAKING

1. Study the material well before the examination and try to employ the knowledge in clinical practice. This will reinforce retention of the information.
2. Reread the sections the week before the examination.
3. Make an effort to feel physically and psychologically strong before the test. Do this by getting a good night's sleep and eating balanced meals before the examination. Do not attempt to study the morning of the test because this usually serves to confuse you.
4. Answer all the questions as you go through the test. Do not leave any blank because this may cause you to misnumber answers. Make a note on a separate paper of any questions you cannot answer. As a rule, however, avoid changing answers. Your first impression is usually correct.
5. During the test, remember you will not answer every question correctly. Do not worry about missing a few questions. A few questions that truly are unknown to you are best answered with a guess; then move on.
6. Review the test in case you misread a question. Change only those answers in which the question was originally misunderstood.

Acknowledgments

This text is a revision of the 2nd edition, which was a combination of Dot Langfitt's original text, *Critical Care Certification: Preparation and Review* (1984) and an update of that text. This current edition is adapted to meet changes in the CCRN examination, primarily through expanding the cardiovascular and pulmonary component, streamlining other chapters that have been reduced in content, and adding chapters on multisystem patient care problems. The authors contributing sections in this text are active practitioners in critical care and are frequent lecturers in CCRN review courses. We wish to thank the contributors for their work, as well as the readers of the past editions, whose comments have resulted in an improved text. We also wish to thank the Nursing Service department at Barnes Hospital for their support during the making of this edition.

PART 1

Cardiovascular

Thomas S. Ahrens, RN, DNS, CCRN
Nelda K. Martin, RN, MSN, CCRN

CHAPTER 1

Cardiac Anatomy

Editor's Note

*As with much of the CCRN test, a good under-
standing of anatomy and physiology will provide
one of the best resources for passing the exam.
The following two chapters are a brief review of
key anatomical and physiological cardiovascular
concepts that should prove useful in taking the
test. These chapters contain a review that addresses background information on cardiovascular
concepts sometimes found on the CCRN exam.
Although basic anatomy is not commonly addressed on a CCRN exam, an understanding of
principles of anatomy may help your perception
of more specific questions regarding cardiovascular concepts. If you do not have a strong background in anatomy and physiology, study this
section closely. You may want to review the cardiovascular sections of physiology textbooks as
well. **In addition, this chapter contains information on physical assessment as it relates to anatomical and clinical conditions. Review this
section carefully, since a few questions may be
drawn from this content area.***

*The CCRN test places the most emphasis on
the cardiovascular component, with approximately 39% of the test questions in this content
area. While many nurses are relatively strong in
cardiovascular concepts, do not take this part of
the exam lightly. The better you perform in any
one area, the greater your chances of overall success on the exam.*

NORMAL LOCATION AND SIZE OF THE HEART

The heart lies in the mediastinum, above the diaphragm
and surrounded on both sides by the lungs. If one looks
at a frontal (anterior) view, the heart resembles a triangle (Fig. 1-1). The base of the heart is parallel to the
right edge of the sternum, whereas the lower right
point of the triangle represents the apex of the heart.
The apex is usually at the left midclavicular line at the
fifth intraclavicular space. The average adult heart is
about 5 inches long and $3^1/_2$ inches wide, about the size
of an average man's clenched fist. The heart weighs
about 2 grams for each pound of ideal body weight.

NORMAL ANATOMY OF THE HEART

The heart is supported by a fibrous skeleton (Fig. 1-2)
composed of dense connective tissue. This fibrous
skeleton connects the four valve rings (annuli) of
the heart: the tricuspid, mitral, pulmonic, and aortic
valves. Attached to the superior (top) surface of this
fibrous skeleton are the right and left atria, the pulmonary artery, and the aorta. Attached to the inferior
(lower) surface of the fibrous skeleton are the right and
left ventricles and the mitral and tricuspid valve cusps.

The heart can be studied as two parallel pumps:
the right pump (right atrium and ventricle) and the left
pump (left atrium and ventricle). Each pump receives
blood into its atrium. The blood flows from atria
through a one-way valve into the ventricles. From each
ventricle, blood is ejected into a circulatory system.
The right ventricle ejects blood into the pulmonary
circulation, while the left ventricle ejects blood into
the systemic circulation. Although the right and left
heart have differences, the gross anatomy of each is
similar. Structural features of each chamber are discussed below.

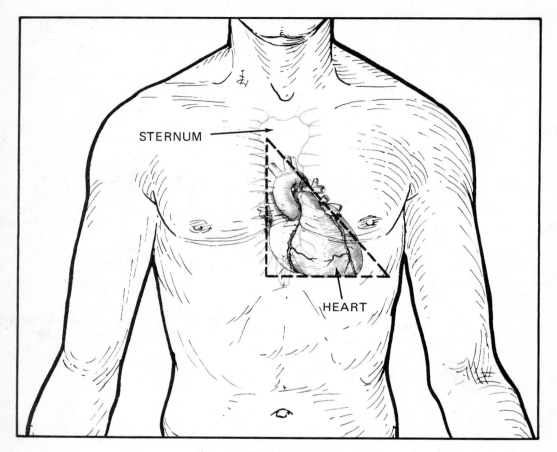

Figure 1-1. Frontal view of the heart.

STRUCTURE OF THE HEART WALL

The heart is enclosed in a fibrous sac called the pericardium. The pericardium is composed of two layers. The fibrous pericardium is the outer layer that helps support the heart. The inside layer is a smooth fibrous membrane called the parietal pericardium.

Next to the parietal serous layer of the pericardium is a visceral layer, which is actually the outer heart surface. It is most often termed the epicardium. Between the epicardium and the parietal pericardium is 10 to 20 milliliters of fluid, which prevents friction during heart contraction and relaxation.

The myocardium is the muscle mass of the heart composed of cardiac muscle, which has characteristics of both smooth and skeletal muscles. The endocardium

is the inner surface of the heart wall. It is a membranous covering that lines all of the heart chambers and the valves.

Papillary muscles originate in the ventricular endocardium and attach to chordae tendineae (Fig. 1-3). The chordae tendineae attach to the inferior surface of the tricuspid and mitral valve cusps to enable the valves to open and close. The papillary muscles are in parallel alignment to the ventricular wall.

CARDIAC MUSCLE CELLS

The information in this section regarding cellular aspects of cardiac muscle anatomy and physiology is not likely to be on the CCRN test. Any questions on this

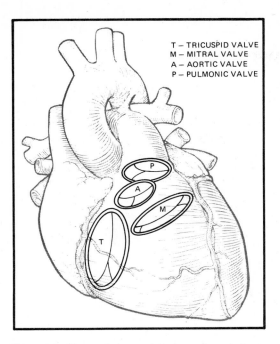

T – TRICUSPID VALVE
M – MITRAL VALVE
A – AORTIC VALVE
P – PULMONIC VALVE

Figure 1-2. Fibrous skeleton of the heart (frontal view).

cium ions) is an intracellular network of channels surrounding the myofibrils. These channels comprise the longitudinal (L-tubule) system of the myofibrils.

Myofibrils are thick and thin parts of the muscle fiber. Thick fibrils are myosin filaments. They have regularly placed projections that form calcium gates to the thick myofibrils. The thin myofibrils are actin. The myosin and actin myofibrils are arranged in specific parallel and hexagonal patterns (Fig. 1-5). This arrangement of fibers forms a syncytium that results in all of the fibers depolarizing when even one fiber is depolarized. This is known as the "all or none" principle—all fibers will depolarize or no fibers depolarize.

Troponin and tropomyosin are regulatory proteins attached to or affecting actin. These thick and thin myofibrils slide back and forth over each other, resulting in contraction and relaxation of the sarcomeres and, thus, the heart.

The study of physiology of the cardiac cycle examines the means by which the heart pumps blood and the various mechanisms that control the heart pump. Before looking at the heart as a whole, let us examine the contraction of a single sarcomere.

area are usually infrequent. However, the concepts addressed in this section form the basis for myocardial dysfunction and pharmacologic intervention. Read this section with the intent of becoming familiar with the concepts but not necessarily focusing on memorizing specific details.

The sarcomere (Fig. 1-4) is the contracting unit of the myocardium. The outer covering of the sarcomere is the sarcolemma, which surrounds the muscle fiber. The sarcolemma covers a muscle fiber that is composed of thick and thin fibers often collectively called myofibrils. Sarcomeres are separated from each other by a thickening of the sarcolemma at the ends of the sarcomere. These thickened ends, called intercalated discs, are actively involved in cardiac contraction. Each sarcomere has a centrally placed nucleus surrounded by sarcoplasma.

The sarcolemma invaginates into the sarcomere at regular intervals, resulting in a vertical penetration through the muscle fibrils coming into contact with both the thick and thin fibrils. These invaginations form the T tubules. Closely related to, but not continuous with, the T-tubule system is the sarcoplasmic reticulum. The sarcoplasmic reticulum (containing cal-

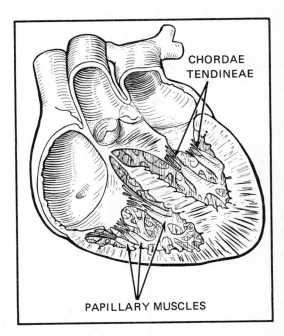

CHORDAE
TENDINEAE

PAPILLARY MUSCLES

Figure 1-3. Papillary muscles and chordae tendineae.

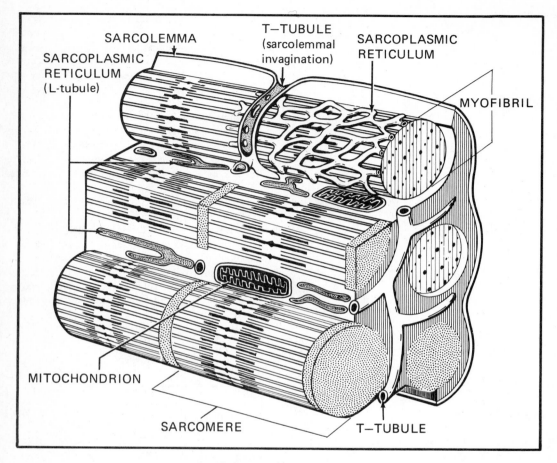

Figure 1-4. The sarcomere.

CONTRACTION OF THE SARCOMERE

The sarcomeres are much like striated muscles, but they have more mitochondria than do striated or smooth muscles. The mitochondria provide the energy

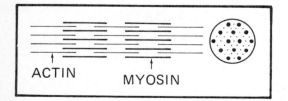

Figure 1-5. Arrangement of myosin and actin myofibrils.

for the sarcomeres to contract. This energy is released by converting adenosine triphosphate (ATP) into adenosine diphosphate (ADP). In addition, the mitochondria are crucial in the storing of energy through the formation of ATP from ADP. The adding of a phosphate molecule to ADP to form ATP is called phosphorylation. This formation of ADP from ATP normally takes place in the presence of oxygen (aerobic metabolism) and is referred to as oxidative phosphorylation. Energy can be produced without oxygen (anaerobic metabolism) but not as efficiently as during aerobic metabolism. Cardiac muscle cells are highly dependent on constant blood flow to maintain adequate supplies of oxygen for the formation of ATP.

In the sarcomere, thick (myosin) and thin (actin)

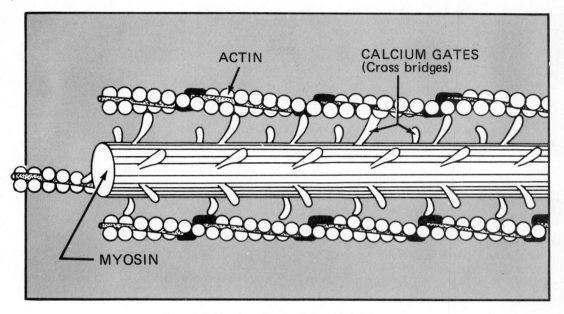

Figure 1-6. Myosin and actin fibrils with calcium gates.

fibrils are arranged side by side in parallel rows. The myosin fibrils have projections that make contact with actin at specific points. These contact points are referred to as calcium gates (Fig. 1-6). During cardiac contraction, the myosin and actin slide together and overlap to as great an extent as possible (Fig. 1-7). (In the normal resting state, there is some overlapping of the myosin and actin fibrils.) Troponin and tropomyo-sin are protein rods interwoven around the actin fibril, having a regulatory effect upon the actin and its ability to connect with the calcium gates in the presence of calcium ions.

At the start of cellular excitation leading to a contraction, calcium ions (Ca^{++}) attach to troponin molecules around the actin fibril. This enables the projections (calcium gates) of the myosin fibril to attach to

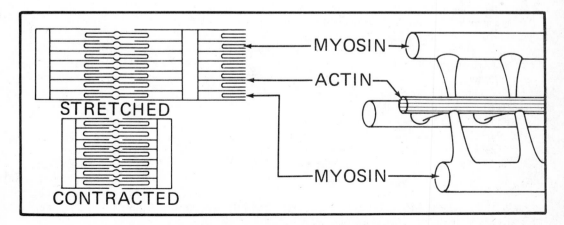

Figure 1-7. Contraction of the myosin and actin fibrils.

the actin. These projections twist around, causing a sliding of the fibers over each other. The calcium is removed from the calcium gates by calcium pumps located throughout the sarcoplasmic reticulum. As soon as the calcium is removed, the myosin and actin fibers slide back to their original position. This process repeats, causing contraction and relaxation of the cardiac cell.

It is important to remember that calcium initiates and regulates the sarcomere depolarization and repolarization. The role of calcium in the contraction and relaxation of the cardiac muscle cell serves as the basis for several cardiac therapies, including the use of calcium channel blocking agents and the potential inotropic (strength) value in administering calcium.

Even though calcium ions initiate the sliding movement of the fibrils, calcium alone is not able to cause the contraction. In addition to the presence of calcium, an exchange of ions (creating electrical energy) must occur during phases of depolarization and repolarization. This ionic exchange is mainly between sodium and potassium, which creates an ionic action potential. The exchange of chemical elements occurs across the semipermeable cell membrane in three ways: filtration, osmosis, and diffusion (active or passing).

ACTION POTENTIAL OF THE CARDIAC CELL

There are five phases of activity during the cardiac cell cycle; each phase is described below. The exchange and concentration of ions differ in each phase. Mainly four ions are involved: sodium (Na^+), potassium (K^+), calcium (Ca^{++}), and chloride (Cl^-). Normally, there is more sodium, calcium, and chloride outside the cell and more potassium inside the cell. Since all ions have an electrical charge, an electrical gradient is established. When a state of ionic electrical neutrality exists, there is a relative impermeability of the cell membrane, a period known as the resting potential. The presence of an electrical and chemical (ion) gradient plus membrane selectively establishes an action potential consisting of five phases, phase 0 through phase 4.

Phase 0

As a result of the presence of sodium and potassium outside and inside the cell, respectively, an electronegative gradient occurs. A depolarizing stimulus is caused by afflux of potassium from the cell, increasing the cell permeability for sodium. Calcium ions in the T-tubule and L-tubule systems of the sarcomere are at Ca^{++} gates on the cell membrane and "open" the gates for the influx of sodium. When this gradient reaches about -90 millivolts (mV) inside the cell, there is a rapid increase of the action potential (zero in Fig. 1-8). The result of the depolarization stimulus is an increase in the cell permeability for sodium. As the sodium threshold (the point at which sodium moves most freely) is reached (about -55 mV), sodium rushes into the cell and depolarizes it. Actually, more sodium rushes in than the amount required to reach electrical neutrality (zero). The cell becomes electropositive at about $+20$ to 30 mV, causing a spike on the action potential diagram.

Phase 1

This is the spike phase of positive electrical charge. There is a brief period of rapid repolarization (tip of spike to #1 in Fig. 1-8), which is probably due to a flow of chloride ions into the cell.

Phase 2

This is a plateau phase of repolarization. Calcium entering the cell and potassium leaving the cell balance each other, so there is no net electrical change and thus a flat line (plateau) appears. Sodium entry into the cell is almost completely inactivated. A slow movement on calcium into the cell begins (phase 2 in Fig. 1-8). Also, a small amount of potassium begins leaving the cell at this point.

Phase 3

This is a rapid decline phase of repolarization (phase 3 in Fig. 1-8). Potassium loss from the cell is greatest in this phase. This potassium loss returns the cell to electronegativity. Sodium and calcium currents are completely inactivated.

Phase 4

This is the resting interval between action potentials (phase 4 in Fig. 1-8). The sodium/potassium pumps (diffusely spread throughout the sarcomere) are the most active here in effecting an exchange of position of potassium for sodium across the cell membrane. Potassium continues to leave the cell, and when electronegativity reaches -90 mV, phase 0 starts again if a stimulus occurs.

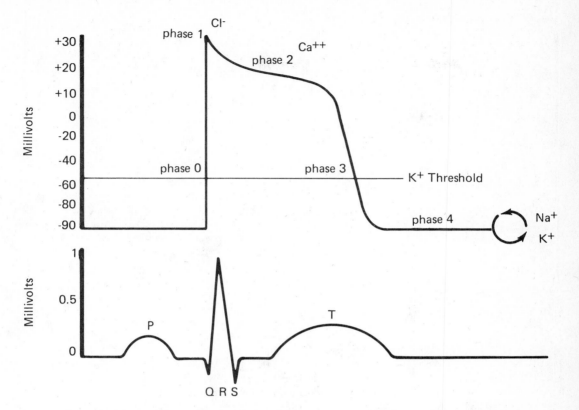

Figure 1-8. Phases of the cardiac potential and ion movement correlated with the ECG tracing.

HEART CHAMBERS

There are four chambers in the heart (Fig. 1-9). The atria are superior to the ventricles and are separated from the ventricles by valves. The right atrium and ventricle are separated from the left atrium and ventricle by the atrial and ventricular septum.

Right Atrium

The right atrium (RA) is a thin-walled chamber exposed to low blood pressures. Systemic venous blood from the head, neck, and thorax enters the right atrium from the superior vena cava. Systemic venous blood from the remainder of the body enters from the inferior vena cava. Venous blood from the heart enters the right atrium through the thebesian veins, which drain into the coronary sinus. The coronary sinus is located on the medial right atrial wall just about the tricuspid valve.

Right Ventricle

The right ventricle (RV) is the pump for the right heart. The right ventricle contracts to pump venous blood into the pulmonary artery and to the lungs. The lungs are normally a low-pressure system. The right ventricle is shaped and functions like a bellows to propel blood out during contraction.

Left Atrium

The left atrium (LA), just like the right, is thin walled. Blood flowing passively from the low-lung-pressure area does not stress the walls of the left atrium. The left atrium receives oxygenated blood from the four pulmonary veins.

Left Ventricle

The left ventricle (LV) is the major pump for the entire body. As such, it must have thick, strong walls. To overcome the high pressure of the systemic circulation,

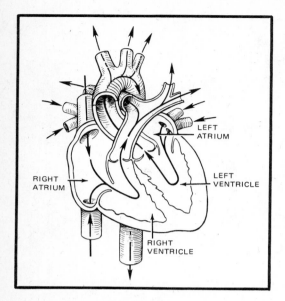

Figure 1-9. Four chambers of the heart.

the left ventricle is shaped like a cylinder. As it contracts (starting from the apex), it also narrows somewhat. This cylindrical shape provides strong physical force to propel blood into the aorta with sufficient force to overcome the high systemic pressure (resulting from the requirement to pump the blood to distant body areas).

HEART VALVES

There are two types of valves in the heart: the atrioventricular and the semilunar valves. All valves in the heart are unidirectional, unless they are diseased or dysfunctional. Normally the valves provide very little resistance to cardiac contractions. If the valves become narrow (stenotic) or allow blood to flow past when the valves should be closed (regurgitation), the work of the heart will substantially increase.

Atrioventricular Valves

The atrioventricular valves of the heart are the tricuspid and the mitral valves. These valves allow blood to flow from the atria into the ventricles during atrial contraction and ventricular diastole. Mnemonics may help you remember which valve is on which side of the heart. Consider the following: "L" and "M" come to-

gether in the alphabet and in the heart. The left heart contains the mitral valve. Likewise, "R" and "T" are close in the alphabet. The right heart contains the tricuspid valve. Both the mitral and the tricuspid valves have two large opposing leaflets and small intermediary leaflets at each end.

Mitral Valve. The mitral valve's two large leaflets are not quite equal in size (Fig. 1-10). The chordae tendineae from adjacent leaflets are inserted upon the same papillary muscles. This physical feature helps to ensure complete closure of the value. When the mitral valve is open, the valve, chordae tendineae, and papillary muscle look like a funnel. Of all the valves, the mitral is most commonly involved in clinical conditions of valvular dysfunction. Mitral regurgitation is the most common clinical valvular disturbance. Clinically, mitral regurgitation may be insignificant (subclinical) or represent a life-threatening situation (papillary muscle rupture). The key factor influencing the significance of any valvular disturbance is the effect on stroke volume (amount of blood the heart pumps with each contraction).

Tricuspid Valve. The tricuspid valve differs from the mitral valve in that it has one larger leaflet than the mitral valve and has three papillary muscles instead of two. Otherwise, the structures and functions of the two

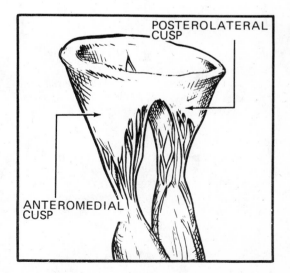

Figure 1-10. Side view of the mitral valve.

valves are similar. Tricuspid dysfunction is not as much of a clinical problem as is mitral dysfunction.

Semilunar (Pulmonic and Aortic) Valves

The semilunar valves (Fig. 1-11) of the heart are the aortic and the pulmonary valves. Each has three symmetrical valve cusps to provide for complete opening without stretching of the valve. The pulmonary valve is located between the right ventricle and the pulmonary artery. The aortic valve is located between the left ventricle and the aorta.

Pulmonary valve dysfunction will potentially affect the performance of the right ventricle. Aortic valve disturbance can affect the performance of the left ventricle.

Physical Assessment of the Cardiac Valves

Cardiac valves can be assessed to some extent through auscultation. Heart sounds can be identified partially based on specific valve functioning. The heart normally generates two sounds, referred to as S_1 and S_2. S_1 is the sound generated through the closure of the mitral (M_1) and tricuspid (T_1) valves. M_1 is best heard at the fifth intercostal space (ICS) in the left midclavicular line. T_1 is best heard the fourth ICS at the

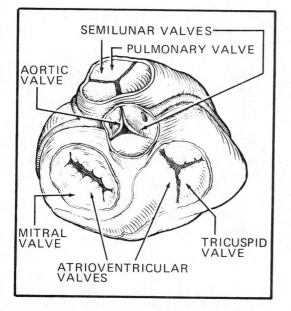

Figure 1-11. The semilunar valves and the atrioventricular valves (posterior view).

left sternal border. S_1 is produced during ventricular contraction. S_1 can be identified by listening (it normally is the loudest of the two cardiac sounds at the fourth ICS, left sternal border or the fifth ICS, left midclavicular line) or by comparing the sounds to the electrocardiogram (ECG). The S_1 sound occurs immediately after the QRS complex (which indicates ventricular depolarization and contraction).

S_2 is produced by the closure of the aortic (A_2) and pulmonic (P_2) valves. A_2 is best heard at the second ICS, just to the right of the sternum. The P_2 sound is heard best at the second ICS, just to the left of the sternum. S_2 can also be identified by listening (it is loudest in the locations described above) or by comparing to the ECG. Normally, the S_2 sound occurs during diastole (when aortic and pulmonary blood pressures are higher than ventricular pressures, forcing the aortic and pulmonary valves to close). The S_2 sound normally appears during the T wave or slightly before the QRS complex.

Abnormal Heart Sounds. Heart valves normally produce sound during closure. Four common abnormal situations exist when other sounds might develop. These situations are valve regurgitation, stenosis, ventricular or atrial failure, or disturbances of electrical conduction.

Valve Regurgitation. When a valve becomes regurgitant (sometimes referred to as insufficient), blood flows past the valve, which is normally closed. This produces a sound usually described as a murmur. Murmurs are sounds that are described in several ways, such as blowing and swishing. Murmurs are graded in degree from I to VI. A grade I murmur (written as I/VI) is a very soft sound. A grade VI murmur (written as VI/VI) is so prominent that it can be heard with the stethoscope held about 1 inch from the chest wall. The other grades of murmurs are subjectively described as between I and VI. It is frequently up to the clinician to grade a murmur, since there are no clear objective criteria for grading murmurs.

Mitral and tricuspid regurgitation will produce a murmur that occurs during systole (normally the mitral and tricuspid valves close during systole). Aortic and pulmonic regurgitation will produce a diastolic murmur.

Valvular Stenosis. A stenosis of a valve produces a murmur that may sound like a regurgitant murmur. However, the reasons for the murmur are different. A mitral or tricuspid stenosis produces a murmur during diastole (normally atrial contraction does not meet resistance to pushing blood past the mitral or tricuspid valve). An aortic or pulmonic stenosis can produce a systolic murmur.

Valves can be dysfunctional in isolation (such as a mitral regurgitation) or in multiples. The clinician attempts to identify the cause of the murmur through auscultation and clinical history.

Ventricular and Atrial Failure. During ventricular failure, an increased pressure builds in the ventricles and atrium. After systole, when blood enters the ventricles from the atrium, the high atrial pressure may force blood into the ventricles with considerable force. This increased flow of blood into the ventricles may produce a sound, the S_3 sound. The S_3 sound occurs immediately after the S_2 sound and can be found after the T wave on the ECG. S_3 sounds are not always abnormal but should be considered significant, particularly in the presence of tachycardia. The combination of a tachycardia and S_3 produces a characteristic "gallop" sound associated with left ventricular (congestive heart) failure.

Another heard sound associated with high pressures is the S_4 sound. The S_4 sound is thought to be an atrial sound, associated with high atrial pressures. It can be found immediately before the QRS complex and after the P wave when compared with an ECG tracing.

Electrical conduction defects. When there is an electrical conduction defect, such as a bundle branch block, the potential exists for the valves to fail to function in unison. When this occurs, a split in the heart sound will occur. For example, a right bundle branch block causes a delay in right ventricular contraction. The result is that the pulmonic valve closes slightly after the aortic valve. The S_2 sound now becomes softer and produces two sounds instead of one. The split S_2 can aid in the diagnosis of a right bundle branch block.

Pulsus Paradoxus and Change in Heart Sounds. Heart sounds can be diminished in intensity in air (as in chronic obstructive pulmonary disease) or fluid (pericardial effusion or tamponade) is between the heart and the stethoscope. In tamponade, fluid fills the pericardial sac and limits sound transmission. In addition, the increased fluid restricts ventricular expansion and can dangerously drop the cardiac output. If tamponade oc-

curs, the inability of the ventricle to distend will produce diminished heart sounds, equalizing chamber pressures (e.g., central venous and pulmonary capillary wedge pressures begin to equalize), venous distension develops, and pulsus paradoxus may occur. Pulsus paradoxus is the decreasing of blood pressure during inspiration. A decrease in systolic blood pressure of more than 10 mm Hg is characteristic of pulsus paradoxus. The blood pressure decreases because of the increase in blood entering the atrium during inspiration, further increasing the pericardial pressure. The added pericardial pressure further decreases stroke volume and systolic blood pressure.

Heart sounds can be useful clinical parameters, but they require frequent practice in order to become proficient. More accurate tests are replacing their clinical use. If valve dysfunction is thought to exist, echocardiography is the test of choice. If conduction defects exist, electrocardiography is more accurate in detecting abnormalities. For the purpose of the CCRN test, the basic information provided above will help identify the essential information. Be prepared for questions in which a heart sound is given and you must then identify a clinical condition. However, be aware of the more accurate methods for assessing cardiac function, as they may also be addressed on the test.

THE NORMAL CONDUCTION SYSTEM OF THE HEART

The conduction of an electrical impulse normally follows an orderly, repetitive pattern from the right atrium, through the ventricles, and into the myocardium, where the impulse usually results in ventricular contraction (Fig. 1-12).

The sinoatrial (SA) node is at the junction of the superior vena cava and the right atrium. The SA node is a group of specialized heart cells that are self-excitatory. All self-excitatory cells have automaticity; that is, if the cells can excite themselves, they require no stimulus and may excite themselves at will. This is termed inherent automaticity or spontaneous depolarization. The SA node excites itself faster than any other cardiac cells under normal conditions. For this reason, the SA node becomes the heart's normal pacemaker.

Once the impulse originates in the SA node, it spreads through the atria along three paths called internodal tracts. The impulse continues from the internodal tracts into the atrioventricular (AV) junction.

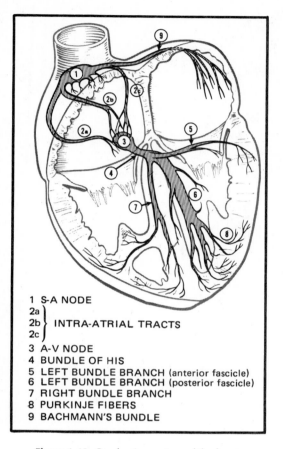

1 S-A NODE
2a ⎫
2b ⎬ INTRA-ATRIAL TRACTS
2c ⎭
3 A-V NODE
4 BUNDLE OF HIS
5 LEFT BUNDLE BRANCH (anterior fascicle)
6 LEFT BUNDLE BRANCH (posterior fascicle)
7 RIGHT BUNDLE BRANCH
8 PURKINJE FIBERS
9 BACHMANN'S BUNDLE

Figure 1-12. Conduction system of the heart.

The AV node is located at the superior end of the junctional tissue, near the tricuspid valve ring just above the ventricular septum. There is a slight pause in the impulse at the upper portion of the AV node to allow for completion of atrial contraction. The impulse traverses the AV node and the junctional tissue, and then reaches the bundle of HIS. The bundle of HIS carries the impulse to the bundle branches. The bundle of HIS divides into right and left bundle branches.

The left bundle branch continues along the ventricular septum, dividing into two subdivisions called fascicles. The anterior fascicle excites the anterior and superior surfaces of the left ventricle. The posterior fascicle excites the posterior and inferior surfaces of the left ventricle. The right bundle branch continues as a single branch to innervate the right ventricle.

Having passed through the bundle of HIS and the bundle branches, the impulse arrives at the Purkinje fibers, which spread into the ventricular myocardium. The impulse spread usually is followed by ventricular contraction, and thus the cycle repeats.

Disturbances in this conduction system will be reviewed as to the specific resulting dysrhythmias. The current CCRN format requires a good understanding of the electrical system of the heart and the ability to interpret dysrhythmias and 12-lead ECGs. While specific sections are provided on dysrhythmias and 12-lead analysis, understanding the basic anatomy and physiology of the electrical conduction system is important.

CIRCULATORY SYSTEMS OF THE BODY

Circulatory paths can be remembered by the mnemonic that "a" for artery means "a" for away. *All* arteries carry blood, either oxygenated or deoxygenated (pulmonary), *away* from the heart. Conversely, all veins carry blood, either oxygenated or deoxygenated, to the heart.

There are two circulatory systems in the body, the pulmonary and the systemic. The heart must pump blood through these two systems in the amount needed by the body to maintain optimal function. In addition, the coronary circulation (a branch of the systemic circulation), the pulmonary circulation, and the systemic circulation have some features helpful to note for the purpose of the CCRN exam.

The Pulmonary Circulation
The pulmonary system is unique in that it is the only system (excluding the fetal) in which the pulmonary artery carries unoxygenated blood away from the heart to the lungs, and the four pulmonary veins carry oxygenated blood from the lungs to the left atrium. The right ventricle sends venous blood into the main pulmonary artery, which divides into the right and left pulmonary arteries. These arteries follow the normal blood vessel path, that is, arteries to arterioles to capillaries (where the blood becomes oxygenated) to venules to veins.

The Systemic Circulation
The aorta is the only artery that the left ventricle normally ejects blood into; it arches over the pulmonary artery. The aorta gives off many branches as it tra-

verses down the body to bifurcate into the iliac arteries. In the capillaries, the blood surrenders oxygen and picks up carbon dioxide. The inferior and superior vanae cavae are the final veins returning blood to the right atrium.

The Coronary Circulation. The coronary circulatory system begins with the inflow of oxygenated blood into the coronary arteries. The openings of these arteries are located near the cusps of the aortic valve. These arteries fill during ventricular diastole.

The right coronary artery supplies the posterior and inferior myocardium with oxygenated blood. The left coronary artery starts at the valve cusp as the left main coronary artery and bifurcates to form the left anterior descending (LAD) and the circumflex arteries. The LAD artery supplies the anterior and septal myocardium. The circumflex artery supplies the lateral myocardium. These arteries then follow the normal sequence of becoming arterioles, capillaries, venules, and veins as they course through the myocardium. The veins empty into thebesian veins, which in turn empty into the coronary sinus. Blood from the coronary sinus joins the venous blood in the right atrium.

CHAPTER 2

Cardiac Physiology

Editor's Note

Physiology is a crucial component of understanding CCRN exam questions. This chapter contains several key concepts that will help in successfully completing the CCRN exam. Direct questions (probably about 10) from this chapter can be expected. Review this chapter carefully in order to prepare for exam questions related to clinical cardiovascular assessment.

All hemodynamic assessments and interventions are based on the following concept:

$$\text{Blood pressure} = \text{Cardiac output (CO)} \times \text{Systemic vascular resistance (SVR)}$$

If the concept of blood pressure regulation through the interaction of CO and SVR is well understood, a clear understanding of cardiovascular principles is much easier to grasp. This chapter presents the key principles necessary to understand regulation of blood pressure.

Cardiac output and SVR work together to maintain blood pressure. Generally, CO and SVR are inversely related; i.e., if one goes up, the other goes down. The inverse relationship is necessary to maintain normal blood pressure. For example, if a patient develops left ventricular failure following a myocardial infarction, the cardiac output will fall. In an attempt to keep the blood pressure normal, the SVR will rise. The rise in the SVR can maintain blood pressure within safe limits for a period of time.

Of the two components that regulate blood pressure, the SVR has the strongest effect. This is why medications that alter SVR have the greatest effect on

the blood pressure. For example, a vasoconstrictor such as norepinephrine (Levophed) has a greater effect on raising the blood pressure than does an inotrope (dobutamine). Medications that affect CO and SVR are listed in Table 2-1. Keep in mind however, that blood pressure does not always equate to blood flow. An adequate blood pressure might exist when blood flow is inadequate. This might happen when a blood vessel is markedly constricted, driving the pressure in the vessel up but limiting blood flow. Although this type of question might not arise on the CCRN exam, keep in mind that blood pressure always must be compared against blood flow, clinical presentation, and oxygenation parameters.

TABLE 2-1. MEDICATIONS THAT CHANGE CO AND SVR

IMPROVE CONTRACTILITY	DEPRESS CONTRACTILITY
Dobutamine	Beta blockers (e.g., Inderal)
Dopamine	Calcium blockers (e.g., Diltiazem)
Amrinone	
REDUCE PRELOAD	**INCREASE PRELOAD**
Diuretics	Colloidal agents (e.g., albumin, hetastarch)
Nitrates (e.g., nitroglycerin)	Crystalloid agents (e.g., normal saline)
Calcium blockers	
REDUCE AFTERLOAD (SVR)	**INCREASE AFTERLOAD (SVR)**
Nitroprusside	Norepinephrine
Apresoline	Dopamine
Prazosin	Phenylephrine
ACE inhibitors (e.g., captopril)	
Calcium blockers (e.g., Nicardipine)	

CARDIAC OUTPUT

Cardiac output components are the most commonly assessed and manipulated aspects in treatment of hemodynamics. Understanding the components of cardiac output simplifies the understanding of hemodynamics. The two major components of cardiac output are stroke volume and heart rate. Normal stroke volume and heart rate parameters are listed in Table 2-2.

STROKE VOLUME

Stroke volume is determined by three factors: preload, afterload, and contractility. Most of the problems with alterations in cardiac output stem from problems with the strength of the heart (contractility). Agents used to alter the strength of the heart are termed inotropes. Positive inotropes increase heart strength, negative inotropes weaken the heart. Preload and afterload contribute to determining contractility. Understanding the interaction of preload, afterload, and contractility is the basis for most of hemodynamic assessment and intervention.

Contractility

Contractility is determined primarily by the inherent structure and abilities of each individual myocardium. There are no currently available methods to accurately measure contractility. Contractility can be inferred, however, from pressure volume relationships involving preload and afterload. The ability to estimate contractility from preload changes is discussed below.

TABLE 2-2. NORMAL CARDIOVASCULAR PRESSURES AND VOLUMES

NORMAL PRESSURES			
Right ventricle	25/0-5	Left Ventricle	110/10
Pulmonary artery	25/10	Aorta	110/80
Mean PA	15	Mean arterial	90
Left atrial	8–12	Right atrial	0–5
PCWP	8–12	CVP	0–5
NORMAL VOLUMES			
Cardiac output	4–8 LPM		
Cardiac output	2.5–4 m²/LPM		
Stroke volume	50–100 cc/beat		
Stroke index	25–45 cc/m²/beat		
Heart rate	60–100 bpm		
Ejection fraction	>60%		

Preload

Preload is a term borrowed from muscle physiology. Cardiac preload can be defined as the stretch of the myocardial muscle prior to contraction. The degree of stretch is partially determined by the pressure in the ventricle just prior to contraction. The point just prior to contraction is left or right ventricular end diastolic pressure (LVEDP or RVEDP). Measurement of LVEDP or RVEDP is possible through cardiac catheterization. Estimation of LVEDP is possible through pulmonary artery catheterization via the left atrial and pulmonary capillary wedge pressure (PCWP). RVEDP is estimated from the right atrial and central venous pressure (CVP). Normal pressures are listed in Table 2-2.

Use of the PCWP to Estimate LVEDP

The PCWP estimates LVEDP due to the relationship of the valveless pulmonary circulation, left atrium, and open mitral valve at end diastole. At end diastole (LVEDP), the mitral valve is open and allows equilibration of ventricular and atrial pressures. The atrial pressure is measurable when a pulmonary artery catheter is inserted and wedged into a pulmonary artery. Once the catheter wedged, right ventricular influence is blocked. A clear communication from the end of the catheter to the left atrium is now possible due to the absence of valves in the pulmonary circulation. The communication from the wedged pulmonary artery catheter to the left atrium allows estimation of LVEDP and, therefore, preload of the left ventricle.

Whereas the PCWP estimates left ventricular pressure, the CVP estimates right ventricular pressure. Right atrial pressure estimates right ventricular pressure through the open tricuspid valve at the end of diastole.

Preload changes are both diagnostic and therapeutic end points. For example, normal preload pressures helps identify normal blood volumes. If preload is low, hypovolemia is assumed. If preload is high, excess volume (usually due to a decreased contractility) is likely. Pressures used to assess hemodynamics are listed in Table 2-3.

The Preload/Contractility Relationship

As the PCWP increases, in theory the strength of the contraction improves. The improved contractility with increasing stretch of muscle is based on Starling's law (Fig. 2-1). As the muscle stretches, the contraction is stronger, similar to a rubber band being stretched further and contracting harder. Obviously, as with a rub-

TABLE 2-3. PRESSURES USED IN HEMODYNAMIC ASSESSMENT

Parameter	Value	Condition Indicated
PCWP	<8	Hypovolemia
PCWP	8–12	Normal
PCWP	12–18	Increasing contractility
PCWP	>18	LV failure
CVP	<5	Normal or potential hypovolemia
CVP	5–10	Increasing contractility
CVP	>10	RV failure

PCWP = pulmonary capillary wedge pressure; CVP = central venous pressure.

ber band, stretching the heart is effective only up to a point. A common end point in hemodynamics is a PCWP of 18 mm Hg. Elevations greater than 18 mm Hg are assumed to be indicative of left ventricular (LV) failure.

As the PCWP increases over 18 mm Hg, the strength of the heart (contractility) is assumed to be inhibited. The PCWP generally would not elevate if the heart had the strength to maintain forward blood flow. As a rule, small increases in the PCWP (between 12 and 18 mm Hg) do not indicate a lessened contractility due to the Starling's law concept. Values in excess of 18 mm Hg, however, are suggestive of loss of contractility and an increased likelihood of LV failure.

Limitations of the PCWP

Always bear in mind that the use of pressures to estimate volumes and contractility is limited. Consequently, use the PCWP only as a guide. Use the PCWP with other parameters, such as stroke volume and cardiac output. In addition, view the PCWP as indicating a trend rather than an absolute single value. For example, some patients (such as those with chronic LV failure) tolerate PCWP values over 18 very well. To assume that a specific value applies to all patients is inaccurate and potentially misleading.

Use of the CVP for Right Ventricular Preload Estimates

The CVP is used to estimate the right ventricular (RV) status in a similar manner as the PCWP is used for the left ventricle. If the CVP is low, venous return to the heart may be low. If the CVP is elevated, RV failure may be present. An extra concern with high CVP values is the inability to estimate LVEDP from CVP levels. A patient can have high CVP levels but low PCWP pressures due to limited blood flow from the RV into the pulmonary circulation.

Afterload

Afterload is defined as the resistance the ventricle faces to eject blood into the circulation. Afterload is estimated by the systemic and pulmonary vascular resistance (SVR and PVR). Normal values and calculations for obtaining SVR and PVR are given in Table 2-4. The SVR does not take into account valvular resistance or blood viscosity. For this and other reasons, the SVR is not an ideal estimate of afterload but is one of the few clinically available measures to estimate afterload. The key concept regarding afterload is related to the myocardial work. The higher the afterload, the greater the myocardial work in overcoming the resistance. If the afterload is too low, the cardiac out-

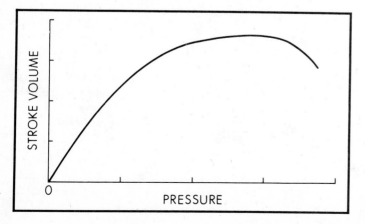

Figure 2-1. Starling's law principle.

TABLE 2-4. CALCULATIONS AND VALUES FOR SVR AND PVR

Parameter	Formula	Normal Values
SVR	$\dfrac{MAP - CVP}{CO} \times 80$	900–1300 dynes/sec/cm
PVR	$\dfrac{MPAP - PCWP}{CO} \times 80$	40–150 dynes/sec/cm
MAP	$\dfrac{(2 \times DBP) + SBP}{3}$	70–110 mm Hg
MPAP	$\dfrac{(2 \times DPAP) + SPAP}{3}$	10–20 mm Hg

SVR = systemic vascular resistance; PVR = pulmonary vascular resistance; MAP = mean arterial pressure; MPAP = mean pulmonary arterial pressure.

put will need to increase in order to maintain blood pressure. Maintaining the afterload at a normal level is crucial to avoid excessive myocardial work.

Effect of Reducing Afterload

Reducing the afterload (SVR) generally lowers the work on the heart unless the SVR decreases to a point where the cardiac output must go to supranormal levels. Myocardial oxygen consumption (MVO_2) is reduced as the SVR fails if the decrease is not excessively abnormal. One method of attempting to improve contractility is to reduce afterload (such as with nitroprusside) alone or in combination with inotropes (dobutamine).

Effect of Increasing Afterload

Increasing the afterload has the opposite effect on myocardial oxygen consumption. In some clinical circumstances, such as hypotension, the risk of increasing MVO_2 is worthwhile. Agents that increase SVR are excellent in elevating the blood pressure but do so at the expense of MVO_2 and perhaps even reducing blood flow. Agents that increase SVR are used with caution in the patient with myocardial ischemia or infarction due to a subsequent rise in MVO_2.

REGULATION OF AFTERLOAD

Afterload is regulated by three known mechanisms: autonomic, baroreceptors, and medullary controls.

Autonomic Regulation of Peripheral Vessels

The sympathetic nervous system has an adrenergic effect upon peripheral vessels. The norepinephrine released by the sympathetic system causes vasoconstriction. This vasoconstriction prevents pooling of blood in the peripheral vessels and augments the return of blood to the heart.

The parasympathetic nervous system has a cholinergic effect upon peripheral vessels. Acetylcholine is released by the parasympathetic nervous system. This causes a vasodilatation of peripheral vessels. With dilation, more blood can remain in the peripheral vessels, and less blood is returned to the heart.

Baroreceptor Control

Baroreceptors are also called pressoreceptors or stretch receptors since these areas respond to a stretching of arterial and venous vessel walls. These receptors are specialized cells located in the aortic arch, carotid sinus, atria, vanae cavae, and pulmonary arteries. These receptor sites are responsive to mean arterial pressure greater than 60 mm Hg. When stimulated by an elevated pressure, these receptors send signals to the medulla oblongata in the brain. The medulla then inhibits sympathetic nervous system activity, which allows the vagus nerve of the parasympathetic nervous system to assume control. This results in vasodilatation of peripheral vessels and a decreased heart rate. Under normal circumstances, this will allow the blood pressure to return to normal.

Conversely, if pressure is low, vagal tone is decreased, which allows the sympathetic nervous system to assume control. This results in vasoconstriction of the peripheral vessels and an increased heart rate. Under normal circumstances, this will allow the blood pressure to return to normal.

Vasomotor Center of Regulation

There are two areas of vasomotor control in the medulla oblongata: a vasoconstrictor area and a vasodilator area. The vasomotor center responds to baroreceptors and chemoreceptors in the aortic arch and carotid sinus.

If the vasoconstrictor area is stimulated, normally an increased heart rate, stroke volume, and cardiac output will result due to peripheral vasoconstriction. As the peripheral vessels constrict, more blood is forced from these vessels and returned to the heart. This normally restores arterial blood pressure.

If the vasodilator area is stimulated (by inhibition of the vasoconstrictor area), a decrease in stroke volume and cardiac output will normally occur. The vasodilatation allows for more blood to remain in peripheral vessels; therefore, less blood is returned to the heart. The normal end result will be a decrease in blood pressure. This partially explains the bradycardia seen in patients who are hypertensive.

Chemoreceptors are activated by a decreased oxygen pressures, an increased carbon dioxide level, and/or a decreased pH. Once activated, the chemoreceptors stimulate the vasoconstrictor area. The events that normally occur with such stimulation are then set into action.

HEART RATE

The other regulator of cardiac output, heart rate, can be used as a guide to therapy and assessments. The heart rate is regulated by the autonomic nervous system through sympathetic (adrenergic) and parasympathetic (cholinergic) mechanisms. Sympathetic regulation occurs through alpha and beta receptors located in the cardiovascular system. There are two types of alpha and beta cells: $alpha_1$ and $alpha_2$, and $beta_1$ and $beta_2$. Parasympathetic effect is primarily through the vagus nerve.

When a bradycardia exists, treatment is based on the factors that control the heart rate. For example, parasympathetic stimulation has a stronger effect on the heart than does sympathetic stimulation. The stronger parasympathetic effect is the reason atropine is the first drug given to treat a bradycardia. Isoproterenol, a sympathetic stimulator, is the second choice.

The heart rate is a valuable diagnostic tool in that it is the first compensatory response to a decrease in stroke volume. A sinus tachycardia frequently heralds a decrease in stroke volume. The other reason an increase in the heart rate may occur is an increase in metabolic rate. The increase in metabolic rate requires an increase in cardiac output, generally met by increasing both heart rate and stroke volume.

Heart rate elevations, e.g., sinus tachycardia, by themselves are not generally dangerous. Although the increase in heart rate will increase MVO2, the reason for the development of the tachycardia is more important. A clinical clue to investigate is the origin of a sinus tachycardia, followed by treating the cause of the tachycardia rather than the tachycardia itself.

RELATIONSHIP OF BLOOD FLOW AND PRESSURE IN CARDIAC CYCLE

The pressure of a fluid in a chamber depends upon the size of the chamber, the amount of fluid, the distensibility of the chamber, and whether the chamber is open or closed.

The atria (both right and left) are open chambers. The venae cavae in the right atrium and the pulmonary veins in the left atrium are always open. Thus, pressures in these chambers will remain low unless something occludes the openings or prevents them from emptying.

The anatomic structure of the right ventricle contributes to its low pressure. The right ventricle normally empties into a low-pressure system, the lungs.

The left ventricle has a high pressure. Its anatomic structure contributes to the high pressure. It empties into a high-pressure, closed system, the aorta. Let us trace the flow of blood through the chambers and examine its relationship to the cardiac valves and the chamber pressures. These relationships are shown in Fig. 2-2.

Atrial Pressure Curve

Throughout diastole, pressure slowly increases in the atria due to the influx of blood. The volume of blood increases in relation to the chamber size (resulting in a V wave on the atrial waveform). With atrial contraction (first curve on the atrial line in Fig. 2-2), there is a sudden increase in pressure (producing an A wave in the atrial waveform) since the contraction decreases the size of the atrium. During atrial contraction, pressure is greater in the atrium than in the ventricle. This higher pressure causes the atrioventricular (AV) valves to open. Atrial blood flows through the open AV valves into the ventricles.

As the ventricles begin the systolic phase, blood flow is reversed. As soon as the blood flow reverses, the blood completely closes the partially closed AV valves. The ventricular pressure increase is so sudden that the AV valves bulge into the atria, increasing the

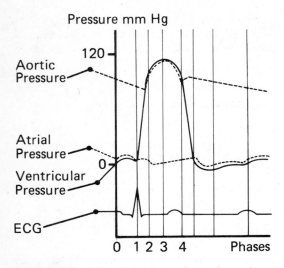

Figure 2-2. Blood flow and pressure during the cardiac cycle.

intra-atrial pressure (second curve on atrial line in Fig. 2-2). Following this second curve, there is a sharp fall in atrial pressure. Gradually, the atrial pressure rises again during the next period of diastole, and the cycle repeats.

The normal atrial pressures generate three waves: A, C, and V (Fig. 2-3). The A wave is the result of atrial contraction and can be found in the PR interval. One exception to the location of the A wave is in regard to the PCWP. The PCWP is found slightly later, in the QRS, because of the time it takes the wave to travel from the left atrium to the pulmonary catheter. The importance of the A wave is that the mean of the A wave is the parameter used to estimate the CVP and PCWP values.

The C wave is due to closure of the tricuspid and mitral valves. The V wave is due to atrial filling and the bulging of the tricuspid and mitral valves into the atrium. Large V waves can develop with noncompliant atria and mitral or tricuspid regurgitation (Fig. 2-4).

Ventricular Pressure Curve

During diastole, the ventricular pressure is less than the atrial pressure. Just before atrial systole occurs, the AV valves open and blood flows into the ventricles. As soon as the ventricles fill, the blood flow reverses and closes the AV valves. At this point, the ventricles become closed chambers. The ventricle walls contract against the volume of blood in the ventricle. Since the ventricle is a closed chamber, pressure rises rapidly. Aortic pressure during diastole has fallen to about 80 mm Hg. The period during which ventricle pressure builds from near zero to 80 mm Hg is termed the isometric contraction phase (ventricle curve between lines 1 and 2 in Fig. 2-2). The left ventricle continues to contract strongly, and the pressure rises to about 110 mm Hg. Since left ventricular pressure exceeds the aortic pressure of 80 mm Hg, the aortic valve is forced open, and blood is ejected into the aorta. These same mechanisms are occurring concurrently in the right ventricle, only under much lower pressures. This is called the rapid ejection phase (ventricle curve between lines 2 and 3 in Fig. 2-2). Pressure begins to

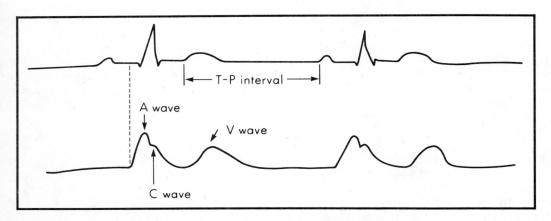

Figure 2-3. Normal atrial waveforms.

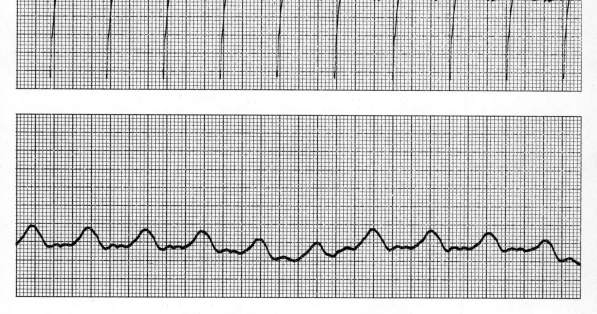

Figure 2-4. Giant V waves in a PCWP tracing.

drop in the ventricle because blood is being ejected faster than the ventricle is contracting. This is called the reduced-ejection phase (ventricular curve between lines 3 and 4 in Fig. 2-2). Ventricular contraction ceases, and the ventricle relaxes. Since the ventricular pressure has dropped rapidly, the blood flow starts to reverse at about 80 mm Hg in the aorta. This backward flow closes the aortic valve. The ventricle again becomes a closed chamber, but since no blood is entering, the pressure does not rise. The fall of pressure in the ventricle continues until it is less than the atrial pressure. Then the cycle begins again.

CHAPTER 3

The Normal ECG

Editor's Note

Generally, the CCRN exam requires interpretation of fewer than three rhythm strips but may have several questions regarding 12-lead ECG analysis. A good basic understanding of dysrhythmia interpretation is generally all that is needed to successfully answer questions regarding dysrhythmia analysis. If you have completed a basic ECG course without difficulty, you should be prepared for the portion of the exam addressing dysrhythmias. This chapter also provides a brief review of all common dysrhythmias to help your review process.

The section in the CCRN exam that addresses 12-lead ECG analysis may be beyond a basic ECG course. If you have completed an ECG course that has a 12-lead ECG component, you should be prepared for this section. If you have not had a 12-lead ECG course, this chapter is important. For the first time in the CCRN exam, you may have to interpret a 12-lead ECG as well as answer questions regarding ECG changes associated with specific clinical conditions.

COMPONENTS OF THE NORMAL ECG

The electrocardiograph is a machine that records the electrical activity of the heart on special paper. The result is an electrocardiogram (ECG or EKG). The electrical activity measured by the ECG is the electrical potential between two points on the body, a positive pole and a negative pole. When one is monitoring patients in critical care, all monitoring leads have one negative and one positive pole. For example, in lead I, the right arm is negative and the left arm is positive. Electrical activity in the heart is monitored by these two poles. Electrical activity that is directed toward the positive pole results in an upright deflection. Activity heading toward the negative pole is upside down. The sum of all cardiac electrical activity (referred to as cardiac vectors) is generally in a direction that is inferior and to the left. The leftward direction of cardiac electrical activity is primarily due to the size and therefore electrical activity of the left ventricle.

The 12-lead ECG is the graphic recording of the electrical output of the heart from 12 different positions. A 12-lead ECG can be diagnostic in drug toxicity, conduction disturbances, electrolyte imbalances, ischemia, infarction, size of the heart chambers, and axis orientation of the heart.

Cardiac monitoring uses rhythm strips to assess heart rate, rhythm, and dysrhythmias. Rhythm strips may be run on any one of the 12 leads used in a 12-lead ECG and several other special leads.

The most common leads used to monitor patients are leads II and MCL_1. Lead II is a standard lead with the negative pole attached to an electrode placed on the upper chest near the right arm and the positive pole attached to an electrode placed on the lower left side of the chest. Lead II normally sees electrical activity in the heart in an upright ECG pattern, since its positive electrode is on the left side of the body. Lead II is especially useful in assessing P waves and QRS complexes that have a small amplitude. It is not, however, the ideal monitoring lead. MCL_1 is a better routine monitoring lead.

MCL_1 is a modified chest lead representative of V_1 of the 12-lead EKG. In MCL_1, the negative pole is attached to an electrode placed on the upper left chest and the positive pole is attached to an electrode placed to the right of the sternum at the fourth intercostal

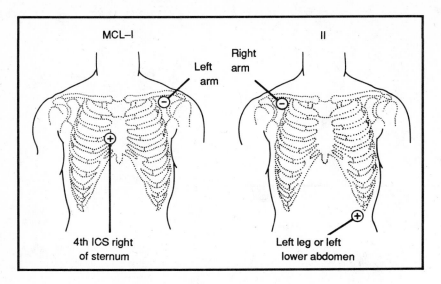

Figure 3-1. Normal placement for MCL$_1$ and lead II.

space. Since the MCL$_1$ positive electrode is placed to the right of the sternum, it views the cardiac electrical activity as heading away from it and therefore sees the QRS complex as primarily upside down.

MCL$_1$ gives more information on conduction defects such as right and left bundle branch blocks than do other routine monitoring leads. As such, it is the routine lead employed to identify most dysrhythmias, particularly aberrant atrial premature contractions from premature ventricular contractions. The one situation for which MCL$_1$ is not as useful is with newer monitoring systems that employ ST segment analysis. ST segment analysis operates better when large R waves are sensed. If large R waves are desired, lead II, MCL$_5$, or MCL$_6$ is employed. Figure 3-1 indicates placement for MCL$_1$ and lead II.

When monitoring dysrhythmias, develop the practice of using multiple leads. Use of a single lead for all situations limits your ability to interpret complex dysrhythmias.

A key ingredient to accurate dysrhythmia analysis is the correct application of lead placement. While the CCRN exam generally does not ask specific questions on lead placement, such questions are possible. More importantly, accurate lead placement has an effect on correct rhythm and 12-lead analysis. Studies have indicated significant changes in QRS morphology with in-

correct lead placement. Follow the examples in the diagram of Fig. 3-1 to aid correct lead placement.

ECG Paper

The CCRN exam will not ask questions about the ECG paper. However, you must know the time grids within the ECG paper to make interpretations of dysrhythmias and 12-lead analysis.

The ECG paper has a series of horizontal lines exactly 1 mm apart (Fig. 3-2).

The horizontal lines represent voltage (or amplitude). ECG paper also has vertical lines that represent time. Each vertical line is 0.04 seconds apart. To help in measuring waveforms, every fifth line is darker than the other lines, both horizontally and vertically. The intersection of these lines produces both small boxes (the lighter lines) and large boxes (the darker, bolder lines). Horizontally, each small box represents 1 mm (0.1 mV) and each large box represents 5 mm (0.5 mV). (Note that each large box is made up of five small boxes.) Vertically, each small box represents 0.04 seconds and each large box represents 0.20 seconds. Because of the design of ECG paper, one can measure the duration of impulses (wavelengths) and the amplitude (height) of impulses. All waves will be either isoelectric (no net electrical activity = flat), positively deflected (upright, toward the positive pole), or

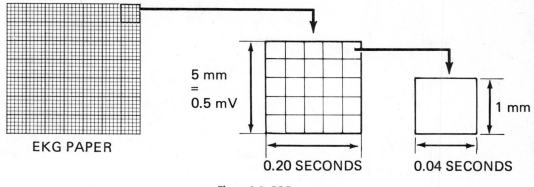

Figure 3-2. ECG paper.

negatively deflected (downward, toward the negative pole).

COMPONENTS OF A CARDIAC CYCLE

Before a rhythm strip can be labeled, a systemic analysis of each portion of the strip and the relation of each wave to the electrical activity in the cardiac cycle is made. The interpretations will be made using lead II or MCL_1 in this text. It is conventional to label the components of the cardiac cycle P, QRS, and T. (There is no reason these specific letters were chosen.)

There are three prominent deflections in the ECG: the P wave, the QRS complex, and the T wave (Fig. 3-3).

P Wave

This represents the generation of an electrical impulse and depolarization of the atria (Fig. 3-4). The P wave is important in determining whether the impulse started in the SA node or elsewhere in the atrium.

QRS Complex

The QRS complex is composed of three separate waveforms which represent ventricular depolarization (Fig. 3-5). Multiple variations exist in the shape of the QRS complex. A Q wave is the first negative deflection and may or may not be present. A large Q wave may be indicative of myocardial death. To be clinically significant, the Q wave should be greater than 0.04 seconds

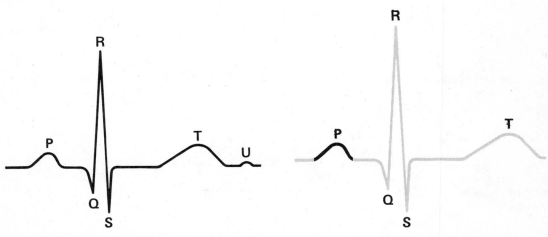

Figure 3-3. The normal PQRST deflections, lead II.

Figure 3-4. The P wave.

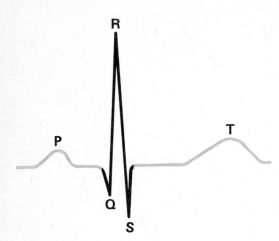

Figure 3-5. The QRS complex.

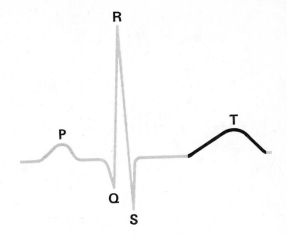

Figure 3-6. The T wave.

and the depth should be greater than one-third the height of the R wave.

The R wave is the first positive deflection in the complex. The R wave is usually large in leads where the positive electrode is on the left (I, II, III, avL, avF, V_5, V_6) and small in leads where the positive electrode is on the right (MCL$_1$, V_1, V_2, avR).

The S wave is the negative deflection following the R wave. The S wave can be useful in interpreting terminal electrical activity in the heart.

T Wave

The T wave is the third major deflection in the ECG (Fig. 3-6). It represents repolarization of the ventricles. In most lead II of a healthy heart, the T wave is positively deflected. In ischemia or infarction, the T wave may be inverted.

Intervals and Segments

There are four other intervals and segments of a rhythm strip and an ECG that must be identified.

PR Interval. The PR interval (Fig. 3-7) represents the time for the electrical impulse to spread from the atrium to the AV node and His bundle. It is measured from the beginning of the P wave to the beginning of the QRS complex. Normally, this interval is 0.12 to 0.20 seconds.

ST Segment. The ST segment (Fig. 3-8) represents the time from complete depolarization of the ventricles

to the beginning of repolarization (recovery) of the ventricles. In the healthy heart, the ST segment is flat or isoelectric. Since no net electrical activity is present during the recovery phase of the cardiac cycle, the wave is not deflected in either direction. In myocardial injury, the segment may be elevated. In ischemia, the ST segment is depressed.

PR Segment. This segment (Fig. 3-9) represents the normal delay in the conduction of the electrical impulse in the AV node. It is normally isoelectric and is measured from the end of the P wave to the beginning

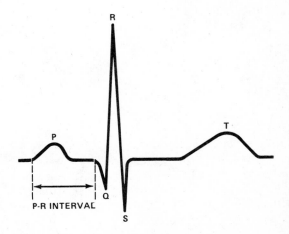

Figure 3-7. The PR interval.

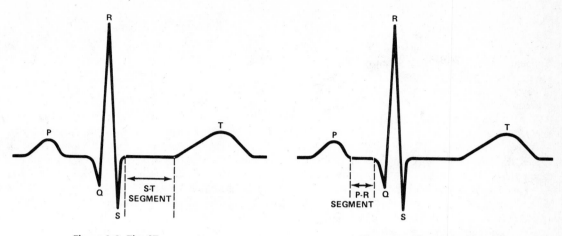

Figure 3-8. The ST segment.

Figure 3-9. The PR segment.

of the R wave. Duration of the PR segment varies. Clinically, the PR segment is not usually addressed.

QT Interval. This interval (Fig. 3-10) represents the total period of time required for depolarization and repolarization (recovery) of the ventricles. It is measured from the beginning of the QRS complex to the end of the T wave. It is normally less than 0.40 seconds, but is dependent upon heart rate, sex, age, and other factors.

Occasionally another wave is seen after the T wave and before the next P wave. This is called a U wave (Fig. 3-11). Some authorities believe that it represents repolarization of the Purkinje fibers. It may or may not be seen.

INTERPRETATION OF A RHYTHM STRIP

Five basic steps are followed in analyzing a rhythm strip (or an ECG) to aid in the interpretation and identification of a rhythm. Each step should be followed in sequence. Eventually this will become a habit and will enable one to identify a strip correctly, accurately, and quickly.

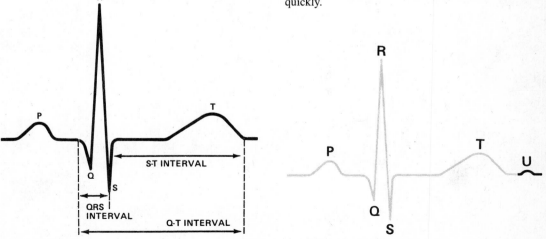

Figure 3-10. The QRS, ST, and QT intervals.

Figure 3-11. The U wave.

Step 1

Determine the rates at which the atria and the ventricles are depolarizing. The rates may not be the same. To count the rate of the atria, count the number of P waves present in the six-second rhythm strip and multiply by ten. (Each mark at the top edge of the ECG paper represents three seconds, and each inch of the ECG paper equals one second.) This gives the atrial rate per minute.

Count the number of QRS complexes in a six-second strip and multiply by ten. This gives the ventricular rate per minute.

For regular rhythms, another method may be used. Determine the rate by counting the number of small boxes between each P wave and divide into 1500 or count the number of large boxes between each P wave and divide into 300. Do the same thing to determine the ventricular rate by counting QRS complexes.

Step 2

Determine whether the rhythm is regular or irregular. The most accurate method is to measure the interval from one R wave to the next R wave. (Set one point of the cardiac calipers on the tip of the first R wave and the other point on the tip of the next R wave.) Then move the cardiac calipers from R to R. If the measurement is the same (or varies less than 0.04 seconds between beats), the rhythm is regular. If the intervals vary by more than 0.04 seconds, the rhythm is irregular. Often one can tell by simply looking at the strip that the rhythm is irregular. However, if it looks regular, it is best to measure the R-to-R intervals to be certain.

Step 3

Analyze the P waves. A P wave should precede every QRS complex. All of the P waves should be identical in shape. The normal P wave is fairly sharply curved, less than 3 mm in height, and less than 0.1 seconds in width in lead II. If the P wave is abnormally shaped or varies in shape from wave to wave, the stimulus may have arisen from somewhere in the atrium other than in the SA node. Almost all impulses that originate in the SA node will meet the "normal" shape and size previously stated if heart function is normal. A biphasic P (a single P wave moves above and below the baseline) may indicate left atrial enlargement; a peaked P may indicate right atrial enlargement, and both of these P waves originate in the SA node. If there is no P wave or if the P wave does not precede the QRS complex, the impulse did not originate in the SA node.

Step 4

Measure the PR interval. This is measured from the beginning of the P wave to the beginning of the QRS complex. It should measure between 0.10 and 0.20 seconds. Intervals outside this range indicate a conduction disturbance between the atria and the ventricles.

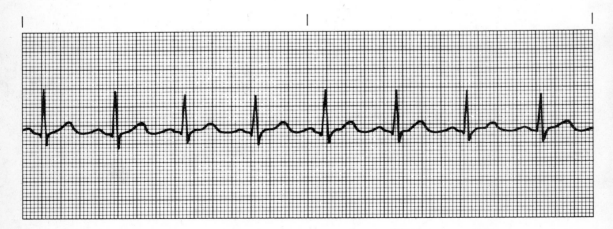

Figure 3-12. Lead II normal sinus rhythm.

Step 5

Measure the width of the QRS complex. This is measured from the beginning of the Q (if present, otherwise the R) to the end of the S wave. The normal duration is 0.06 to 0.12 seconds. A QRS measurement of greater than 0.12 seconds indicates an intraventricular conduction abnormality.

Figure 3-12 is a six-second, lead II rhythm strip. Let us analyze this rhythm strip by applying the five steps just mentioned.

- Step 1: The atrial rate is 80 (eight P waves in six seconds). The ventricular rate is 80 (eight R waves in six seconds). The heart rate is 80.

- Step 2: There is less than a 0.04-second variation from R wave to R wave, so the rhythm is regular.
- Step 3: The P waves are all the same shape, size (in height), and duration. Each P wave appears immediately before a QRS complex. These factors indicate that the impulse starts in the SA node.
- Step 4: The PR interval is about 0.16 seconds. This is within the normal duration range, indicating normal conduction of the impulse from the SA node to the AV node.
- Step 5: Each QRS complex is less than 0.10 seconds in duration, which is normal.
- Interpretation of the strip: Normal sinus rhythm.

CHAPTER 4

Sinus and Atrial Dysrhythmias

Editor's Note

The CCRN exam can be expected to directly address either the interpretation or treatment of sinus and atrial dysrhythmias. There may be few or many questions, depending on the type of test. The most important concepts in this area are the correct interpretation of dysrhythmias and the treatment each would require. Most of this information is included in a basic ECG course, something most of us have already had. However, if dysrhythmia interpretation is not a strength for you, review this chapter carefully.

All dysrhythmias are caused by a disturbance in the formation of the cardiac impulse or a disturbance in the conduction of the impulse. Classification of the dysrhythmias is shown in Table 4-1.

Every dysrhythmia has specific identifying characteristics. The first four dysrhythmias discussed in this chapter originate in the SA node. The next six dysrhythmias originate in the atrium, but not in the SA node. (*Note:* All rhythm strips are six seconds, lead II.)

SINUS ARRHYTHMIA (OR SINUS DYSRHYTHMIA)

Etiology

Variations of impulse formation in the SA node are caused by the vagus nerve and changes in venous return to the heart. This results in an irregular rhythm with alternating fast and slow rates (Fig. 4-1).

Identifying Characteristics

The rate varies, usually between 60 and 100 beats per minute. The rate increases with inspiration and decreases with expiration. Both atrial and ventricular rhythms are regularly irregular if the variation is due to a regular breathing pattern. The P waves are normal and the PR interval is within normal limits. The QRS complex is normal. The difference between normal sinus rhythm and sinus arrhythmia is the variation of the R-to-R intervals. In sinus arrhythmia, the variation is at least 0.04 seconds between the shortest and the longest R-to-R intervals. The variation in normal sinus rhythm is less than 0.04 seconds.

Risk

No risk exists for the patient because this dysrhythmia is a normal variant and causes no hemodynamic compromise.

Treatment

No treatment is needed.

Nursing Intervention

Document the dysrhythmia with a rhythm strip. This interpretation can be substantiated if the patient holds his or her breath and the rate stabilizes.

SINUS BRADYCARDIA

Etiology

Parasympathetic (vagal) control over the SA node due to ischemia, pain, drugs, sleep, or athletic conditioning decreases the formation of electrical impulses (Fig. 4-2).

Identifying Characteristics

The rate is less than 60 but usually more than 40. Both atrial and ventricular rhythms are usually regular. P

TABLE 4-1. CLASSIFICATION OF DYSRHYTHMIAS

Dysrhythmias Due to Disorders in Impulse Foundation or Accessory Pathway	Dysrhythmias Due to Conduction Disturbances

SA node dysrhythmias
  Sinus tachycardia
  Sinus bradycardia
  Sinus arrhythmia
  Wandering pacemaker
  SA arrest
	SA block
	AV blocks
	  First-degree AV block
	  Second-degree Type I AV block
	  Second-degree Type II AV block
	  Third-degree (complete) AV block

Atrial dysrhythmias
  Premature atrial contractions
  Paroxysmal atrial tachycardia
  Atrial flutter
  Atrial fibrillation
	Intraventricular blocks
	  Left bundle branch blocks
	  Right bundle branch blocks
	  Bilateral bundle branch blocks

AV nodal area (junctional) dysrhythmias
  Premature junctional contractions
  Junctional escape rhythm
  Paroxysmal junctional tachycardia
  Junctional tachycardia	

Ventricular dysrhythmias
  Premature ventricular contractions
  Ventricular tachycardia
  Ventricular fibrillation
  Ventricular Asystole	

waves are normal. The PR interval is within the upper limits or is slightly prolonged. The QRS complex in normal. Conduction is normal.

Risk

This dysrhythmia may lead to syncopal attacks, angina, premature beats, ventricular tachycardia, congestive heart failure (CHF), and cardiac arrest. This is a serious warning dysrhythmia if the rate is low (about 40) and accompanied by hypotension (P < 90/60). Sinus bradycardia is generally benign but should be assessed for its effect on hemodynamics.

Treatment

No treatment may be necessary if the rate is close to 60 or if the patient is asymptomatic. If the rate is low and/or the patient is symptomatic (hypotensive or showing signs of CHF), atropine given intravenously is

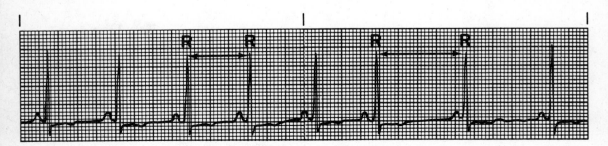

Figure 4-1. Sinus arrhythmia.

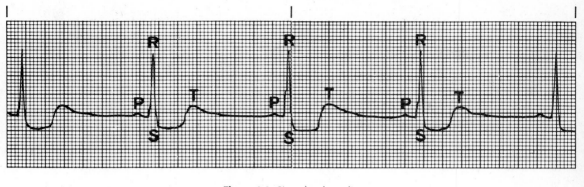

Figure 4-2. Sinus bradycardia.

the drug of choice to increase the heart rate. If this treatment is unsuccessful, isoproterenol hydrochloride (Isuprel) by intravenous drip may be tried. An external or temporary pacemaker may be required if pharmacologic management is unsuccessful.

Nursing Intervention
Document the dysrhythmia with a rhythm strip. Monitor and document the effectiveness of drug therapy. Do not administer drugs such as digitalis or propranolol (Inderal) that may further slow the heart rate. Be especially alert for premature ventricular contractions (PVCs). If PVCs occur, obtain a rhythm strip and notify the physician; do not treat with lidocaine or other agents that may eliminate the PVCs. PVCs associated with a bradycardia are generally treated with atropine or isoproterenol. As the heart rate increases, the PVCs usually disappear.

SINUS TACHYCARDIA

Etiology
Cardiac decompensation (CHF) is the most serious cause of sinus tachycardia. The increase in heart rate during CHF is a compensatory response due to a reduced stroke volume. Sinus tachycardia may also be caused by any factor that stimulates the sympathetic nervous system, such as anxiety, exertion (physical), and fever (Fig. 4-3).

Identifying Characteristics
The rate is greater than 100 and is usually between 100 and 160. Both atrial and ventricular rhythms are regular. The P wave is normal but may be difficult to identify because of the rapid rate. (*Note:* Look for the P wave superimposed on the T wave with fast rates.) The PR interval is usually at the lower limits of normal.

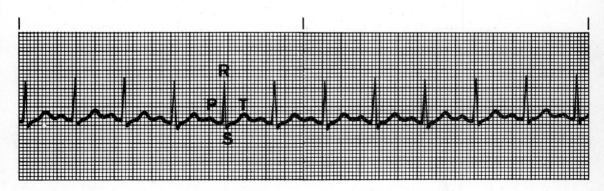

Figure 4-3. Sinus tachycardia.

Risk

Regardless of the etiology, prolonged sinus tachycardia may precipitate CHF in patients with borderline cardiac function. The ability to tolerate a prolonged sinus tachycardia is dependent on the underlying cardiac function of the patient.

Treatment

Effective treatment depends upon controlling the underlying cause. Normally sinus tachycardia does not in itself require treatment. In a persistent sinus tachycardia that is compromising the cardiac output, pharmacologic treatment may be required with therapies such as calcium channel blockers (e.g., verapamil), beta blockers (e.g., esmolol), or adenosine or digitalis preparations (e.g., digoxin).

Nursing Intervention

Document the dysrhythmia with a rhythm strip. Monitor the patient for signs of left ventricular failure (restlessness, orthopnea, cough, shortness of breath). Attempts to calm the patient and to decrease the patient's stress may be helpful.

SINUS PAUSE/ARREST, SA BLOCK

Etiology

Ischemic injury to the SA node is the most common and important cause of SA block. A technical, but not clinical, difference exists between sinus pause/arrest and SA block. In the pause/arrest, the SA node does not form an electrical impulse. In SA block, the node initiates an impulse, but the impulse is prevented from leaving the node and thus it cannot be visualized. Regardless of this difference, the end result is that no impulse stimulates the atria or the ventricles. The terms pause and block are often used interchangeably. Sinus disease, vagal effect, digitalis toxicity, quinidine sulfate (Quinidine), and sympathetic stimulation such as with isoproterenol hydrochloride (Isuprel) may be causes of SA block (Fig. 4-4).

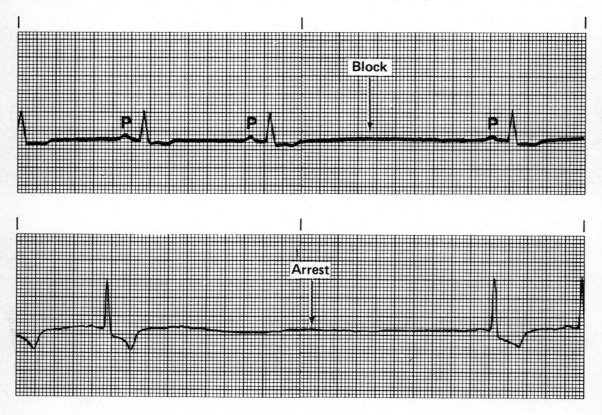

Figure 4-4. SA arrest or block.

Identifying Characteristics

The rate is usually slower than normal. Rhythm (both atrial and ventricular) is generally regular except for the arrest/block complex. P waves are absent in arrest and block for a specific time period. Otherwise, P waves are normal. The PR interval is absent in the arrest/block complex. The QRS complex may be normal or abnormal in arrest, depending on the escape site. No QRS complexes are seen during the block. Conduction depends on the escape site in arrest and is absent in sinus block for that specific interval.

Risk

The greatest risk is that both sinus pause/arrest and sinus block may proceed to a reduced cardiac output if the arrest or block is frequent. If the arrest or block is infrequent and self-limiting, it is not dangerous.

Treatment

If the arrest or block is rare, it does not require treatment. If the arrest is frequent, treatment is essential. If drugs are the underlying cause, they should be evaluated and stopped. Atropine and isoproterenol may be effective in increasing the heart rate. If these are not effective and the patient is symptomatic, initially an external pacemaker could be applied, but long-term treatment will require a permanent pacemaker.

Nursing Intervention

Document the dysrhythmia with a rhythm strip. If a drug is the possible underlying cause, withhold the drug until reordered. Monitor the patient closely to determine whether the frequency of arrest or block is increasing. If it is, document with rhythm strips and notify the physician; a pacemaker may be indicated.

PAROXYSMAL ATRIAL TACHYCARDIA

Etiology

Paroxysmal atrial tachycardia (PAT) is the term to describe several causes for a rapid atrial heart rate (Fig. 4-5). Another term, paroxysmal supraventricular tachycardia, is also used to describe this rhythm. In PAT, excessive sympathetic stimulation or abnormal conduction situations are present. Abnormal conduction situations include AV nodal reentry problems or the presence of accessory pathways.

Identifying Characteristics

Three characteristics are associated with PAT:

1. It starts suddenly.
2. It ends abruptly.
3. The ventricles respond to either every impulse created by the focus (1:1 conduction) or most impulses, creating a rapid ventricular response.

Both atrial and ventricular rates are usually between 150 and 250. The rhythm is regular. P waves are present but may be very difficult to identify. The P wave will not have the normal, smooth, rounded shape of a sinus P wave, since this impulse originates in the atrium. The PR interval varies. It may be within normal limits and is frequently greater than one expects for the rate. However, in some accessory pathway situations, the PR interval may be shortened. The QRS complex is usually normal. Once again, however, if the problem is due to an accessory pathway, an initial distortion in the QRS complex may be present. This distortion is sometimes seen as a delta wave, causing a slurring of the upstroke on the R wave of the QRS complex.

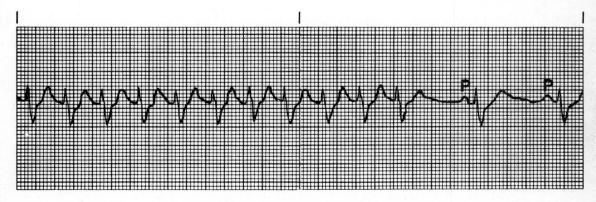

Figure 4-5. Paroxysmal atrial tachycardia.

Risk

PAT frequently stops spontaneously. If it does not, the rapid rate may lead to myocardial ischemia and, eventually, cardiac decompensation. If PAT occurs post-myocardial infarction or in the patient with limited cardiac function, it may rapidly lead to increased myocardial ischemia and injury and left ventricular failure.

Treatment

Vagal stimulation and other vagal maneuvers such as coughing and pressure on the eyes may terminate the dysrhythmia. Having the patient perform a Valsalva maneuver stimulates the vagus nerve. If this fails to terminate the rhythm, carotid massage by the doctor (or nurse, if allowed) often terminates PAT. If this fails and the patient is asymptomatic, drug therapy may be tried. Beta blockers such as esmolol or propanolol, digoxin, calcium channel blockers (verapamil or diltiazem) or adenosine intravenously may terminate PAT. If the patient is symptomatic (complains of angina, becomes diaphoretic, short of breath, and hypotensive), synchronized cardioversion may be used immediately. Cardioversion usually terminates PAT.

Surgical interventions and radiofrequency ablation are increasingly options for the patient with PAT. In order to surgically cut the accessory pathway (or eliminate the path with radiofrequency ablation), extensive electrical mapping of the heart in an electrophysiology lab is required in order to locate the origin of the abnormal pathway.

Nursing Intervention

Document the dysrhythmia with a rhythm strip. Assess and monitor the patient for signs of ischemia and decompensation. Medicate as ordered by the physician. Be prepared for synchronized cardioversion.

ATRIAL TACHYCARDIA

The impulse of atrial tachycardia originates in the atrium. The rate of atrial tachycardia is constant. The difference between PAT and atrial tachycardia is only that PAT starts and stops suddenly. Atrial tachycardia is a constant rhythm, not irregular. All other parameters of PAT apply to atrial tachycardia (Fig. 4-6).

PREMATURE ATRIAL CONTRACTION

Note: Premature atrial contractions (PACs) are also called atrial premature beats.

Etiology

On occasion, an irritable focus in the atrium or an impulse through an accessory pathway causes an unexpected complex initiating depolarization. The irritable focus does not become the heart's pacemaker except for this single beat (Fig. 4-7).

Identifying Characteristics

The underlying rate is usually normal. The rhythm has an occasional irregularity due to the premature nature of the beat and a brief pause after the premature beat. The P wave is abnormally shaped for only the premature beat. The PR interval is usually prolonged but may be normal or shortened. The QRS complex is normal. PACs may be blocked or may have an aberrant (abnormal or wide QRS) conduction. Conduction below the atria (junctional and ventricular) is usually normal.

Risk

If PACs occur infrequently, there is no risk. If they occur six or more times per minute, they indicate atrial flutter, atrial fibrillation, or atrial tachycardia.

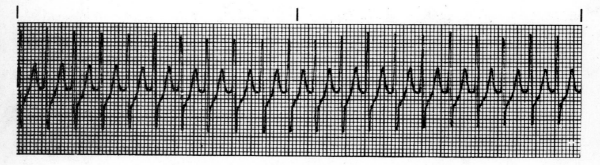

Figure 4-6. Atrial tachycardia.

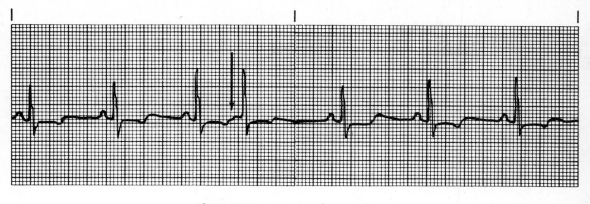

Figure 4-7. Premature atrial contraction.

Treatment

PACs of fewer than six per minute do not need treatment. With more than six PACs per minute, the physician may elect to control them with digitalis or with calcium channel or beta blockers.

Nursing Intervention

Document the dysrhythmia with a rhythm strip. Monitor the patient for increasing frequency of PACs. Increasing PACs may cause anxiety, some hemodynamic compromise, hypotension, and dyspnea. Document an increase in frequency with rhythm strips and notify the physician of the increase.

WANDERING ATRIAL PACEMAKER

Etiology

Various foci within the atrium or from the AV node supersede the SA node as the pacemaker for a variable number of beats (Fig. 4-8).

Identifying Characteristics

Rate is usually normal but may be slow. Rhythm is frequently regular. P waves are abnormal and change in size, shape, and deflection. The PR interval may vary or may be constant. The QRS complex is normal. Conduction is abnormal in the atrium and sometimes in the AV node. Below the AV node, conduction is normal.

Risk

Generally there is no risk. The presence of a wandering atrial pacemaker is normally insignificant, although it may indicate the presence of SA disease.

Treatment

Usually no treatment is necessary. If the rhythm produced symptoms, the symptoms would be treated. For example, a bradycardia could be treated with atropine.

Nursing Intervention

Document the dysrhythmia with a rhythm strip. Monitor for an unacceptably low ventricular rate (below 50 beats per minute) and treat as necessary.

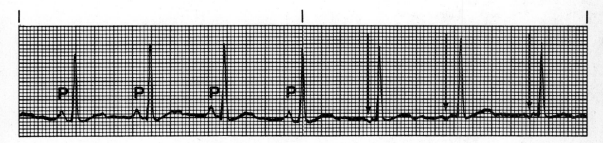

Figure 4-8. Wandering atrial pacemaker.

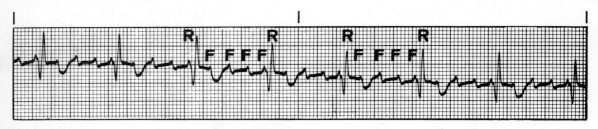

Figure 4-9. Atrial flutter.

ATRIAL FLUTTER

Etiology
An irritable atrial focus or accessory pathway may supersede the SA node and produce atrial flutter. This is a fairly common dysrhythmia in atherosclerotic heart disease and some congenital heart diseases (Fig. 4-9).

Identifying Characteristics
The atrial rate is rapid, usually 250 to 350 beats per minute. Atrial rhythm is regular, and ventricular rhythm varies with the number of impulses transmitted through the AV node. The P wave is replaced by a flutter wave (F wave). Flutter waves have no isoelectric interval between the waves. The PR interval is usually prolonged although difficult to measure from a rhythm strip. The QRS complex is usually normal. Conduction is abnormal in the atria, and the AV node normally blocks many of the F waves.

Risk
Congestive heart failure may occur quickly if the patient has limited cardiac function and if the AV node conducts almost all of the F waves. There is the possibility of severe hemodynamic compromise. If the ventricular response is rapid, there is insufficient filling time for the ventricle. The rapid rate can cause a reduction in cardiac output. Rapid response of the ventricle increases myocardial oxygen demand, which cannot be met due to the decreased cardiac output. If severe, the hemodynamic compromise may lead to CHF.

Treatment
Digitalis preparations may be used in treating this dysrhythmia if the ventricular response is slow. If the ventricular response is rapid, synchronized cardioversion with low voltage is the preferred treatment.

Nursing Intervention
Document the dysrhythmia with a rhythm strip. Monitor the patient closely for signs of hemodynamic compromise. The physician should be notified when this dysrhythmia develops.

ATRIAL FIBRILLATION

Etiology
Many irritable foci develop in the atrium to the extent that normal atrial contraction is an impossibility. This condition may be caused by rheumatic heart disease, coronary disease, hypertension, thyrotoxicosis, and congenital heart disease (Fig. 4-10).

Identifying Characteristics
The atrial rate is not measurable but is probably greater than 300. The atrial rate is so high that the AV node cannot accept all of the stimuli it receives. Consequently, the atrial and ventricular rates are markedly different. The atrial and ventricular rhythms are irregular. P waves are nonexistent and are replaced by fibrillatory waves. There is no true PR interval. The QRS complex may be normal or abnormal. Ventricular response may be slow, normal, or very rapid. Conduction is abnormal in both the atria and the AV node. The number of impulses that the AV node transmits determines the degree of AV block.

Risk
There may be a rapid development of CHF. Atrial thrombi may form, leading to embolization. Marked hemodynamic disturbance is common if the rhythm is of recent onset. Angina and increased myocardial ischemia may occur.

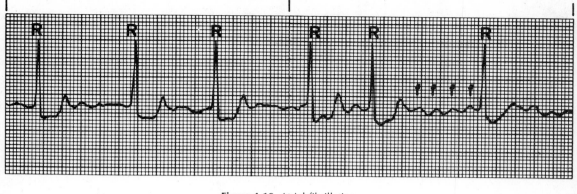

Figure 4-10. Atrial fibrillation.

Treatment

If the dysrhythmia is not causing hemodynamic compromise, digitalis preparations (digoxin) are commonly employed. If hemodynamic compromise develops, synchronized cardioversion is essential to reduce and control the ventricular response, provided the dysrhythmia has not been present for 72 or more hours. The risk of atrial thrombus development after 72 hours contraindicates the use of cardioversion to terminate the dysrhythmia, since it may produce embolization.

If there is hemodynamic compromise within the first 72 hours, synchronized cardioversion is essential to reduce and control a rapid ventricular response. This is considered an acute form of atrial fibrillation.

A chronic form of atrial fibrillation is considered to exist if there is no hemodynamic compromise, if the dysrhythmia has been present for more than 72 hours, and if the patient is asymptomatic and has a ventricular response of greater than 50 complexes per minute but less than 100 complexes per minute. In these instances, treatment may not be needed.

Nursing Intervention

Document the dysrhythmia with a rhythm strip. Notify the physician if atrial fibrillation develops suddenly. Monitor the patient carefully for hemodynamic compromise and embolization. Contact the physician if rapid ventricular response develops or if an unacceptably low ventricular response develops (less than 50 beats per minute).

CHAPTER 5

AV Node and
Ventricular Dysrhythmias

Editor's Note

The most common dysrhythmias likely to be addressed on the CCRN exam involve disturbances of the AV node (junctional rhythms and conduction blocks) and ventricular ectopy (premature ventricular contractions, ventricular tachycardia, and fibrillation). This chapter contains information that addresses several questions from the exam. In addition, information regarding 12-lead ECG analysis and pacemakers is provided. Each of these areas can also be expected to contain information addressed on the CCRN exam. Once again, if dysrhythmias are not a strength for you, review this chapter carefully.

It was once thought that the AV node itself could initiate impulses. Such rhythms were termed nodal rhythms. Research has shown that the AV node itself does not initiate an electrical impulse but that an electrical impulse is initiated in the junctional tissue around the AV node. This finding has resulted in changing the term nodal rhythm to the more accurate term of junctional rhythm. All rhythm strips in this chapter are six seconds, lead II or MCL_1.

JUNCTIONAL RHYTHM

Etiology

This dysrhythmia is often due to an acute myocardial infarction, an SA block, digitalis toxicity, or treatment with drugs that slow the atrial rate (e.g., digitalis and procainamide) (Fig. 5-1).

Identifying Characteristics

The rate is usually 40 to 60 beats per minute. The rhythm is usually regular. P waves are abnormal in shape and size and may precede or follow the QRS complex or be buried in it. If seen, the P wave is usually inverted (negatively deflected). This inversion is caused by the electrical impulse originating in junctional tissue and moving both down into the ventricles (a normal path) and back up into the atrium (retrograde movement, which is an abnormal path). The PR interval, if present, is less than 0.10 seconds and often is immeasurable. The QRS complex is normal, unless a P wave is buried in it. Conduction to the atria is abnormal due to its retrograde depolarization of the atria.

Risk

The junctional impulse formation is slow. The junctional rhythm is normally a protective rhythm, taking over as the pacemaker of the heart when the SA node slows to rates below 40 to 60 beats per minute. Hemodynamic balance may be compromised by a slow ventricular rate, leading to poor cardiac output and perhaps ventricular failure.

Treatment

Medications that increase the heart rate, such as atropine, would be considered if the bradycardia was associated with hypotension or CHF. If medications fail to work, pacemakers can be used to override the slow rate. If drug toxicity is the underlying cause, the drug should be stopped immediately.

Nursing Intervention

Document the dysrhythmia with a rhythm strip. Monitor the patient closely. PVCs may occur and do not respond well to lidocaine or other ventricular antidysrhythmic agents, since the PVCs are usually a result of decreased cardiac output. Increasing the heart

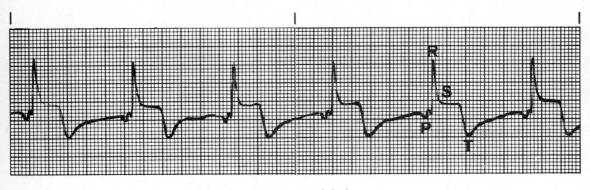

Figure 5-1. Junctional rhythm.

rate is a more effective method for eliminating the PVCs. Monitor for signs of hemodynamic compromise. Notify the physician immediately if compromise occurs.

PREMATURE JUNCTIONAL CONTRACTION

Etiology
An irritable focus in the junctional tissue initiates an impulse early. The impulse depolarizes the ventricles normally and the atria in a retrograde fashion. Coronary artery disease, acute myocardial infarction, and digitalis toxicity are frequent causes. Any factor that increases junctional ischemia may produce a premature junctional contraction (PJC) (Fig. 5-2).

Identifying Characteristics
The underlying rate may be normal or slow. The rhythm is regular except for the premature (early) beat. P waves are abnormal, inverted, and may precede,

follow, or be buried in the QRS complex of the PJC. The PR interval varies with the position of the pacemaker and is frequently immeasurable. The QRS complex is normal unless the P wave is buried in it or aberration occurs. Conduction is normal through the ventricles and retrograde through the atria.

Risk
PJCs may lead to a supraventricular tachycardia if frequent. If rare, PJCs do not pose a threat for the patient.

Treatment
If PJCs are infrequent or the patient is asymptomatic, no treatment is necessary. If frequent, PJCs may be controlled by digitalis preparations or other atrial antidysrhythmics such as pronestyl.

Nursing Intervention
Document the dysrhythmia with a rhythm strip (to justify junctional origin rather than ventricular origin). Monitor the patient for increasing frequency of PJCs and notify the physician if the frequency does increase.

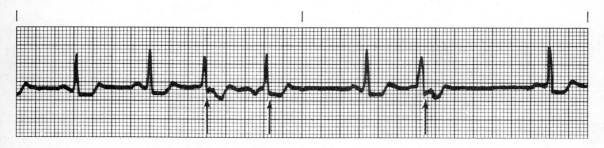

Figure 5-2. Premature junctional contraction.

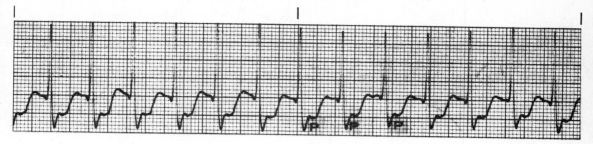

Figure 5-3. Paroxysmal junctional tachycardia (PJT).

PAROXYSMAL JUNCTION TACHYCARDIA

Etiology

Paroxysmal junction tachycardia (PJT) is probably similar to PAT, both in origin and in treatment. The cause may be disease of the AV node or abnormal pathways, either anatomic or physiologic (Fig. 5-3).

Identifying Characteristics

The rate is usually 150 to 250 beats per minute. The rhythm is usually regular. P waves are abnormal and inverted, and they may precede, follow, or be buried in the QRS complex. The PR interval, if present, is shortened or not measurable. The QRS complex is normal unless the P wave is buried in it or it is aberrantly conducted. Conduction of the QRS may be normal. Atrial conduction is retrograde. PJT may be difficult to distinguish from PAT. They are often called SVT (supraventricular tachycardia).

Risk

The danger associated with PJT is the same as for PAT. The faster the rate, the greater the likelihood of a de-

creased cardiac output. If the cardiac output is reduced enough, left ventricular failure will result.

Treatment

The treatment is similar to that for PAT.

Nursing Intervention

Document the dysrhythmia with a rhythm strip. Assess the patient for hemodynamic compromise. If compromise occurs, notify the physician and medicate as the situation dictates.

FIRST-DEGREE BLOCK

Etiology

First-degree AV junctional block may be caused by arteriosclerotic heart disease (ASHD), acute myocardial infarction, AV node ischemia, and drugs that act at the AV node (e.g., digitalis). The AV node delays the progression of the impulse from the SA node for an abnormal length of time (Fig. 5-4).

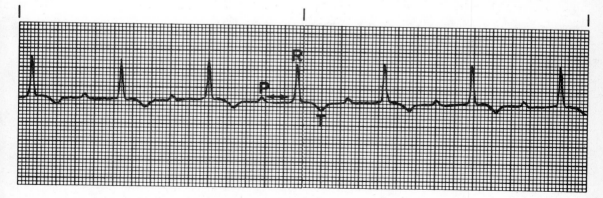

Figure 5-4. First-degree AV heart block.

Identifying Characteristics

The rate is normal. The rhythm is regular. P waves are normal. The PR interval is prolonged beyond 0.20 seconds. The QRS complex is normal. Conduction is normal except for the prolonged delay at the AV node.

Risk

First-degree block is not a serious dysrhythmia itself. It may progress to a second-degree type I block and less commonly to a second-degree type II or third-degree block.

Treatment

If the PR interval is less than 0.25 seconds and if it does not increase, no treatment may be required. The length of the PR interval is not as significant as the effect on stroke volume and heart rate. No treatment is indicated unless a bradycardia results.

Nursing Intervention

Document the dysrhythmia with a rhythm strip. Monitor the patient closely for progression to a slower heart rate or a worsening block. If progression develops, document with a rhythm strip and notify the physician immediately.

SECOND-DEGREE BLOCK—TYPE I AND TYPE II

The terms Mobitz I and Wenckebach (named after cardiac physiologists in the early twentieth century) are frequently used instead of type I. Mobitz II is also used in place of type II. These terms will not be used in this section, although it is helpful to remember that you may see them on the exam or in clinical practice.

Both type I and type II are AV junctional blocks. The AV node delays the progression of the SA node impulse for a longer than normal time. The characteristics, treatment, and prognosis in these two forms of second-degree AV block differ. The type I form of second-degree block will be considered first.

SECOND-DEGREE TYPE I

Etiology

Conduction arises normally from the SA node and progresses to the AV node. With each succeeding impulse, it becomes more difficult for the AV node to conduct the impulse. Eventually, one impulse is not conducted and a QRS complex does not occur. The progression then begins again. Ischemia or injury to the AV node is the cause of this progression (Fig. 5-5).

Identifying Characteristics

The following are the key components of the second-degree type I heart block:

1. Progressive prolongation of the PR interval
2. Increment of conduction delay that is greatest between the first and second sinus beat in each cycle
3. Progressive decrease in succeeding increments of delay
4. Progressive shortening of the PR interval before each pause
5. Pause in the ventricular rhythm that is less than twice the PP interval or sinus cycle length

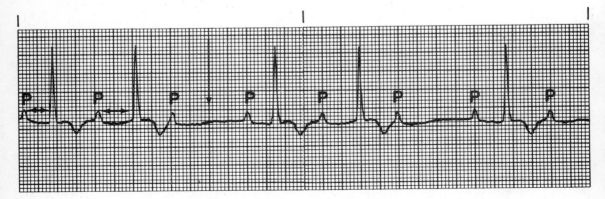

Figure 5-5. Second-degree AV block—type I (Wenckebach).

Risk

Second-degree type I is often a temporary block following an acute myocardial infarction. It may, however, progress to a complete (third-degree) block. For this reason, second-degree type I is considered a potentially dangerous dysrhythmia, although by itself it usually does not produce a clinical problem.

Treatment

Frequently, no treatment is indicated. If the ventricular rate is slow, atropine may increase AV conduction. Isoproterenol is the second drug of choice to increase the SA node rate and thus the overall rate. On occasion, an external pacemaker or temporary transvenous pacemaker may be inserted.

Nursing Intervention

Document the dysrhythmia with a rhythm strip. Monitor the patient, although this dysrhythmia is normally not clinically significant. If the ventricular rate slows enough to produce symptoms, document it with a rhythm strip and notify the physician.

SECOND-DEGREE TYPE II

Etiology

An impulse originates in the SA node and progresses normally to the AV node. Below the AV node in the common bundle or bundle branches, impulses are blocked on a regular basis with every second, third, or fourth impulse not being conducted. In this block, a QRS complex is regularly missing. More than one P wave is present for every QRS complex. This dysrhythmia is due to disease of the AV node, the AV junctional tissue, or the His-Purkinje system (Fig. 5-6).

Identifying Characteristics

Atrial rate may be normal. The ventricular rate is usually one-half or one-third of the atrial rate (referred to as 2:1 or 3:1 block). At times, the block rate may be even greater than 3:1. The ventricular rate depends on the frequency of the block. (In 4:1 block, there are four atrial beats to every one QRS complex.) The atrial rhythm is regular. Ventricular rhythm is regular or irregular, but slow. P waves are normal. The PR interval is constant. The QRS complex may be normal or widened. Conduction is normal in the atria and may be abnormal in the ventricles.

Risk

Type II block is unpredictable and may suddenly advance to complete heart block or ventricular standstill, especially common after inferior infarction. This is a dangerous warning dysrhythmia.

Treatment

If the ventricular response is slow, atropine or isoproterenol may be tried. Because the condition is so unpredictable, a temporary pacemaker is often the treatment of choice. A permanent pacemaker is frequently necessary.

Nursing Intervention

Document the dysrhythmia with a rhythm strip. Determine the width of the QRS complex. The greater the width, the more dangerous the dysrhythmia. Monitor

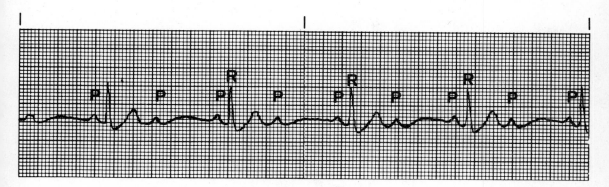

Figure 5-6. Second-degree AV block—type II.

the patient closely for a widening of the QRS complex. The width of the QRS complex indicates the location in the conduction system of the block. The wider the complex, the lower the block is in the bundle branch system. Document the widening, if it occurs, with a rhythm strip, notify the physician immediately, and prepare for the insertion of a transvenous pacemaker or use of an external pacemaker. Assess the patient frequently for hemodynamic compromise if the ventricular response is slow (3:1 and 4:1 block).

While type I and II heart blocks are differentiated by the PR interval changes, another feature is important to bear in mind with these two types of dysrhythmias. Consider that the right coronary artery (RCA) is responsible for feeding the AV node in 90% of the population. In addition, the RCA supplies the inferior region of the left ventricle. Therefore, in inferior myocardial infarctions (MIs), a common dysrhythmia is AV blocks, specifically type I blocks. Clinically this is relevant since type I blocks may appear like II blocks, i.e., in 2:1 patterns. These 2:1 blocks generally are less dangerous, though, because the bundle branches remain intact. If a pacemaker is required, a temporary will usually suffice.

Anterior MIs are different, however, in their effect on producing type II blocks. An anterior MI is usually the result of obstruction of the left anterior descending artery. This artery also feeds the left and right bundle branches. In the presence of an anterior MI, a type II block may also appear in a 2:1 pattern. This pattern is more dangerous with an anterior MI since the block is due to loss of ventricular conduction system, i.e., the left and/or right bundle system. Type II blocks in the presence of an anterior MI require more

attention. Pacemakers for this dysrhythmia usually need to be permanent.

THIRD-DEGREE BLOCK—COMPLETE HEART BLOCK

Etiology
Ischemia or injury to the AV node, junctional tissue, or His-Purkinje tissue is the cause of complete heart block. The ischemia may be secondary to ASHD, acute myocardial infarction, drug use (e.g., digitalis toxicity), systemic disease, or electrolyte imbalances (especially in renal patients) (Fig. 5-7).

Identifying Characteristics
Atrial rates are faster than ventricular rates. P waves are not conducted. The ventricular rate is 30 to 40 (unless there is a junctional escape mechanism). The rhythm is regular for both the atria and the ventricles even though they are depolarizing completely independently of each other. P waves are normal and not associated with a QRS complex. The PR interval is not constant. QRS complexes are close to normal if they arise near the AV node. The QRS complex may be wide and bizarre if the impulse arises from the ventricles. There is no AV conduction. The atrial pacemaker controls the atria, and the ventricular pacemaker controls the ventricles.

Risk
The main danger of third-degree heart block is the potential bradycardia producing a decrease in cardiac output, leading to hypotension and myocardial ische-

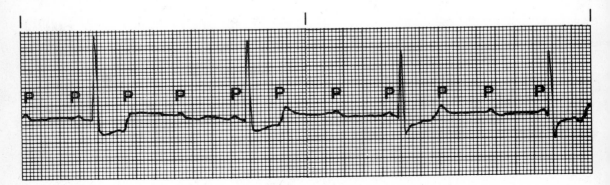

Figure 5-7. Third-degree (complete) AV block.

mia. Third-degree heart block is a potentially lethal dysrhythmia.

Treatment

Immediate pacemaker insertion is the treatment of choice. A temporary pacemaker may be tried initially until the presence of the block has been determined to be permanent. Complete heart block may be temporary after a myocardial infarction, and pacing should be available for several days after the return of a normal sinus rhythm.

Nursing Intervention

Document the dysrhythmia with a rhythm strip and notify the physician immediately. Monitor the patient for signs of ventricular failure and hypotension. Hemodynamic status is compromised by the slow ventricular rate, and circulatory collapse is not uncommon.

AV DISSOCIATION

Many conditions can be termed AV dissociation. Ventricular tachycardia and conduction defects where the atrial and ventricular rhythms do not match can all be examples of AV dissociation. Some clinicians make the mistake of using the term third-degree block synonymously with AV dissociation; however, third-degree block is only one form of AV dissociation.

Etiology

The many causes of AV dissociation include anesthesia, medications, infections, acute myocardial infarction, and ischemic heart disease (Fig. 5-8).

Identifying Characteristics

The relationship in AV dissociation is from P to P, which is regular, and from R to R, which is regular. The PR interval is inconsistent since the atrial and ventricular pacemakers are independent of each other. The P wave, usually normal in form, may vary slightly in measurements. The P wave may fall immediately before, during, or after a QRS complex during the absolute refractory period of the ventricles (the period in which they cannot depolarize). The QRS complex may be normal or abnormal, depending on whether the ventricular pacemaker is at or below the bundle of His.

Risk

AV dissociation by itself is significant since atrial and ventricular contractions are not in synchrony. The loss of synchrony can produce a substantial reduction in cardiac output. However, rather than treat AV dissociation, the underlying rhythm producing AV dissociation should be addressed.

Treatment

Treatment is dependent on the underlying rhythm and the effect on hemodynamics. Treatments range from

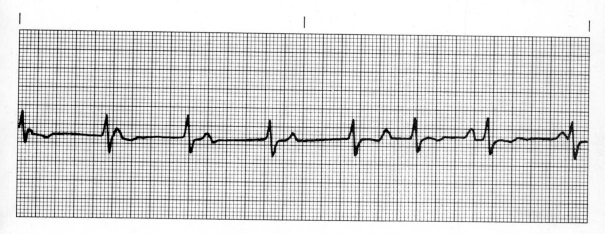

Figure 5-8. One type of AV dissociation.

pacemakers for bradycardias to antidysrhythmics for ventricular tachycardia.

Nursing Intervention

Monitor the patient closely for signs of cardiac decompensation and progression of the dysrhythmia. Document the dysrhythmia with a rhythm strip and notify the physician.

THE 12-LEAD ECG

The CCRN exam can include questions that require an understanding of the 12-lead ECG. With the recent increased emphasis on cardiovascular concepts, the CCRN exam now includes 12-lead electrocardiograms for you to interpret. Other typical questions involving the 12-lead ECG usually focus on conditions such as left and right ventricular hypertrophy, left and right bundle branch blocks, differentiation of aberrant APCs from PVCs, and identification of myocardial infarction patterns. This section provides the information necessary to interpret these conditions.

Basics of 12-Lead Interpretation

The 12 monitoring leads used to assess myocardial conduction patterns are listed in Table 5-1. When assessing patterns of injury, hypertrophy, or axis deviations, noting the views of the heart from different leads is essential. Whenever possible, a prior 12-lead ECG can help interpret questionable results.

Left and Right Ventricular Hypertrophy

Left ventricular hypertrophy (LVH) causes more electrical forces to be generated on the left side of the

TABLE 5-1. 12-LEAD ECG LEADS

Lead	View of the heart
I	Lateral wall
II	Inferior wall
III	Inferior wall
avR (augmented vector of the right)	
avL (augmented vector of the left)	Lateral wall
avF (augmented vector of the foot)	Inferior wall
V_1	Ventricular septum
V_2	Anterior wall
V_3	Anterior wall
V_4	Anterior wall
V_5	Lateral wall
V_6	Lateral wall

heart. This can understandably lead to left axis deviation. The leads viewing the heart on the left side (such as V_5 and V_6), will reflect the increased electrical activity by having large R waves. Leads on the right side show large S waves, the opposite of large R waves. The most common criterion for diagnosing LVH is a combination of right and left precordial chest leads. For example, if the height of the R wave in V_5 combined with the depth of the S wave in V_1 exceeds 35 mm, then the voltage criterion for LVH is present.

Right ventricular hypertrophy (RVH) is better noted from right precordial leads. Leads V_{3R} and V_{4R} are better able to pick out changes in right ventricular size through the presence of large R waves (R:S ratio > 1). Figure 5-9 illustrates right precordial leads. In addition to possible right axis deviation, the best criteria for RVH include a large R wave in V_1 and V_2 and a deep S in V_5 and V_6. Table 5-2 lists criteria for left and right ventricular hypertrophy.

BUNDLE BRANCH BLOCKS

Bundle branch blocks are also termed intraventricular conduction defects. There may be a right or left bundle branch block. In addition, the left bundle has two divisions, referred to as fascicles. These fascicles may also become blocked. Obstructions of the fascicles are termed hemiblocks. There may be a left anterior hemiblock of the anterior fascicle of the left bundle branch or there may be a left posterior hemiblock of the posterior fascicle of the left bundle branch. Trifascicular blocks involve both left bundle fascicles and the right bundle branch. Bifascicular blocks usually involve the right bundle branch and one fascicle of the left bundle branch, or both fascicles of the left branch. Bundle branch blocks *cannot* be diagnosed by a rhythm strip, only suspected. A 12-lead ECG is essential.

Criteria for diagnosing conduction defects are listed in Table 5-3. Identification of conduction defects is useful for several reasons, ranging from identifying areas of disease in the heart to assessing the significance of injury patterns. In addition, interpretation of conduction defects, particularly right bundle branch blocks, is helpful in differentiating APCs with aberrant conduction from PVCs.

Etiology

Three different factors may cause a bundle branch block. First, an acute myocardial infarction may cause

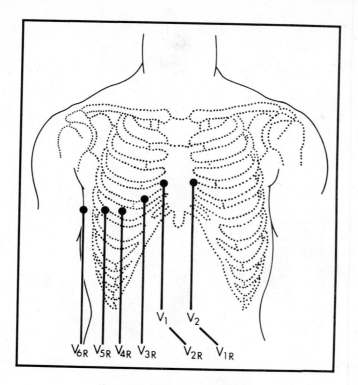

Figure 5-9. Right precordial leads.

ischemia in the intraventricular conduction system. Second, chronic degeneration with fibrous scarring may permanently block the bundle branches. Third, bundle branch blocks may be congenital or rate dependent (i.e., they appear only at certain heart rates).

Identifying Characteristics
Bundle branch blocks cannot be diagnosed by a rhythm strip. Rate is usually normal, although it may vary if the bundle branch block varies. Rhythm is regular. P waves may be normal. The PR interval is normal. The QRS complex is wide (greater than 0.12) and may be notched, depending upon the lead viewed.

Risk
The development of bundle branch blocks indicates marked ischemia of the intraventricular conduction system, and bundle branch blocks are potentially more dangerous than AV blocks since these blocks are subjunctional. The involvement of more than one fascicle often progresses to complete heart block. In these instances, the prognosis is poor.

Treatment
It is not uncommon for the bundle branch block to cause no symptoms. Because of the lack of symptoms, most bundle branch blocks require no direct treatment.

TABLE 5-2. CRITERIA FOR LEFT AND RIGHT VENTRICULAR HYPERTROPHY

Condition	Leads and Criteria
Left ventricular hypertrophy	S wave in V_1 + R wave in V_5 > 35 mm
	R_1 + S_3 > 26 mm
Right ventricular hypertrophy	V_{3R} and V_{4R}, R:S ratio > 1:1

TABLE 5-3. CRITERIA FOR VENTRICULAR CONDUCTION DEFECTS

Condition	Lead	QRS Appearance
Right bundle branch block	V_1 (MCL$_1$)	rSR'
	I & V_6	Deep S wave
Left bundle branch block	I & V_6	Wide QRS (>0.12)
	I & V_6	Notched QRS
Anterior hemiblock	I, avF	Left axis > 30 degrees
	I, avL	Initial Q wave
	II, III, avL	Small R wave, deep S wave
Posterior hemiblock	I	Large S wave
		Right axis
	I, avL	Initial R wave
	II, III, avF	Large R wave

Many patients tolerate conduction defects such as bundle branch blocks for long periods of time without developing any problems. The potential danger of the bundle branch block, however, is that it can deteriorate into a more severe obstruction such as complete heart block. In this case, the treatment is focused on improving the heart rate, as with atropine or a pacemaker.

Nursing Intervention

The primary consideration is to identify the conduction defect and document the type of block. Notify the physician if the block is new. Monitor the rhythm and be aware of the potential for a bradycardia, such as complete heart block, to develop.

IDIOVENTRICULAR RHYTHM

Etiology

In this rhythm, there is no functioning pacemaker above the ventricles. A secondary pacemaker in the ventricles initiates an impulse in order to generate a heart rate. Normally, a ventricular pacemaker is very slow, generally less than 40 beats per minute. The terms idioventricular pacemaker (which means unknown ventricular pacemaker) and ventricular escape rhythm both apply to this dysrhythmia. All diseases and injuries that cause loss of function from the SA node down are etiologic factors (Fig. 5-10).

Identifying Characteristics

The ventricles initiate a rate at their inherent ability, usually 20 to 40 beats per minute. The rhythm is regular but may slow as a "dying heart syndrome" pro-

gresses. There is no P wave. There is no PR interval. The QRS complex is wide and bizarre, measuring 0.12 or more.

Risk

The imminent danger is ventricular standstill. It is possible that the electrical event is not leading to an effective contraction, which means that electrical mechanical dissociation has developed. This rhythm is normally a protective or compensatory response. It may be the last natural pacemaker in the heart, so treatment becomes urgent.

Treatment

A pacemaker is the only reliable and totally effective form of treatment. In a crisis until a transvenous or external pacemaker can be applied, atropine or isoproterenol hydrochloride (Isuprel) may accelerate the heart rate.

Nursing Intervention

Document the dysrhythmia with a rhythm strip. Notify the physician immediately. Assess and treat the patient continuously for hypotension or signs of CHF. Prepare an external pacemaker for use or be prepared to assist in the insertion of a transvenous pacemaker.

ACCELERATED IDIOVENTRICULAR RHYTHM

Etiology

The etiology is the same as for the idioventricular rhythm (Fig. 5-11).

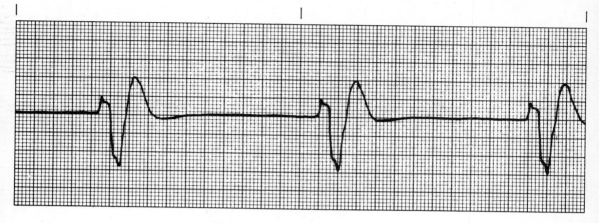

Figure 5-10. Idioventricular rhythm.

Identifying Characteristics
These are the same as for an idioventricular rhythm with the exception that the rate is usually 60 to 100 beats per minute.

Risk
The immediate risk is that the accelerated focus may cease and the dysrhythmia may convert to an idioventricular rate or cardiac standstill. The accelerated idioventricular rhythm is generally of no danger by itself.

Treatment
No treatment is indicated unless the patient demonstrates signs of hemodynamic compromise. Since the rate is normal, this dysrhythmia may generate an adequate cardiac output.

Nursing Intervention
Monitor the patient for signs of hypotension or CHF.

PREMATURE VENTRICULAR CONTRACTION (PVC, PVB, VPC)

Etiology
An irritable focus in the ventricle initiates a contraction before the normally expected beat. The irritability may be due to acute myocardial infarction (most common), ASHD, CHF, drug toxicity, hypoxia, electrolytes, acidosis, or bradycardia (Fig. 5-12).

Identifying Characteristics
The rate is variable. Rhythm is irregular due to the premature beat. P waves are present but frequently not

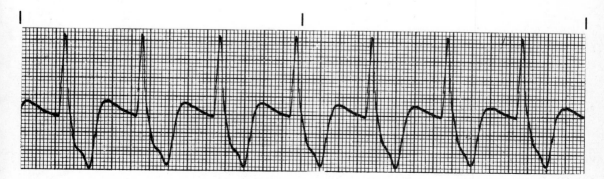

Figure 5-11. Accelerated idioventricular rhythm.

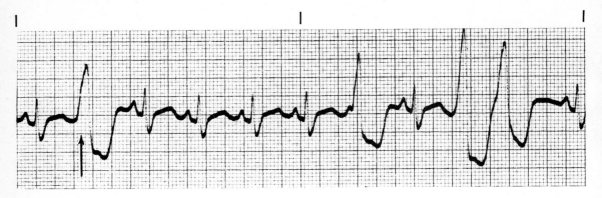

Figure 5-12. Premature ventricular contraction (PVC, PVB, or VPC).

visible. P waves are most commonly lost in the QRS complex of the PVC. However, they may be slightly before or after the PVC. The PR interval is not present, since the atrial impulse does not conduct the PVC. The QRS complex is wide and bizarre, exceeding 0.12 and frequently being greater than 0.14. It usually has a compensatory pause that is equal to two PP distances following the PVC.

Risk

The danger of a PVC is the possibility of increasing myocardial irritability leading to an increasing frequency of PVCs. With an increased occurrence of PVCs, ventricular tachycardia and/or ventricular fibrillation may occur. There is an increased potential for problems when any of the following occur:

1. PVCs occur from more than one focus (multiform PVCs).
2. PVCs occur more often than six per minute, including rhythms such as bigeminy (every other beat is a PVC), or short runs of PVCs occur frequently (two to three sequential PVCs) every few beats.
3. There are variable coupling intervals (the period between the beginning of a normal QRS and the beginning of the QRS of the PVC).
4. The PVC occurs on the T wave of the preceding complex (described as the R-on-T phenomenon). If the PVC occurs on the T wave, it may precipitate ventricular fibrillation.

Treatment

Lidocaine bolus followed by a lidocaine drip is the treatment of choice. (*Note:* If a lidocaine bolus has

been given and 10 to 15 minutes have elapsed, another bolus must be administered before the drip is hung to establish and maintain therapeutic blood levels of the drug.) If hypokalemia is present, potassium may terminate the PVCs. If lidocaine is an unsuccessful treatment, procainamide or bretylium may be tried.

Chronic PVC control is usually with oral preparations, such as tocainide or mexilitine. Many agents are available for the control of chronic PVCs. If PVCs are not controlled by conventional therapies, amniodorone may be required. Amniodorone is usually used as an end-stage treatment because of the multiple side effects associated with this agent.

Nursing Intervention

Document the dysrhythmia with a rhythm strip. Differentiate the PVC from an APC with aberrant conduction. Monitor the patient closely for increasing frequency of PVCs or the development of multiform PVCs. Bolus with lidocaine or another antidysrhythmic agent and document the effect. Prepare a continuous drip to maintain control over the PVC frequency. Notify the physician. Observe the patient and monitor closely for ventricular tachycardia and ventricular fibrillation.

Differentiating APCs with Aberrant Conduction from PVCs

APCs with abnormal (aberrant) conduction can mimic PVCs. Criteria that help different APCs with aberrant conduction from PVCs have been described in both medical and nursing research articles. Table 5-4 provides the criteria necessary to aid differentiation. The key to identifying an aberrantly conducted APC cen-

TABLE 5-4. DIFFERENTIATING APCs WITH ABERRANT CONDUCTION FROM PVCs

Criteria for PVCs	Criteria for APCs
Extreme right axis	rSR' in V_1
Rr' in V_1	Bi- or triphasic QRS
rS in V_6	Normal Axis
Precordial concordance (all V leads show same axis pattern, i.e., upright or inverted)	

ters around two features. First, identify any characteristics of an APC that are different from those of a PVC. For example, in Fig. 5-13, note the P wave on the downstroke of the T wave. This is suggestive of an APC. Second, note the shape of the QRS complex. The morphology or appearance of the QRS complex is a key factor in differentiating APCs with aberrancy from PVCs. Table 5-4 provides clues to QRS complex appearances in the two dysrhythmias. The CCRN exam frequently has a question, and sometimes a rhythm strip, on differentiating between the two, so it is wise to be familiar with the differences.

VENTRICULAR TACHYCARDIA

Etiology
Advanced irritability of the ventricles allows a ventricular focus to become the heart's pacemaker. The myocardial irritability may be due to ASHD, CHF, acute myocardial infarction, electrolyte imbalance, hypoxia, acidosis, or occasionally drugs (Fig. 5-14).

Identifying Characteristics
The rate is greater than 100, often 120 to 220 beats per minute. The rhythm is regular or only slightly irregular. P waves are usually not discernible, although it is important to try to identify them. If P waves are present, they will not be related to the QRS complex (AV dissociation exists). No measurable PR interval exists. The QRS complex is wide and bizarre, resembling essentially a salvo (or burst) of premature ventricular contractions. A ventricular focus initiates ventricular depolarization.

Risk
The risk with ventricular tachycardia is the potential to develop dangerous or lethal reductions in cardiac output.

Treatment
According to the American Heart Association (AHA), three or four types of ventricular tachycardia exist. Treatment is dependent on the type of ventricular tachycardia. The types of ventricular tachycardia and treatments are listed in Table 5-5.

Nursing Intervention
Document this dysrhythmia with a rhythm strip. If the patient is unconscious, immediate defibrillation and institution of cardiac arrest procedures are essential.

VENTRICULAR FIBRILLATION

Etiology
Due to extensive ventricular irritability, ventricular fibers fail to depolarize in sequence; instead, they depolarize individually, creating an uncoordinated series of

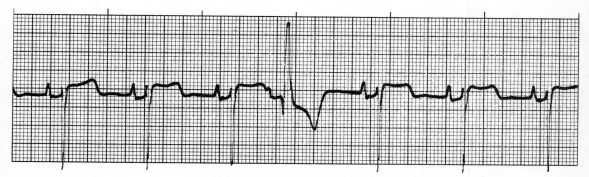

Figure 5-13. Aberrantly conducted APC.

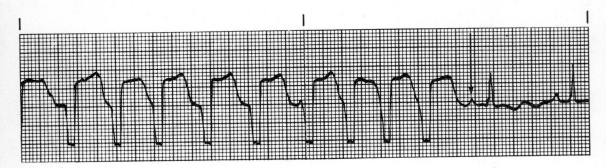

Figure 5-14. Ventricular tachycardia terminating spontaneously.

muscle depolarization. No substantial cardiac output is generated. Ventricular fibrillation may occur after an acute myocardial infarction. It may, however, occur as a result of ASHD, CHF, digitalis or other drug toxicity, and electrolyte imbalance (Fig. 5-15).

Identifying Characteristics
There is no identifiable rate. The rhythm is irregular and immeasurable. P waves are replaced by undulating waves as the baseline. The PR interval is nonexistent or immeasurable. The QRS complex is an undulating, asymmetrical line.

Risk
The development of cardiac standstill may occur within seconds. Circulatory collapse occurs within approximately two minutes and is followed by death.

Treatment
Immediate defibrillation is the only possible means of establishing a viable cardiac rhythm. The AHA has recommended a series of actions to occur when ventricular fibrillation occurs. Essentially, these actions are as follows:

1. Defibrillate initially at 200 joules. If unsuccessful (determined by assessing for the return of a pulse), repeat the defibrillation at 300 joules. If still unsuccessful, repeat at 360 joules.
2. If initial defibrillations are unsuccessful, begin cardiopulmonary resuscitation (CPR) and establish artificial airway and venous access.
3. Administer epinephrine (10 mg). Epinephrine can be repeated every five minutes.
4. Defibrillate at 360 joules.

5. If unsuccessful, restart CPR and give lidocaine (1 mg/kg). Lidocaine can be repeated up to a total of 3 mg/kg, although usually the repeat doses are at 0.5 mg/kg.
6. Defibrillate at 360 joules.
7. If unsuccessful, restart CPR and administer bretylium (5 mg/kg). Bretylium can be given to a total dose of 30 mg/kg.
8. Defibrillate at 360 joules.

During the sequence, sodium bicarbonate can be considered to correct an acidosis. If the rhythm terminates, start a drip of whichever drug (lidocaine or bretylium) was likely responsible for aiding in the termination of the rhythm.

TABLE 5-5. VENTRICULAR TACHYCARDIA CATEGORIES AND TREATMENT

Type	Characteristics	Treatment
Stable	No symptoms	Lidocaine Pronestyl Bretylium
Unstable I	Mild symptoms (chest pain, shortness of breath (SOB))	Synchronized Cardioversion, beginning at 50 joules and progressing to 360 joules
Unstable II	Serious symptoms (pulmonary edema, hypotension)	Defibrillation, beginning at 50 joules and progressing to 360 joules
Unstable III	No pulse	Treat as ventricular fibrillation

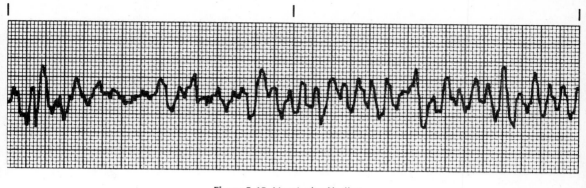

Figure 5-15. Ventricular fibrillation.

Nursing Intervention

Document the dysrhythmia with a rhythm strip and keep the monitor recorder running throughout the dysrhythmia. Initiate cardiac arrest procedures and follow the above guidelines.

ESCAPE BEATS

A dominant rhythm, essentially regular but with intermittent interruptions, may contain escape beats. This results in an occasional prolonged RR interval. Several areas may produce escape beats.

Atrial escape beats have an abnormal P wave, a normal PR interval, and a normal QRS complex. Junctional escape beats have an abnormal P wave, a short PR interval, and usually a normal QRS complex. Ventricular escape beats have an abnormal QRS complex without a preceding P wave.

Escape beats usually occur with an associated prolonged RR interval (but not long enough to be compensatory).

Escape beats are of minor significance and usually require no treatment. It is important not to suppress an escape beat; this might allow ventricular foci of a more serious nature to develop.

PACEMAKERS

There are many pathologic states that may be most efficiently treated by the use of an artificial pacemaker. Pacemakers may be particularly useful in the treatment of symptomatic bradycardias that have not responded to atropine or isoproterenol.

Definition

A pacemaker is a system consisting of a lead and a pulse generator. The generator is capable of producing repeated, short (three to five milliseconds), and rhythmic bursts of electric current for a prolonged period of time. The bursts of electric current are of sufficient magnitude to initiate depolarization of the heart.

Modes of Pacing

There are two modes of pacing. Temporary pacing is one mode used mainly to manage emergencies such as acute heart block and cardiac arrest. Two types of temporary pacemakers exist: transvenous or transthoracic and transcutaneous (external). In the transvenous or transthoracic mode, the lead is inserted into the right atrium or ventricle. The pulse generator is external. Insertion routes include the transvenous (brachial via cutdown), subclavian, femoral, or jugular (via percutaneous entry), postsurgery (endocardial), and transthoracic (needle through chest into heart muscle). The power supply for temporary pacing is external batteries (the pulse generator). For a specific insertion procedure, the nurse is referred to his or her institution policy.

Transcutaneous cardiac pacing has gained increasing acceptance in recent years. The principle of transcutaneous pacing is based on sending direct current transcutaneously between electrodes placed on the skin. The advantages of transcutaneous pacing are the ease of use (it can be applied in a matter of minutes) and the fact that no invasive equipment is necessary. The benefit of pacing is obtained through this method without the difficulty of inserting the transvenous or transthoracic pacing mode.

In the transcutaneous mode of pacing, the nurse must be aware of the potential for some discomfort for the patient due to the electrical stimulation. The electrical stimulation will cause superficial, as well as cardiac, muscle contraction. Some conscious patients, particularly if the milliampere setting is high, may complain of pain upon stimulation. Sedatives or analgesics may be required.

Permanent pacing with a fully implantable system is a second mode of pacing the heart. The pulse generator is implanted into the patient. The pulse generator contains the circuit for the specific pacing mode selected and a battery that provides energy to the circuit. The components are encased in a nonconductive plastic material that does not react with body tissue.

Indications for Pacing

The major indication for pacing is the development of second-degree type II or third-degree heart block. Pacemakers can be used for any bradycardia that is producing hypotension or signs of reduced cardiac output.

Chronic heart block of varied degrees may be treated by pacing if the patient has syncopal episodes, congestive heart failure, convulsions, or evidence of cerebral dysfunction.

Intermittent complete heart block (third degree) is often treated with a pacemaker. Usually, there is evidence of block in one or two of the three bundle branches (fascicles). Thus, these patients rely solely on the third fascicle, which may become dysfunctional at any time.

Complete heart block that develops in conjunction with an acute myocardial infarction may be an indication for pacing. If the infarction is anterior, the involved artery is usually the left anterior descending. This results in ischemia or necrosis of part of the ventricular septum, with damage to the intraventricular conduction system below the His bundle. These patients frequently die despite the insertion of a pacemaker because of the extent of myocardial damage. If the infarction is posterior or inferior, the artery involved is usually the right coronary (90% of the time) or the circumflex (10% of the time). The area of damage is the AV node area. Types I and II may be indications for pacing. Type I may progress into a type II (2:1) or higher block. Type II, due to the block occurring below the AV node, often progresses into third-degree heart block. A block that develops postinfarction is usually transient and responds to atropine or a brief period of time with a temporary pacemaker.

Conduction defects may occur after a cardiac surgical procedure. For this reason, most cardiac surgeries (e.g., coronary artery bypass grafting) have pacing wires attached to the epicardium for postoperative management. Some centers also use a pacing port through a pulmonary artery catheter.

Pacemakers may be used in other rhythm disturbances if bradycardia is a component of the dysrhythmia. Sick sinus syndrome indicates dysfunction of the SA node. This may occur as sinus bradycardia, sinus arrest, and/or brady-tachy syndromes.

Pacemakers may also be used to treat tachydysrhythmias, such as atrial or ventricular tachycardia. In these rhythmias, the pacemaker rate is increased to a level higher than the tachycardia. Once the pacemaker is controlling the rate, the rate is slowed to a more acceptable level.

Pacemakers may be used as a diagnostic aid to evaluate SA node function and AV node function. They may be used to eliminate multiple ectopic foci by overriding the rate of the foci, or they may be used to abolish reentry phenomena by delivering a premature stimulus that breaks the reentry pattern.

Types of Pacing Modes

Several types of pacing modes exist. These are categorized according to the Inter-Society Commission on Heart Disease (ICHD) nomenclature in Table 5-6. There are two codes, a simplified three-letter and more comprehensive five-letter code. Table 5-6 contains the five-letter code. As a rule, the CCRN exam requires one to remember only the simpler three-letter code.

The major concept to remember is that the pacemaker electrically paces a cardiac chamber (the first letter), senses an electrical impulse in a cardiac chamber (the second letter), and discharges the impulse in either a triggered or inhibited manner (the third letter). In critical care, the inhibited manner is almost always used.

If a patient had a transvenous pacemaker inserted that would pace and sense only in the ventricle, the ICHD description would be a VVI. If the pacemaker paced both atrium and ventricle, but sensed only in the ventricle, then the pacemaker would be a DVI (AV sequential) pacemaker.

Nursing Care

The patient with a temporary pacemaker will need documentation as to the effectiveness of rhythm capture and sensing. The electrical signal indicating that a

TABLE 5-6. FIVE-POSITION PACEMAKER CODE (ICHD)

I. Chamber Paced	II. Chamber Sensed	III. Mode of Response	IV. Programmability	V. Tachyrhythmia Functions
V = Ventricle		I = Inhibited	P = Programmable rate and/or output	B = Burst
A = Atrium		T = Triggered		N = Normal rate completion
D = Atrium and ventricle		D = Atrial triggered and ventricular inhibited	M = Multiprogram- mability	S = Scanning
O = None		O = None	O = None	E = External
			C = Programmable with telemetry	

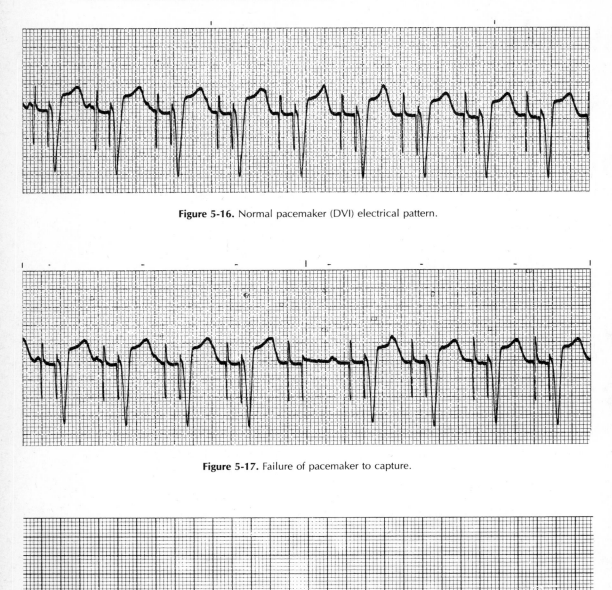

Figure 5-16. Normal pacemaker (DVI) electrical pattern.

Figure 5-17. Failure of pacemaker to capture.

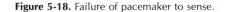

Figure 5-18. Failure of pacemaker to sense.

pacemaker impulse has occurred should be evident only immediately prior to capturing a paced beat (Fig. 5-16). If a pacemaker signal is present and the heart is not in a refractory mode, a captured beat should follow. If no beat occurs, this would be called failure to capture (Fig. 5-17). Failure to sense would be a paced beat or pacemaker artifact occurring too soon after a spontaneous beat. The spontaneous beat should inhibit the next paced impulse; if it does not, failure to sense is present (Fig. 5-18). Notify the physician if either of these conditions occurs more than once.

Care of the pacemaker insertion site is the same as for any central intravenous catheter. Careful explanation of the purpose and duration of the pacemaker to the patient is important in order to avoid unnecessary anxiety.

CHAPTER 6

Angina Pectoris and Myocardial Infarction

The CCRN exam can be expected to contain questions on assessing and treating coronary artery disease. This chapter provides brief but key concepts in the area of coronary artery disease. Expect several questions in the CCRN exam on the assessment, diagnosis, and treatment of angina and myocardial infarctions.

Angina (including coronary artery vasospasm) and myocardial infarction (MI), are common test items on the CCRN exam. Fortunately, if one works in a coronary area, the assessments and interventions may be familiar. This chapter emphasizes the main features of the origin, symptomatology and medical and nursing interventions associated with angina and MI. An understanding of the concepts in this chapter should aid in successfully answering questions regarding these conditions.

A series of physiologic changes within the body and heart starts with arteriosclerosis and advances (without intervention) to coronary artery disease. A combination of lipid accumulation and endothelial injury with subsequent thrombosis formation probably forms the basis for obstruction of blood flow. While obstruction of blood flow is responsible for symptoms associated with coronary artery disease, the symptoms will vary depending on the development of collateral circulation. The first symptoms of coronary artery disease may be those of angina pectoris, but they may also be myocardial infarction or sudden death.

ARTERIOSCLEROSIS/ATHEROSCLEROSIS

Arteriosclerosis is the name applied to a group of three chronic disease states, one of which is termed atherosclerosis. Frequently, the terms arteriosclerosis and atherosclerosis are used interchangeably to mean that fatty acid plaques have adhered to the intimal layer of the arteries. Although atherosclerosis occurs throughout the body, the focus in this chapter is on the effect of atherosclerosis upon the heart and the coronary arteries.

Classification

The degree of atherosclerosis can be described in several ways. A recent review presented a three-step description. The CCRN exam has not traditionally asked questions regarding the classification of atherosclerosis. For the purpose of this chapter, a four-step process will be used for illustration (Fig. 6-1). Normally (i.e., ideally), significant atherosclerosis is not present. However, almost all blood vessels have some degree of atherosclerosis.

1. Grade one atherosclerosis is minimal; that is, less than 25% of the lumen of the coronary artery is occluded.
2. Grade two atherosclerosis is present when 50% of the lumen of the coronary artery is occluded.
3. Grade three is severe atherosclerosis with 75% of the lumen of the coronary artery occluded.
4. Grade four is complete occlusion of the coronary artery, resulting in MI unless collateral circulation has developed.

Obstruction by atherosclerotic plaques may occur in any or all of the coronary arteries. It is thought that grade three atherosclerosis must be present before significant symptoms develop. Specific factors tend to be related to the development of atherosclerosis.

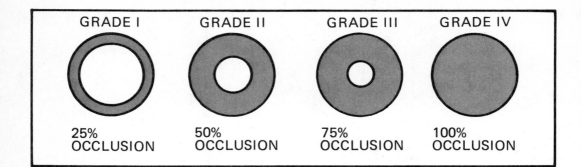

Figure 6-1. The four grades of coronary artery occlusion.

Etiology

Four Unalterable Risk Factors

1. Hereditary predisposition to the development of atherosclerosis seems to be a prime factor in developing atherosclerosis.
2. Age appears to influence the development of atherosclerosis, since it is more prevalent in older persons than in younger persons.
3. Sex seems to be a factor in the development of atherosclerosis, since the condition is more prevalent in men than in women (at least prior to menopause). Recent evidence suggests that postmenopausal women may have a higher incidence of myocardial disease than was previously estimated.
4. Race may influence atherosclerosis. It appears to be more common in Caucasians, although other factors, such as diet, may obscure the influence of race.

Medically Alterable Risk Factors

1. Hypertension has been shown to be related to the development of atherosclerosis. Close medical treatment of hypertension may retard the development of atherosclerosis.
2. Diabetics develop atherosclerosis more often than nondiabetics. Close medical treatment and control of diabetes may reduce the atherosclerotic process.
3. Hyperlipidemia, when accompanied by high serum cholesterol levels, may have a bearing on the development and/or progression of atherosclerosis. The presence of low-density lipoproteins appears to be a precursor to the development of atherosclerosis. Medical treatment of hyperlipidemia may help retard the atherosclerotic process.

Personal Alterable Risk Factors. These factors can be altered by the individual to decrease the possibility or progression of atherosclerosis.

1. Weight control can be beneficial in reducing the risk of coronary artery disease.
2. Cigarette smokers have an higher incidence of heart disease than do nonsmokers. Elimination of smoking will reduce the risk of MI.
3. Emotional tension and stress, such as experienced by type A personalities, may be influential in the development of myocardial disease. The exact role of emotional stress is not as clear as the physical factors contributing to coronary disease.
4. Sedentary life styles predispose one to developing atherosclerosis. Exercising three to four times per week for 30 minutes of activity that pushes the heart rate into the target heart rate zone for aerobic exercise will reduce the rate of coronary artery disease.
5. Moderate alcohol intake may reduce the risk of coronary artery disease. However, the limitation to moderate intake is difficult in many people, and the risk of alcoholism may outweigh the benefit of this factor.

If an individual is sufficiently motivated, these last five risk factors can be incorporated into a personal life style.

Prognosis

One cannot change some risk factors, one can alter other risk factors with medical treatment, and one can eliminate some risk factors if so motivated. If risk factors are not modified, atherosclerosis may progress from the development of angina and ischemia to myocardial infarction, congestive heart failure, or sudden death. Despite the prognosis with alterable risk factors, coronary atherosclerosis is still one of the leading causes of deaths in the United States.

ANGINA PECTORIS

Angina can result from a reduced blood flow, low oxygen content, or myocardial oxygen demand in excess of supply. No actual injury to the myocardial muscle occurs during most types of angina. Autopsy results of patients with angina have demonstrated frequent total occlusion of coronary vessels with subsequent development of extensive collateral circulation. The development of collateral circulation has allowed maintenance of coronary perfusion and no permanent injury to the myocardium even when cardiac catheterization results have indicated total occlusion.

Causes of reduced blood flow to the myocardium include atherosclerosis, valvular dysfunction, hypotension, and coronary vasospasm. Low oxygen content can also precipitate anginal episodes. Causes of low oxygen content include reduced hemoglobin and low PaO_2/SaO_2 levels. Causes of excessive oxygen demands relative to perfusion include hypertension, exercise, and increased metabolic rates. Many predisposing factors can precipitate a reduced blood flow, decreased oxygen content, or increased myocardial oxygen demands.

The occurrence of angina is variable, depending substantially on the degree of collateral circulation that has developed to reduce blood and oxygen flow. Angina can be suddenly precipitated by any event that increases oxygen demand (such as anxiety, stress, eating, or exercise) or reduces blood flow (smoking or sleeping).

Clinical Presentation

Pain is the primary symptom. It may be described as burning, squeezing in a tight band, or extreme heaviness or pressure on the lower sternum. It may radiate to the neck, jaws, shoulders, arms, and stomach.

Characteristically, the pain begins after eating or physical activity and subsides with rest. The pain usually lasts one to four minutes, but it may require as long as ten minutes to subside completely. Anginal pain should always last less than 30 minutes. Pain for more than 30 minutes suggests MI and the need for immediate treatment. Not all coronary artery disease will present with anginal symptoms. Some patients can have evidence of ischemia without symptoms. This possibility of ischemia without pain serves as a clue in the education of patients with angina and MI. Frequent evaluation of cardiac status, such as with exercise testing, can detect symptoms earlier than waiting for an anginal episode to indicate ischemia.

Diagnosis

Diagnosis of angina is based on history and ECG findings. Cardiac isoenzymes are usually normal. The 12-lead ECG usually has depressed ST segments over the affected area. ST segment elevation (Prinzmetal's angina) can occur but is less common.

Treatment

Vasodilators, such as sublingual nitroglycerin, usually relieve the angina within $1\frac{1}{2}$ minutes. Nitroglycerin taken before an activity may prevent an attack. Alteration of one's life style to eliminate the alterable risk factors may help decrease the severity and frequency of attacks. If the angina attacks increase in frequency or intensity (crescendo angina), stress testing and/or cardiac catheterization to determine the extent of the disease is indicated. Nitrates, beta blockers, and calcium channel blockers may be used alone or in combination to resolve anginal episodes. The patient may be a candidate for transluminal angioplasty or coronary bypass surgery, which will stop the angina and decrease the risk of myocardial infarction. The patient is advised to exercise within the limits of pain and obtain adequate rest. Coronary artery bypass grafting (CABG) is the treatment for failure of medical intervention. CABG has demonstrated the potential for alleviating symptoms of angina although not necessarily prolonging life.

Variants

Several variations of angina exist. The most prevalent is unstable angina, which accounts for approximately 20% of all cardiac care unit admissions. Unstable angina differs from stable angina in that it is more easily initiated. Unstable angina usually involves crescendo angina, may occur at rest, and is characterized by increasing severity in the past few months. Clinically, the patient may complain of reduction in activities that precipitate anginal episodes and an increase in severity of symptoms.

Treatment of unstable angina usually requires additional medical therapy. Beta blockers (propanolol) are helpful in reducing myocardial oxygen consumption. Calcium channel blockers (nifedipine) may be useful in reducing afterload and myocardial oxygen use.

Another type of angina, Prinzmetal's angina, was identified in 1959. In this form of angina, the origin is thought to be both coronary vasospasm and stenosis. The patient presents with symptoms most often including pain at rest and other symptoms of angina. The ECG shows reversible ST segment elevation rather than depression.

Calcium channel blockers have much more effect in reducing the anginal episode than do beta blockers, probably because they reduce vasospasm to a greater extent. Diltiazem and nifedipine are both effective in reducing episodes of Prinzmetal's angina. If medical therapy fails, both unstable angina and Prinzmetal's angina may require CABG or angioplasty.

Coronary Artery Vasospasm. Coronary artery vasospasm, a form of variant angina, is a transient narrowing of a large coronary artery. The origins are unclear but could include sympathetic stimulation, prostaglandin mediation, or pharmacologic stimulation. Treatment is similar to that for angina, with more emphasis on calcium channel blockers as well as nitroglycerin.

ACUTE MYOCARDIAL INFARCTION

Myocardial infarction is the actual necrosis or death of myocardial tissue because of reduced blood supply (loss of oxygen) to a specific area of the heart (Fig. 6-2).

Etiology

In most MIs, atherosclerotic heart disease is present. The remaining incidences of MIs are likely due to coronary artery spasm in which the artery spasms sufficiently to prevent blood from reaching the myocardium.

Most MIs have been demonstrated to be the result of coronary thrombosis formation on top of an atherosclerotic plaque. The rapid identification of myocardial infarction is crucial to treatment. Within six hours of onset, myocardial muscle becomes generally

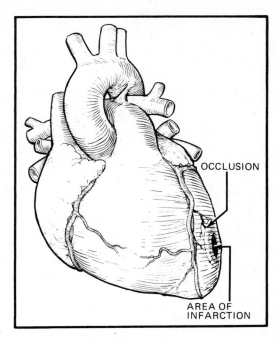

Figure 6-2. Myocardial infarction.

irreversibly damaged. While this time period can vary and some tissue can be salvaged at later times, the earlier the treatment, the more likely recovery will take place.

Diagnosis and Clinical Presentation

Chest pain with nausea (and maybe vomiting), diaphoresis, and weakness are the most common symptoms of an MI. The infarct pain differs from anginal pain. With an MI, the chest pain is constant, severe, and not relieved with nitroglycerin. The location of the pain is similar to that for anginal pain. It is, however, not relieved with rest or lying down. In fact, it often occurs at rest without a clear precipitating event. As the pain, nausea, weakness, and diaphoresis continue, patients become dyspneic and often develop severe apprehension that may be accompanied by a sense of impending doom.

The 12-lead ECG reveals initial T-wave inversion followed quickly by ST segment elevation in the affected area. Q-wave formation, indicating cellular death, occurs after 24 hours and is considered more diagnostic of myocardial infarction. Areas of the heart and their corresponding ECG leads for MI interpreta-

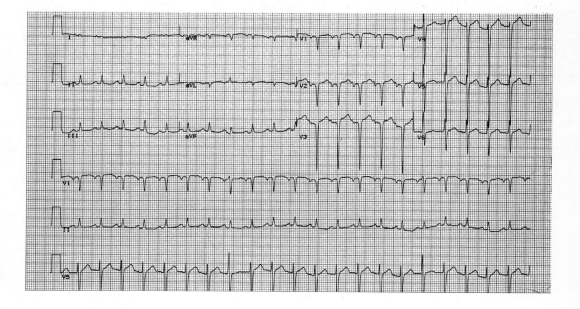

Figure 6-3. Anterior-septal myocardial infarction.

tion are presented in Table 5-1. Figure 6-3 contains an example of myocardial infarction of the anterior-septal region, Fig.6-4 shows an example of an inferior MI, and Fig. 6-5 illustrates a lateral MI.

Cardiac isoenzymes are the most diagnostic criteria for MIs. Specifically, creatine phosphokinase (CPK) and lactic dehydrogenase (LDH) isoenzymes are used, with CPK isoenzymes possessing enough accuracy to be used without LDH isoenzymes. CPK isoenzymes include MM, MB, and BB bands. The CPK-MB band is more specific for cardiac muscle. If the CPK-MB band elevates more than 12 IU, a myocardial infarction can be diagnosed with 95% accuracy. When LDH isoenzymes are used, the LDH 1 isoenzyme, indicative of cardiac muscle, elevates. LDH 1 is normally lower than LDH 2; in an MI, LDH 1 exceeds LDH 2, resulting in a "flip" of LDH 1 and 2.

The potential value of LDH in MI is the slower elevation of the LDH isoenzymes. CPK isoenzymes elevate within hours of injury, peaking within 24 hours. LDH rises more slowly and may not peak until 48 to 72 hours. The slower rise in LDH may be useful in the patient who delays coming to the hospital after the onset of symptoms.

Occlusion of the right coronary artery results in an inferior MI. Inferior MIs have a lower mortality rate than anterior MIs. Symptoms associated with an inferior MI include more mild AV node dysrhythmias, such as first- and second-degree type I blocks.

Occlusion of the left anterior descending coronary artery results in an anterior MI. Anterior MIs have higher mortality rates and are associated with more serious dysrhythmias. Rhythm disturbances are more likely to include second- and third-degree blocks.

Less serious MIs are lateral and posterior, each with lower mortality rates than inferior or posterior MIs. More dangerous MIs are those with multiple regions affected, such as anterior-lateral MIs. When more than 40% of the left ventricle is acutely damaged, mortality is extremely high.

Right ventricular MIs are less common and are commonly associated with obstruction of the right coronary or left circumflex artery. Mortality is less with right ventricular MIs. Diagnosis is made from the ECG, indicating a posterior MI pattern (large R waves in V_1 and V_2) and ST segment elevation in the right precordial leads, e.g., V_{4R} and V_{6R}.

Symptoms include elevated CVP values although

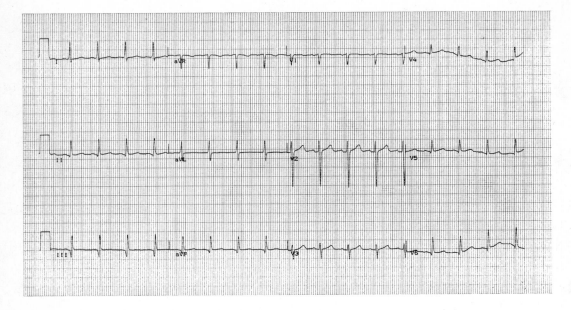

Figure 6-4. Inferior myocardial infarction.

PCWP levels may be normal. Venous congestion, the result of the high CVP from RV failure, is the primary symptom. Treatment centers on maintaining CVP values higher than normal, up to 25 mm Hg, in order to improve blood flow through the right ventricle. In severe RV failure, less blood is pumped into the lungs, and a drop in PCWP results.

Treatment and Complications

The goals of treating an infarction are to increase coronary blood flow and decrease oxygen demand. These goals should prevent death or extension of injury to the myocardium and control or correct dysrhythmias that occur.

Pain relief is a prime objective and is usually accomplished with intravenous analgesics, i.e., morphine sulfate (drug of choice), hydromorphone hydrochloride (Dilaudid), or meperidine hydrochloride (Demerol). Vasodilators such as nitroglycerin are also likely to reduce pain.

Thrombolytic Therapy. If the patient presents within four hours of onset of symptoms, thrombolysis is the treatment of choice. Controversy exists as to the agent of choice, either a tissue plasminogen activator (TPA) or streptokinase. TPA has more specific clot

resolution activity than streptokinase but is much more expensive.

Nursing care of the patient with thrombolytic therapy centers around reducing potential episodes of bleeding. Only arterial punctures and venipunctures that are absolutely necessary should be performed. Finger oximetry should be employed, for example, rather than drawing blood gases to obtain a PaO_2 level. If venipuncture has been performed, extra time in holding the site is necessary to achieve hemostasis.

Assessment of the patient for signs of bleeding is important. Hypotension, tachycardia, or specific organ changes (i.e., reduced level of consciousness) are indicators of possible bleeding.

Reperfusion dysrhythmias are common. Bradycardias are frequently seen after infusion of thrombolytic agents. Ventricular tachycardias are also common. Treatment of dysrhythmias is discussed in Chapter 5.

Cardiac catheterization is performed as soon as possible, perhaps even during the acute MI episode. Angioplasty, athrectomy, or surgery (CABG) may be performed at this time.

Angioplasty. Angioplasty is the dilatation of a stenotic coronary artery through the insertion of a catheter into the coronary artery. Once the catheter is inserted, the stenotic area (identified by cardiac catheterization) is compressed through expanding a balloon on the end of the catheter. Angioplasty has the benefit of avoiding CABG while maintaining good results with expanding the stenotic area.

Several criteria for angioplasty are present. Criteria for angioplasty include one-vessel coronary artery disease, stable angina of less than one year, no prior MI, lesion that is easy to reach (proximal) and discrete, and normal LV function; a patient meeting these criteria is a candidate for CABG if necessary.

Nursing care of the patient with angioplasty includes care of the cardiac catheterization insertion site (bedrest and site compression for several hours) and observation for signs of reperfusion (dysrhythmias). If the stenosis recurs, chest pain or symptoms of decreased cardiac output may occur.

Athrectomy

A newer therapy is athrectomy, or the removal of the atherosclerotic plaque by excision. This technique is still developing, but essentially involves cutting the narrowed area after it has been identified from cardiac catheterization. While reocclusion still occurs, the technique has the potential for improving long-term patency of the coronary artery.

Medical Therapy. If cardiac support is necessary, dobutamine is the therapy of choice to improve inotropic (strength) properties of the heart. Dopamine would be reserved for episodes of hypotension or at low doses (less than 5 mcg/kg/min) to improve renal blood flow. If medical support is not adequate, intra-aortic balloon pumping has been demonstrated to effectively increase hemodynamic performance.

Vasodilators, such as nitroglycerin or nitroprusside, may be cautiously employed in an attempt to reduce preload and afterload. Continuous hemodynamic monitoring is necessary to accurately manipulate many of the cardiac medications.

Continuous cardiac monitoring is used to provide for the early identification and intervention of dysrhythmias. If the patient survives the initial infarction and subsequently dies, death is usually due to a shock

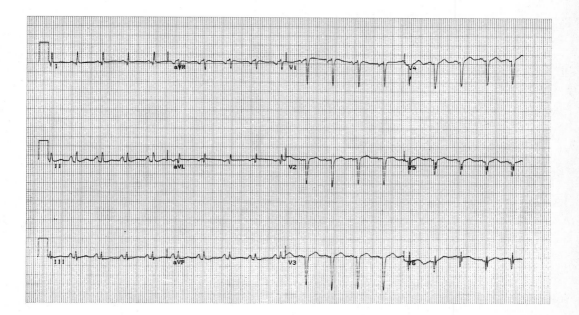

Figure 6-5. Lateral myocardial infarction.

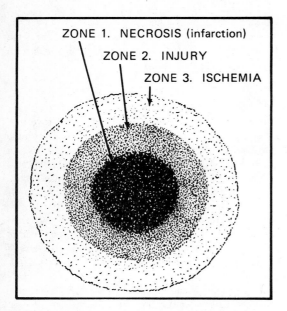

ZONE 1. NECROSIS (infarction)

ZONE 2. INJURY

ZONE 3. ISCHEMIA

Figure 6-6. The development of scar tissue following myocardial infarction.

syndrome. Dysrhythmias of all types, including conduction disturbances, occur.

Oxygen therapy is usually started to ensure that sufficient oxygen content is available for myocardial needs. An intravenous line is started for use in emergency situations. Food, usually low in sodium, is given as tolerated. Many cardiac care units prohibit foods containing caffeine (a mild cardiac stimulant).

Hemodynamic monitoring must be continuous for early intervention in congestive failure, ventricular failure with pulmonary edema, and cardiogenic shock. Bedrest and emotional support of the patient are necessary for healing the injured myocardium.

Long-term immobility may result in venous pooling, with an increased risk of thromboembolism. Passive and active range-of-motion exercises and support hose help reduce this risk.

Less common but equally lethal complications of an MI include pericarditis, papillary muscle rupture, ventricular aneurysm, and ventricular rupture. Sudden death commonly occurs with the last three of these complications.

Recovery

Recovery begins as soon as myocardial injury and necrosis stop. Scar tissue develops (Fig. 6-6) at the necrotic area. This process takes six to eight weeks to complete.

Emotional support of the patient and family is a key factor in recovery. Patients often feel that their active and productive lives are over. It is not uncommon to see the patient and family members going through the stages of grief following an MI. Education of the patient and family in ways of changing their life styles to eliminate alterable risk factors is an essential role of the nurse and helps the patient and family work through the emotional grieving process.

CHAPTER 7

Congestive Heart Failure, Pulmonary Edema, and Pericarditis

Editor's Note

The assessment of abnormal hemodynamics, particularly in regard to left and right ventricular failure, is a common topic for questions in the CCRN exam. This chapter reviews the major concepts normally employed in the assessment, as well as diagnosis and interventions associated with ventricular dysfunction. Expect several questions on the CCRN exam from this content area.

TABLE 7-1. METHODS TO ASSESS LEFT AND RIGHT VENTRICULAR PERFORMANCE

Parameter	Right Ventricle	Left Ventricle
Preload	CVP	PCWP
Afterload	PVR	SVR
Contractility	Stroke volume	Stroke volume

CVP = central venous pressure; PCWP = pulmonary capillary wedge pressure; PVR = pulmonary vascular resistance; SVR = systemic vascular resistance.

All forms of myocardial failure are based upon a disturbance in the relation BP = CO × SVR, where BP is blood pressure, CO is cardiac output, and SVR is systemic vascular resistance. Specifically, the problem lies in a disturbance of the CO, although the SVR can affect the output. When studying the concept of myocardial failure, keep in mind the factors that regulate cardiac output, i.e., preload, afterload, and contractility. All myocardial failure can be assessed and treated through these three components. While ventricular failure can be assessed by noting each component of cardiac output, each ventricle is assessed slightly differently. For example, preload of the left ventricle is partially assessed by the pulmonary capillary wedge pressure (PCWP), while preload of the right ventricle is assessed by the central venous pressure (CVP). Other factors used to differentiate left and right ventricular influences are listed in Table 7-1.

The specific pressures frequently used in the assessment of ventricular preload are listed in the guidelines of Table 7-2. While these guidelines are general examples, the CCRN exam is likely to utilize values such as these when clinical scenarios are provided in situations describing ventricular failure. More sophisticated measures to estimate cardiac performance, such

as radionucleotide ventriculogram and echocardiography, are available. However, the basic guidelines listed in Tables 7-1 and 7-2 are fundamental to assessing cardiac performance in most clinical practice settings. Because of the common application of these concepts, it is helpful to understand their role in clinical assessment.

CONGESTIVE HEART FAILURE

Congestive heart failure (CHF) is the inability of the heart to pump blood through the systemic circulation in an amount sufficient to meet the body's needs. CHF

TABLE 7-2. USE OF THE PULMONARY CAPILLARY WEDGE PRESSURE (PCWP) AND CVP

Value	Condition Indicated
PCWP	
<8	Hypovolemia
8–12	Normal
12–18	Beginning failure or fluid overload
>18	Left ventricular failure
CVP	
0–5	Normal or hypovolemia
5–10	Beginning failure or fluid overload
>10	Right ventricular failure

normally refers to biventricular failure, although it is important to understand that each ventricle can fail independently of the other. Left ventricular failure is a common precursor to right ventricular failure and can precede right ventricular dysfunction. Right ventricular failure is frequently associated with lung disease or dysfunction, or it may be the result of ischemia of the right-sided coronary circulation. Right ventricular failure is unlikely to produce left ventricular failure.

Chronic heart failure is the gradual inability of the heart to pump sufficient blood to meet the body's demands. Chronic heart failure can become acute without an obvious cause or may be precipitated by an acute ischemic cardiac event. The presence of right ventricular failure in the face of left ventricular failure usually indicates a more advanced disease state and worse prognosis.

Etiology

Unless specified otherwise, assume that the term CHF implies biventricular failure. On the CCRN exam, if only one ventricle is involved, the term CHF will not likely be employed. Signs and symptoms of CHF result from both ventricles failing. However, even though signs and symptoms of CHF are biventricular in nature, the origin of the failure is usually the left ventricle. Factors commonly influencing the development of left ventricular dysfunction and eventually causing CHF are listed in Table 7-3.

Left ventricular pump failure usually occurs before right ventricular pump failure. The left ventricular myocardium weakens to the extent that it cannot eject blood in the normal amount. This reduces the cardiac output secondary to a reduction in stroke volume. Before stroke volume decreases, however, two changes in myocardial function may take place. First, if the failure is slow, the left ventricle enlarges in both capacity (measured by end diastolic volume [EDV]) and muscle size. Second, the ability of the heart to eject blood

TABLE 7-3. CAUSES OF CHF

Systemic hypertension
Coronary artery disease
   Myocardial infarction
   Angina
Aortic stenosis
Mitral regurgitation
Cardiomyopathy
Atrial and ventricular tachydysrhythmias

(measured by ejection fraction [EF]) is reduced but offset by the increased end diastolic volume.

Normally, about 70% of the end diastolic volume is ejected with each beat. The amount of blood ejected with each beat is the stroke volume. The amount of blood ejected (stroke volume [SV]) in comparison with the EDV is termed the ejection fraction (SV/EDV = EF). As the contractile ability of the heart worsens, EF falls. As EF levels decrease to below 40%, exercise limitations become evident and progress to interfere with activities of daily living.

If the left ventricle cannot pump all the blood it receives from the atrium, a buildup of blood and pressure occurs in the left atrium. As the pressure increases in the left atrium, it becomes more difficult for blood to enter the atrium from the pulmonary veins. As the blood in the pulmonary veins becomes unable to flow into the left atrium, blood backs up in the lung vessels. When pressure in the pulmonary capillaries exceeds 18 to 25 mm Hg, fluid from the capillaries leaks into the interstitial spaces. Once this leaking of fluid into the pulmonary interstitial space exceeds the ability of the pulmonary lymphatics to drain the fluid, pulmonary edema may develop.

Since the lung vasculature is distensible, it can accept a moderate amount of increased pressure and volume. However, without intervention, the pressure in the pulmonary capillaries increases to the point that the right ventricle cannot eject its blood into the lungs for oxygenation. As the backflow pressure increases, the right ventricle fails and the CVP increases. Then blood from the right atrium cannot drain completely, and consequently the right atrium cannot accommodate all of the blood entering from the venae cavae. Since venous blood flow to the heart is impeded, venous pooling and eventual organ congestion with venous blood occur.

Left Versus Right Heart Failure

Right heart failure is most commonly caused by left heart failure and then by all the factors that cause left heart failure. Right failure may also be caused by isolated right coronary ischemia, pulmonary emboli, essential pulmonary hypertension, and chronic obstructive pulmonary disease.

Left heart failure alone can occur from the same factors that cause CHF. Since left heart failure occurs before right heart failure in these cases, initial symptoms of left heart failure differ from those of CHF. Due to the potential for left heart before right heart failure, measures that formerly were used to estimate left heart function by right-sided measures (such as CVP) have been demonstrated to be inaccurate.

Clinical Presentation
Symptoms of left and right heart failure are presented in Table 7-4.

Complications
The major complications of heart failure are the progression of failure and loss of cardiac output and oxygen delivery. In addition, progression of cardiac failure can lead to the development of lethal dysrhythmias. It is also important to keep in mind that therapies to treat heart failure may cause drug toxicity (including oxygen toxicity) and fluid and electrolyte imbalances.

Treatment and Nursing Intervention
The goal of treating CHF is to improve ventricular function and to prevent the progression to right heart failure. Three methods of treatment exist, based on the factors regulating stroke volume.

1. Improve contractility of the ventricle. This is attempted by drug therapy with positive inotropic agents such as dobutamine. Within the limits of Starling's law, this method of treatment is very effective. Only three inotropes are commonly used in acute clinical settings: dobutamine, dopamine, and amrinone. Indications for use of these inotropes are centered around low cardiac indices (less than 2.2 LPM/m^2) and high PCWP (over 18 mm Hg). In theory, these agents are the ideal treatment choice due to the ability to directly improve stroke volume, ejection fraction, and cardiac output. Unfortunately, no consistently effective oral inotrope has been demonstrated to be effective. Several oral inotropes are under clinical trials. Digitalis preparations, such

as digoxin, have been used in the chronic control of CHF. However, the role of digitalis preparations in CHF is controversial. Recent research has supported the chronic use of digitalis. Its role in acute CHF is less clear.

Part of the reason for the less than optimal effectiveness of oral inotropes may involve a concept called down regulation. Down regulation refers to the lack of responsiveness of cardiac muscle to sympathetic stimulation. In chronic heart failure, sympathetic stimulation has been occurring for a long time. This chronic stimulation leads eventually to failure of the cardiac muscle to respond to further stimulation. Due to the failure of long-term oral inotropes in the presence of CHF, the current therapy emphasizes manipulation of preload and afterload to improve contractility.

2. Decrease afterload. Afterload is the resistance of the blood, valves, and blood vessels that the left ventricle must overcome to eject blood. Decreasing any of these factors will decrease afterload. Reduction in afterload (estimated by the SVR) eases the work of the left ventricle. Reduced work may allow for improved contractility, thereby increasing stroke volume and cardiac output. Afterload agents include vasodilators of several different pharmacologic types, including nitroprusside, angiotensin-converting enzyme inhibitors (captopril and enalapril), calcium channel blockers (nifedipine and nicardipine), and many other agents.

3. Decrease preload. If one can lower the volume of blood entering the left atrium, the stress on the left ventricle is reduced. Diuretic therapy (e.g., furosemide and thiazides), venodilators (nitroglycerin), and fluid and sodium restrictions are examples of treatment of preload.

Close monitoring of the patient and his or her response to these treatments is very important in early detection of a deteriorating state requiring more aggressive therapy.

PULMONARY EDEMA

Pulmonary edema is the most serious progression of CHF. Pulmonary edema may occur when pressure in the pulmonary vasculature exceeds 18 to 25 mm Hg.

TABLE 7-4. SYMPTOMS OF LEFT AND RIGHT VENTRICULAR FAILURE

Left Ventricle	Right Ventricle
Orthopnea	Distended neck veins
Dyspnea of exertion	Dependent edema
Crackles	Hepatic engorgement
Low PaO$_2$/SaO$_2$/SpO$_2$	Hepatojugular reflux
S$_3$, S$_4$	
Systolic murmur	

This results in extravasation of fluid from pulmonary capillaries into interstitial tissue and intra-alveolar spaces.

Etiology

Acute pulmonary edema is usually the result of left ventricular failure although noncardiac forms of pulmonary edema (e.g., adult respiratory distress syndrome) exist. Symptoms of CHF are exacerbated in pulmonary edema. Dyspnea and orthopnea become markedly pronounced; crackles may be heard throughout the lungs and be accompanied by blood-tinged, frothy sputum. Hypoxemia will worsen as lung function deteriorates from the increased fluid. The patient becomes restless and anxious before changing level of consciousness as cerebral oxygenation falls.

X-Ray Changes

Changes due to pulmonary edema occur on x-rays in stages equal to the progression and/or severity of the pulmonary edema. The first change is an enlargement of the pulmonary veins. As interstitial edema occurs, the vessels become poorly outlined and foggy. This is frequently referred to as hilar haze. As intra-alveolar edema develops, the x ray shows a density in the inner middle zone. This gives the appearance of a "bat wing" or "butterfly" at the hilum.

Treatment and Nursing Intervention

The treatment for pulmonary edema is the same as for CHF, with a few exceptions. The goal of therapy is to resolve the pulmonary edema by improving cardiac function, which will improve renal function while supporting respiratory needs. The goal is to decrease preload, decrease afterload, and increase contractility.

Preload is reduced by diuretic therapy. Furosemide (Lasix) and ethacrynic acid are potent, fast-acting diuretics that may be used. Pulmonary edema responds well to Lasix, possibly due to a vasodilatory effect as much as a diuretic action. Morphine sulfate intravenously is used to both relieve anxiety and cause a vasodilation to occur, resulting in a reduced afterload.

Cardiac function is immediately supported with dobutamine. If hypotension exists, mid-dose dopamine may be given. If no response from dobutamine is seen, amrinone can be given.

Normally, hypoxemia is aggressively treated. Hypoxemia can be treated by increasing the FIO_2 (fraction of inspired oxygen). Oxygen therapy is usually administered by a high-flow face mask system, with oxygen concentrations from 40 to 100% sometimes required. The addition of continuous positive airway pressure or intubation and implementation of positive end expiratory pressure may be necessary for patients whose hypoxemia (PaO_2 levels below 60 mm Hg) does not respond to oxygen therapy. However, when positive pressure is applied, care must be taken to avoid a decrease in cardiac output.

Nursing intervention focuses on monitoring significant changes in preload, afterload, and contractility. If the preload (PCWP) changes, the nurse must observe whether other parameters e.g., stroke volume and cardiac output, have changed. Trends in data analysis are more important than absolute numbers. Monitoring treatments over several readings as opposed to a single data point is very important for accurately assessing clinical conditions.

Emotional support of the patient with pulmonary edema is made difficult by the patient's fear of shortness of breath. It is important to decrease this fear concurrently with providing treatment.

PERICARDITIS

Etiology

Pericarditis may be present or may develop in essentially any disease process. It may be infectious (most common) due to a virus or bacteria, metabolic such as seen in uremia, or related to such drugs as hydralazine and procainamide. The exact cause of pericarditis may not be known. It may be secondary to systemic disease or myocardial trauma, or it may follow acute myocardial infarction.

Clinical Presentation

Symptoms vary with the etiology of the pericarditis. Most commonly, pain is present. The pain may mimic an acute MI, angina, or pleurisy. Pain usually increases with deep respiration and when the patient is lying supine. Sitting up and leaning forward usually diminishes the pain. Fever is commonly present due to the infectious or inflammation process. Pericardial friction rub may be present for only a few days (post-MI) or prolonged for many days (uremia). The pericardial friction rub is a scratchy, superficial sound with three components best heard at the lower left sternum. Classical ECG changes are ST segment elevation in all leads except avR.

Complications

Complications of pericarditis include dysrhythmias, tamponade, and restriction of ventricular contraction. Each complication must be treated promptly. Hemodynamic monitoring with a pulmonary artery catheter is useful in early detection of tamponade. Equalization of pressures in the heart, particularly the CVP and the PCWP, may signal the presence of tamponade. Auscultation of heart sounds is essential on a regular and frequent schedule, with the clinician attempting to identify whether a muffling of the heart sounds has occurred.

Treatment

Pain relief is essential to promote normal and adequate ventilation. Anti-inflammatory and steroid therapies may be tried. Treatment of the underlying cause is imperative. Antipyretic agents will control the fever if the patient is uncomfortable. Pericardiocentesis or a pericardial window may be performed if the possibility of developing a tamponade is present. Anticoagulants are contraindicated in order to avoid an increase in pericardial fluid.

Nursing Intervention

Perform continuous ECG monitoring for signs of dysrhythmias that may indicate the early development of cardiac tamponade. The most dangerous dysrhythmia is electromechanical dissociation (an ECG pattern is present but there is no pulse). Monitoring with a pulmonary artery catheter is more sensitive to early changes. The standard nursing interventions involved with pulmonary artery monitoring are employed in these instances. The nurse should be prepared to assist with an emergency pericardiocentesis if it becomes warranted. Especially close auscultation of cardiac sounds is imperative for early intervention. Medications to relieve pain and fever are administered as ordered.

Arterial blood gases or pulse oximetry should be monitored at regular intervals to determine ventilatory status and to allow early intervention if hypoxemia develops. Emotional support of the patient and explanations of the close monitoring will help to alleviate some of the patient's anxiety.

CHAPTER 8

Hemorrhagic (Hypovolemic) and Cardiogenic Shock

Editor's Note

The CCRN exam is likely to ask several questions that test your knowledge of treatment of the major forms of shock. In this chapter, a simple approach to understanding the forms of shock is presented. This approach should provide you with the information necessary to successfully answer questions on the concepts of shock.

HYPOVOLEMIC SHOCK

Two major syndromes producing shock, hemorrhagic and cardiogenic shock, are both due to loss of cardiac output. One other syndrome commonly produces shock: a low SVR as in sepsis. In low-SVR shock, high cardiac outputs are more likely than low outputs. In this chapter, the emphasis is placed on identifying low cardiac output states and the symptoms associated with hemorrhagic and cardiogenic shock. The hemodynamic changes associated with sepsis are discussed briefly in this chapter and also in Chapter 37.

The CCRN exam can be anticipated to contain questions on each type of shock. The review presented here is designed to build on previous chapters and improve your ability to recognize and differentiate the types of shock that produce a low cardiac output state.

Shock occurs when a low mean arterial pressure (MAP) (<60 mm Hg) produces clinical symptoms of cellular hypoxia. Two common types of shock that can be readily identified based on differences in preload are hemorrhagic and cardiogenic. While causes of the various types of shock are markedly different, clinical differentiation is possible based on understanding the principles involved in the regulation of blood pressure.

Hemorrhagic shock is basically characterized by loss of blood volume due to active bleeding or chronic loss of vascular volume. For clinical purposes, the concept of hemorrhagic shock can also include hypovolemia from a number of causes. In the rest of this section, hypovolemic shock will replace the term hemorrhagic shock.

The causes of the loss of blood volume are wide ranging, including trauma, postoperative bleeding, and third spacing of fluid. Specific causes of hypovolemic shock are listed in Table 8-1. Both medical and surgical units are likely to see hypovolemic shock. Loss of vascular volume is probably the most common cause for loss of blood pressure, making this the most common reason for hypotension. When a patient is admitted with hypotension of unknown origin, hypovolemia must be suspected and treated before other forms of therapy are instituted.

Etiology

The loss of circulating blood volume leads to reduction in preload and eventually to reduction in stroke volume and cardiac output. The loss of stroke volume can be

TABLE 8-1. CAUSES OF HYPOVOLEMIC AND CARDIOGENIC SHOCK

Hypovolemic	Cardiogenic
Trauma	Myocardial infarction
Postoperative bleeding	Atrial tachydysrhythmias (atrial tachycardia, flutter, fibrillation)
Gastrointestinal bleeding	Ventricular tachycardia fibrillation
Burns	CHF
Capillary leak syndromes	Papillary muscle rupture
	Septal or ventricular wall rupture
	Tension pneumothorax
	Pericardial tamponade

compensated for by an increase in heart rate. The increase in heart rate can be substantial enough to prevent reduction in blood pressure (BP). The compensating increase in heart rate may result in early phases of hypovolemic shock not being reflected in BP changes.

As the heart rate increase fails to compensate for the loss of stroke volume and cardiac output falls, SVR increases as a second compensatory mechanism. Again, the BP does not change markedly until the SVR cannot regulate the BP. At the same time that heart rate and SVR are compensating for loss of stroke volume, microcirculation changes are occurring in an attempt to maintain organ blood flow.

The microcirculation is a group of blood vessels that act as an independent organic unit to regulate blood supply to the tissues. The microcirculation (Fig. 8-1) consists of vessels having a unique function. Each functioning unit is interactive with the others to maintain the balance between blood flow and tissue demand. The microcirculation is capable of adjusting blood flow in relation to tissue metabolic needs. It also plays a significant role in maintaining oncotic balance, in facilitating the movement of large molecules through the interstitium, and in regulating total blood volume.

The components of the microcirculation are capillaries, which form the vascular system between arterioles and venules. The arterioles bifurcate at points called metarterioles or precapillary arterioles. Smooth muscle cells cover the metarterioles at the bifurcation but disappear as each metarteriole becomes a true capillary.

At the point of metarteriole bifurcation into true

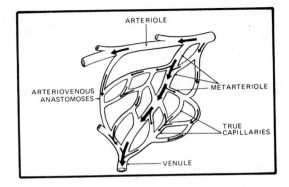

Figure 8-1. Microcirculation.

capillaries, there is a muscle sphincter. This precapillary sphincter acts as an autoregulatory system, dilating to allow increased perfusion when blood pressure is low or constricting when blood pressure is increased to adjust to the metabolic needs of the tissues in normal states.

The precapillary sphincter constricts in cases of shock and sympathetic nervous system stimulation to maintain perfusion of the vital organs. This constriction directs the available blood from nonessential tissues, such as the stomach, to vital organs, especially the heart and brain. This is a first major compensatory mechanism with the onset of shock.

Many chemical and humoral factors alter the regulation in the microcirculatory system. Some of these factors are listed in Table 8-2. Neurochemical controls provide a negative feedback response that results in adaptive responses to maintain cellular oxygenation. If

TABLE 8-2. REGULATION OF THE MICROCIRCULATORY SYSTEM

Chemical	C	D	Humoral	C	D
Hypoxemia		+	Catecholamines		
Hydrogen		+	Epinephrine	+	+
Potassium		+	Norepinephrine	+	
Hypercapnea	+		Dopamine	+	+
Hyperosmolarity	+		Amines		
			Serotonin	+	+
			Acetylcholine		+
			Histamine		+
			Polypeptides		
			Angiotensin	+	
			Kinins	+	
			Vasopressin		+

C = vasoconstriction; D = vasodilatation.

the shock is mild and or slow in developing, the negative feedback of the microcirculatory system will reverse the shock state. If the shock is severe or rapid in developing, this negative feedback of the microcirculatory system may not reverse the shock state. Failure to restore a hemostatic state allows a positive feedback system to develop. In this vicious cycle of positive feedback, an inadequate tissue perfusion leads to a deterioration in cardiovascular function, which decreases tissue perfusion even more. Consequently, in these instances, the shock state precipitates an even more severe shock state leading to death if not reversed.

The release of catecholamines (epinephrine and norepinephrine) in early shock results in vasoconstriction of the microcirculatory vessels at the precapillary sphincter level. The precapillary sphincter constriction is an attempt to increase venous return to the heart (by preventing blood flow in unnecessary tissues), which in turn improves cardiac output and tissue perfusion.

The hemodynamic mechanism to resolve shock is movement of fluid from the interstitial space into the vascular tree, causing an increase in plasma volume. This fluid shift occurs because a change in the hydrostatic pressure in the capillaries alters fluid exchange across the capillary membrane. With increased fluid shifting into the vascular tree, the plasma is diluted, decreasing plasma oncotic pressure and fostering more fluid movement into capillary beds. After hemorrhage, the liver synthesizes new proteins immediately to replace the lost plasma proteins in an attempt to force the fluid shift from the interstitium to the vascular tree and thus maintain adequate intravascular volume.

The renin-angiotensin-aldosterone cascade is activated by decreased renal blood flow. The renin is acted upon in several stages to convert it to angiotensin II. Angiotensin II is one of the most potent vasoconstrictors known. It augments the blood pressure and ideally increases blood flow in the process. Angiotensin II and the catecholamines (epinephrine and norepinephrine) increase vasoconstriction in all organs except the brain and heart. At the same time, aldosterone secretion is stimulated by angiotensin II. Aldosterone increases sodium retention by the kidneys, thereby increasing water reabsorption in the convoluted tubular system of the nephron. This additional retention of water helps increase intravascular volume.

A low cardiac output, secondary to hypovolemia, stimulates the neurohypophysis to increase release of the antidiuretic hormone (ADH). ADH promotes water reabsorption through its actions on the convoluted tubules and collecting ducts of the kidneys. ADH also has a vasoconstricting effect that further increases arterial pressure. Because of this action, ADH is sometimes called vasopressin.

Chronic hypovolemia can manifest physically in many ways. Acute hypovolemia, however, may be difficult to detect until hypotension develops. One method for assessing physical symptoms of hypovolemia is to apply the concept of preload. Preload (PCWP) in hypovolemia is low, differentiating hypovolemic shock from CHF and cardiogenic shock. The low preload does not produce any of the pulmonary or vascular congestion symptoms seen in CHF and cardiogenic shock. Specific symptoms of hypovolemic shock are given in Table 8-3.

Orthostatic blood pressure changes can indicate hypovolemia. These changes, which are measured by changing positions from supine to sitting, are defined by an increased heart rate (>10 bpm) and a fall in systolic (<25 mm Hg) and diastolic blood pressure (<10 mm Hg).

Since initial symptoms of any shock are minimal, observation to detect subtle changes is important. A gradually increasing heart rate coupled with a downward trend in BP may be a clue of impending hypovolemia. Initial intervention can result in much more favorable outcomes. If intervention is delayed, enough cellular damage may occur that the shock becomes irreversible. Measurement of oxygenation principles will give an idea of the severity of the shock state. Lactate levels, for example, have been correlated with survival in patients with hemorrhagic shock. If lactate levels exceed 4 mmol/L and are associated with a pH decrease, the likelihood of survival drops markedly.

Systemic signs of hypovolemia include possible decrease in urine output (less than 30 cc/hour or 0.5 cc/kg), change in level of consciousness (LOC) or behavior (cerebral ischemia may develop when the cerebral perfusion pressure drops below 60 mm Hg), increase in respiratory rate, and change in pulse quality. These symptoms are highly variable in the initial stages of shock. As shock progresses, severe depression in LOC, cool clammy skin, oliguria, hypotension, and tachycardia are common symptoms.

Complications

Sustained tissue hypoxia will lead to tissue necrosis and release of endotoxins into the system. Brain damage secondary to stagnation or prolonged hypoperfusion occurs as glucose, the only substrate available for

TABLE 8-3. SYMPTOMS OF HYPOVOLEMIC AND CARDIOGENIC SHOCK

Symptoms	Hypovolemic	Cardiogenic
Common		
BP	Low	Low
P	Tachycardia	Tachycardia
Urine output	Low (<0.5 cc/kg)	Low
LOC	Altered	Altered
Skin	Cool, clammy	Cool, clammy
Pulse quality	Weak	Weak
Differentiating		
Pao2	Normal	Low
Sao$_2$	Normal	Low
Cyanosis	Absent	May be present
a/A ratio	Normal	Low
PCWP	Low (<10)	High (>18)
Orthopnea	Minimal	Present
Crackles	Minimal	Present
Dependent edema	Absent	Present

cerebral metabolism, is consumed. Coma, seizures, and intracerebral hemorrhage may occur.

Electrolyte disarrangement and acid-base alterations are a result of both the shock state and renal failure. Cardiac dysrhythmia may herald the onset of irreversible shock resulting in death. Systemic disturbances, such as ARDS, are possible complications as cellular hypoxia develops.

Treatment

The primary focus in hypovolemic shock is the replacement of lost vascular volume. The treatment modalities are controversial in the correction of hypovolemic shock, with the controversy centering on which type of plasma expander, i.e., crystalloid or colloid infusion, to use. This question is addressed below. In addition, if the patient has a decreased LOC, intubation and protection of the airway is the highest priority.

Often, whole blood and a crystalloid solution (e.g., normal saline or Lactated Ringer's solution) are used to provide a balance between infusion of red blood cells, electrolytes, and fluid that would affect all three compartments (intravascular, intracellular, and extracellular). Interstitial and intracellular compartments are not replenished by blood or other colloidal agents. Blood administration increases vascular volume, osmotic pressure, and oxygen-carrying capacity.

Colloidal therapy is based on the administration of fluids that contain large-molecular-weight solutes, such as albumin or a glucose polymer (hetastarch). The proponents of colloidal agents claim that increasing the colloid osmotic pressure in the vascular tree will either "pull" interstitial fluids back into the vascular system or at least provide for a rapid volume expansion, since fluid will not leak out of the vascular compartment. Many authorities believe that acute hypovolemia can best be managed with use of colloidal agents; others feel that there is a greater risk of overtransfusion with colloids, which remain in the intact vascular tree, than with crystalloids, which can be absorbed into intracellular and interstitial spaces.

Nursing Intervention

Monitoring hemodynamic parameters of shock usually involves a central venous pressure (CVP) line or ideally a pulmonary artery catheter in order to guide the effectiveness of treatment. Nursing procedures related to any CVP or pulmonary artery catheter are applicable to the shock patient.

Patients traditionally have been placed in the Trendelenburg position or positioned with use of "shock blocks." Recent research indicates that a supine position or elevation of only the legs provides adequate circulation to the brain. If a concurrent head injury exists, the head of the bed may be placed in a low

Fowler's position. In cases of severe shock, a supine position with legs elevated 20 to 30 degrees by pillows may increase venous return.

Cardiovascular status, in addition to hemodynamic monitoring, is continuously monitored for signs of dysrhythmias. Dysrhythmias due to electrolyte disturbance are common with massive blood transfusions and with inadequate vascular volume.

Vasomotor tone is normally controlled by constriction secondary to sympathetic and catecholamine factors. Sympathetic stimulants such as norepinephrine (Levophed) and dopamine may need to be administered to maintain blood pressure.

Acid-base disturbances may be severe, and mixed metabolic and respiratory acidosis is common. Respiratory acidosis is corrected by adequate ventilation. Metabolic acidosis may be corrected by reversing decreased organ blood flow. If the pH is severely reduced, i.e., <7.20, sodium bicarbonate ($NaHCO_3$) may be used to raise the pH to tolerable levels (>7.20). One milliequivalent per kilogram of body weight is an initial loading dose for $NaHCO_3$. Additional doses depend upon the arterial blood gas values. The use of sodium bicarbonate is controversial, however, and changes in the guidelines for its application may alter the above recommendations.

Renal function is monitored hourly, usually with an indwelling Foley catheter. Severe or sustained hypovolemia may result in acute tubular necrosis, although prerenal azotemia is the first renal response. The blood urea nitrogen (BUN) may rise disproportionately to the creatinine, creating an increased BUN/creatinine ratio (greater than 15:1).

Nutritional support is essential, since a shock state rapidly depletes glucose storage with a resulting negative nitrogen balance, and protein catabolism increases acidotic states. Hyperalimentation (total parenteral nutrition) may be instituted to provide adequate nutrition. If the shock state was not caused by gastrointestinal or esophageal bleeding, a small-bore duodenal tube may be inserted and a continuous drip infusion of commercial food substitutes (e.g., Ensure, Osmolite, and Jevity) is started.

Stress ulcers may occur secondary to necrosis of the gastric mucosa during the hypovolemic period. Intravenous H_2 blockers (e.g., Ranididine and Tagamet) are often used to help reduce the incidence of gastric ulcers.

Emotional support consists of reassurance and explanation of procedures. Short brief comments regard-ing the patient's condition and the use of monitoring equipment will help decrease anxiety. Explanations to family members about the patient's current status and nursing procedures usually console the family and the patient.

CARDIOGENIC SHOCK

Etiology

Cardiogenic shock produces the same cellular disruption of oxygen as does hypovolemic shock but with different causes. In cardiogenic shock, mortality is frequently greater than 80%. As with hypovolemic shock, MAP is less than 60 mm Hg and the cardiac index is less than 1.8. However, preload is elevated, characterized by PCWP of greater than 18 to 25 mm Hg. As the left ventricle is unable to maintain forward flow of blood, pressure builds in the ventricle, causing an increased left ventricular end diastolic pressure (preload). Two primary manifestations of the reduced cardiac output are seen. The most dangerous manifestation is the development of systemic hypotension. In addition, pulmonary congestion secondary to the increased preload will occur, with a resulting increase in the intrapulmonary shunt (decrease in PaO_2 and SaO_2 levels).

Compensation Mechanisms

Cardiogenic shock produces compensation mechanisms similar to those for hypovolemic shock (see above). To review, in an attempt to maintain tissue perfusion, several compensation mechanisms are activated. Two key compensation mechanisms for shock are as follows:

1. Sympathetic stimulation. Release of epinephrine acts to increase heart rate, improve contractility, and improve impulse transmission. Epinephrine has a mild vasoconstriction effect as well. Norepinephrine is released, which has strong vasoconstricting effects, with a mild increase in heart rate, strength, and impulse transmission. The increased contractility and heart rate serve to increase the cardiac output. The increased vasoconstriction acts to maintain perfusion pressures and improve core organ blood flow.
2. Decrease of renal perfusion. Decreased renal perfusion activates the renin-angiotensin sys-

tem, promoting sodium and water retention. This mechanism acts to increase an already normal or elevated total vascular volume compartment.

Identifying Characteristics

The patient in cardiogenic shock will present with the symptoms listed in Table 8-3. In addition, the patient may present with hyperventilation brought on in an attempt to compensate for a lactic acidosis. The nurse should attempt to identify any potential risk factors (such as those that may lead to the causes in Table 8-1) to aid in identifying the types of shock involved.

Treatment

In a patient who presents with cardiogenic shock, the nurse must act to improve myocardial function as rapidly as possible. Much of the current treatment centers on pharmacologic or mechanical support of the heart.

Pharmacologic Treatment

Improving Cardiac Output—Contractility. Improvement in cardiac output is most often achieved with the use of dobutamine, although amrinone and mid-dose dopamine may also be used.

Improving Cardiac Output—Preload Reduction. Diuretics and vasodilators (nitroglycerin, diltiazem) may be employed. The use of a pulmonary artery catheter may facilitate assessment of the effectiveness of these agents. The goal of preload reduction is to reduce preload and improve myocardial contractility while reducing pulmonary congestion.

Improving Blood Pressure. In the patient with severe hypotension, vasoconstrictors such as norepinephrine, phenylephrine, or dopamine may be employed. Use of these drugs is not without risk, due to the increased myocardial oxygen consumptions associated with their vasoconstriction properties, but if the improvement in blood pressure is accomplished, an improved myocardial blood flow may offset the increased myocardial oxygen consumption. However, an improved blood pressure does not always cause an improved blood flow. Use of oxygenation parameters, such as SvO_2 values and lactate levels, will help determine whether an improvement in blood pressure has improved blood flow.

Adjuncts to Pharmacologic Support. If the cardiogenic shock is due to a recent MI, thrombolytic therapy may also be employed. In addition, angioplasty coupled with thrombolysis may reestablish blood flow and improve LV function. While this form of therapy is not standard, it does emphasize the importance of reestablishing blood flow rather than treating symptoms.

Use of mechanical support of the heart is increasing for the patient with cardiogenic shock. Mechanical support ranges from intra-aortic balloon pumping to left and right ventricular assist devices.

Protecting Ventilation. Intubation and aggressive oxygen therapy are frequently necessary in cardiogenic shock. Positive end expiratory pressure (PEEP) should be used cautiously, and the nurse should monitor cardiac output changes if PEEP is employed.

Treating Lactic Acidosis. Lactic acidosis will resolve if perfusion is reestablished. In the case of severe systemic pH disturbances (<7.20), small doses of sodium bicarbonate may be necessary. Despite the controversy over this measure, if the pH is below 7.20, bicarbonate administration to maintain pH levels over 7.20 may buy time in reestablishing blood flow.

Intra-Aortic Balloon Pump. Use of the aortic counterpulsation balloon, or the intra-aortic balloon pump (IABP), is increasingly available. The IABP reduces afterload of the left ventricle and increases blood flow into the coronary arteries, which makes it useful in treating refractive cardiac failure and cardiogenic shock and setup. IABP may be used as a supplement to medical treatment for cardiogenic shock or as a presurgery cardiac augmentation mechanism.

Insertion of the IABP. The IABP is inserted in the femoral artery (rarely a subclavian artery) after local anesthesia is achieved. It is advanced up the artery until it is in the descending thoracic aorta (Fig. 8-2). The IABP is synchronized with the patient's own heart rate and is timed to inflate immediately after aortic valve closure. Deflation occurs at variable points prior to the next QRS. The exact point varies from patient to patient to optimize afterload reduction.

Inflation should not occur until after the aortic valve closes due to the increased resistance the LV would encounter. Blood may also be forced back into the LV.

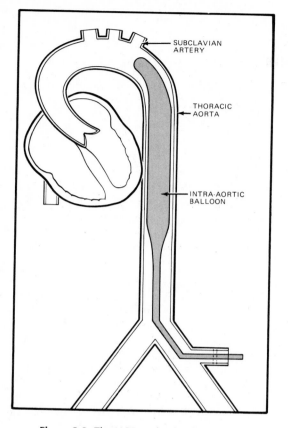

Figure 8-2. The IABP in the thoracic aorta.

Complications of the IABP. There are two major issues associated with the use of the IABP.

1. Circulation to the leg inferior to the insertion site is compromised to varied degrees. Monitoring and documenting the pulses, temperature, and appearance of the leg below the insertion site is extremely important. A comparison with the opposite extremity should be made.

2. The patient is weaned off the IABP usually by changing the ratio of IABP function to cardiac function. The ratio with insertion is normally 1:1. To effect weaning, the ratio first becomes 2:1, then 4:1, and then 8:1, as the patient tolerates it. Weaning may also be achieved by decreasing balloon volume, depending upon the model of the IABP machine in use. There are times when the left myocardium is so severely damaged that it cannot function adequately without the support of the IABP. In any event, use of the IABP must be terminated at some point.

A complication of IABP therapy is balloon rupture. For this reason, a rapid-exchanging gas (e.g., helium) is used for the balloon.

Contraindications of IABP include the presence of aortic or ventricular aneurysms, ventricular septal defects, or aortic regurgitation.

Deflation must occur before the end of the QRS to avoid balloon inflation during ventriculation contraction. Proper deflation will result in a reduction in afterload due to a "windkessel" effect.

Principles of the IABP. The IABP decreases strain on the left ventricle by lowering afterload in the aorta. With a reduced afterload, the ventricle does not have to contract as forcibly to expel its blood into the aorta.

During ventricular diastole, the balloon inflates to improve coronary blood flow. Blood is forced back into the coronary arteries with proper inflation (Fig. 8-3). The proper point for inflation is frequently near the dicrotic notch. Closure of the aortic valve is the event that produces the dicrotic notch on the arterial wave (Fig. 8-4). As discussed earlier, prior to ventricular systole (Fig. 8-5), the balloon deflates, decreasing the aortic afterload.

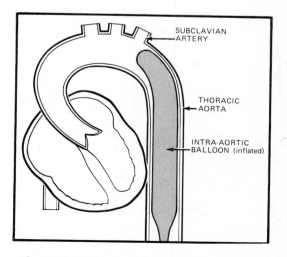

Figure 8-3. IABP inflated during ventricular diastole.

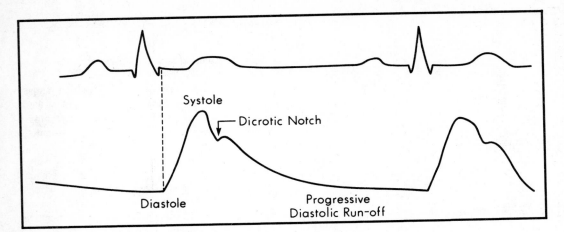

Figure 8-4. Normal arterial waveform.

HYPERTENSIVE CRISIS

Hypertension is not a disease but rather a symptom of a disease. The "normal" blood pressure range is 110 to 140/60 to 80. Hypertension is considered present if systolic pressure is 140 mm Hg or higher (in the adult) and/or if the diastolic pressure is greater than 90 mm Hg.

Primary hypertension (idiopathic, or of unknown cause) is common in the general population, with up to 30% of the population being affected. Hypertensive crises, however, occur only in a small percentage of the hypertensive population.

MAP is routinely lower in normal populations (MAP of between 60 and 120 mm Hg) than in chronic hypertensive patients (MAP commonly between 120 and 160). The fact that hypertensive patients have higher mean pressures is important when therapeutic end points are identified. The chronic hypertensive patient may tolerate a higher MAP, and rapid reduction to normal levels is generally not necessary.

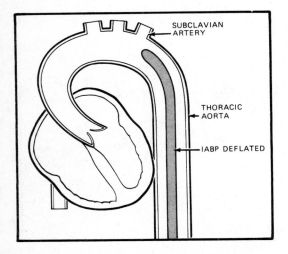

Figure 8-5. IABP deflated prior to ventricular systole.

TABLE 8-4. CHARACTERISTICS OF EMERGENCY HYPERTENSION

DBP > 120 mm Hg
One of the following is present:
    Acute aortic dissection
    Left ventricular failure with or without pulmonary edema
    Myocardial ischemia
    Acute renal failure
    Cerebrovascular or subarachnoid bleed
    Hypertensive encephalopathy
    Head injuries
    Grade 3–4 Keith-Wagener-Barker retinopathy
    Toxemia of pregnancy
    Burns
    Medication interaction
    Pheochromocytoma crisis

TABLE 8-5. MEDICATIONS TO TREAT HYPERTENSIVE CRISIS

Most Common	Less Common	Chronic
Nitroprusside (Nipride)	Trimethaphan (Arfonad)	Clonidine
Esmolol (Brevibloc)	Diazoxide (Hyperstat)	Propanolol
Labetalol	Hydralazine (Apresoline)	Captopril (Capoten)
Nifedipine (Procardia)	Phentoloamine (Regitine)	Prazosin (Minipress)
Nitroglycerin		Hydralazine
		Nicardipine
		Enalapril

The severity of the hypertensive disturbance can be identified along the guidelines of the Joint National Committee on Detection, Evaluation and Treatment of High Blood Pressure, published in 1984. Emergencies are BPs that need treatment within one hour; urgencies are BPs that need treatment within one day. Characteristics of emergencies are listed in Table 8-4.

Etiology

There are several major classifications of hypertension by etiology.

1. Unknown origin accounts for 90% of all cases of hypertension identified. This is termed essential hypertension.
2. Adrenal origin results from a tumor (pheochromocytoma) secreting epinephrine and norepinephrine, Cushing's disease, or a brain tumor.
3. Renal origin is due either to an interruption of blood supply or to a disease state of the kidney itself (e.g., pyelonephritis).
4. Cardiovascular hypertension can either be in response to a CHF or myocardial ischemia or act as their cause. Postoperative hypertension is common, particularly early in CABG recovery. The postoperative hypertension is probably due to excess catecholamine release.
5. The origin of obstetrical hypertension is unclear, but the condition usually presents in the second trimester of pregnancy.
6. Medications that cause vasoconstriction.

7. Lack of compliance with medical therapy in "known" hypertension or inadequate treatment in "known" hypertension. Also, certain drugs may cause hypertension.

Clinical Presentation

The most common symptom is severe headache accompanied by nausea, vomiting, restlessness, and mental confusion, which may rapidly advance to coma and/or convulsions. Signs of a specific organ injury may be present. For example, myocardial ischemia, cerebral vascular accident, hematuria, or retinopathy may become evident. Sudden elevations in blood pressure are more likely than gradual elevations to present with symptoms.

Treatment

Treatment of hypertensive crisis centers around reduction of blood pressure to safe levels without producing a subsequent hypotension. Remember, hypotensive symptoms can appear at higher than expected pressures in the patient with chronic hypertension. Gradual reduction of the MAP to below 85 is generally safe. Therapeutic modalities to achieve the MAP reduction generally initially involve a rapidly acting agent, with conversion to an oral agent as soon as possible. A diuretic is frequently added to counter potential water and sodium disturbances resulting from normal renal compensatory mechanisms of the hypertension. Examples of rapidly acting and oral maintenance agents are listed in Table 8-5.

CHAPTER 9

Cardiac and Vascular Surgery

Editor's Note

Cardiovascular surgery has assumed a greater role in critical care over the past decade, and the CCRN exam reflects this trend. Expect several questions on topics of cardiovascular surgery, including a few (usually only one or two) on cardiac transplantation. Use this chapter in conjunction with the preceding chapters in order to be able to apply hemodynamic analysis to the concept of cardiovascular surgery. This will help in understanding the assessment of and need for surgical treatment of cardiovascular disorders.

Cardiovascular surgery in the critical care environment can include many procedures, although the key surgical interventions generally center around cardiac or vascular circulation problems. The cardiac disturbances that require emergency surgery include acute coronary artery obstruction, ventricular septal rupture, pericardial tamponade, and papillary muscle rupture. Other than acute coronary artery obstruction, the problems present with symptoms similar to those of cardiogenic shock and will not be discussed here. While this chapter will not specifically address emergent problems except for the acute obstructed artery, the principles discussed cover most essential information related to cardiovascular surgery. This chapter does not address all possible surgical interventions but rather focuses on the common major cardiac and vascular surgeries of coronary artery bypass grafting (CABG), vascular aneurysm, and occlusive disease interventions. An introduction to the principles of cardiac transplantation will round out this chapter.

Knowledge of these common problems and the associated nursing care will prepare you for most CCRN questions on this content area, including the emergent surgical procedures. With the greater emphasis on the cardiovascular component of the CCRN exam, understanding cardiovascular surgical concepts has increased in importance.

CORONARY ARTERY BYPASS GRAFTING

Coronary artery bypass grafting is the technique of using blood vessels obtained from another part of the body to replace obstructed coronary arteries. Generally, the saphenous vein is utilized to bypass the obstructed coronary artery, although other techniques such as internal mammary artery bypass have also been used. Nursing care postoperatively differs somewhat for the different types of grafts; with saphenous vein removal, for example, one must care for the wound created by removal of the graft. Otherwise, postoperative care does not markedly change.

Determination of the Need for CABG

The need for CABG is determined from cardiac catheterization studies and the patient's symptoms. General criteria for CABG are presented in Table 9-1. Cardiac catheterization indicates the need for surgery when one or more coronary arteries are more than 75% obstructed and there is a patent vessel below the obstruction. If there are multiple obstructions in a single artery, making bypass difficult, surgery is generally not indicated or helpful. Pain relief from bypass surgery is individualized, since bypass surgery is effective primarily if blood flow to viable cardiac muscle is reestablished.

Questions have been raised as to the need for CABG versus medical treatment, although the dominant practice is to perform the surgery on patients meeting the criteria listed in Table 9-1. Since collateral circulation is common in patients with obstructions in

TABLE 9-1. CRITERIA FOR CORONARY ARTERY BYPASS GRAFTING

Chronic stable angina, left main disease on angiography, ejection fraction >20%.

Chronic stable angina, three-vessel disease on angiography, class III or IV angina with maximal medical therapy, ejection fraction >50%.

Chronic stable angina, three-vessel disease on angiography, class I or II angina with maximal medical therapy, ejection fraction >50%.

Unstable angina that responded to maximal medical therapy, three-vessel disease on angiography, ejection fraction >20%.

Chronic stable angina, three-vessel disease on angiography, class I or II angina with less than maximal medical therapy, ejection fraction >50%.

Chronic stable angina, two-vessel disease with left anterior descending coronary artery disease, less than a very positive exercise stress test, class I or II angina with less than maximal medical therapy, ejection fraction >50%.

Chronic stable angina, two-vessel disease with left anterior descending coronary artery disease, less than a very positive exercise stress test, class I or II angina with maximal medical therapy, ejection fraction >50%.

Asymptomatic or chest pain of uncertain origin in patients younger than 65 years with three-vessel disease, less than a very positive exercise stress test.

the coronary artery, the severity of the patient's symptoms will also dictate the need for surgery. A patient who has multivessel coronary artery disease with angina and is unresponsive to medical therapy will be a prime candidate for CABG. A patient with recurrent stenotic lesions after angioplasty is also a candidate for CABG.

Once the need for CABG is identified, the patient is classified as emergent or elective. The emergent CABG patient has either unstable hemodynamics (hypotension), unremitting chest pain despite maximal medical treatment, or the potential to become unstable (subjective assessment). Any of these emergent classifications requires immediate CABG. Elective surgeries are utilized for those patients with hemodynamic stability and symptoms partially controlled through medical therapy.

Surgical Procedure

The surgical techniques utilized during CABG are unlikely to be covered on the CCRN exam. However, this section contains information that provides a useful background on the surgical procedure.

During CABG, several surgical techniques are employed to improve success rates. The patient is typically cooled to near 34°C (to reduce oxygen demands) and is placed on cardiopulmonary bypass (CPB). CPB is a technique for diverting blood from the heart during surgery while simultaneously oxygenating the blood and removing carbon dioxide. During CPB, three maneuvers help achieve safe and successful extracorporeal oxygenation: hemodilution, hypothermia, and anticoagulation. While these techniques help reduce complications, they also form the basis for many of the postoperative observations by the critical care nurse. Nursing measures primarily include observing for side effects of hemodilution and coagulation.

The hemodilution that occurs reduces colloidal osmotic pressure and makes capillary leaking more likely. As fluid leads from the blood vessels, the nurse should be alert for the need to give volume (generally osmotic agents such as albumin or hetastarch) to maintain fluid status. Patients may gain several pounds following CPB due to the loss of vascular volume into the interstitial space. Careful observation of urine output to assess vascular volume is helpful. Impaired gas exchange as manifested by low PaO_2 and SaO_2 levels also indicates excess capillary leaking. Improved blood gases can indicate clearing of third space volume.

Postoperative bleeding is usually not due to CPB. Measurement of the partial thromboplastin time will best detect an excessive heparin effect from CPB. Administration of protamine sulfate will usually correct bleeding due to CPB.

Postoperative Measures

The primary postoperative assessments following CABG involve hemodynamic monitoring, pain relief, dysrhythmia control, and recovery from surgical techniques such as CPB. Hemodynamic monitoring centers on maintaining adequate blood pressure, cardiac indices (greater than 2.2 LPM/m^2), and tissue oxygenation ($SvO_2 > 0.60$). Acceptable blood pressure and cardiac index are achieved through maintaining acceptable vascular volumes (commonly obtained via titrating the PCWP to between 12 and 18 mm Hg) and the use of inotropes such as dobutamine or dopamine to maintain normal stroke volumes. As the patient warms postoperative, vasopressors may initially need to be used to maintain blood pressure.

More aggressive measures to maintain cardiac output such as left ventricular and or right ventricular assist devices may be required. However, few if any questions on the CCRN exam cover these aggressive measures at this time. One assist method that is covered on the exam in intra-aortic balloon pumping, which may be used to maintain acceptable cardiac indices. This subject is covered in Chapter 8.

Postoperative blood loss should not exceed 300 cc/hour in the first several hours after bypass. After this time period, bleeding should be less than 150 to 200 cc/hour. The physician should be notified when blood loss is excessive. Autotransfusion may be employed to aid replacement of normal blood loss. Autotransfusion usually is done when blood loss reaches 300 cc/hour.

Monitoring of temperatures is typically indicated by pulmonary artery and rectal (or bladder) temperature probes. The patient will attempt to rewarm through shivering; although this reflex is effective, the increase in oxygen consumption is undesirable. The nurse can aid in rewarming the patient through external methods (blankets, radiant lights) and internal methods (warmed blood, warmed inspired gases). Some institutions advocate the administration of paralytic agents to avoid the muscle activity associated with shivering. Avoidance of marked shivering is one key goal in the rewarming therapy.

During rewarming, the patient appears to be hypovolemic as vasodilation occurs. Volume replacement and vasopressors may be required to initially combat the loss of PCWP and CVP.

The nurse needs to maintain pain reduction while simultaneously allowing for recovery of ventilatory function. Aggressive pulmonary toilet via suctioning initially and then encouraging coughing will aid in reducing pulmonary complications. The nurse's support in pain reduction and the sensitivity shown for the patient's adjustment to temporary dependence on nursing will aid adaptation to the immediate postoperative recovery.

Dysrhythmia control centers on two factors. First, any metabolic disturbance that may precipitate either atrial or ventricular dysrhythmias should be corrected. For example, potassium (K^+) levels should be monitored when dysrhythmias, particularly ventricular ectopy (PVCs), exist. Second, pharmacologic or electrical therapy can be utilized to control dysrhythmias. Pharmacologic treatments are dictated by the type of dysrhythmia. For example, atrial tachycardias are treated with agents such as digoxin, beta blockers (esmolol), calcium channel blockers (verapamil), adenosine, or a combination of these agents. Ventricular tachycardias and PVCs are treated with lidocaine, pronestyl, or bretylium.

Electrical therapy is usually performed through the pacing wires placed on the right atrium and ventricle near the end of the CABG procedure. These pacing wires can be used postoperatively to manage both supraventricular tachycardias and bradycardias. Postoperative bradycardia is the most common indication for use of the pacing wires. Simple ventricular demand pacing (VVI) or AV sequential pacing (DVI) can be used. Newer pacemakers, such as more sophisticated DDD pacemakers, allow for improving cardiac output to a greater extent than is currently available.

Cardiac Tamponade

Cardiac tamponade is a potential complication following CABG. Tamponade occurs when fluid fills the pericardial sac and limits the ability of the ventricles to fill with blood. Clinical signs of tamponade include an increase in an equalization of venous pressures (due to resistance of ventricular expansion), decreased blood pressure (due to a drop in cardiac output), and diminished heart sounds. Pulsus paradoxus is a common clinical finding in tamponade. Ejection fractions fall as the tamponade restricts ventricular contraction.

Treatment for tamponade is a pericardiocentesis. If the accumulation of fluid is rapid, surgery may be required to locate the source of the bleeding.

CARDIAC TRANSPLANTATION

Heart transplantation is generally not covered on the CCRN exam. Nonetheless, transplantation may be an option for patients with cardiomyopathy, and you should be familiar with the procedure.

In patients with cardiomyopathies or reduced cardiac function from coronary artery disease, CABG will not improve cardiac performance. Replacement of the heart is indicated in patients with end-stage heart disease untreatable by medical or CABG intervention. Once identified as a candidate for transplantation and no contraindications to the transplant are present (Table 9-2), the patient is categorized as to severity. The patient typically has less than one year of expected survival without transplantation. The time between being placed on the list and undergoing transplantation is

TABLE 9-2. ELIGIBILITY CRITERIA FOR CARDIAC TRANSPLANTATION

1. End-stage, ischemic, valvular, or congenital heart disease with maximal medical therapy, not amenable to conventional or high-risk surgery.
2. NYHA functional class III-IV congestive heart failure with maximal medical therapy.
3. Intractable, recurrent, malignant ventricular arrhythmias.
4. Age generally younger than 60 years.
5. Psychologically stable, compliant, reliable. Patient should be able to understand the procedure and risks involved.
6. Absence of the following contraindicating factors:
   Systemic disease or infection
   Serious, irreversible impairment of hepatic, renal, or pulmonary functions
   Recent cerebrovascular accident or neurologic deficits
   Recent pulmonary embolization
   Active ulcer or bleeding diathesis
   Current smoking, alcohol abuse, or drug abuse
   Insulin-dependent diabetes
   Pulmonary vascular resistance greater than 6 to 8 Wood units

highly variable and can serve as a major source of anxiety to the potential recipient.

The success rate for transplantation is very good, with five- and ten-year survival rates of 73%. However, the shortage of donors means that not all patients who might benefit from transplantation actually undergo the procedure.

The surgical procedure has been improved since the time of the first transplantation in 1967, but the prime difference has been in the area of immunosuppression. Suppression of rejection through such agents as cyclosporine has been the major factor in improving outcome following transplantation.

Postoperative care is similar to that for CABG surgery with the exception of medications for immunosuppression. The ECG has two sinus nodes initially (due to the retention of the recipient sinus node), and the recipient sinus node gives P waves unrelated to the QRS complex. Since the transplanted heart has been denervated, the patient will feel no anginal pain. Because of the denervation, sympathetic stimulants such as isoproterenol may be necessary to maintain a safe heart rate.

VASCULAR SURGERY

The two most common problems requiring vascular surgery are aneurysms and occlusions. Aneurysms are more problematic when they occur in major arteries. Occlusions are problematic when they occur in major arteries or veins.

Aortic Aneurysms

The two common types of aortic aneurysms are thoracic and abdominal. Abdominal aneurysms are more common (65% of aneurysms) than thoracic aneurysms. The aneurysm can typically take on one of two patterns: a weakness and bulging of the entire vessel wall, or a weakness within the vessel wall (intimal tear or dissection).

Aortic Dissection

Aortic dissection is potentially life threatening due to rapid progression, loss of vascular volume, potential bleeding into the pericardial sac (tamponade resulting), and disruption of the aortic valve with resultant left ventricular failure. Ascending aortic involvement is more difficult to surgically correct than descending aortic dissecting aneurysms due to the proximity of the major cardiac structures.

The origin of aortic dissection is usually hypertension. The presentation is one of hypertension with severe chest pain frequently radiating to the back. Immediate surgical treatment is necessary. Medical management with antihypertensives can take place but may be unsuccessful.

Abdominal Aneurysms

Abdominal aneurysms may occasionally be identified by noting a palpable mass on physical exam. Symptoms may include abdominal or back pain with tenderness on palpation.

Diagnosis of Aneurysms

The use of computerized tomography (CT) and magnetic resonance imaging (MRI) to identify abdominal and thoracic vascular structures is common practice. Routine chest and abdominal x-rays and ultrasound may detect the aneurysm, although the detail is not as great as with CT or MRI. Angiography is a good test to demarcate the boundaries of the blood vessels.

Treatment of Aneurysms

Replacement of the aneurysm with a graft is the most common surgical intervention. Figure 9-1 contains an example of the surgical replacement technique. The closer the aneurysm is to the heart, the more difficult the surgery will be. Thoracic aneurysms of the descending aorta and abdominal aneurysms offer the surgeon a better operative field and reduce postoperative complications.

Postoperative Considerations

The most serious complication following aortic surgery is myocardial infarction, accounting for almost half of the postoperative mortality from aortic surgery. Monitoring cardiovascular performance such as cardiac index, stroke index or volume, PCWP, CVP, and ECG rhythms is helpful in assessing cardiac performance.

Common postoperative problems include acute renal tubular necrosis due to potential loss of renal blood flow during surgery and bleeding due to leakage of the graft. The nurse must be aware of symptoms of hypovolemia (Chapter 8) indicating a potential bleed. The presence of a strong pulse on palpation of the femoral artery gives an indication of adequate patency of the aorta. Renal function is assessed through measurement urine volume, intake and output and serum and urine creatinine and electrolytes.

Bowel and spinal cord ischemias are less common complications but when they occur have high incidences of morbidity and mortality. Respiratory complications may be avoided through routine postoperative therapy, i.e., incentive spirometry, early ambulation and, if necessary, postural drainage and percussion.

Occlusive Disorders

Obstruction of arterial or venous flow due to atherosclerosis is the most common cardiovascular disturbance. Obstruction can occur anywhere along the major arterial tree, although in critical care settings, aortofemoral obstructions are most likely to bring the patient to the intensive care unit setting.

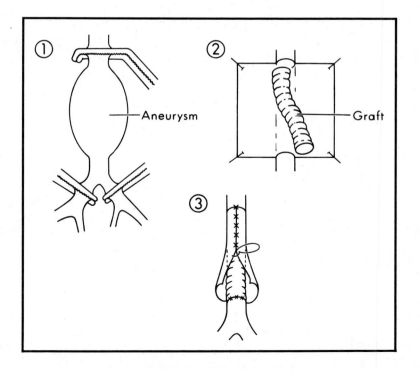

Figure 9-1. Aneurysm graft technique.

Obstruction due to arterial flow usually results in pain on exercise. Lower-extremity obstruction is more common than upper-extremity obstruction. Pain in the legs upon activity due to obstruction is called intermittent claudication. Arterial obstructions are potentially more dangerous due to the loss of oxygen and substrates necessary for energy generation. Venous obstructions tend to be more chronic and are less likely to be seen in the critical care settings.

Clinical indications of decreased arterial blood flow include diminished pulses, loss of temperature (cool skin), change in color (cyanosis reflects venous obstruction, pallor reflects arterial obstruction), and diminished sensation. If the obstruction is sudden, severe pain distal to the obstruction is a common symptom.

Assessment of the need for surgery generally includes Doppler ultrasound studies and possibly abdominal aortic ultrasound and CT exams. Surgery is indicated when the patient has symptoms severe enough to restrict activities of daily living.

Surgical Intervention

The optimal surgical method to relieve obstruction to blood flow is dependent on the location of the obstruction. Figure 9-2 illustrates the most common types of surgical procedures to bypass obstructions of the aorta and femoral arteries.

A rapidly expanding area of surgical intervention is the use of endovascular therapies. Application of balloon angioplasties, atherectomy, and laser angioplasties are quickly expanding. The use of these techniques will reduce the incidence of surgery and the subsequent postoperative problems. The nursing management is similar to that for surgical techniques in many ways. Postoperative considerations for both surgical techniques and endovascular therapies are covered together below.

Postoperative Considerations

Assessment of blood flow is an important nursing measure both pre- and postoperatively. Blood flow assessment includes pulse quality, capillary refill, and sensation. Pulse presence does not necessarily mean that the graft has good patency. Doppler assessment is a better parameter to measure flow than is palpation.

Loss of flow following surgery can be due to failure of the bypass graft or obstruction as a result of clot formation. In the case of clot formation, the danger for potential embolization exists. In arterial surgery, the emboli will obstruct a site beyond the site of surgery and may result in loss of a portion of the extremity involved. If obstruction is on the venous side, the emboli will result in pulmonary embolization. Symptoms of pulmonary emboli are chest pain, shortness of breath, decreased PaO_2/SaO_2, and elevation of pulmonary artery pressures.

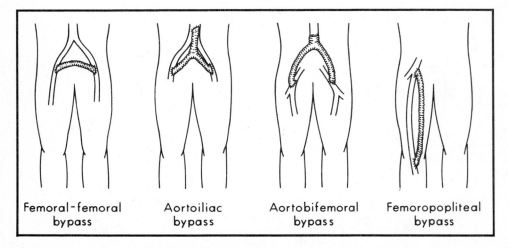

Femoral-femoral bypass   Aortoiliac bypass   Aortobifemoral bypass   Femoropopliteal bypass

Figure 9-2. Femoral vascular bypass techniques.

BIBLIOGRAPHY

Abedin, Z., & Conner, R.P. (1989). *12 Lead ECG Interpretation*. Philadelphia: W.B. Saunders.

Ahrens, T.S., & Taylor, L. (1992). *Hemodynamic waveform analysis*. Philadelphia: W.B. Saunders.

Appel-Hardin, S. (1992). The role of the critical care nurse in noninvasive temporary pacing. *Crit Care Nurse, 12,* 10–19.

Ayres, S.M., Schlichtig, R., & Sterling, M.J. (1988). *Care of the Critically Ill*. Chicago: Yearbook Medical Publishers.

Beare, P.G. (1989). Calcium channel blockers: Nursing care for hypertension. *Crit Care Nurse, 9,* 37–44.

Benedict, C.R., Mueller, S., Anderson, H.V., & Willerson, J.T. (1992). Thrombolytic therapy: A state of the art review. *Hosp Pract, 27,* 61–72.

Cooper, J., & Marriott, J.L. (1989). Why are so many critical care nurses unable to recognize ventricular tachycardia in the 12-lead electrocardiogram? *Heart Lung, 18,* 3, 243–247.

Dalsing, M.C., & Sawchuk, A.P. (1988). Surgery of the aorta. In *Vascular Nursing*. Ed. Fahey, V.A. Philadelphia: W.B. Saunders, 202.

Disler, L., Haitas, B., Benjamin, J., Steingo, L., & McKibbin, J. (1987). Cardiogenic shock in evolving myocardial infarction: Treatment by angioplasty and streptokinase. *Heart Lung, 16,* 649–652.

Drew, B.J. (1991). Beside electrocardiographic monitoring: State of the art for the 1990's. *Heart Lung, 20,* 610–623.

Dubin, D. (1989). *Rapid Interpretation of ECG's*. Tampa: Cover Publishing Co.

Ewer, M.S., & Naccarilli, G.V. (1989). Cardiac critical care. *Crit Care Clin, 5,* 3.

Funk, M. (1986). Diagnosis of right ventricular infarction with right precordial ECG leads. *Heart Lung, 15,* 6, 562–572.

Futterman, L.B. (1988). Cardiac transplantation: A comprehensive nursing perspective. Part 1. *Heart Lung, 17,* 5, 499–510.

Houston, M.C. (1986). Hypertensive urgencies and emergencies: Pathophysiology, clinical aspects and treatment. In *Critical Care - State of the Art*. Ed. Chernow, B. & Shoemaker, W.C. Fullerton, CA: Society of Critical Care Medicine.

Imperial, F.A., Cordova-Manigbas, L., & Ward, C.R. (1989). Cardiac transplantation. *Crit Care Nurs Clin North Am, 1,* 2, 399–416.

Jansen, K.J., & McFadden, P.M. (1986). Postoperative nursing management in patients undergoing myocardial revascularization with the internal mammary artery bypass. *Heart Lung, 15,* 1, 48–54.

Joint National Committee on Detection, Evaluation and Treatment of High Blood Pressure. (1984). The 1984 Report of the Joint National Committee. *Arch Intern Med, 144,* 1045.

Khan, A.H. (1992). The postcardiac injury syndrome. *Clin Cardiol, 15,* 67–72.

Lefor, N., Cardello, F.P., & Felicetta, J.V. (1992). Recognizing and treating Torsade de Pointes. *Crit Care Nurse, 12,* 20–29.

Ley, S.J., Miller, K., Skov, P., & Preisig, P. (1990). Crystalloid versus colloid fluid therapy after cardiac surgery. *Heart Lung, 19,* 31–40.

McCarthy, W.J., & Williams, L.R. (1985). Femoral artery reconstruction. *Crit Care Q, 8,* 2, 39–50.

Memmer, M.K. (1988). Acute orthostatic hypotension. *Heart Lung, 17,* 2 134–141.

Notterman, D.A. (1991). Inotropic agents. Catecholamines, digoxin, amrinone. *Crit Care Clin, 7,* 583–613.

Pape, L.A. (1985). Dissection of the aorta. In *Intensive Care Medicine*. Ed. Rippe, J.M., Irwin, R.S., Alpert, J.S., Dalen, & J.E. Boston: Little, Brown & Co., 234–243.

Passmore, J.M., & Goldstein, R.A. (1989). Acute recognition and management of congestive heart failure. *Crit Care Clin, 5,* 497–532.

Phillips, R., & Skov, P. (1988). Rewarming and cardiac surgery: A review. *Heart Lung, 17,* 511–520.

Pierce, C.D. (1989). Transcutaneous cardiac pacing: Expanding clinical applications. *Crit Care Nurs Clin North Am, 1,* 423–435.

Prolux, R., Guidetti, K., Bagg, A.M., & Marchette, L. (1992). Detection of right ventricular myocardial infarction in patients with inferior wall myocardial infarction. *Crit Care Nurse, 12,* 50–59.

Roberts, R. (1981). Diagnostic assessment of myocardial infarction based on lactate dehydrogenase and creatinine kinase isoenzymes. *Heart Lung, 10,* 3, 486–506.

Rossignol, M., Mickles, L., & Rock, S. (1985). Assessment and treatment of right ventricular infraction. *Focus Crit Care, 12,* 6, 20–25.

Schiro, A.G., & Curtis, D.G. (1988). Asymptomatic coronary artery disease. *Heart Lung, 17,* 2, 144–149.

Schott, K.E. (1991). Intra-aortic balloon counterpulsation as a therapy for shock. *Crit Care Nurs Clin North Am, 2,* 187–193.

Smith, T.W., & Kelly, R.A. (1992). Therapeutic strategies for CHF in the 1990s. *Hosp Pract, 26,* 127–150.

Sobel, B. (1987). Fibrinolysis and activators of plasminogen. *Heart Lung, 16,* 6, 775–779.

Stier, F. (1992). Antidysrhythmic agents. *AACN Clin Issues Crit Care, 3,* 483–493.

Sulzbach, L.M. (1989). Measurement of pulsus paradoxus. *Focus Crit Care, 16,* 2, 142–145.

Symbas, P.N. (1989). *Cardiothoracic Trauma*. Philadelphia: W.B. Saunders.

Weeks, L. (1986). Care of the patient post cardiothoracic surgery. *Advanced Cardiovasc Nursing*. Boston: Boston Press, 601.

Weiland, A.P., & Walker, W.E. (1986). Physiologic principles and clinical sequelae of cardiopulmonary bypass. *Heart Lung, 15,* 1, 34–39.

Part 2

Pulmonary

Pamela Becker-Weilitz, RN, MSN

CHAPTER 10

Pulmonary Anatomy

Editor's Note

The CCRN exam will have a few questions that are directly related to the anatomy of the pulmonary system. However, as you read this chapter, concentrate on understanding the major pulmonary features rather than minute details. For example, the CCRN exam is not likely to ask what the larynx is composed of (e.g., cartilage), but it may give a clinical scenario involving right mainstem intubation secondary to the anatomy of the tracheobronchial tree that facilitates right mainstem entry by an endotracheal tube. Try to understand the anatomy as it relates to clinical application rather than memorizing details of anatomy.

The pulmonary anatomy includes the upper airway, consisting of the mouth, nose, oral pharynx, and larynx, and the lower airway, consisting of the tracheobronchial tree and the lung parenchyma. Discussion of the pulmonary anatomy also includes the thoracic cage and the musculature of the thorax.

THORACIC CAGE

The thoracic cage (Fig. 10-1) is the bony frame of the chest. The sternum makes up the anterior portion of the thoracic cage. The sternum is actually three connected flat bones: the manubrium, the body, and the xiphoid process (Fig. 10-2). Seven pairs of ribs attach to the sternum, called the true ribs. The remaining five pairs of ribs form the anterior bony portion of the thoracic cage. Each is attached to the rib above it by intercostal muscles. Each of the 12 pairs of ribs has cartilage and muscle attached to it.

The posterior thoracic cage is formed by the vertebrae and each of the 12 pairs of ribs that are attached to the vertebrae. Since the ribs are C shaped, they serve as the bony protective side borders of the thoracic cage. The thorax is shaped like an inverted cone with the apex about 2.5 cm above the clavicles. The clavicles and first rib form the protective barrier of the superior portion of the thoracic cage. The diaphragm is the inferior portion of the thoracic cage (Fig. 10-3). The diaphragm is a muscle that contracts and flattens, enlarging the thoracic cage. When the diaphragm relaxes, it becomes dome shaped and decreases the space of the thoracic cage. The diaphragm is the major muscle of respiration. On inspiration, the diaphragm contracts (Fig. 10-4), which lengthens the chest cavity, while the external intercostal muscles contract to raise the ribs, thus enlarging the diameter of the chest.

Expiration is a passive act accomplished by relax-

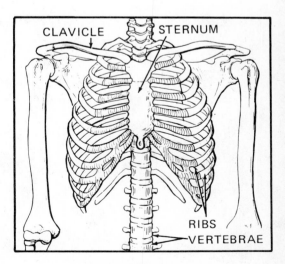

Figure 10-1. The thoracic cage.

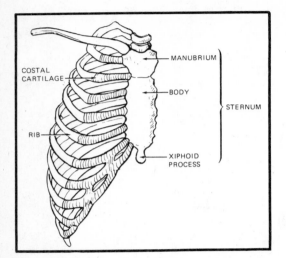

Figure 10-2. The sternum.

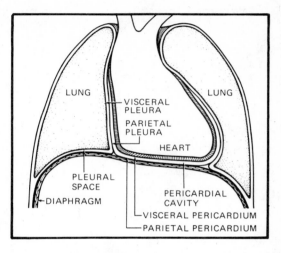

Figure 10-3. The diaphragm.

ing the diaphragm and the external intercostal muscles. The lungs have a normal tendency to collapse. Relaxation of the musculature provides the major mechanism for the passive act of exhalation.

The intercostal muscles are composed of two layers, internal and external. Any change in the musculature of the chest alters normal thoracic pressures and affects ventilation. The internal intercostal muscles, which pull the ribs down and inward, play a role in forceful expiration, coughing, and sneezing. The intercostal muscles are used mostly during stressful states and exertional activities. The intercostal muscles may facilitate a smooth transition from inspiration to expiration. In cases of pulmonary distress or disease,

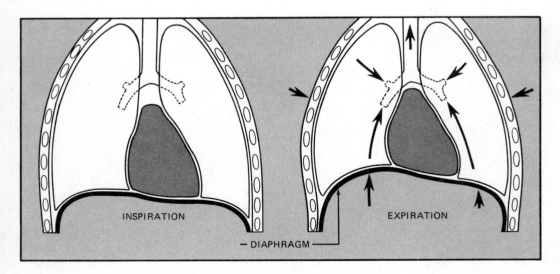

Figure 10-4. The diaphragm on inspiration and expiration.

accessory muscles may be used to help inspiration. The accessory muscles of respiration include the scalene, sternocleidomastoid, trapezius, and pectoral muscles.

MEDIASTINUM

The lung parenchyma and the mediastinum are contained within the bony thoracic cage. The mediastinum is a space midline in the chest and contains the heart, great vessels, trachea, major bronchi, esophagus, thymus gland, lymphatics, and various nerves.

PLEURA

Each lung lies free in its own pleural cavity except at its single point of attachment, the hilum (Fig. 10-5). One lung can collapse but not the other because the lung cavities are independent from each other. The pleural covering of lung is composed of two layers. The visceral layer is contiguous with the lung and does not have pain nerve fibers. The parietal layer is the outer pleural layer that lines the inside of the thoracic cage. The parietal layer of the pleura contains pain nerve fibers.

The two pleural layers are separated by a small amount of fluid known as the pleural fluid. This fluid allows the two pleurae to slide easily over each other during inspiration and expiration. If the pleurae become inflamed, there is restriction of normal pleural movement. Irritation of the parietal pleura accounts for the pleuritic pain.

The diaphragm is the inferior border for each pleural space. The chest wall is the lateral border, and the mediastinum is the medial border for each pleural space.

LUNG

Each lung is composed of divisions or segments of the bronchial tree and the lung parenchyma. There are ten segments in the right lung and eight in the left lung. These 18 bronchial segments are grouped into lobes. Three lobes form the right lung, and two lobes form the left lung (Fig. 10-6). Each lobe of the lung is separated from the adjacent lobe by fissures. The left lung also has an upper and lower division of its superior lobe, separated by a fissure called the lingula. The lingula is equal in size to or smaller than the middle lobe of the right lung.

UPPER AIRWAY

The upper airway consists of the nose and pharynx. The larynx is included as part of the upper airway but functions in part as a transitional structure between the upper and lower airways.

Nose

The first part of the upper airway (Fig. 10-7) is the nose. Air normally enters the respiratory system through the nose. The nose has skeletal rigidity, which maintains patency during inspiration.

The first two-thirds of the nose is cartilaginous, and the last one-third is bony. The cartilaginous septum, straight at birth, frequently becomes deviated during life for many reasons. Unless the deviation is severe enough to obstruct air flow, no medical treatment is necessary. The nasal septum divides the nose into two fossae, with the lateral border known as the alae. The opening between the alae and the nasal septum is known as the nostril or the naris (plural, nares). The nose has a small inlet and a large outlet. Anatomically, this feature allows inspired air to have maximum contact with the upper airway mucosa. By sniffing through

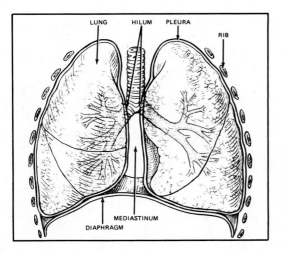

Figure 10-5. The hilum.

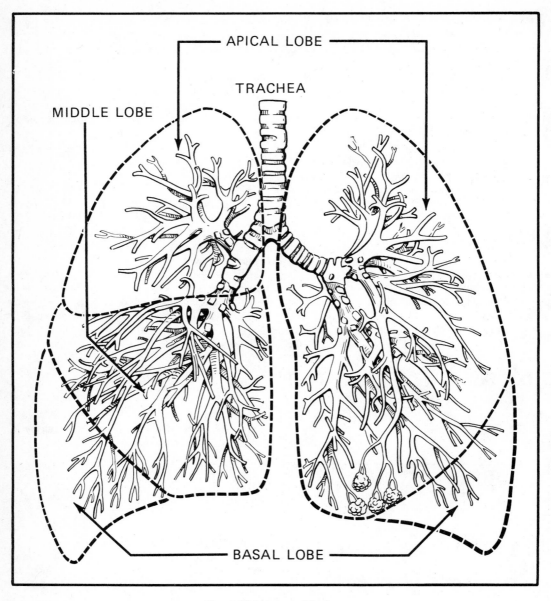

Figure 10-6. Lobes of the lungs.

the nose, we direct inhaled air toward the superior turbinates, where the olfactory area is located.

Pharynx

The main function of the pharynx is to collect incoming air from the mouth and nose and project it down-

ward to the trachea. Anatomically, the pharynx is subdivided into the nasopharynx, the oropharynx, and the laryngopharynx (Fig. 10-8). The nasopharynx is the space behind the oral and nasal cavities and above the soft palate. It contains the orifices of the eustachian tubes. The eustachian tubes maintain proper air pres-

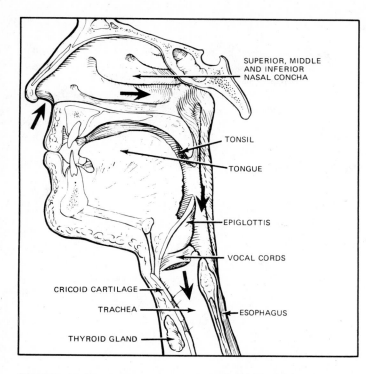

SUPERIOR, MIDDLE
AND INFERIOR
NASAL CONCHA

TONSIL

TONGUE

EPIGLOTTIS

VOCAL CORDS

CRICOID CARTILAGE

TRACHEA

ESOPHAGUS

THYROID GLAND

Figure 10-7. The upper airway.

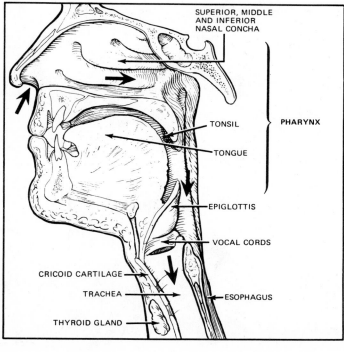

SUPERIOR, MIDDLE
AND INFERIOR
NASAL CONCHA

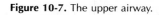

TONSIL

PHARYNX

TONGUE

EPIGLOTTIS

VOCAL CORDS

CRICOID CARTILAGE

TRACHEA

ESOPHAGUS

THYROID GLAND

Figure 10-8. The pharynx.

sure in the middle ear, for normal tympanic membrane function. The pharyngeal tonsils (adenoids) are located in the superior nasopharynx. This lymphatic tissue is an important defense mechanism of the pulmonary system.

The oropharynx is that portion of the pharynx from the soft palate to the base of the tongue. It receives air from the mouth and nose, and food from the mouth. The faucial tonsils are located at the anterolateral borders of the oropharynx.

The laryngopharynx is the lower portion of the pharynx, located from the base of the tongue to the opening of the esophagus. The laryngopharynx contains muscles within its wall called pharyngeal constrictors. These muscles aid in the mechanism of swallowing.

Larynx

The larynx is the upper portion of the trachea and connects the upper and lower airways (Fig. 10-9). It lies in the anterior portion of the neck extending from C-4 through C-6. The larynx protects the lower airway

against foreign material, aids in speech, and is an essential part of the mechanism of coughing.

The glottis is the opening into the larynx. The epiglottis, a flexible cartilage attached to the thyroid cartilage, functions primarily to prevent entry of foreign material into the airway by covering the glottis when a person swallows.

The larynx is composed of cartilage, connected by membranes, and muscle. One cartilage is a complete ring and is called the cricoid cartilage. It is located just below the thyroid cartilage. The vocal cords lie inside the thyroid cartilage.

In the adult, the thyroid cartilage (Fig. 10-10), housing the vocal cords, is the narrowest part of the air passage of the larynx. As muscles in the larynx contract, the vocal cords change shape and vibrate. This vibrating of the vocal cords produces sound.

In children, the cricoid cartilage (Fig. 10-10) is the narrowest part of the laryngeal airway. Therefore, children do not need a cuffed endotracheal tube. The cricothyroid membrane is an avascular structure that connects the thyroid cartilage and cricoid cartilage. It

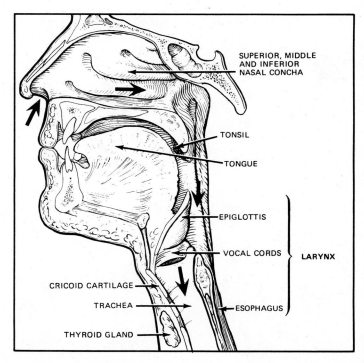

Figure 10-9. The larynx.

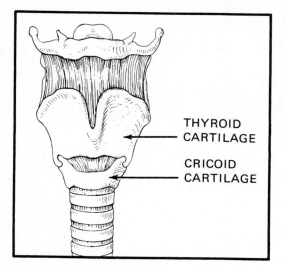

Figure 10-10. The thyroid-cricoid cartilages.

is through this membrane that an airway may be established in an emergency. The posterior wall of the larynx and the vocal cords will not be injured.

Linings of the Upper Airway
The first one-third of the nose is lined with nonciliated, squamous epithelium. The remaining two-thirds of the nose is lined with ciliated, pseudostratified epithelium. Coarse particles larger than 4 microns are entrapped by nasal hairs. The nasopharynx is lined with ciliated, pseudostratified epithelium. The laryngeal mucosa is stratified squamous epithelium above the vocal cords, and pseudostratified columnar epithelium below. The entire upper airway is lined with a mucous membrane. This membrane is essential for accomplishing the functions of the upper airway. The ciliated portions of mucosa in the upper airway filter pollutants and irritants. Fine particles from 1 to 4 microns come in contact with the respiratory mucosa and become trapped; these are eventually carried to the pharynx by the mucociliary escalator and finally swallowed.

The mucous membrane of the upper airway moisturizes and warms the inspired air because of the vast blood supply in the mucosa and the thick layer of mucus present from secretions of both serous glands and goblet cells. Serous glands in the mucosa secrete a watery mucus. Goblet cells in the epithelium secrete a thick, tenacious mucus.

The functions of the upper airway are to warm, humidify, and filter the respiratory passageways. These functions are essential to protect the alveoli so that they may function to their fullest capacity and be guarded against erosion and hemorrhage from dry air. In a patient with an endotracheal or tracheostomy tube, the upper functions are bypassed. The nurse must be aware of the need to provide these functions for the patient with proper respiratory therapy equipment and principles of aseptic technique.

Coughing and Sneezing
The sneeze reflex is a reaction to irritation in the nose, and the cough reflex is a reaction to irritation in the upper airway distal to the nose. Both processes are complex mechanisms that require the integration of increased intrathoracic pressure, complete and tight closure of the epiglottis and vocal cords, and strong contraction of the abdominal musculature, diaphragm, and intercostal muscles.

LOWER AIRWAY

The lower airway consists of two divisions, the tracheobronchial tree and the lung parenchyma.

Tracheobronchial Tree
The tracheobronchial tree is a system of conducting tubes allowing air to reach the alveoli. The large airways in the tracheobronchial tree are called bronchi. The smaller airways are called bronchioles.

The trachea is the portion of the airway that extends from approximately C-6 to the point of bifurcation of the right and left main-stem bronchi, which is called the carina. The second intercostal space (ICS) is found by locating the sternomanibrial junction (Angle of Louis). The sternomanibrial junction is a spot about 7 cm below the sternal clavicular junction. The second ICS is found slightly below and to the side of the sternomanibrial junction.

The trachea is composed of C-shaped cartilaginous rings. The C-shaped cartilaginous rings have a posterior muscle that is membranous and friable. On inspiration, this muscle relaxes and the diameter of the trachea increases. On exhalation, this muscle contracts and the diameter of the trachea decreases. Occasionally, the muscle relaxes and then bows in on exhalation, decreasing the effectiveness of the mucociliary

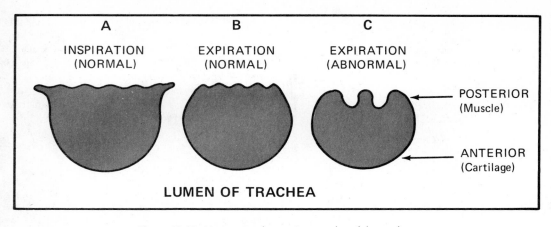

Figure 10-11. Movement of posterior muscles of the trachea.

stream in clearing secretions from the lungs. This is seen in Fig. 10-11.

The carina is the bifurcation of the trachea into the right and left main-stem bronchi. The right main-stem bronchus comes off the trachea in almost a straight line, whereas the left main-stem bronchus angles more acutely to the left (Fig. 10-12). The right main stem bronchus is wider in diameter than the left. Foreign matter tends to lodge in the right main-stem bronchus

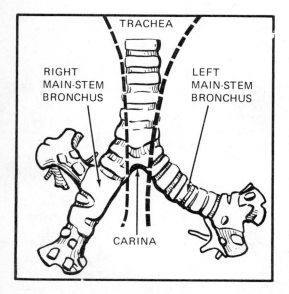

Figure 10-12. The carina.

due to its size and the angle it takes off the trachea. On physical exam, the carina is located near the second ICS.

The right and left main-stem bronchi separate into 22 divisions before the terminal respiratory bronchioles are reached. These divisions are cartilaginous, whereas the respiratory bronchioles are small tubes with no cartilage. Only smooth muscle surrounds the respiratory epithelium. Contraction of this smooth muscle results in bronchospasms.

The respiratory bronchioles branch directly into alveolar ducts, which give rise to the alveoli, the bulk of lung parenchyma. This is possible only because many alveoli and alveolar ducts have common walls, termed septa. These septa play an important role in elastic recoil. The septal wall is composed of smooth muscle and is thought to contract to narrow the alveolar duct lumen.

Alveolar sacs are the terminal end of the respiratory tree (Fig. 10-13). These sacs are dead-end structures in that inhaled ambient air can go no farther. The sacs are found in groups numbering 15 to 20 alveoli per sac. Alveolar sacs share a common wall with adjacent sacs.

Lung Parenchyma

The lung parenchyma (lung tissues) consists of primary lobules, which are the functioning units of the lung. Lobules are composed of alveolar ducts and sacs. The 200 to 600 million alveoli in the normal lung have an average total surface area of 40 to 100 m^2 (approximately the size of a football field). The surface area is

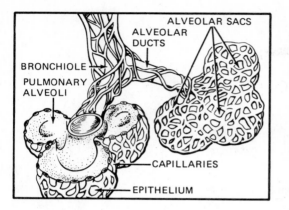

Figure 10-13. Alveolar sacs.

directly related to body length and decreases by about 5% per decade.

Epithelium lines the entire lung parenchyma. The alveolar epithelium is lined with a fluid. The origin of the fluid is unknown. It is believed that this fluid mixes with the mucous blanket and helps to protect the parenchyma.

Alveolar Airways

Alveolar sacs are lined with epithelium. The alveolar epithelium is composed of three types of cells. Type I cells are characterized by cytoplasmic extensions and are the cells that make up most of the lung. Type II alveolar cells are found where one extension interfaces with another. Type II cells are active metabolic cells that contain organelles to synthesize surfactant. Type III alveolar cells are phagocytes that arise from bone marrow or may be from Type II cells.

Pulmonary Surfactant

Alveolar epithelium is lined with a fluid that contains a phospholipid protein called surfactant. Surfactant functions to reduce surface tension in the alveoli. The phospholipid is insoluble but is highly permeable to all gases. Normal alveolar function is dependent upon this surfactant. Two pathologic states that are complicated by insufficient or absent surfactant are (1) hyaline membrane disease in the neonate and (2) adult respiratory distress syndrome. The pulmonary surfactant contains large amounts of dipalmitoyl lecithin, a phospholipid that decreases the surface tension of the fluid lining the alveoli. Surfactant functions by forming a thin, monomolecular layer at the interface of the air

and fluid in the alveoli. Normally, an interface of air and fluid produces surface tension that forces collapse of the small alveoli. Surfactant decreases the surface tension in the alveoli by preventing the development of the air-fluid interface.

The pulmonary surfactant serves two additional functions. Pulmonary surfactant counters the instability of smaller alveoli that have a greater pressure and tend to collapse. Second, the absence of pulmonary surfactant alters the surface tension of the alveoli. Without the proper amount of surfactant, there is a filtration of fluid from the alveolar wall capillaries into the alveoli, leading to development of pulmonary edema and/or adult respiratory distress syndrome.

Mucociliary Escalator

The mucociliary escalator is the primary protective mechanism for the entire respiratory system (Fig. 10-14). The entire respiratory tree is lined with various types of epithelial cells. The airway is lined with cilia, which are fine, hairlike filaments projecting into the airway lumen. Goblet cells in the epithelium produce watery and thick mucus that covers the inside of the airway lumen. The mucous lining is called the mucous blanket. Various mechanisms move the mucous blanket to the pharynx, where it will be swallowed, to the larynx, where coughing will expel it, and to the nose, where it will be expelled by blowing and sneezing. Cilia lining the larger airways help to move the mucous blanket up the respiratory tract by the cilia's continuous undulating movement, referred to as the mucociliary escalator.

Gas Exchange Pathways

The alveoli are the areas in which gas exchange actually occurs. Consider that oxygen has been inhaled and has traveled through all the conducting tubes and is now in the alveolus. The oxygen must diffuse across the alveolar epithelium and the basement membrane and move across the small interstitial space. Oxygen continues the diffusion process through the capillary membrane, the plasma fluid, and the erythrocyte membrane. The capillary endothelium is very sensitive and easily damaged by endotoxins, oxygen, or other noxious substances. At this point, the capillary is so small that the erythrocytes are lined up in a single column to move through the capillary. Oxygen diffuses rapidly through the erythrocyte membrane and attaches to the hemoglobin molecule of the erythrocyte. Carbon dioxide molecules diffuse across the alveolar capillary

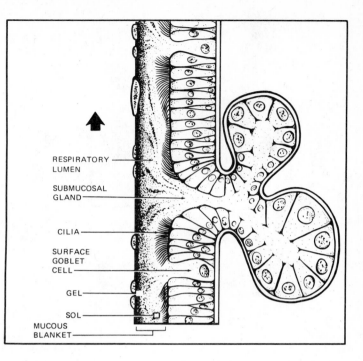

RESPIRATORY LUMEN

SUBMUCOSAL GLAND

CILIA

SURFACE GOBLET CELL

GEL

SOL

MUCOUS BLANKET

Figure 10-14. The mucociliary escalator.

membrane in the opposite direction at a rate 20 times faster than oxygen.

Pulmonary Circulation of the Lung Parenchyma

As with all tissues in the body, the lung tissue must receive oxygenated blood and dispose of its own waste products. The lungs' arterial system follows the bronchial tree, bifurcating at each bronchial division and following close to the bronchus or its subdivisions. As the bronchioles become smaller, some arteries fail to bifurcate. Nearby arteries send out branches from their stems to provide oxygenated blood to the central part (Fig. 10-15) of the alveolar tissue (lobule). Venous blood flows through the capillaries and venules to the periphery of the alveolus and then reenters the venous circulation to be directed back to the right atrium.

Pulmonary Circulation of the Alveolar System

The total volume and rate of pulmonary blood circulation is about 5 liters per minute. Blood flow is greatest to the dependent portions of the lung, due to gravity. Thus, in an erect person, the apex of the lung will have the least circulating blood volume. When the person is lying down, the anterior lung surfaces will have the least circulating blood volume.

The erythrocyte completes the pulmonary circulation very rapidly (0.75 seconds at rest). This rapid circulation helps maintain adequate perfusion. The total volume of blood in the pulmonary arteries, veins, and capillaries is about 500 to 750 mL in the average adult male or about 10 to 15% of the total blood vol-

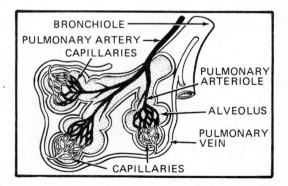

BRONCHIOLE

PULMONARY ARTERY CAPILLARIES

PULMONARY ARTERIOLE

ALVEOLUS

PULMONARY VEIN

CAPILLARIES

Figure 10-15. Entrance of freshly oxygenated blood of the lung parenchyma.

ume. Thus, the pulmonary circulation functions as a reservoir in times of increased need of cardiac output.

CONTROL OF VENTILATION

Three major factors control ventilation: neural, central chemical, and peripheral chemical control mechanisms.

Neural Control

The respiratory center is in the medullary portion of the brain stem. Neurons initiate impulses that result in inspiration. An increase in the rate of impulses results in an increase in respiratory rate. An increase in the amplitude (strength) of impulses increase the tidal volume.

Normally, chemical factors keep the inspiratory and the expiratory centers in balance, providing normal ventilation patterns. A spirometer pattern for normal ventilation is shown in Fig. 10-16.

The inspiratory center is in the dorsal aspect of the medulla oblongata, in close association to the vagus nerve and the glossopharyngeal nerves. There appears to be an inherent automaticity in the electrical impulse release for inspiration. The apneustic center (located in the pons) acts to prevent the interruption of these inspiratory impulses.

If the apneustic center takes control over the normally balanced ventilation pattern, apneustic breathing patterns would be established. Apneustic breathing consists of slight pauses following some expirations in an otherwise normal breathing pattern. An apneustic spirometer pattern is shown in Fig. 10-17.

Expiration control is in the pneumotaxic center located in the upper pons. The neurons located there transmit impulses to limit inspiration. When the pneumotaxic center takes control over ventilation, there is irregular, deep, and shallow breathing with randomly spaced pauses of apnea of varying length. The pneumotaxic or ataxic breathing spirometer pattern is

shown in Fig. 10-18. If all three neural centers, medullary, apneustic, and pneumotaxic, become nonfunctional, respiration ceases.

Five basic terms are used to describe breathing patterns:

1. Eupnea—regular rhythm and a respiratory rate of 12 to 20 breaths per minute
2. Tachypnea—increased respiratory rate of >24 breaths per minute with normal depth of respiration
3. Hyperpnea—increased depth of respiration at a normal respiratory rate
4. Bradypnea—decreased respiratory rate of <10 breaths per minute with normal depth of respiration
5. Apnea—the absence of breathing

There are four common patterns of respiration seen in critical care areas. Central neurogenic hyperventilation is regular, deep, and rapid respirations without periods of apnea. Neurogenic dysfunction causes this pattern of breathing. A central neurogenic hyperventilation spirometer pattern is shown in Fig. 10-19.

Cheyne-Stokes is a pattern in which respirations start from apnea, reach a maximum in depth and rate, and then fade back to apnea. Cheyne-Stokes respirations are caused by alterations in acid-base status, an underlying metabolic problem, or neurocerebral insult. The crescendo-decrescendo pattern of Cheyne-Stokes respiration is shown in Fig. 10-20.

Kussmaul breathing is a tachypnea pattern of labored, deep breaths. Most often seen in diabetic ketoacidosis, Kussmaul respirations are also associated with metabolic acidosis and renal failure (Fig. 10-21).

Biot's respirations are regular, fast, and shallow breaths with irregular, abrupt periods of apnea. This pattern of breathing is caused by central nervous system disorders but may be found in healthy patients. Figure 10-22 illustrates the Biot's respiration pattern.

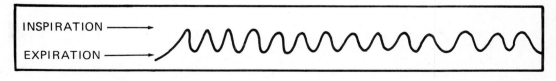

Figure 10-16. Spirometer pattern of normal ventilation.

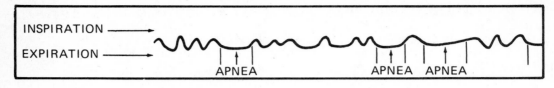

INSPIRATION ⟶

EXPIRATION ⟶

APNEA   APNEA   APNEA

Figure 10-17. Spirometer pattern of apneustic breathing.

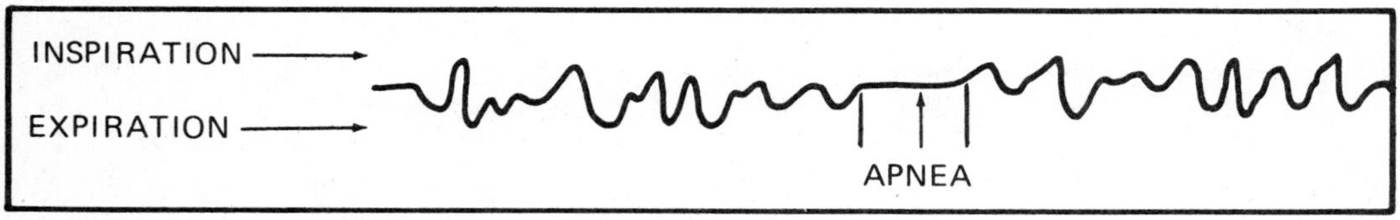

INSPIRATION ⟶

EXPIRATION ⟶

APNEA

Figure 10-18. Spirometer pattern of pneumotaxic (ataxic) breathing.

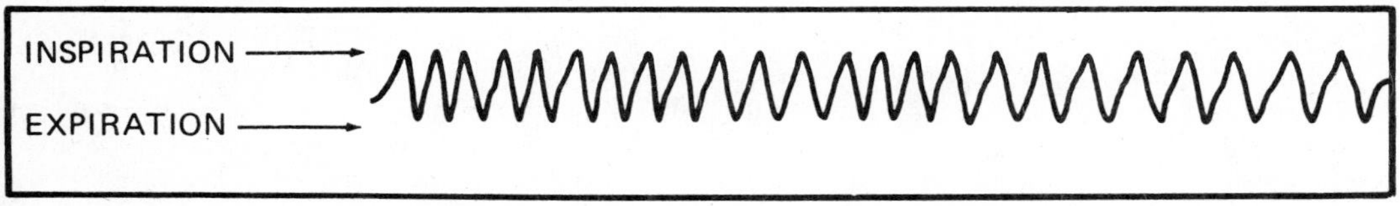

INSPIRATION ⟶

EXPIRATION ⟶

Figure 10-19. Spirometer pattern of central neurogenic hyperventilation.

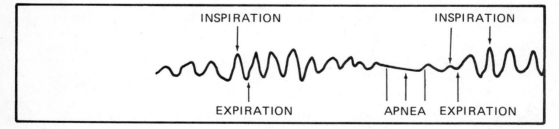

INSPIRATION

INSPIRATION

EXPIRATION   APNEA   EXPIRATION

Figure 10-20. Spirometer pattern of Cheyne-Stokes breathing.

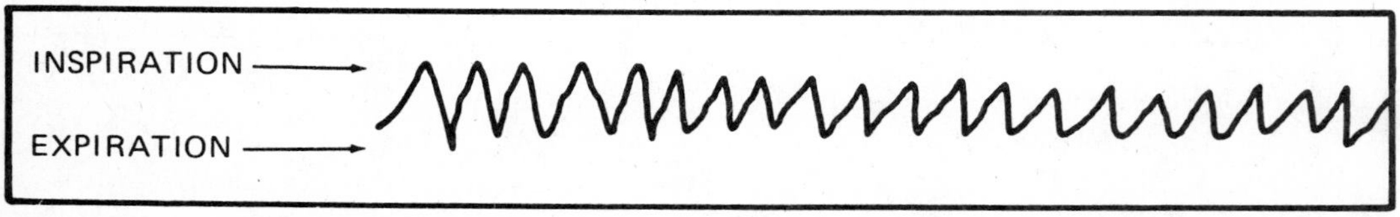

INSPIRATION ⟶

EXPIRATION ⟶

Figure 10-21. Spirometer pattern of Kussmaul breathing.

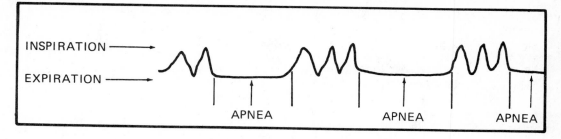

Figure 10-22. Spirometer pattern of Biot's (cluster) breathing.

Central Chemical Control

Cerebrospinal fluid (CSF) pH is the primary control of respiratory center stimulation. A change in the CSF hydrogen ion concentration occurs very quickly in relation to arterial PCO_2. The change in the CSF hydrogen ion concentration will result in the appropriate change in stimulation of the neural respiratory center. Acidosis, a rise in CSF hydrogen ion concentration, increases stimulation to respiratory centers. Alkalosis, a drop in CSF hydrogen ion concentration, decreases stimulation to neural respiratory centers.

Arterial PCO_2 is the normal neurochemical control of the respiratory cycle because of its effect on the CSF pH. A rise in CSF hydrogen ion concentration will first increase respiratory depth and then increase the respiratory rate.

Peripheral Chemical Control

Chemoreceptors are located at the bifurcation of the internal and external carotid arteries, at the carotid bodies, and at the aortic arch (aortic body). These highly vascular, neural bodies are stimulated by any decrease in oxygen supply, e.g., decreased blood flow, decreased hemoglobin, increased pH, or increased PCO_2. Stimulation of the carotid or aortic bodies will increase cerebral cortex activity, causing tachycardia, hypertension, increased respiratory rate, tidal volume, pulmonary resistance, bronchial smooth muscle tone, and adrenal gland secretions.

Hering-Breuer (Stretch) Reflex

The walls of the pulmonary bronchi and bronchioles have stretch receptors that interact with the vagus nerve when they become overstretched. This seems to be a feedback mechanism to prevent overinflation of the lungs. It functions like the pneumotaxic center in limiting the extent of inspiration and thereby protects the lungs from hyperinflation.

Factors That Alter Ventilation

Certain drugs may depress the respiratory center. The mechanisms of depression are related to decreased alveolar ventilation or central respiratory center block. Decreased alveolar ventilation is characterized by shallow respirations and a respiratory rate of less than 12 breaths per minute. Normally, an increase in PCO_2 results in an increase in respirations. Drugs that depress the respiratory center block this normal, protective mechanism.

Chronic respiratory disease may modify the normal respiratory patterns. In patients with chronic CO_2 retention, a change in the respiratory drive occurs. The constantly elevated $PaCO_2$ decreases the ability of the peripheral chemoreceptors to sense changes in hydrogen ion concentration. Instead of an increase in PCO_2 levels initiating the respiratory drive, a decrease in PO_2 levels initiates ventilation. High-flow oxygen therapy may result in apnea.

LUNG SOUNDS

Lung sounds have been utilized for assessment of both the heart and lungs since Laennec developed the stethoscope early in the nineteenth century. The exact origin of lung sounds remains unclear, although a general consensus is developing on how to describe lung sounds. The following section reviews the key principles involved in the application of lung sounds to clinical assessment.

Lung sounds are frequently described in general terms regarding the quality of sound heard over each anatomical region. Tracheal and bronchial sounds reflect the air flow in the major airways. Bronchovesicular and vesicular sounds reflect the progression of air flow in more distal airways. The presence of bronchial sounds in the periphery or anywhere other than the bronchial area may reflect an abnormality. Any abnormal sound is referred to as an adventitious sound.

Crackles, formally termed rales, describes the reopening of airways secondary to change in forces surrounding the airways. Crackles can be of pulmonary or cardiac origin. Pulmonary crackles are thought to be due to airway collapse, primarily on expiration. Their sounds can be heard throughout the lungs. Pulmonary crackles are generally not gravity dependent. Cardiac crackles are thought to be due to increasing fluid in the lungs, promoting collapse of small airways. Cardiac crackles are more gravity dependent. Clinicians describe, for example, basilar crackles or crackles up the lungs as a method of assessing left ventricular failure.

Wheezes are thought to be due to either partial or complete airway obstruction. Wheezes can be high or low pitched. Low-pitched wheezes have also been referred to as rhonchi. The presence of a wheeze is further assessed by identifying where the wheeze is loudest and listening to the air flow distal to this point. The presence of air flow distal to the loudest wheeze location indicates air flow past the obstruction. If a wheeze disappears, the obstruction may be either lessening or worsening, indicating complete obstruction and lack of air movement. If air flow is more easily heard as the wheeze diminishes, then the lung is improving. If air flow diminishes, then the patient is worsening.

Lung sounds can be diminished by the presence of fluid or air between the lung and the stethoscope. For example, a pneumothorax or pleural effusion will diminish the intensity of lung sounds. On the other hand, consolidation of fluid in the lung itself will accentuate sound transmission. A pneumonia, for example, may accentuate the sound heard in the location of the pneumonia. A bronchial sound would be heard instead of the expected vesicular sound. Loss of air flow, such as with bronchoconstriction or obstruction, differs from consolidation in that reduction in air flow generally diminishes breath sounds. For example, atelectasis or airway obstruction will reduce the intensity of breath sounds. The clinician must determine whether the loss of breath sound is due to intrapulmonary (atelectasis, mucous plugs) or extrapulmonary (pneumothorax) causes.

When listening to lung sounds, remember these key anatomic landmarks:

1. The lungs extend over the inner third of the clavicles.
2. The lower border of the lungs are the 6th intercostal space (ICS) anteriorly and the 10th ICS posteriorly.

CHAPTER 11

Pulmonary Physiology

Editor's Note

Understanding concepts in pulmonary physiology is crucial to applying the clinical concepts necessary in the CCRN exam section on pulmonary critical care. While much of this chapter is explanatory and somewhat theoretical, it is important to be familiar with most of the concepts presented. As you read this chapter, focus on understanding key principles rather than on minute details. This is a long chapter, and it may be useful to read it sections in order to improve understanding of the key concepts. You can expect the CCRN exam to have several questions addressing major concepts in pulmonary physiology, so be familiar with the information in this chapter.

The physiological basis of pulmonary function is the key to understanding all pulmonary disturbances, including both assessment and interventions. This chapter presents key critical care concepts in pulmonary physiology, emphasizing gas exchange principles and blood gas analysis.

LUNG FUNCTIONS

There are four major functions of the lungs:

1. Gas exchange. The main function is the exchange of gases to oxygenate the blood. The main gases exchanged are carbon dioxide and oxygen. The functional reserve of the lung is eight times the amount needed to perform normal activities.

2. Reservoir. The lungs are a reservoir storing 1 to 2 liters of blood that is available for increasing cardiac output.

3. Filter. The lungs filter out bacteria and microaggregates. These microemboli are phagocytized by macrophage cells of the lung (Type III cells).

4. Endocrine Organ. The lungs may function as an endocrine organ, altering certain compounds that pass through its system. Most cancers of the lung have endocrine producing insulin, antidiuretic hormone, and cortisol.

RESPIRATORY PROCESSES

The process of respiration has four phases. Phase 1 is pulmonary ventilation, which is the movement of ambient air (room air) into and out of the lungs. Phase 2 is the diffusion of oxygen and carbon dioxide in the alveoli. Phase 3 is the transport of oxygen to the cells and carbon dioxide away from the cells. Phase 4 is the regulation of ventilation.

Mechanical Process of Phase 1 (Pulmonary Ventilation)

Normal atmospheric (barometric) pressure at sea level is 760 mm Hg. For the average, healthy person at rest, the intrapleural pressure is slightly subatmospheric, or about 755 mm Hg. If the pressures were equal, there would be no flow of air into or out of the lung.

As the mechanics of inspiration begin, the thoracic cage increases in size. This size increase produces a negative intrapleural inspiratory pressure, as compared with atmospheric pressure, resulting in air flowing into the lungs. If one considers atmospheric pressure to be zero, then resting intrapleural pressure is -5 and inspiratory intrapleural pressure is -10.

It is possible under extreme physical exertion, especially for athletes, to reduce the intrapleural inspiratory pressure to as low as -50 to -80 mm Hg. The intrapleural expiratory pressure does not exist in terms of negative pressures. As inspiratory muscle activity ends, the normal elastic recoil of the lung tissue and muscles decreases the size of the thoracic cage. Gas flows out of the lungs and back into the atmosphere. The repetition of this process establishes the breathing pattern and pulmonary ventilation.

Lung Pressures

The low-pressure system that exists in the right heart pumps blood into the pulmonary arterial system, where there is also a low pressure or resistance. The right heart circulation pressures are lower than the pressures of the left heart and the systemic circulatory system. This low-pressure system in the lungs allows the capillaries to distend easily to accommodate increased volumes from the systemic circulatory system in times of distress or exertion. This distensibility helps regulate resistance to blood flow through the pulmonary system.

In the normal disease-free lung, the average pulmonary artery systolic pressure is 15 to 30 mm Hg and the average diastolic pressure is 5 to 15 mm Hg. The pressure necessary to overcome to move blood from the right heart to the left heart is the left atrial pressure (or the pulmonary capillary wedge pressure [PCWP]). The normal left atrial pressure (and PCWP) is 8 to 12 mm Hg. The mean pulmonary artery pressure must always be higher than the left atrial pressure in order to move blood from the right heart, through the lungs, and to the left atrium.

Compliance

Compliance is a measurement of the distensibility of the lungs and the thorax. If the lungs were removed from the bony thorax, their expansion would be almost doubled. Compliance is expressed as the volume change in the lungs for each unit of pressure change in the intra-alveolar pressure (V/P). The respiratory symbol for volume is "V," and the symbol for pressure or partial pressure is "P." Greater compliance means that there is a larger volume change in the lung for each pressure change. Reduced compliance means that there is less volume change in the lung for each pressure change. In other words, the more pressure needed to change the volume in the lung, the less compliance.

Intrathoracic Causes (Obstructive) of Compliance Changes

Any disease that stiffens the lungs will decrease compliance. Diseases that increase congestion in the lungs result in an increase in the distance that oxygen molecules must travel to exchange places with carbon dioxide molecules. This makes it more difficult for gas molecules to penetrate this congestion. Diseases that may decrease compliance are listed in Table 11-1.

Space-occupying neoplasms, infections, or increased extravascular lung water decrease lung compliance. The area of increased weight or consolidation is stiff and noncompliant. Gas molecules cannot readily penetrate a consolidated mass. For example, flail chest decreases the lung compliance in the area of the flail segment. Every time the patient inhales, the flail segment is pulled in toward the lung instead of expanding outward. Simultaneously, every time the patient exhales, the flail segment expands outward, decreasing the effective ventilation of that portion of the lung.

Extrathoracic Causes (Restrictive) of Decreased Compliance

Any condition that limits the ability of the bony thorax to expand will decrease lung compliance. Table 11-2 lists some of the extrathoracic causes of decreased lung compliance. An example of a restrictive cause of decreased compliance is third-trimester pregnancy. During the third trimester of pregnancy, abdominal contents are displaced upward and prevent the diaphragm from descending fully, thus decreasing the extent of chest wall expansion.

Morbid obesity and abdominal distension present the same deterrent on the diaphragm. Obesity presents one other problem in lung compliance. If the patient is morbidly obese, the sheer burden of excess weight on

TABLE 11-1. SOME INTRATHORACIC CAUSES OF DECREASED COMPLIANCE

Atelectasis
Pneumonia
Pleural effusion
Empyema and lung abcesses
Bronchospasm
Pulmonary edema
Bronchitis
Asthma
Adult respiratory distress syndrome
Closed tension pneumothorax

TABLE 11-2. SOME EXTRATHORACIC CAUSES OF DECREASED COMPLIANCE

Flail chest
Pectus excavatum (funnel chest)
Pectus carinatum (pigeon chest)
Kyphosis
Scoliosis
Kyphoscoliosis

the upper torso strains the intercostal muscles in attempting to lift the massive weight. The muscles cannot function efficiently, and lung compliance is decreased. Postoperative binders and/or chest splints decrease the ability of the bony thorax to expand, resulting in a decreased lung compliance over a large segment of the thorax.

Types of Compliance

There are two types of compliance, static and dynamic.

Static compliance (C_{st}) is the change in lung volume per unit airway pressure change when the lungs are motionless. Static compliance can be measured only when there is no flow of gases, that is, at the end of inspiration or expiration. Static compliance is normally about 100 mL of pressure per cm of water pressure. Static compliance measurements are a reliable index of lung compliance when no airway disease is present. Airway disease alters the rate of gas flow from the mouth to the alveoli, resulting in inaccurate static compliance values.

If airway disease is present, most of the resistance to air flow will be in the medium-size bronchi. The massive number of airways accounts for the lack of decreased resistance to air flow through them, but this massive number also makes the small airways capable of developing rather extensive disease before static compliance measurement reveals the disease.

Dynamic compliance (C_{dyn}) can be easily tested in the critical care areas. For patients receiving mechanical ventilation, divide the tidal volume (VT) by the peak airway pressure. This gives an estimate of dynamic compliance. Normal dynamic compliance is about 35 to 55 mL/cm H_2O. A measure of airway resistance can be made by comparing the C_{st} and the C_{dyn}.

Airway resistance results from friction caused by gas molecules trying to flow in one direction and the flow being impeded by the walls of the airway or obstruction. This impediment changes the ratio of alveolar pressure against the rate of air flow.

Airway resistance is increased by the collection of secretions, artificial airways, endotracheal tubes, bronchospasms, laryngeal or tracheal strictures, edema, emphysema, or space-occupying lesions.

Elasticity (Recoil Tendency)

Intra-alveolar septa are a major factor in the elastic recoil of the interstitial parenchyma. The thorax, pleura, and lung parenchyma have opposing elastic forces. The fluid lining the alveoli and the interstitial parenchymal tissues are elastic fibers trying to collapse the lungs, while the thoracic cage and pleura are trying to expand the lungs.

The critical volume is the specific volume below which the elastic forces overcome other factors, and the alveolus will collapse. As long as the volume remains above this critical volume, a state of equilibrium is maintained between the surface-acting substances. The balance between surface tension trying to collapse the alveolus and the expanding pressures of inhalation keeps the alveolus open.

As long as the thoracic cage and pleura are patent, these elastic forces tend to balance each other. If the integrity of the pleura is compromised, the parenchymal forces become greater, and the lung collapses.

Air Flow

There are three basic types of air flow within the lung airways: turbulent, transitional and laminar.

Turbulent air flow occurs in large chambers such as the nose and oral pharynx. Figure 11-1 illustrates turbulent air flow.

Transitional air flow occurs in large to medium airways at points of bifurcation or narrowing. As inspired air flows down the respiratory tree, it branches into smaller and smaller tubes, creating transitional air flow. Transitional air flow is seen in Fig. 11-2.

Laminar air flow is flow occurring in thin, flat, continuous sheets. The outermost layer of air has minimal contact with the air passage walls, providing slight filtering in the small peripheral airways. Laminar air flow is seen in Fig. 11-3.

Lung Volumes

The total lung capacity (TLC) is the maximum amount of gas that the lungs can hold. The TLC is composed of

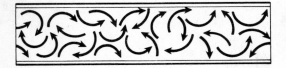

Figure 11-1. Turbulent air flow.

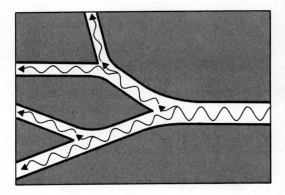

Figure 11-2. Transitional air flow.

four discrete lung volumes. These volumes can be measured by spirometry (Fig. 11-4).

1. Inspiratory reserve volume (IRV) is the amount of reserve or extra gas that can be inhaled at the end of a normal inspiration. It is not usually used in normal breathing at rest. Normal IRV may be as much as 3000 mL.
2. Tidal volume (VT) is the amount of gas that is exhaled or inhaled during normal breathing. Normal VT is 5 to 10 mL/kg or about 350 to 600 mL in a young adult.
3. Expiratory reserve volume (ERV) is the amount of gas that can be exhaled after a normal expiration. Normal ERV is about 1000 to 1500 mL.
4. Residual volume (RV) is the amount of gas that always remains in the lungs and cannot be exhaled.

There are four lung capacities that represent the combination of two or more lung volumes.

1. TLC = IRV + VT + ERV + RV. Normal is about 4000 to 7000 mL.
2. Vital capacity (VC) is the amount of gas that can be forcefully exhaled after a maximum inspiration. VC = VT + IRV + ERV. Normal is about 4000 to 5000 mL.
3. Inspiratory capacity (IC) is the amount of gas that can be inhaled after a normal exhalation. IC = VT + IRV. Normal is about 3500 mL.
4. Functional residual capacity (FRC), also

called the resting lung volume, is the amount of air left in the lungs after normal expiration. FRC = ERV + RV. Normal is about 2000 to 3000 mL.

The values listed for lung capacities are averages and will differ according to body size, weight, and age.

Early in a critical illness, these respiratory volumes and capacities can be used to prevent respiratory deterioration. Throughout the patient's illness, monitor the effectiveness of treatment modalities by measuring these components. Vital capacity, inspiratory force, and tidal volume are the most frequently measured parameters of respiratory muscle function.

Measuring the flow of gas being exhaled and the time of exhaling helps distinguish between restrictive and obstructive lung diseases. Forced vital capacity (FVC) measures the vital capacity that the patient can forcibly exhale. The FVC is important because it reveals the maximum volume of air that the patient will have under stress for ventilation.

FEV_1 is the forced expiratory volume over one second. The patient inhales as much as possible, holds his or her breath briefly, and then exhales as forcibly as possible. Obstructive lung diseases decrease the FEV_1. In restrictive lung diseases, the FVC will be decreased, but the FEV_1 will be normal.

Lung function tests used to assess readiness to wean include tidal volume, vital capacity, minute ventilation ($\dot{V}E$), respiratory rate (RR), and negative inspiratory force (NIF) or peak inspiratory pressure (PIP). Minute ventilation ($\dot{V}E$) is the amount of air exchanged in one minute. Normal minute ventilation is 5 to 10 LPM. NIF or PIP is the maximal inspiratory effort

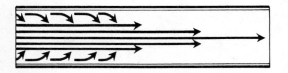

Figure 11-3. Laminar air flow.

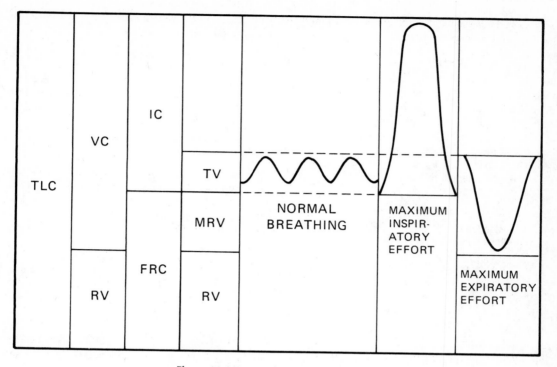

Figure 11-4. Lung volumes and capacities.

the patient can generate, measured by an inspiratory manometer. Normal PIP or NIF is −70 to −90 cm H_2O.

Mechanical Process of Phase 2 (Diffusion of the Alveoli)

Up to this point, oxygen has not reached the erythrocyte to be transported throughout the body. Only the mechanics of getting the oxygen from the atmosphere into the alveolus so that the oxygen can be consumed have been discussed.

Dead Space

Not all of the gas inhaled reaches the alveoli. Gas exchange does not occur until the area of the respiratory tree at the bronchiole and alveoli. The area where no gas exchange takes place is called the anatomic dead space. It is difficult to measure but is estimated to be 150 mL (or 1 mL per pound of ideal body weight). If the tidal volume is about 500 mL in normal breathing, approximately 350 mL of each inhalation will reach the alveolar areas. Each time one exhales, a similar volume of gas remains in the airway passages.

Volume of dead space is abbreviated V_{DS}. It can be calculated by the following formula (where $\dot{V}_E$ is minute ventilation):

$$\frac{(P_{aCO_2} - P_{ECO_2})}{P_{aCO_2}} \times \dot{V}_E$$

The amount of inhaled air that is not anatomic dead space but also does not participate in gas exchange is called physiologic dead space. Physiologic dead space is more helpful than anatomic dead space in assessing effective pulmonary ventilation. It can be calculated by the Bohr equation:

$$\frac{P_{aCO_2} - P_{ECO_2}}{P_{aCO_2}}$$

The amount of inhaled air that reaches the alveoli and takes part in gas exchange is termed alveolar ventilation (V_A). Note the capital "A," which stands for alveolar; the lowercase "a" stands for arterial. V_A can be estimated by P_{aCO_2} (arterial carbon dioxide pressure), which is inversely related to V_A. Physiologic dead space is that amount of the available 350 mL of gas that does not become involved in oxygen and carbon dioxide exchange. If the person is in a fairly stable state, the arterial carbon dioxide is inversely related to alveolar ventilation. Arterial carbon dioxide can be measured, and the value obtained will indicate whether the amount of alveolar ventilation is adequate for the body's demands. Arterial carbon dioxide is abbreviated $PaCO_2$, which stands for the partial pressure of carbon dioxide in the arterial blood.

The following key formula describes the relationship of dead space and minute ventilation.

- $\dot{V}E$ = inspired or expired air in one minute
- VDS = amount of air not participating in gas exchange
- $VA = VE - VDS$
- If VDS increases, VE must increase to maintain VA
- If VA decreases, $PaCO_2$ levels will rise as a reflection of inadequate clearance of alveolar gas

Gas Diffusion Principles

The entire purpose of the second phase of respiration is the diffusion of oxygen into the erythrocyte and the diffusion of carbon dioxide out of the erythrocyte. There are three major components of the diffusion of gases.

The first component is partial pressure of individual gases (Dalton's law). Every gas has a pressure determined by its molecular weight. Atmospheric pressure (PB) at sea level is equal to the sum of all gases that compose atmosphere, mainly oxygen, nitrogen, carbon dioxide, and a few others in minute amounts. Atmospheric gas contains some water vapor that adds to the total gas tensions. The only thing that affects the water pressure is temperature. At body temperature (37°C), the water pressure is equal to 47 mm Hg. Dalton's law says that the total pressure is equal to the sum of the individual gas pressures, as if they occupied the same space corrected for water pressure. So each gas has its own pressure or tension (P) and is present in a certain concentration (C) or fractional concentration (F).

Dalton's law is the basis for understanding alveolar and arterial gas levels. For example, the normal PaO_2 is 80 to 100 mm Hg. The normal PaO_2 is derived from alveolar oxygen tensions (PAO_2). Alveolar oxygen tensions are computed from Dalton's law. Clini-

cally, the PaO_2 tensions are estimated from the alveolar air equation. For example:

Room air FIO_2 =	0.21
PB	760 mm Hg
PH_2O	47 mm Hg
$PACO_2$	$PaCO_2/0.8$
$PAO_2 = 0.21 (760-47) - PaCO_2/0.8$	
$PaO_2 = 100$ mm Hg	

The difference between arterial and alveolar gas tensions is the basis for estimating lung dysfunction secondary to intrapulmonary shunts. Concepts such as the arterial/alveolar (a/A) ratio, the PaO_2/FIO_2 ratio, and the alveolar-arterial (A-a) gradient gives estimates of the intrapulmonary shunt.

On inspiration, the oxygen concentration or pressure is greater in the alveolus compared with the oxygen concentration in the area of the erythrocyte. At exactly the same time, the carbon dioxide concentration is greater in the erythrocyte, so it diffuses toward the low-concentration area of the alveolus.

The second component is diffusion through the respiratory membrane. In addition to the pressure and concentration gradients, a few other factors affect the ability and speed of gas molecules to diffuse through membranes. The actual area of space across which gases have to diffuse is very thin (0.2 to 0.5 microns). The alveoli and capillaries are so small and thin that they look like a single sheet of blood. In fact, they are made up of six layers: the alveolus, alveolar membrane, interstitial space, capillary membrane, plasma, and erythrocyte membrane. Exhaled carbon dioxide moves through the same layers in reverse order. These six layers are collectively called the respiratory membrane. If it becomes thickened as in pulmonary edema or interstitial pulmonary fibrosis, the diffusion of gases will be slowed.

Another factor affecting diffusion through the respiratory membrane is the amount of membrane surface area available. If a lobe of the lung is filled with pus, that portion of the respiratory membrane is not available for diffusion and will cause it to be slowed or stopped completely. In emphysema, when tiny alveoli collapse and disintegrate, the amount of surface area of the respiratory membrane decreases and diffusion slows.

The solubility of gases (Henry's law) will affect the speed of diffusion. Henry's law states that the vol-

TABLE 11-3. COMPOSITION OF GASES IN THE ALVEOLAR, ARTERIAL, VENOUS, AND ATMOSPHERIC COMPONENTS

Alveolar	Arterial	Venous	Atmospheric
$P_{H_2O} = 47$	$P_{H_2O} = 47$	$P_{H_2O} = 47$	$P_{H_2O} = 47$
$P_{ACO_2} = 40$	$Pa_{CO_2} = 40$	$Pv_{CO_2} = 46$	$P_{ICO_2} = 0$
$P_{AO_2} = 100-110$	$Pa_{O_2} = 92$	$Pv_{O_2} = 40$	$P_{IO_2} = 150$
$P_{AN_2} = 563$	$Pa_{N_2} = 563$	$Pv_{N_2} = 563$	$P_{IN_2} = 563$
			$\overline{760 \text{ mm Hg}}$

Remember the respiratory abbreviations? P = pressure or partial pressure; H_2O = water; A = alveolar; O_2 = oxygen; a = arterial; CO_2 = carbon dioxide; v = venous; N_2 = nitrogen; I = inspired.

ume of a gas dissolved in a liquid is proportional to its partial pressure. The structure of some gas molecules is such that they dissolve more easily in some fluid such as water or plasma than in others.

Graham's law states that in the gas phase, the rate of diffusion of gas is inversely proportional to the molecular weight of that gas. This simply means that the lighter the weight of a gas, the slower it will diffuse; and the heavier the gas, the faster it will diffuse.

The third component is diffusion in relation to composition. The specific composition of the alveolar, arterial, and venous compartments will directly affect the diffusibility of gases (Table 11-3).

Intrapulmonary Shunting

Shunting is the final segment in phase 2 of respiratory ventilation. A shunt exists when blood bypasses the alveolus without participating in gas exchange. Intrapulmonary shunting is the most common cause of low Pa_{O_2} and important in understanding the reasons for hypoxemia.

CAUSES OF HYPOXEMIA

Hypoventilation (decreased V_A) can cause hypoxemia. As V_A decreases, P_{ACO_2} values will rise. The rise in P_{ACO_2} levels cause displacement of oxygen, lowering the Pa_{O_2} values. Hypoventilation induced hypoxemia is easily treated with oxygen therapy. However, the decreased V_A must be improved or respiratory failure will occur.

Normally, about 2 to 5% of the blood flowing through the lungs does not come in contact with inspired air for gas exchange (shunt). This is due to the anatomic arrangement of the circulatory system of the lungs. Any shunting that occurs (outside of the normal 2 to 5%) may be classified as one of two types: physiologic shunt and anatomic shunt.

Physiologic, or intrapulmonary shunt is an obstruction of inspired air. The air cannot pass through the respiratory membrane to diffuse into the erythrocyte. Physiologic shunt (Fig. 11-5) results in no increase in physiologic dead space. Accumulated secretions, atelectasis, pulmonary edema, neoplasms, and foreign objects are only a few of many causes of obstruction. Physiologic shunts are also referred to as low ventilation/perfusion (V/Q) ratios. As ventilation is reduced to an alveolar area, without a subsequent reduction in perfusion, venous blood is not completely oxygenated. Since normal venous oxygen levels are low (Pv_{O_2} 35 to 45 mm Hg and Sv_{O_2} 0.60 to 0.75), less oxygenated blood becomes mixed with normally oxygenated blood. The problem produced by low V/Q ratios is hypoxemia, or Pa_{O_2} values below 60 mm Hg. Physiologic shunts are measured by shunt equations or estimated from oxygen tension indices such as the a/A ratio or A-a gradient.

Normal pulmonary anatomy accounts for 2 to 5% of anatomic shunts due to anomalies in the pulmonary vasculature, which channel unoxygenated blood into the left atrium through thebesian, pleural, and bronchial veins. Pathological conditions causing anatomic shunts include states of pulmonary embolisms, thrombi, neoplasms, and intracardiac septal defect (Fig. 11-6).

Oxygen Transport

Once oxygen has penetrated the erythrocyte membrane, it will be carried through the systemic circulatory system to all body tissues. Oxygen is transported in only two possible forms in the body: either dissolved in plasma or combined with hemoglobin. Very limited

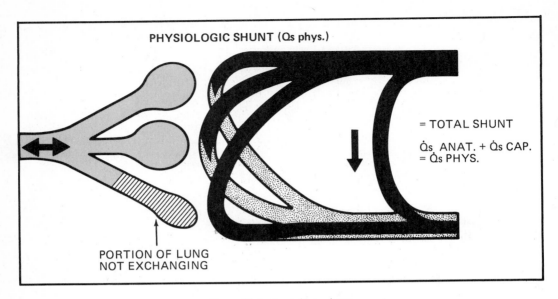

Figure 11-5. Physiologic shunt.

amounts of oxygen are dissolved in plasma. The amount is determined by Henry's law; that is, the amount dissolved is proportional to the partial pressure. This amounts to 0.003 mL of O_2 per mL of blood, which means that about 3% of the total body oxygen is in the dissolved state. When arterial blood gas measurements are performed, the value for Po_2 measures the dissolved oxygen.

The remaining 97% of oxygen being transported through the system's circulation is in combination with

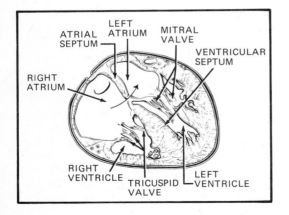

Figure 11-6. Anatomic shunt.

hemoglobin (Hgb). If the hemoglobin were chemically pure, a gram could combine with 1.39 mL of oxygen. Usually, the body hemoglobin is not pure, containing an estimated 2 to 4% of impurities such as methemoglobin and sulfhemoglobin. Therefore, a more practical estimate would be that each gram of hemoglobin can combine with 1.34 mL of oxygen. The transport of oxygen to body tissues is influenced most by cardiac output, by hemoglobin concentration, and by oxygen-hemoglobin binding and releasing factors.

Cardiac output is usually 4 to 8 liters per minute. As the cardiac output varies, the quantity of blood being oxygenated in the lungs will be altered. With normal, healthy lungs, a somewhat decreased cardiac output will not greatly alter oxygen content. The dynamics of the gas pressures allow for rapid oxygen equilibration between the alveolus and the erythrocyte. A markedly decreased cardiac output will alter the oxygen content, but what blood is available will have its maximum amount of oxygen. If hemoglobin is abnormally low, the cardiac output will increase to help compensate and, to maintain adequate oxygen content. The amount of oxygen transported per minute is determined basically by the cardiac output, even though other factors will contribute some effect.

Oxygen content (Cao_2) is the maximum potential amount of oxygen that blood can carry. It is expressed as milliliters of oxygen per 100 mL of blood. In oxygen capacity, the dissolved oxygen in plasma (PaO_2) is virtually ignored since it is so small an amount.

Oxygen content = Hgb × 1.34 (mL of O_2) × SaO_2). Remember, only pure Hgb can be combined with 1.34 mL of oxygen. Oxygen content = Hgb × 1.34 (oxygen capacity) SaO_2 + (PO_2 × 0.003). Oxygen content is equal to the actual amount of oxygen in both the plasma and the erythrocytes.

Oxygen saturation (SaO_2) is the ratio comparing the actual amount of oxygen that could be carried with the amount actually carried, expressed as a percentage.

O_2 Capacity

Hemoglobin is like a magnet and has a natural affinity for oxygen. Once the oxygen diffuses through the erythrocyte membrane, it readily attaches to a site on the hemoglobin molecule. Under ideal conditions, 100 mL of blood will have enough hemoglobin to carry 20 mL of oxygen. (Patient Hgb = 15 gm%). If this amount of oxygen is in fact present, the hemoglobin is said to be 100% saturated. Hemoglobin cannot be oversaturated. One hundred percent is the maximum under human physiologic conditions. However, it may not always be 100% saturated. This is important when one remembers that hemoglobin is a major factor that determines how much total oxygen will be carried in the blood. Oxygen that is attached to hemoglobin (oxyhemoglobin) is not dissolved. Therefore, it does not directly exert a gas pressure.

O_2 Transport

Oxygen transport is the amount of oxygen delivered to the cells, expressed as milliliters of oxygen per minute. O_2 transport = O_2 content × 10 × cardiac output, in liters per minute. Normal oxygen transport is between 600 and 1000 cc/minute or 10 to 12 cc/kg.

Oxygen content and oxygen transport are a more reliable index of hypoxia than the PaO_2 alone. The oxygen content and transport take into consideration the Hgb level and cardiac output. Considering both the oxygen content and cardiac output helps prevent underestimation of the presence and severity of hypoxemia.

Oxygen Consumption

Cellular oxygenation is based partially on oxygen transport. Oxygen transport is the most commonly applied measure to estimate oxygenation, although accurate assessment of oxygenation cannot occur without an oxygen consumption measurement. Normal oxygen consumption (VO_2) is approximately 3.5 cc/kg/min-

ute. A 70-kg man would use 245 cc of oxygen per minute.

Under normal circumstances, only 25 to 30% of the transported oxygen is used by the cells. If oxygen transport is 1000 cc/minute and VO_2 is 250 cc, 25% of the oxygen transported was used. The comparison of oxygen transport and consumption is referred to as the oxygen extraction rate. As the oxygen extraction rate increases, cellular oxygenation is threatened. Extraction rates over 40% require investigation of the adequacy of oxygen transport and consumption components.

Hemoglobin Binding

Oxygen-hemoglobin binding and releasing factors affect the oxygenation of blood even in the presence of marked disease. The effects of these factors are seen on the oxyhemoglobin dissociation curve (Fig. 11-7). The oxyhemoglobin curve is an S-shaped curve representing the nonlinear relationship of the PaO_2 and the SaO_2. Physiologically, the mechanisms for oxygen-binding and oxygen-releasing factors are fascinating.

The amount of oxygen dissolved in the plasma provides the "driving pressure" that forces oxygen to combine with hemoglobin. The dissolved oxygen is directly proportional to its partial pressure and is termed the arterial oxygen tension. The driving pressure of dissolved oxygen exists until the alveolar (PAO_2) and the arterial (PaO_2) pressures are almost equal. The oxygen pressure gradient between the alveolus and the erythrocyte is now almost in equilibrium. This is the point of the normal curve in the upper right of Fig. 11-7. In the normal healthy person, the oxygen tension is 95 to 97 mm Hg with a hemoglobin saturation (SaO_2) of about 97%.

There is a steep down-slope portion to the curve indicating a move from the lungs into the systemic circulation. The hemoglobin saturation and the oxygen pressure are dropping because the hemoglobin is readily giving oxygen up to the tissue capillaries. Each hemoglobin molecule has four sites to which an oxygen molecule can attach. As the hemoglobin moves through the body, the arterial oxygen tension drops and hemoglobin loses its affinity for oxygen, readily releasing it into the tissues. When hemoglobin saturation drops to 50%, the hemoglobin begins to give up its oxygen much less readily. This point is known as the P50 (Fig. 11-7). At the P50, the partial pressure of oxygen is about 27 mm Hg.

The normal curve can be shifted to the right or to

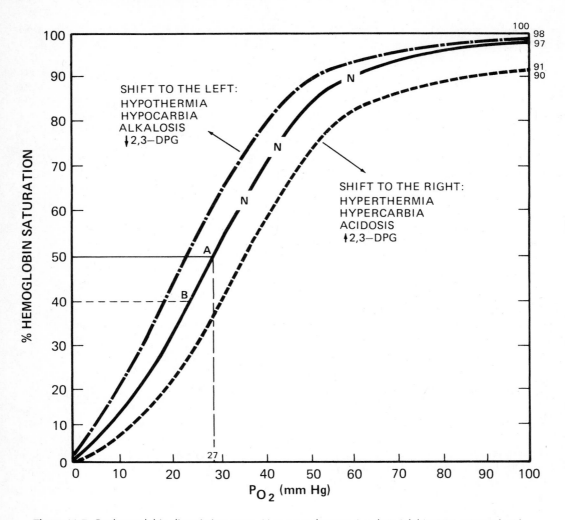

Figure 11-7. Oxyhemoglobin dissociation curve. N = normal curve; A = hemoglobin 50% saturated with O_2; B = hemoglobin bound tightly with O_2, refusing to release the O_2 to the tissues, leading to hypoxia.

the left by many factors. A shift in either direction indicates a change from the normal hemoglobin saturation and oxygen tension.

A shift to the right will occur in acidosis, hypercarbia, increased carbon dioxide, and fever. As one can tell from the change in the normal slope to the slope of a right shift in Fig. 11-7, the arterial oxygen tension and hemoglobin saturation are less than the normal curve. This means that there is less oxygen content of the blood; however, it also means that the hemoglobin will more readily give oxygen up to the tissues, preventing hypoxia. Physiologically, this is an advantage only within certain limits. If the shift is not returned toward normal, eventually the decreased oxygen content will not prevent tissue hypoxia. If the oxygen is not there, it simply does not matter how easily hemoglobin gives it up.

A shift of the curve to the left occurs in alkalosis, hypocarbia, and hypothermia. Note on Fig. 11-7 that the arterial oxygen tension and hemoglobin saturation are only very slightly changed from the normal curve. In a shift to the left, hemoglobin binds oxygen much more tightly and releases less oxygen to the tissues.

2,3-Diphosphoglycerate (2,3-DPG) is an important organic phosphate that will shift the normal curve to the right and left. 2,3-DPG is a phosphate-type enzyme that is present in the erythrocyte. An increase of 2,3-DPG in the hemoglobin of the erythrocyte shifts the curve to the right and facilitates release of oxygen in the tissues. A decrease of 2,3-DPG in the hemoglobin of the erythrocyte shifts the curve to the left and hinders the release of oxygen into the tissues.

Oximetry

Pulse Oximetry (Spo$_2$) is commonly used to estimate Sao$_2$ values. Oximetry does not measure fractional hemoglobin saturation, but rather a functional Sao$_2$. Functional Sao$_2$ differs from laboratory fractional Sao$_2$ only slightly, usually overestimating the real Sao$_2$. Oximetry devices have been demonstrated to be excellent indicators of arterial hemoglobin saturation values.

Oximetry does decrease the need to obtain blood gases to assess Sao$_2$ and Pao$_2$ values. It is most useful in trending saturations during weaning from oxygen. Altering oxygen therapy or positive end expiratory pressure and continuous positive airway pressure levels can be done with oximetry rather than blood gases.

Venous oximetry (Svo$_2$) utilizing blood from the pulmonary artery has been employed for over ten years to estimate overall oxygenation. The balance between oxygen transport and consumption is estimated by Svo$_2$ levels. Normal Svo$_2$ values, between 0.60 and 0.75, indicate safe oxygenation. If the Svo$_2$ falls to less than 0.60, either oxygen transport has decreased or oxygen consumption has increased. While limitations exist with Svo$_2$ use, it remains one of the more valuable tools in the assessment of oxygenation.

TRANSPORT OF CARBON DIOXIDE

As long as life processes are functioning, carbon dioxide is formed as a by-product of metabolism. It is produced in large quantities, averaging 2 pounds per day. Carbon dioxide is effectively eliminated only through respiration. Changes in Paco$_2$ values reflect some change in respiration. Carbon dioxide is transported in the blood in five different states: (1) dissolved in plasma, (2) as bicarbonate ion, (3) as carbonic acid, (4) in combination with hemoglobin, and (5) in an extremely small amount as the carbonate ion.

Much like oxygen, only a very small amount of carbon dioxide is transported in the dissolved state, making up about 7% of the total carbon dioxide. The presence of carbon dioxide in a dissolved state creates a pressure gradient or driving force measured as carbon dioxide tension, or Pco$_2$. Since carbon dioxide is a gas in solution, it follows Henry's law. The pressure gradient of the dissolved CO$_2$ at the tissue level continues until the blood reaches the pulmonary capillaries. Since no CO$_2$ is normally inhaled, the pressure gradient is almost completely one-sided, pushing carbon dioxide from the capillary into the alveolus.

The dissolved carbon dioxide in the blood reacts with water to form carbonic acid. The amount of carbon dioxide that diffuses into the erythrocyte comes into contact with carbonic anhydrase, an enzyme that is a strong catalyst enabling dissolved carbon dioxide to convert to carbonic acid rapidly. The actual rate of the reaction is about 5000 times faster than in the plasma portion. About 70% of the body's carbon dioxide waste is handled this way; therefore, this is the body's most important means of transporting carbon dioxide to the lungs for exhalation. As soon as carbonic acid is formed, it immediately is broken down into hydrogen and bicarbonate ions through the process of dissociation. The hydrogen ions combine with hemoglobin, the bicarbonate ions diffuse into the plasma, and chloride ions diffuse into the red blood cells to maintain homeostasis. Movement of the bicarbonate ion results in a chloride shift, allowing chloride to move into the erythrocyte. Since this is the body's most important way of transporting carbon dioxide, it is important to review the steps of the chemical reactions:

a. Carbon dioxide enters the erythrocyte and does two things:
1. Combines with hemoglobin:

$$CO_2 + Hgb \rightarrow Hgb\ CO_2$$

2. Combines with water:

$$Co_2 + H_2O$$
(carbon dioxide + water)

$$CA \leftrightarrow H_2CO_3$$
(carbon anhydrase $\leftrightarrow$ carbonic acid)

b. The carbonic acid of step b dissociates:

$$H_2CO_3 \leftrightarrow HCO_3 + H^+$$
(carbonic acid $\leftrightarrow$ bicarbonate ion
+ hydrogen ion)

c. HCO_3 leaves the erythrocyte and enters the plasma, allowing the Cl^- to enter the erythrocyte (the chloride shift).

d. The H^+ from step c binds with hemoglobin:

$$H^+ + Hgb \leftrightarrow HHgb$$

VENTILATION PHYSIOLOGY

Life processes continue only as long as the acid-base state in the body is kept within a very narrow range. An acid state that is not corrected will eventually result in a coma and then death. A base or alkalotic state that is not corrected will eventually result in convulsion, tetany, or eventually death.

An acid is a chemical substance that dissociates into positive or negative electrically charged ions. The positive ion is a cation, and the negative ion is an anion. An acid is a substance that dissociates and gives up a proton to the solution. The electrical charge placed as a superscript, e.g., Cl^-, indicates that the substance is an ion. A base is a substance that can and will accept a proton while in solution. Water is the most common and abundant base in the body.

The pH is an expression of the hydrogen ion concentration as a negative logarithm. The hydrogen ion concentration indicates the intensity with which the hydrogen ion will react with bases in solution.

Acid-Base Balance

Two types of acids, volatile and nonvolatile (fixed), are formed in the body. These acids are formed by the metabolism of food and by anaerobic glycolysis.

Volatile Acids

Carbonic acid is the major volatile acid in the body. It is made by the combination of carbon dioxide and water:

$$Co_2 + H_2O \leftrightarrow H_2CO_3$$

The double-headed arrow indicates that the reaction readily moves in either direction. Volatile acids are those acids that can form a gas and, because of an open system, can be eliminated in the gas form. All volatile acids can therefore be eliminated by the lungs. The two main sources of volatile acids are the body's metabolism of glucose and fat.

Nonvolatile (Fixed) Acids

Acids that cannot be converted into the gas form for elimination are termed nonvolatile or fixed acids. Nonvolatile acids are excreted mainly by the kidneys via the urine and in the stool. Nonvolatile acid sources are anaerobic glycolysis, amino acid metabolism, and phosphoprotein/phospholipid metabolism. The kidneys excrete these fixed acids in amounts totaling about 50 mEq per day. Disease can also produce nonvolatile acids.

Acid-Base Disturbance

When there is any disruption in the acid-base balance of the arterial blood toward acidosis, the body has three main defense mechanisms: buffering, increasing alveolar ventilation, and increasing hydrogen ion elimination along with increasing bicarbonate reabsorption. These three defense mechanisms begin to operate in the order listed.

Buffering is the immediate response to an acid-base disturbance in an attempt to prevent changes in hydrogen ion concentration. Increasing alveolar ventilation begins in one to two minutes. As the hydrogen ion concentration builds up, the lungs attempt to reduce the amount of hydrogen ions by increasing ventilation to excrete more carbon dioxide. The kidneys provide the strongest defense against acid-base disturbances by increasing hydrogen ion elimination and increasing bicarbonate ion reabsorption. Unfortunately, it takes from several hours to several days for the kidneys to rebalance the hydrogen ion concentration.

Buffering

There are three major buffering systems: the bicarbonate buffer system, the phosphate buffer system, and the protein buffer system. The bicarbonate buffer system is by far the most important system because the end products of the chemical buffer are regulated by both the kidneys and the lungs. The chemical reaction in this system is reversible and occurs extremely rapidly. The reaction is:

$$H^+ + HCO_3 \leftrightarrow H_2CO_3 \leftrightarrow CO_2 + H^+$$

If the buffering moves toward the left, bicarbonate ion is the end product, regulated by the kidneys. If the buffering moves toward the right, the end product is carbon dioxide, regulated by the lungs. Since one end product is regulated by the kidneys and the other end product is regulated by the lungs, and because buffering must occur by the lungs or the kidneys, this system is especially important. It means that the pH can be shifted up or down by either or both the renal system and the respiratory system. With so many possible controls, even though this is a weak chemical reaction, it is a very important and easily manipulated system.

The phosphate buffer system is similar to the bicarbonate system in function. The phosphate system buffers best at a slightly different pH than the bicarbonate system. It buffers mainly in the tubular fluids of the kidney. This system buffers strong acids (e.g., hydrochloric acid) and strong bases (e.g., sodium hydroxide) into weak acids and bases that will have little effect upon the blood pH.

The protein buffer system is the most inexhaustible buffering system in the body. All the plasma proteins and intracellular proteins, such as hemoglobin, buffer. Proteins buffer carbon dioxide quickly and bicarbonate ions over a period of several hours. The extreme importance of the system is that it helps to buffer the extracellular fluids through the diffusion of carbon dioxide and bicarbonate ion. The supply of protein is infinite.

Changes in Alveolar Ventilation

Assuming that buffering has not rectified an acid-base disturbance within one to two minutes, the respiratory system will become active. Alveolar hyperventilation increases the rate at which the body excretes carbon dioxide, compensating for a metabolically generated acidosis. Alveolar hypoventilation does the opposite, compensating for a metabolic alkalosis. Changes in alveolar ventilation alter the relationship between pH, $Paco_2$, and the bicarbonate ion. As alveolar ventilation increases the $Paco_2$ decreases. The decreased $Paco_2$ results in a respiratory-induced alkalosis, reducing the availability of hydrogen by combining the hydrogen with HCO_3. If alveolar ventilation decreases, the $Paco_2$ level increases, resulting in a respiratory acidosis due to the increased availability of hydrogen. The respiratory system reacts within minutes to compensate for metabolically induced change in hydrogen ion concentration.

Hydrogen Ion Concentrations

Normal hydrogen ion concentration of blood is 0.0000001 to 0.00000001 moles/liter of blood, or 10^{-7} moles/liter. It is difficult to comprehend such tiny numbers. In the early twentieth century, Sorenson

eliminated the zeros by redefining the hydrogen ion concentration in 10^{-7} moles/liter as seven puissance hydrogen. The term puissance was a French word expressing logarithm in a specific way. Hasselbalch simplified all of this by referring to the hydrogen ion concentration simply as pH. In equation form, pH = log H^+. Hasselbalch also determined that pK = log K, where K is the constant ratio of the release of protons from acids to the bonding of protons to bases. The final version of Henderson and Hasselbalch's combined equations is base pH = pK + log acid. This means that the behavior of the hydrogen ion in a solution is equal to its chemical energy or potential. This potential is dependent upon or results from the activity of the substance.

Blood has a major acid (carbonic acid) and a major base (bicarbonate ion). The pK, or dissociation reaction constant, has been calculated to be 6.10 in blood. The ratio of bicarbonate to carbonic acid in the blood is 20:1. The log of 20 is 1.30. These figures are expressed in the Henderson-Hasselbalch equation as:

$$pH = pK\ (6.10) + \log acid\ (1.30) = 7.4$$

The pH expresses the driving pressure of the acid-base balance. The pH is a negative logarithm; therefore, the smaller the value of the pH, the greater the concentration of hydrogen ions and the more acidic the solution. Conversely, the larger the value of the pH, the smaller the concentration of hydrogen ions and the less acidic the solution.

Increased Hydrogen Ion Elimination Along with Increased Bicarbonate Ion Reabsorption

The final mechanism that the body can utilize to alter acid-base disturbances is to increase the hydrogen ion elimination and increase bicarbonate ion reabsorption. This defense mechanism involves both the lungs and the kidneys:

$$pH = \frac{HCO_3}{Paco_2} = \frac{(kidney\ function)}{(lung\ function)}$$

The kidney function of acid-base disturbances reacts within a few hours of the disturbance. However, it is a slowly acting defense mechanism and may take several days to rebalance the acids and bases. The kidneys are able to excrete some hydrogen ions in relation to excretion of nonvolatile acids. This is a very small additional percentage of hydrogen ion elimination, since the lungs excrete most of hydrogen ions. At the same time, the kidneys reabsorb bicarbonate ions in the proximal tubule to equal the excessive number of hydrogen ions. As this reabsorption proceeds, carbon dioxide and water are formed:

$$H^+ + HCO_3 \leftrightarrow H_2CO_3 \leftrightarrow CO_2 + H_2O$$

If this reabsorption is not adequate to restore the acid-base balance, then sodium and hydrogen ions will trade places to maintain electrical neutrality. The sodium bicarbonate then returns from the kidney tubules to the plasma.

If this defense does not reestablish acid-base balance, the kidneys will conserve still more bicarbonate by substituting ammonium ions (NH_4) for bicarbonate ions. If the acid-base disturbance continues and all of the possible bicarbonate ions have been retained, hydrogen ions will reach the distal tubules and combine with phosphates. These phosphates, with the added hydrogen ions, will then be excreted in the urine. Alterations in potassium and in extracellular fluid volume are final efforts of the kidney to restore acid-base balance.

ARTERIAL BLOOD GASES

There are five values of importance in interpreting arterial blood gases (Table 11-4).

Acidosis is an acid-base disturbance with a predominant quantity of acid. Acidemia is a state of increased hydrogen ions reflected in an arterial blood pH below 7.35. Alkalosis is an acid-base disturbance in which acids are insufficient in quantity or base is in excess. Acid insufficiency is more commonly a cause than is base excess. Alkalemia is a state of decreased hydrogen ions reflected in an arterial blood pH above 7.45.

Altering Acid-Base Abnormalities

There are only two ways in which the pH may be returned toward the normal 7.40 in acid-base disturbances, compensation and correction. Compensation occurs when the body attempts to respond to the acid-base abnormality. If the primary disturbance is respiratory, the kidneys will respond to shift the pH toward normal. If the primary disturbance is metabolic, the respiratory system will attempt to compensate for the alteration.

In respiratory acidosis, the lungs are responsible for the altered state. The kidneys will try to compensate by excreting more acid in the urine and increasing reabsorption of the bicarbonate ion. These two concurrent actions will move the pH nearly back to the normal value of 7.40. In respiratory alkalosis, the kidneys will try to compensate by increasing the amount of bicarbonate excreted.

In metabolic acidosis, the respiratory system is stimulated to increase alveolar ventilation. The hyperventilation increases the excretion of carbon dioxide as an acid waste product of metabolic processes. This is an effective and rapid way to decrease arterial carbon dioxide ($Paco_2$) levels. The respiratory system can compensate in metabolic acidosis in just a few minutes. In metabolic alkalosis, the respiratory system will hypoventilate, retaining carbon dioxide and shifting the pH toward normal. The body cannot fully compensate for metabolic alkalosis. The hypoventilation necessary for compensation causes a decrease in the arterial oxygen (Pao_2) level. When the oxygen level becomes too low, the respiratory system will respond to the decreased oxygen by increasing ventilation. Although this compensation effort is rapid, it is not a complete compensation.

Many authorities agree that the most significant fact about compensation as a defense mechanism in acid-base disturbance is that the body never overcom-

TABLE 11-4. NORMAL ADULT BLOOD GAS VALUES AT SEA LEVEL

| Determination | Arterial[a] | | Mixed Venous[v] |
		Midpoint	Range
pH	7.35–7.45	7.40	7.36–7.41
Po_2	80–100 mm Hg	93	35–40 mm Hg
Pco_2	35–45 mm Hg	40	41–51 mm Hg
HCO_3	22–26 mEq/L	24	22–26 mEq/L
SO_2	95–100%	97%	70–75%
Base excess	+2	0	+2

pensates. Compensation will return the body pH to near normal (7.40), but it will never "overshoot the mark."

Interventions to Aid pH Correction

If the primary acid-base disturbance is respiratory acidosis, it is corrected by increasing ventilation. The increase will enable more carbon dioxide (acid) to be "blown off." For the patient on mechanical ventilation, the respiratory rate is increased to decrease the $Paco_2$ and maintain effective ventilation, or the tidal volume may be increased.

If the primary acid-base disturbance is respiratory alkalosis, correcting the cause of excessive breathing is necessary (e.g., calming an anxious patient). If the patient is on mechanical ventilation, decreasing the respiratory rate, decreasing the tidal volume, or adding additional tubing (dead space) may correct the imbalance.

A primary acid-base disturbance of metabolic acidosis is treated with intravenous sodium bicarbonate when the pH has fallen below 7.25. If given judiciously, bicarbonate will begin to return the pH toward normal while the underlying cause of the imbalance is identified and treated.

If the primary acid-base disturbance is metabolic alkalosis, the imbalance is corrected by giving the patient acetazolamide (Diamox), ammonium chloride, hydrochloric acid, or potassium chloride (KCl). The pH usually is greater than 7.55 before these aggressive measures are taken.

Respiratory Disturbances

A look at the respiratory parameter will help determine some of the clinical conditions that may precipitate a respiratory acid-base imbalance. It is known that the $Paco_2$ represents a measurement of the effective alveolar ventilation. The $Paco_2$ is used to determine the presence of respiratory acidosis or alkalosis.

Respiratory Acidosis. If the $Paco_2$ is elevated (>45 mm Hg) and the pH decreased (<7.35), respiratory acidosis is present, indicating hypoventilation. Hypoventilation may be of an acute or chronic nature. Regardless, the clinical cause must be determined and treated. Pathologic conditions usually cause respiratory acidosis. A pure respiratory acidosis is an extremely dangerous situation since it implies inadequate alveolar ventilation.

Obstructive lung diseases may result in a degree of V/Q disturbance, increasing the risk for developing both acute and chronic CO_2 retention. Since obstructive lung diseases tend to be progressive and chronic, one can anticipate elevated $Paco_2$ values in the arterial blood gas studies. Eventually, the $Paco_2$ becomes ineffective as a means of stimulating ventilation, and the PaO_2 becomes the primary drive to breathe.

Any clinical condition that depresses the respiratory center in the medulla oblongata may precipitate hypoventilation and result in respiratory acidosis. These conditions include head trauma, oversedation, and general anesthesia. More rarely, neoplasms in the medulla oblongata or nearby areas with increasing intracranial mass, size, and pressure may cause a respiratory acidosis. Neuromuscular diseases, including myasthenia gravis, Guillain-Barré syndrome, multiple sclerosis, and amyotrophic lateral sclerosis, and trauma to the cervical spinal cord may cause hypoventilation resulting in respiratory acidosis. Inappropriate mechanical ventilation may cause respiratory acidosis. Too low a respiratory rate or tidal volume and too much dead space in the tubing may result in respiratory acidosis.

Respiratory Alkalosis. When the $Paco_2$ is decreased (<35 mm Hg) and the pH is increased (>7.45), respiratory alkalosis is present, indicating hyperventilation. Restrictive lung diseases are common pathologic causes of respiratory alkalosis. Other causes include anxiety, nervousness, agitation, hyperventilation via mechanical ventilation, and excessive ambu-bagging during a cardiopulmonary arrest.

Metabolic Disturbances

The bicarbonate ion (HCO_3) and base excess are the parameters of the arterial blood gases used to identify nonrespiratory imbalances. Base excess is an easy guide to use in identifying metabolic acidosis versus alkalosis. Base excess is the amount of base above the normal level, after adjusting the level for hemoglobin. The normal midpoint value is zero. If the base excess is above +2, there is an excess of metabolic base in the body fluids and a metabolic alkalosis exists. If the base excess is below −2, there is not enough metabolic base in the body fluids and a metabolic acidosis exists.

Metabolic Acidosis (HCO_3; Negative Base Excess). Metabolic acidosis occurs in the body when there is an increase of any metabolic acid except carbon dioxide. Although carbon dioxide is an acid end product of body metabolism, it is excreted by the lungs and therefore classified as a respiratory acidosis when elevated. Metabolic acidosis may occur with an excess loss of body alkali (bicarbonate ion), with certain medications, with retention of hydrogen ions, and in prolonged vomiting and diarrhea of small intestine fluids.

Metabolic acidosis is classified in two major groups: those with an increase in unmeasurable anions and those with no increase in unmeasurable anions. Understanding which causes of metabolic acidosis result from an increase in unmeasurable anions and which result from no increase in unmeasurable anions helps to alert us to possible problems for which the patient needs monitoring.

Anion Gap—Increase in Unmeasurable Anions. To calculate unmeasurable anions, add the serum chloride and the bicarbonate ion values, then subtract this sum from the serum sodium level. If the difference is greater than 15 mEq/liter, there is an increase in unmeasurable anions known as the anion gap. No real anion gap exists, since positive (cations) and negative (anions) ions must always be present in equal numbers. However, it appears as if the anion gap is present because only the major ions (sodium, chloride and bicarbonate) are measured.

Common etiologies of metabolic acidosis with an increase in unmeasurable anions include (the specific anion is in parentheses): diabetes mellitus (ketone bodies), uremia (phosphates and sulfates), lactic acidosis (lactate), aspirin poisonings (salicylate), methyl poisoning (formic acid), ethylene glycol poisoning (oxalic acid and formic acid), and paraldehyde.

Absence of Anion Gap—No Increase in Unmeasurable Anions. There are several common etiologies of metabolic acidosis with no increase in unmeasurable anions. Diarrhea is probably the most common cause. Large amounts of bicarbonate ion are in the intestines and are washed out in cases of diarrhea. The more severe the diarrhea, the greater the likelihood of metabolic acidosis. A general guide for the possible development of metabolic acidosis with no increase in unmeasurable anion is the presence of a drainage tube, except a Foley catheter, below the umbilicus. This includes drainage of pancreatic juices, ureterosigmoidostomies, and any other drainage tubes.

A final major category is uremia. With severe renal failure, the kidneys cannot excrete the normal acids formed daily by the body. As the acids build up,

uremia develops, resulting in an increase in unmeasurable anions.

Metabolic acidosis is the most difficult acid-base disturbance to correct. The high hydrogen ion concentration stimulates the body to attempt compensation by increasing both the depth and the rate of respiration. Compensation is not usually enough by itself. The electrolytes are often quite abnormal and complicate the correcting acid-base disturbance.

Metabolic Alkalosis (HCO_3; Positive Base Excess). Any condition that increases metabolic processes beyond the ability of the body to eliminate or neutralize the waste products results in an increase in bicarbonate ions. Metabolic alkalosis is less common than metabolic acidosis, except in the surgical patient with nasogastric suctioning.

Metabolic alkalosis is a condition with an excess base. The three most common causes are diuretic therapy, excessive vomiting of stomach contents, and excessive ingestion of alkaline drugs. Less commonly, treatment with corticosteroids, hyperaldosteronism, and, rarely, Cushing's syndrome result in a metabolic alkalosis. These conditions result in a loss of hydrogen ions (diuretics), chloride ions (vomiting), and potassium ions (hyperaldosteronism) through the kidneys. The effect is increased bicarbonate ion (HCO_3) reabsorption in the kidneys, which forces excretion of the hydrogen, chloride, and potassium ions in the urine. Excessive ingestion of alkaline drugs such as antacids and soda bicarbonate may lead to metabolic alkalosis. The other cause of metabolic alkalosis is excessive loss of gastric acids. This can be from excessive vomiting or nasogastric suctioning. Since nasogastric suctioning is a common and often lengthy treatment in critical care units, patients with nasogastric tubes should be monitored closely for acid-base disturbances. Corrective therapy is far easier in the early stages of the disorder, before electrolyte imbalances become markedly abnormal.

Interpreting Normal Arterial Blood Gases

Basic acid-base disturbances can be identified by following a step-by-step procedure of analyzing arterial blood gases.

When the pH and the P_{CO_2} move in opposite directions, the primary cause of acid-base disturbance is respiratory. If the pH and the P_{CO_2} move in the same direction, the primary cause is metabolic.

Step 1: Look at the pH.

- A pH of 7.35 to 7.45 is normal.
- If the pH is less than 7.35, an acidosis exists.
- If the pH is greater than 7.45, an alkalosis exists.

Step 1 identifies the presence of an acidosis or alkalosis. The mitochondria in cells are unable to function adequately if the pH falls below 6.9 to 7.2 or rises above 7.6 to 7.7.

Step 2: Look at the $Paco_2$.

- If the $Paco_2$ is between 35 to 45, it is normal. If the value is below 35, a respiratory alkalosis exists. If the value is above 45, a respiratory acidosis exist.
- If the $Paco_2$ moves in the same direction as the pH, the primary cause is metabolic. If the $Paco_2$ moves in the opposite direction of the pH, the primary cause is respiratory.

Look at the following two examples.

Example 1

pH	7.25
$Paco_2$	26

Since the $Paco_2$ and pH moved in the same direction, the primary problem is a metabolic one. Since the pH is acidotic, a metabolic acidosis exists. A respiratory alkalosis exists as well, as evidenced by the low $Paco_2$. The respiratory alkalosis is an attempt to compensate for the metabolic acidosis, but is unable to correct the acidosis.

Example 2

pH	7.24
$Paco_2$	59

Since the $Paco_2$ and pH moved in opposite directions, the primary problem is respiratory. As the $Paco_2$ is elevated and the pH is depressed, a pure respiratory acidosis exists.

Step 3: Look at the bicarbonate ion (HCO_3) value.

- If it is 22 to 26, consider it normal.
- If it is less than 22, a metabolic acidosis exists.
- If it is greater than 26, a metabolic alkalosis exists.

Step 2 is the real key. Step 3 confirms step 2 or identifies a secondary imbalance.

Consider the first blood gas given above and add a HCO_3 value to see how to apply the HCO_3.

pH	7.25
$Paco_2$	26
HCO_3	17

We determined that a metabolic acidosis existed because the pH and $Paco_2$ moved in the same direction. The low HCO_3 level confirms a metabolic acidosis.

Applying the principles of blood gas interpretation listed above usually will provide the information needed to interpret blood gases. To help review the principles, three examples are given below. Try to interpret these values before reading the answers to test your skill.

	Example 1	Example 2	Example 3
pH	7.19	7.35	7.52
P_{aCO2}	30	62	25
HCO_3	14	40	25

In example 1, since the $Paco_2$ and pH moved in the same direction, the primary problem is metabolic. The pH and HCO_3 confirm a metabolic acidosis. The low $Paco_2$, a respiratory alkalosis, is an attempt to correct for the metabolic acidosis. Since the pH is very low, this situation requires intervention to correct the metabolic acidosis.

In example 2, the $Paco_2$ is elevated, indicating a respiratory acidosis, but the pH is normal. This could happen only if a compensation had occurred to offset the acidosis. The high HCO_3 confirms that a metabolic alkalosis exists. The interpretation is respiratory acidosis compensated for by a metabolic alkalosis. Since the pH is normal, no acute danger exists in this patient.

In example 3, since the $Paco_2$ and pH moved in opposite directions, the primary problem is respiratory. Due to the low $Paco_2$ and high pH, a respiratory alkalosis exists. No compensation has occurred, as evidenced by the normal HCO_3 level. In this case, a pure respiratory alkalosis exists.

The combination of an acidosis and an alkalosis is tolerated better by the body than is the combination of two acidoses or two alkaloses. The combination of two acidoses or two alkaloses tends to block compensation for each other. The result is severe acid-base and electrolyte disturbances. The combination of an acidosis and an alkalosis tends toward a more normal pH, since the two conditions have opposite effects on the carbonic acid/bicarbonate ion ratio.

TREATMENT CONSIDERATIONS IN ACID-BASE DISTURBANCES

Respiratory Acidosis

Respiratory acidosis can best be treated by improving ventilation. This includes nursing measures such as protecting the airway through positioning or creating artificial airways. Mechanical ventilation may be necessary. The key to treatment is to find the cause of the respiratory depression and correct it. A respiratory acidosis requires active treatment only if the rise in $Paco_2$, has produced a pH decrease to the level of about 7.25. The more alert the patient, the longer intubation and mechanical ventilation can be delayed.

Respiratory Alkalosis

A respiratory alkalosis is treated by finding the cause of the excessive breathing, such as anxiety, pain, fear, hypoxemia compensation for a metabolic acidosis, or central nervous system disturbance. Correcting the cause will correct the respiratory alkalosis.

Metabolic Acidosis

A metabolic acidosis is treated by correcting the cause of the acidosis. Correcting the underlying cause will reverse the metabolic acidosis. If the pH is less than 7.25, sodium bicarbonate ($NaHCO_3$) may be ordered in a dose of 1 mcg/kg.

Metabolic Alkalosis

A metabolic alkalosis is corrected by finding and treating the underlying cause. Most instances of metabolic alkalosis in the critical care setting are due to electrolyte disturbances, such as a low potassium or high chloride level. In severe disturbances where the pH is greater than 7.60, hydrochloric acid or ammonium chloride may be administered.

CHAPTER 12

Acute Respiratory Failure and Adult Respiratory Distress

Several questions on the CCRN exam can be expected to address the concepts of acute respiratory failure and adult respiratory distress syndrome. It is important to understand key physiological events that produce clinical symptoms of these conditions as well as the likely therapeutic events that might improve pulmonary function. It is important to understand concepts of mechanical ventilation, positive end respiratory pressure/continuous positive airway pressure therapy, and oxygen therapy. This chapter provides a concise review of the major areas that the CCRN exam is likely to cover with respect to these topics.

ACUTE RESPIRATORY FAILURE

Acute respiratory failure (ARF) is the inability of the lungs to maintain adequate oxygenation (Pao_2 and Sao_2 levels) and/or carbon dioxide elimination ($Paco_2$ values). Reasons for oxygenation and carbon dioxide elimination disturbances vary. Identification of the origin of the problem is required to correctly initiate supportive and definitive therapies.

Etiology

ARF presents with a disturbance of either oxygenation or ventilation. The severity and difficulty in treating the cause of respiratory failure vary substantially between the types of failure. Table 12-1 contains common causes of respiratory failure. ARF may be life threatening. Ventilation disturbances, i.e., a respiratory acidosis, is more serious due to the potential to quickly cause a systemic acidosis. If the $Paco_2$ rises and produces an uncompensated decrease in the pH,

the patient can quickly succumb to the cellular disruption associated with the acidosis. Oxygenation disturbances are potentially dangerous, yet the ability of the cardiac output to offset Pao_2 and Sao_2 levels prolongs the time a patient can tolerate low oxygenation values. When one is prioritizing the severity of a disturbance, an uncompensated respiratory acidosis is one of the most dangerous clinical signs. Low Pao_2 and Sao_2 levels are dangerous but are more likely to be better tolerated over the short-term course of respiratory failure.

Two points are important to remember in the patient with ARF: (1) identify the type of disturbance, i.e., oxygenation, ventilation, or both, that is present, and (2) isolate possible causes in order to establish curative therapy.

Ventilation Failure—Respiratory Acidosis ARF with a primary ventilation problem can result from several factors. Problems that are primarily oxygenation disturbances can also develop into ventilation

TABLE 12-1. CAUSES OF RESPIRATORY FAILURE

Disturbances in oxygenation
  Adult respiratory distress syndrome
  Infections, e.g., pneumonia
  Pulmonary edema, cardiac or noncardiac origin
  Lung trauma
    Pulmonary bleeding
    Inhalation injury
  Pneumonitis
Disturbances in ventilation
  CNS depression
  Medication or anesthetic effect
  Head or cervical cord trauma
  Cardiovascular accident
Disturbances affecting both oxygenation and ventilation
  Chronic obstructive lung disease
  Pulmonary emboli

problems as the disorder worsens. If the patient presents with respiratory acidosis, a pH below 7.25, and a decreased level of consciousness, the treatment of choice is to establish a patent airway and adequate ventilation.

Ventilation-induced respiratory failure can be due to a depressed central nervous system (CNS) or ventilation markedly in excess of perfusion (high V/Q ratio). The net result is inadequate alveolar ventilation and a failure to eliminate carbon dioxide. The failure to eliminate CO_2 results in an acute rise in arterial CO_2 values. If the depressed CNS is due to medications, reversal of the medication effect is the treatment of choice. When respiratory depression is due to trauma or an increase in intracranial pressure, treatment is focused on relieving the increased intracranial pressure.

A more complicated situation exists when the problem is due to high V/Q ratios. High V/Q ratios can also be referred to as increased physiologic deadspace. The patient increases $\dot{V}E$ in an attempt to offset the VDS in order to maintain alveolar ventilation. The increased $\dot{V}E$ results in a markedly increased work of breathing. Identification of the patient with an increased deadspace is relatively easy. If the $Paco_2$ is normal, the $\dot{V}E$ would be normal. If the $Paco_2$ is normal but the $\dot{V}E$ is increased, deadspace must be increased. Under normal circumstances, any increase in $\dot{V}E$ would decrease the $Paco_2$.

Clinical Presentation. If the ventilation failure is due to CNS depression, the rate of breathing is slowed, causing increased $Paco_2$ levels. Few other obvious physical symptoms may exist. If the ventilation failure is due to increased deadspace, the respiratory rate and depth may be markedly increased and the patient may complain of shortness of breath and appear anxious.

Treatment. Supportive treatment involves protecting the airway and establishing ventilation. Endotracheal intubation and mechanical ventilation may be necessary. Treatment of ventilation failure is to correct the underlying problem. When medication is the cause of respiratory failure, discontinuation of the medication may reverse the respiratory depression. The problem is more difficult when the cause is a high V/Q ratio. Reestablishing perfusion is the key to high V/Q ratios. If a pulmonary embolism exists, thrombolytic therapy, such as with streptokinase or tissue plasminogen activator, may be indicated. If low perfusion is due to a low cardiac output, improving the cardiac output is necessary.

Oxygenation Failure—Low Pao_2/SAo_2 Values. ARF due to an oxygenation problem is the most common form of respiratory failure. Oxygenation disturbances can be traced to low V/Q ratios. Perfusion exceeds ventilation, resulting in decreased oxygenation of the venous blood and the mixing of the less oxygenated blood with the arterialized blood. The effect is a reduced Pao_2 value. Many causes exist for oxygenation failure.

Adult Respiratory Distress Syndrome

Adult respiratory distress syndrome (ARDS) is a common form of respiratory failure in the critical care unit. The origin of ARDS is unclear, although potential causes have been narrowed since the syndrome was first identified. Current theories are listed in Table 12-2.

ARDS is a response to some systemic insult resulting in an increase in pulmonary capillary permeability. Normally, the pulmonary capillary allows only small amounts of fluid to leak into the interstitial compartment that is readily drained by the pulmonary lymphatic system. In ARDS, capillary leakage results in a tremendous loss of fluid from the vascular space primarily due to the loss of vascular proteins. As the proteins leave the capillaries, they pull large amounts of fluid into the pulmonary interstitial space. The large fluid leak overwhelms the pulmonary lymphatic drainage capability, causing alveolar flooding. Oxygen transfer is impaired by the alveolar flooding. The result is severe hypoxemia, a cardinal symptom of ARDS.

Prognosis. Mortality from ARDS remains high, within the 40 to 70% range. The severe hypoxemia associated with ARDS, however, is usually not the cause of death. Mortality is multifactorial, with the

---

TABLE 12-2. POTENTIAL CAUSES AND CONDITIONS ASSOCIATED WITH ARDS

Potential causes
   Polymorphonuclear leukocyte release
   Metabolites of arachidonic acid
   Complement activation
Conditions associated with ARDS
   Long-bone fractures
   Excessive fluid administration
   Sepsis
   Inhalation injury
   Pulmonary infection or trauma
   Multisystem organ failure or injury

TABLE 12-3. SYMPTOMS OF OXYGENATION INDUCED RESPIRATORY FAILURE

Shortness of breath
Orthopnea
$Pao_2 < 60$ mm Hg
$SaO_2 < 0.90$
Anxiety
Increased respiratory rate (>30 bpm)
Possible labored breathing
Increased intrapulmonary shunt
   Qs/Qt > 20%
   a/A ratio < 25%
   Pao_2/Fio_2 ratio < 200
   A-a gradient > 350 on 100% oxygen

primary problem usually acting as the major cause of death.

Clinical Presentation. ARDS presents with symptoms similar to those of oxygenation-induced respiratory failure (Table 12-3). Rapid deterioration of pulmonary function is a hallmark of ARDS. The chest X ray can change within a hour from relatively normal to a "white-out," reflecting large accumulation of lung water in a short period of time. Hemodynamic parameters are used to differentiate ARDS from pulmonary edema due to left ventricular failure. The pulmonary capillary wedge pressure (PCWP) is generally less than 18 mm Hg in ARDS. Left ventricular failure presents with a high PCWP.

Treatment. Treatment of ARDS is supportive, primarily centering on supporting oxygenation through use of high oxygen concentrations, positive end expiratory pressure (PEEP), continuous positive airway pressure (CPAP), or inverse ratio ventilation (IRV). Fluid administration is kept to a minimum, allowing for a PCWP as low as possible to avoid further increases in lung water. Some centers have advocated the use of extracorporeal membrane oxygenation (ECMO) as a therapy for ARDS. ECMO therapy is not yet widely used in the treatment of ARDS.

Other Forms of Oxygenation-Induced Respiratory Failure

Oxygenation-induced respiratory failure can result from conditions other than ARDS. Chronic lung disease complicated by a pneumonia is a common form of respiratory failure. Left ventricular failure producing pulmonary edema, head injuries producing noncar-

diogenic pulmonary edema, inhalation injuries, and sepsis can all produce respiratory failure of the oxygenation type. Supportive treatment is the same for all of these conditions. Oxygen therapy, PEEP, and mechanical ventilation are included in the treatment plan. Curative therapy is determined by the origin of the problem. For example, left ventricular failure producing pulmonary edema focuses on resolving the cardiac dysfunction. In a pulmonary infection, antibiotic support is indicated.

OXYGENATION SUPPORT

Oxygen Therapy

Oxygen therapy is one of the most common support measures in critical care. Oxygen therapy is not curative and is used to support oxygen transport until curative measures can be applied.

    There are two methods of delivering oxygen therapy, low- and high-flow systems. Low-flow systems do not meet all inspiratory volume needs, requiring patients to entrain room air to meet their inspiratory needs. Examples of low-flow oxygen systems are listed in Table 12-4. The advantage of a low-flow oxygen system is the ease of use. The problem with a low-flow system is that the Fio_2 fluctuates with varying depths of inspiration. A shallow breath will have a higher Fio_2 than a deep breath, even though the liter flow is the same. A shallow breath has a higher Fio_2 level because less room air is entrained during inspiration. Low-flow systems cannot provide high Fio_2 levels. The nasal cannula can provide between 40 and 60% Fio_2 at a liter flow of 6 LPM. Rebreathing masks can provide higher levels of inspired oxygen but are not as reliable as high-flow systems.

TABLE 12-4. EXAMPLES OF LOW- AND HIGH-FLOW OXYGEN THERAPY

Low flow
   Nasal cannula
   Nasal catheter
   Simple face masks
   Rebreather masks
   Nonrebreather masks
High flow
   Venturi masks
   Nebulizer-regulated Fio_2 systems
   Ventilator circuits

Low-flow oxygen systems are useful in the less acutely ill patient and with mouth-breathing patients. The oral inspiration of air draws nasal gases simultaneously into the lungs, allowing for effective oxygen therapy.

High-flow oxygen systems meet all inspiratory volume and flow requirements independent of inspiratory changes. Examples of high-flow systems are given in Table 12-4. High-flow systems are more difficult to apply, requiring face masks or ventilator circuits. High-flow oxygen systems provide stable FIO_2 levels. With a high-flow oxygen system, high oxygen concentrations are possible with FIO_2 levels of from 24 to 100%. Critically ill patients with oxygenation disturbances will almost always use high-flow oxygen systems.

Oxygen Toxicity. Oxygen therapy is not without risk. When oxygen concentrations in excess of 50% are inspired for more than 24 hours, lung damage can occur. Alveolar Type II cells, responsible for producing surfactant, are impaired by high oxygen levels. The potential result is worsening oxygenation due to atelectasis from surfactant loss.

Reabsorption Atelectasis. One of the factors promoting alveolar expansion is the presence of nitrogen, the dominant gas in the atmosphere and alveoli, making up approximately 79% of the barometric pressure. When 100% oxygen therapy is employed, nitrogen is completely displaced or washed out by oxygen. If perfusion exceeds ventilation, such as in oxygenation problems, all oxygen can be absorbed from the alveoli, resulting in alveolar collapse. As long as oxygen therapy generates a PaO_2 level greater than 60 mm Hg or an SaO_2 level greater than 0.90, no further increases in oxygen therapy should be instituted.

Positive End Expiratory Pressure and Continuous Positive Airway Pressure. PEEP and CPAP are therapies used to treat oxygenation problems. PEEP is the application of a positive airway pressure at end exhalation while the patient is on mechanical ventilation. CPAP is positive airway pressure above atmospheric levels applied throughout the respiratory cycle for spontaneous breaths.

PEEP is effective in raising PaO_2 and SaO_2 levels by maintaining alveolar air flow during expiration. Airways have a tendency to collapse during expiration due to increasing pressures outside the airway. PEEP and CPAP stabilize the airways during the expiratory phase. The functional residual capacity (FRC) is the key capacity to improve when trying to change gas tensions. PaO_2 values can be increased if the FRC can be increased and prolong the time for gas exchange to occur. The actions of PEEP and CPAP are to increase FRC, improve distribution of ventilation, recruit alveoli, and open smaller airways, thereby improving oxygenation.

Some clinicians believe in "physiologic PEEP," a concept that assumes that some PEEP is present in all people due to resistance of the airways. Physicians may order low levels of PEEP, such as 3 to 5 cm H_2O, even in patients without oxygenation problems, in order to simulate physiologic PEEP.

"Auto-PEEP" is a term used when describing the trapping of air that may occur during rapid breathing. Auto-PEEP is the result of airway closure or insufficient exhalation time, resulting in the trapping of positive pressure in the airways. The effect of auto-PEEP is the same as the effect of PEEP. However, auto-PEEP is usually inadvertent and is not normally a part of the plan of care. Auto-PEEP is usually measured by obstructing the exhalation port of a ventilator immediately prior to an inspiratory effort.

Indications for PEEP and CPAP. PEEP or CPAP is indicated to help reduce FIO_2 levels or to elevate PaO_2/SaO_2 values when high FIO_2 levels are unsuccessful. PEEP has been advocated for other reasons, such as driving lung water back into the vascular system or reducing mediastinal bleeding postoperatively. Use for these purposes has not been well substantiated in research.

The optimal PEEP level is the lowest level of PEEP needed to raise the PaO_2/SaO_2 levels without producing serious complications. The optimal PEEP level varies from patient to patient, although levels of PEEP higher than 20 cm H_2O are uncommon. PEEP values between 9 and 15 cm of H_2O are common in support of the patient with oxygenation problems.

Complications of PEEP and CPAP. PEEP and CPAP have potential side effects related to the increased airway pressures. The most obvious side effect is barotrauma and pneumothorax. The nurse should be aware to check breath sounds, monitor peak airway pressures, and percuss the thorax to check for potential pneumothorax development. A less obvious but just as serious problem is the loss of cardiac output and stroke volume. Cardiac outputs can fall due to the increased intrathoracic pressure with PEEP and CPAP. The increased pressures impede venous blood return and produce a pseudohypovolemia. When PEEP or CPAP is applied, monitor the cardiac output carefully. If no cardiac outputs are available, the heart rate and systolic blood pressure are monitored. Increases in the heart rate and decreases in systolic blood pressure may signal a reduction in cardiac output and stroke volume.

Other Forms of Oxygenation Support.
Therapies slightly different from PEEP and CPAP have been proposed to attempt to improve arterial oxygen levels. One such therapy is airway pressure release ventilation (APRV). In this therapy, the patient is not intubated but uses a tightly fitting face mask. However, positive pressure is applied throughout the respiratory cycle with short periods of airway pressure release. The release of pressure is designed to improve the elimination of carbon dioxide. APRV is not widely used at this time but has potential for avoiding intubation if applied to an alert, cooperative patient.

Inverse Ratio Ventilation.
In severe, refractory hypoxemia, a more aggressive form of oxygenation support may be required. One of the most aggressive forms of support is inverse ratio ventilation. The patient must be intubated for this therapy. In inverse ratio ventilation, the inspiratory time from the ventilator is prolonged until it equals or exceeds expiratory time (the opposite of normal). The primary advantage of inverse ratio ventilation is an elevation of mean airway pressure. The elevation of mean airway pressure causes an opening of airways and a subsequent elevation of the Pao_2 and Sao_2. Inverse ratio ventilation is usually given via a pressure-controlled mode of ventilation in an attempt to reduce high airway pressures. The term used to describe pressure-controlled inverse ration ventilation is PC-IRV.

When inverse ratio ventilation is used several nursing considerations are essential. First, the patient is usually sedated and paralyzed in order to decrease resistance to the ventilation and to reduce oxygen consumption. The patient and family must be advised as to what is involved with sedation and paralyzation therapy. Second, the risk of barotrauma is increased with inverse ratio ventilation. Both a reduction in cardiac output and increased risk of lung injury (including pneumothorax) are present and should be monitored.

Mechanical Ventilation
Mechanical ventilation is indicated for one of three reasons. The most common is to improve or support alveolar ventilation. Improving V_A is most obvious

when $Paco_2$ levels are decreasing along with a rising pH. A second reason is to reduce the work of breathing. Reducing the work of breathing may be necessary when respiratory rates are in excess of 30 breaths per minute. A third reason is to aid in supporting oxygenation, either directly or indirectly through the use of PEEP. All modes of mechanical ventilation are designed to support one of these three functions.

Methods of Delivering Volumes. Mechanical ventilation is delivered by either negative or positive pressure. Negative-pressure ventilators are devices such as the iron lung and thoracic cuirass. Neither of these devices is common in the support of acute respiratory failure. Positive-pressure ventilators force air into the lungs, reversing normal breathing pressures but successfully supplying alveolar ventilation support. A complication of positive-pressure ventilation is pulmonary barotrauma. The nurse should check the peak airway pressure manometer on the ventilator to assess excessive airway pressures. High peak airway pressures can be monitored through dynamic compliance by dividing peak airway pressure into the tidal volume. Normal dynamic compliance is 40 to 55 cm/mL. Values less than 30 cm/mL place the patient at increased risk for barotrauma.

Modes of Ventilation. Ventilator breaths can be delivered by several modes. The most common modes are assisted mandatory ventilation (AMV or assist/control), intermittent mandatory ventilation (IMV), and pressure support ventilation (PSV). Each type has specific advantages and limitations. Tidal volumes on all modes are generally set initially at 10 to 15 mL/kg, with the respiratory rate between 10 and 20 beats per minute. Respiratory rates and tidal volumes are manipulated to achieve specific end points presented under each mode of ventilation. No one mode of ventilation is best. The proper mode depends on which end point is desired. Properly set, AMV and IMV can be used almost interchangeably. PSV generally is not used in acute respiratory failure but rather is used for weaning patients from mechanical ventilation.

Assisted Mandatory Ventilation. AMV delivers constant preset tidal volumes. The patient will receive a minimum number of breaths as determined by the preset respiratory rate. The patient can initiate more breaths by attempting to breathe spontaneously. The patient-initiated breaths will be delivered to the patient at the preset tidal volume. The patient can alter the respiratory rate but not the tidal volume. AMV's advantage is a reduction in the work of breathing. If the goal or end point in therapy is to reduce the work of breathing, AMV is the most appropriate mode of ventilation. AMV can be used in weaning from mechanical ventilation by incorporating spontaneous breathing (T-piece) trials. In T-piece trials, the patient is removed from the ventilator for progressively increasing periods of time. If the patient can successfully breathe for about one hour, extubation is more likely to be successful. The time off the ventilator before extubating is controversial and variable, being dependent on other factors such as respiratory muscle strength, nutrition, and gas exchange.

Intermittent Mandatory Ventilation (IMV). IMV delivers a preset respiratory rate and tidal volume but allows the patient to breathe spontaneously between the preset tidal volume and rate. IMV was developed to prevent respiratory muscle atrophy and aid in the weaning from mechanical ventilation. Although much has been written about the application of IMV, it can be used both as a weaning tool and as a primary method of delivering mechanical ventilation. If IMV is used as a weaning tool, the IMV rate is reduced slowly (e.g., one to two breaths) until the patient is weaned or shows signs of failure to breathe successfully (Table 12-5). The rate of reducing the IMV rate varies from hours to days, depending on the patient tolerance of the rate reduction.

Pressure Support Ventilation. PSV differs from IMV and AMV in that the delivered ventilation is regulated by pressure rather than volume. During PSV, the patient initiates a breath. During the inspiratory cycle, positive pressure is delivered to the patient, assisting the inspiration. When the patient ceases to inspire, the pressure support drops to zero. The goal of pressure support is to provide enough pressure to achieve a tidal

volume of 10 to 15 mL/kg. If high PSV levels are necessary, more than 30 cm H_2O, IMV, or AMV may be used to provide a backup of consistent tidal volumes. PSV is valuable as an adjunct to overcoming endotracheal tube resistance and weaning from mechanical ventilation. PSV is used in weaning by slowly reducing PSV levels (e.g., 1 to 3 cm H_2O) until levels of 3 to 5 cm are reached. The key is patient tolerance of the rate reduction.

Weaning from Mechanical Ventilation. Weaning from mechanical ventilation can occur when the problem causing the need for intubation and ventilation has been corrected. Assessment of spontaneous breathing abilities can be checked by measuring weaning parameters (Table 12-6). Achievement of successful weaning parameters means that the patient has a good chance of weaning safely. Good weaning parameters do not, however, guarantee success in extubation. Adequate weaning parameters are a minimum starting point in deciding when to begin weaning.

Artificial Airways

In order to use a ventilator, the patient must have an artificial airway such as an endotracheal tube or a tracheostomy tube.

TABLE 12-5. SIGNS OF FAILURE OF SPONTANEOUS BREATHING

Respiratory rate	>35 bpm
Tidal volume	<2 cc/kg
Minute ventilation	<5 or >12 LPM
$Paco_2$	Increasing by more than 10 mm Hg from baseline
pH	< 7.30 with a rising $Paco_2$
BP	Increase in systolic of 20 mm Hg
HR	Increase of >20 bpm over resting heart rate

TABLE 12-6. PARAMETERS FOR WEANING FROM MECHANICAL VENTILATION

Muscle efficiency	
V_T	4–5 cc/kg
$\dot{V}_E$	5–10 LPM
VC	>10 cc/kg
RR	<30 bpm
NIF/PIP	>−20 cm H_2O
Oxygenation	
Pao_2	>60 mm Hg on Fio_2 < 0.40
Hgb	>10 g/dL
CI	>2.5 LPM
a/A	>30%
Carbon dioxide elimination	
$Paco_2$	35–45 mm Hg or at the patient's baseline level to maintain pH between 7.35 and 7.45
V_D/V_T	<60%

V_T = tidal volume; $\dot{V}_E$ = minute ventilation; VC = vital capacity; RR = respiratory rate; PIP = peak inspiratory pressure, also called negative inspiratory pressure, also called negative inspiratory force (NIF); Hgb = hemoglobin; CI = cardiac index; a/A = arterial/alveolar ratio; V_D/V_T = deadspace/tidal volume ratio.

Endotracheal Tubes. Endotracheal tubes may be inserted nasally or orally. Only trained and experienced persons should intubate a patient. Immediately after intubation, auscultation of peripheral chest fields is essential to ascertain that both lungs are being ventilated. Chest x- ray is important to determine that the tip of the endotracheal tube is about 1 inch or 2 to 3 cm above the carina.

The advantage of nasotracheal intubation is that it allows the patient to eat and drink, and mouth care is simplified. Disadvantages are the possibility of tissue necrosis, nosebleed, rupture of nasal polyps, and submucosal dissection. Increased mucus production as a result of the irritant properties of the tube increases the patient's susceptibility to infection. Stabilization of the tube is difficult if the patient is diaphoretic.

The advantages of orotracheal intubation are direct visualization and rapid intubation. Some feel that orotracheal tubes are easier to stabilize than nasotracheal tubes. Oral tubes should be moved to the opposite side of the mouth at least every 24 hours or when the tape becomes soiled. Precautions relating to nasal intubation apply also to oral intubation. Disadvantages of oral intubation include increased drying of oral mucosa, increased mucus production, increased gagging, and increased susceptibility to infection. Complications of intubation are laryngeal trauma, intubation of the right main-stem bronchus, and infection.

Suctioning the Patient with Artificial Airway. Maintaining patency of the airway can be facilitated through suctioning. Hyperoxygenation and ventilation of the patient prior to suctioning may reduce hypoxemia accompanying suctioning. Suction pressures of less than 200 mm Hg are generally adequate to remove secretions. Removing viscous, thick secretions is difficult, however, even with adequate suction. Adding saline in an attempt to reduce viscosity has not demonstrated consistent improvement in secretion removal.

Cuffs of Endotracheal Tubes. Most endotracheal tubes have inflatable cuffs. The cuff provides a closed system with a seal and prevents aspiration of fluids into the lungs. Soft, low-pressure (<25 cm water pressure, 20 mm Hg pressure) cuffs are preferred. Cuff leaks are associated with increased mortality. Soft cuffs minimize tracheal necrosis and fistula development. Pressure is distributed over a large area, and only pressure sufficient to provide a seal is necessary.

Policies vary from hospital to hospital regarding the deflation of cuffs. Precautions to prevent aspiration are necessary when the cuff is deflated. Cuff pressure should be checked every four to eight hours, regardless of policies on inflation-deflation and minimal leak procedure.

Tracheostomy

Tracheostomy, the formation of an opening into the trachea, may be performed if ventilatory support may be long term. Tracheostomies bypass upper airway obstruction, decrease dead space, may help prevent aspiration, and may decrease the possibilities of necrosis and/or tracheoesophageal (TE) fistula formation. A sterile tracheostomy tube of the same size as that in the patient should be taped to the head of the bed for as long as the patient is dependent upon a tracheostomy. When changing the tracheostomy tube, be sure to have a tube one size smaller in case difficulty arises during the insertion. An endotracheal tube of the same or smaller size is also acceptable for maintaining the airway in an emergency.

Complications of Endotracheal Tubes and Tracheostomies

The major complication of cuffed tubes is obstruction caused by dried secretions. The patient appears to be in acute respiratory distress. Mucus production is increased by the foreign body. Endotracheal tubes become displaced rather easily, leading to carinal rupture, ventilation of only one lung, tension pneumothorax, and atelectasis. Signs of tube misplacement into a bronchus include diminished or absent lung sounds on the contralateral side, little if any chest excursion on the contralateral side, expiratory wheezing, and sometimes uncontrollable coughing. Pneumothorax may occur in the lung that has become intubated. This is one of the most serious complications of ventilatory support. The only treatment is a chest tube to bleed out the air of the pneumothorax. Without adequate treatment, pneumothorax can be rapidly fatal.

If a tracheostomy tube fluctuates with the patient's pulse, suspect that the tube is rubbing against the innominate artery and notify the physician immediately. Erosion of the artery usually results in exsanguination. A tracheostomy tube may become misplaced, causing subcutaneous and/or mediastinal emphysema or pneumothorax. Progressively deteriorating blood gases, poor air movement throughout lung fields, or difficulty in suctioning the patient should alert one to a possible shift in the tracheostomy tube.

Tracheal dilatation, ischemia, and necrosis may occur because tracheostomy tubes and endotracheal tubes are round, whereas the trachea is oval. If ischemia and necrosis progress, a TE fistula may occur. Whether a TE fistula has occurred can be easily tested by instilling methylene blue or cranberry juice into the mouth. If it is suctioned from the endotracheal tube or tracheostomy, a TE fistula may have developed. This risk may be minimized by the use of low-pressure cuffs.

The longer an endotracheal tube or tracheostomy tube is in place, the greater the danger of infection. Sputum cultures may be routine with fever. As soon as the infecting microorganisms is identified, appropriate antibiotic therapy is started. Proper, frequent, and correct oral hygiene is of paramount importance, both for the patient's comfort and as an aid to prevention of infection.

Complications of Ventilator Support

Hypotension may occur secondary to decreased cardiac output when a patient is put on a ventilator or when ventilator adjustments are increased. All positive-pressure ventilators exert a continuous positive pressure that decreases venous return to the heart, decreasing cardiac output. The decreased cardiac output may result in a decreased urine output and cardiac dysrhythmias. Cardiac monitoring is essential. Hypotension may be caused by hypovolemia, and intravenous fluids may correct the problem. Vasopressors are indicated if the PCWP is increased and the cardiac output is decreased.

Infection is a most common complication of mechanical ventilation. Strict adherence to sterile technique, ventilator tubing changes every 48 hours, and sputum culture will help to prevent and detect infection. As soon as a culture identifies an infecting organism, specific antibiotic therapy is started. Broad-spectrum antibiotics are not used prophylactically, since many organisms are resistant to them. The excessive use of broad-spectrum antibiotics may allow opportunistic organisms to invade the patient's system. Aggressive pulmonary hygiene procedures are vital nursing interventions in preventing infection.

Atelectasis often occurs with mechanical ventilation. The use of the sigh control to administer deep inspirations up to one and one-half to two times the normal tidal volume may help to open alveoli. Bronchial hygiene is extremely important to prevent further complications once atelectasis has developed. Atelectasis leads to alveolar hypoventilation, the most common medical complication associated with increased mortality.

Pneumothorax is not unusual when PEEP is used with mechanical ventilation. Treatment is insertion of a chest tube. Without adequate treatment, pneumothorax can be rapidly fatal.

Emotional Support

Patients requiring intubation and mechanical ventilation need emotional support from the nurse. The patient needs to be assured that the inability to talk is temporary and related to the intubation. Explain to the patient and family the purpose of the ventilator and the alarms that assist the nurse and respiratory therapist in providing care for the patient. Be sure to establish a method of communication for the patient. The use of nods, blinks, and an alphabet or letter board is helpful. When the patient and family understand the purpose for the interventions and are offered a method to cope with the changes, the experience on the ventilator can be less stressful.

Chronic Obstructive Pulmonary Disease and Status Asthmaticus

Editor's Note

The CCRN exam is likely to address how chronic lung disease might affect an admission to the unit or complicate an acute respiratory event. To understand how chronic lung disease may be presented on the CCRN exam, it is important to understand the basics of obstructive lung disease (chronic bronchitis, emphysema, and asthma). This chapter should provide you with the information necessary to understand the types of concepts presented on the CCRN exam.

CHRONIC OBSTRUCTIVE PULMONARY DISEASE

Chronic obstructive pulmonary disease (COPD) is characterized by airway obstruction and decreased expiratory flow. Asthma, bronchitis, and emphysema are the three major obstructive diseases. The two reversible components in COPD are airway size and the expiratory flow rates through the use of bronchodilators and aggressive pulmonary hygiene measures.

Etiology

There are five major causes of COPD:

1. Cigarette smoking. Cigarette smoking, the leading cause effectively (1) stops ciliary action so the lungs cannot clear themselves, (2) prevents surfactant production, which results in areas of microatelectasis, and (3) increases the production of digestive substances, with resulting loss of elasticity and eventual breakdown in the alveolar capillary wall.
2. Pollution. Auto exhausts are the worst pollu-

tants because of insufficient combustion of sulfur and nitrates. Smog, regardless of its cause, may increase bronchospasm.
3. Pesticides. Exposure results in actual destruction of pulmonary tissue; however, one needs a fairly heavy, long-term exposure.
4. Industrial exposure. Prolonged exposure to inhalants results in permanent damage to the lung. Cotton dust eventually causes brown lung, and coal dust causes black lung.
5. Hereditary factors such as α_1-antitrypsin deficiencies. Trypsin is a proteolytic enzyme that dissolves small thrombi and microaggregates. If trypsin increases sufficiently, it will actually dissolve blood vessel walls, the alveolar membrane, and cell walls. Antitrypsin controls the body's trypsin level. About 0.1% of the population has no α-antitrypsin factor. There are two types of α-antitrypsin deficiencies. Type one includes the homozygous deficiencies. Homozygous-deficient people have less than 10% of the normal α_1-antitrypsin level. These people develop COPD in the early twenties, are very sick in the mid-thirties, and die by the mid-forties. Type two includes the heterozygous deficiencies. Heterozygous-deficient people have less than 60% of the normal α_1-antitrypsin level and may be the group with a propensity for COPD.

Diagnosis

A patient's history of exertional dyspnea, smoking, frequent upper respiratory infections, chronic productive cough, and a family history of COPD are very suggestive of the diagnosis of COPD. Upon physical examination, decreased chest excursion, adventitious lung sounds, cyanosis, jugular venous distension, and symptoms of cor pulmonale may be present. The chest x-ray is of little value in diagnosing COPD; however, if it is hyperlucent and the diaphragm is depressed, COPD is suggested. Patients with COPD often have polycythemia. The bone marrow produces more red blood cells to carry oxygen in an oxygen-deprived body. Sputum cultures are of value to determine secondary bacterial infection. *Streptococcus pneumoniae* and *Haemophilus influenzae* are the microorganisms most often found outside the hospital. Nosocomial infections can present with many more resistant infectious agents.

Obstructive Disease

Asthma. Asthma is defined as an increased airway responsiveness to internal or external stimuli. The increased responsiveness is manifested by narrowing of airways secondary to bronchial constriction and excessive mucous obstruction. The increased mucus production and bronchial constriction increase the work of breathing and interfere with gas exchange, most notably producing hypoxemia. Air trapping with resulting hyperinflation of the lungs is a common clinical feature in acute asthmatic episodes. Asthma is a condition of recurrent episodes of bronchospasm manifested by symptoms of dyspnea, wheezing, and a sensation of chest tightness. Between periods of bronchospasm, pulmonary function is normal or near normal. Asthma is classified as mild, moderate, or severe (Table 13-1).

Asthma is a disease characterized by airway hyperreactivity or hyperresponsiveness, airway obstruction, and airway inflammation. Asthma can result as a reaction to an allergen or to a nonallergen, such as exercise. It can be precipitated by irritants such as cold air, odors, chemicals, or changes in the weather.

When an antigen to which the patient is sensitive is inhaled, a pattern of airway obstruction occurs. This airway obstruction results within 15 to 20 minutes and is manifested by bronchospasm caused by smooth muscle contraction. Following the immediate response, there is a late-phase response of airway obstruction that develops four to six hours after exposure to the antigen presenting as airway edema, inflammation, and mucous plugging (Fig. 13-1). This results in dyspnea and inspiratory and expiratory wheezing. The expiratory phase is prolonged as the patient tries to exhale the trapped air through narrow airways.

Initial arterial blood gases for an asthmatic patient may appear to be normal or reflect respiratory alkalosis as the patient increases the respiratory rate. The most critical time is when the $PaCO_2$ begins to rise and the pH begins to fall. This indicates that the work of breathing has become too great and the patient is tiring. At this point, the decision to provide respiratory support through intubation and mechanical ventilation may be considered.

Status Asthmaticus. This is a severe continuing attack of asthma that fails to respond to conventional drugs. Initially, the same pathologic changes as occur

TABLE 13-1. CLASSIFICATION OF ASTHMA

	Mild	Moderate	Severe
Symptoms	Cough and/or chest tightness 1–2 times/week	Cough, wheeze, and/or chest tightness on most days Significant exacerbations 1–2 times/year Nocturnal symptoms 2–3 times/week	Significant daily symptoms Frequent exacerbations, >2 hospitalizations
Physical activity	Normal between episodes	Mild to moderate reduction	Major limitation
Peak expiratory flows	80% or greater than predicted	60–80% of predicted 20% variability from a.m. to p.m.	<60% of predicted 30% variability from a.m. to p.m.
Treatment	Inhaled beta agonists prn	Beta agonist, inhaled corticosteroids	Beta agonist, inhaled and systemic corticosteroids

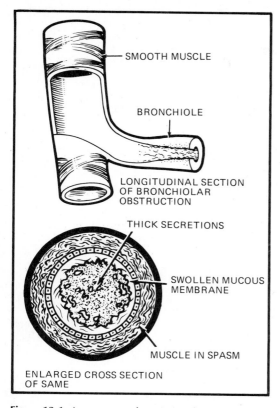

SMOOTH MUSCLE

BRONCHIOLE

LONGITUDINAL SECTION
OF BRONCHIOLAR
OBSTRUCTION

THICK SECRETIONS

SWOLLEN MUCOUS
MEMBRANE

MUSCLE IN SPASM

ENLARGED CROSS SECTION
OF SAME

Figure 13-1. Appearance of respiratory bronchioles in asthma (bronchiole obstruction on expiration by muscle spasm, swelling of mucosa, and thick secretions).

in asthma occur in status asthmaticus. However, as the attack continues unabated, the bronchial walls hypertrophy and secretion clearance is diminished, causing a bronchiolar obstruction. This obstruction reduces alveolar ventilation and results in hyperinflation of alveoli.

The three most common causes of status asthmaticus are (1) exposure to allergens, (2) noncompliance with the medication regimen, and (3) respiratory infections. Environments that become unusually hot, cold, or dusty often trigger status asthmaticus because of the effect of inspired air on the lungs.

Patients in status asthmaticus are physically exhausted from the work of breathing. They are extremely dyspneic. Their respiratory pattern is hyperpneic, which may result in the development of a dehydrated state. Inspiratory and expiratory wheezing is present, with a prolonged expiratory phase.

Diagnosis. All of the symptoms of asthma may be present. In addition, the history may reveal noncompliance with the medical regimen. Symptoms of upper respiratory infection may be present. Dyspnea, cough, wheezing, and an inability to sleep are common complaints.

Physical examination revealing tachypnea, tachycardia, use of accessory respiratory muscles, dyspnea, pallor, cyanosis, and abnormal breath sounds will help confirm status asthmaticus. The disappearance of wheezing may not be a good sign. If the wheeze disappears, the airway may have become completely obstructed rather than opened.

Arterial blood gases usually reveal a decreased Pao_2 and an increased $Paco_2$ with respiratory failure. If the status asthmaticus has reached this point, the patient is critically ill and may require respirator assistance. Chest X ray will probably not be helpful. It may be normal or translucent.

Nursing Intervention. The nursing interventions for status asthmaticus are the same as those for COPD. The objective is to support ventilation and respirations to prevent respiratory failure and pneumothorax. Because of the extreme life-threatening aspects of status asthmaticus, treatment with continuous intravenous theophyllines, usually aminophylline, in addition to aggressive respiratory therapies is usually instituted.

Bronchodilators, antibiotics, oxygen therapy, physical therapy, hydration, nourishment, corticosteroid use, exercise, psychotherapy, and patient and family education were discussed earlier in this chapter in the section on COPD and are applicable to status asthmaticus. Mechanical ventilation may be necessary to support respiration while these therapies take effect.

Bronchitis. Bronchitis is diagnosed by sputum production, cough, and wheezing. Chronic bronchitis is an inflammation of the tracheobronchial tree characterized by fibrotic and atopic changes in the bronchial mucosa.

Chronic bronchitis is accompanied by right heart failure, pulmonary hypertension, hypoxemia, and compensated hypercarbia (elevated $Paco_2$ with normal pH). Symptoms are a result of low V/Q ratios, the result of reduced ventilation from excessive secretions, ineffective secretion removal, and bronchoconstriction. The low V/Q ratio produces regional vasoconstriction in an attempt to shunt blood away from the low-ventilation areas. The vasoconstriction produces pulmonary hypertension, eventually causing right ventricular failure. The hypoxemia and hypercarbia are a result of chronic V/Q imbalances.

Bronchitis is an inflammation usually caused by an infectious agent, such as *Haemophilus influenzae* or pneumococcus, that penetrates the bronchial wall. The inflammatory response results in hypertrophy and hyperplasia of the bronchial glands and goblet cells, producing an overabundance of mucus. With repeated attacks of bronchitis, metaplasia of bronchial and bronchiolar epithelium eventually occurs, resulting in a loss of cilia and excessive mucus production. Frequent attacks cause distortion and scarring of the bronchial wall, decreasing the size of the airway lumen (Fig. 13-2). The excessive mucus production in the bronchi causes the chronic or recurrent productive cough. Since the airway lumen is decreased, some secretions are trapped in the alveoli and smaller air passages.

Emphysema. Emphysema is actual destruction of pulmonary tissue by the breakdown of the alveolar wall. Lungs become hyperinflated due to decreased elasticity. The main symptom is an increase in the work of breathing. In eupnea (normal breathing), 63% of the work of breathing is in overcoming the elastic resistance of the lungs and chest wall. This is greatly increased in emphysema. Emphysematous patients generally have normal blood gases, although pulmon-

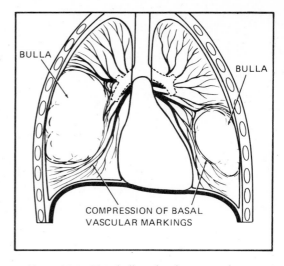

Figure 13-3. Giant bullae of end-stage emphysema.

ary hypertension may exist. Emphysema and bronchitis occur together 85% of the time.

Emphysema is an enlargement of the air spaces distal to the terminal nonrespiratory bronchiole, with destruction of alveolar walls. There are usually blebs and bullae in the lungs (Fig. 13-3). A bleb is an air-filled space in the visceral pleura. Bullae are air-filled spaces in the parenchyma greater than 1 cm in diameter. This results in overinflation of alveoli and loss of the elastic recoil property of the lung. Table 13-2 is a comparison of the major symptoms of bronchitis and emphysema.

Complications

COPD is a progressive disease. The rate of progression may be controlled, but COPD cannot be cured. The most common complications are pneumonia, respiratory failure, spontaneous pneumothorax, cor pulmonale, pulmonary embolism, and peptic ulcer with or without hemorrhage. The use of sedative and tranquilizers is avoided in patients with COPD. The respiratory centers are relatively insensitive to oxygen stimuli. If the patient is chronically hypoxic and is given oxygen in high concentrations, the patient may decrease ventilation and suffer a respiratory arrest.

Nursing Intervention and Treatment

Bronchodilators are effective in relieving bronchospasm associated with asthma and bronchitis. Among the compounds that can be used are alpha-beta stimula-

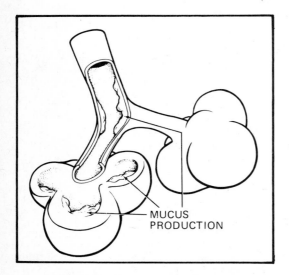

Figure 13-2. Airway lumen in bronchitis.

TABLE 13-2. COMPARISON BETWEEN BRONCHITIS AND EMPHYSEMA

Symptoms	Bronchitis	Emphysema
Cough	4+	No
Shortness of breath (SOB)	2+	4+
CO_2 retention	Due to V/Q disturbance	0 (until end-stage disease)
Arterial hypoxemia	Due to 2+ relative shunt	0 (until end-stage disease)
Weight loss	No	Yes
CHF	Yes	No
Cyanosis	Yes	No
VC	Unchanged	Unchanged
FEV_1	Decreased	Decreased
TLC	Normal	Increased
FRC	Normal or increased	Increased
RV	Normal or increased	Increased
With bronchodilator being given	Improvement	Little improvement measured

tors (epinephrine), beta agnoists (albuterol, meta-proterenol sulfate, terbutaline sulfate, isoproterenol), and methyl xanthine theophyllines (aminophylline). If severe bronchospasm is present, aminophylline may be used as a continuous drip or epinephrine may be given subcutaneously. Use of nebulizing beta stimulators is an effective way to deliver medication directly to the lung. Antibiotics can be given to control infection.

Patient education includes physical therapy, postural drainage, and abdominal breathing exercises to increase vital capacity and decrease functional residual capacity by exhaling with pursed lips.

Hydration is used to keep secretions thin, white and watery. A balanced diet is very important to improve efficiency of the respiratory muscles. Small meals taken six or eight times a day may reduce breathlessness associated with eating.

Systemic corticosteroids are used to reduce the inflammatory reaction in the lung. Inhaled corticosteroids are useful in reducing airway inflammation.

RESTRICTIVE LUNG DISEASE

A restrictive lung disease results in impaired inhalation and restriction of lung expansion such that there is decreased total lung capacity and vital capacity. Restriction may be the result of interstitial lung disease such as pulmonary fibrosis. Interstitial pulmonary fibrosis is a diffuse process resulting in cellular thickening of the alveolar walls and a decrease in lung compliance. Extrapulmonary causes of restrictive lung disease include obesity, pregnancy, and musculoskeletal deformities. Diminished lung compliance results in increased work of breathing.

CHAPTER 14

Pulmonary Embolism and Chest Trauma

Editor's Note

Pulmonary embolism and chest trauma are both likely content areas for questions in the CCRN exam. Pulmonary emboli are best understood when applied to concepts in pulmonary physiology relative to disturbances of ventilation and perfusion (Chapter 11). However, the physical presentation and treatment discussed in this chapter are necessary to remember for purposes of the test. Chest trauma is reviewed in this chapter to provide adequate information about the assessment and treatment of chest injuries. Chest trauma, particularly from an assessment point of view, is also better understood if considered along with concepts in pulmonary physiology. The goal of this chapter is to provide enough information to help you understand how to assess and treat key pulmonary and cardiac injuries but not overwhelm you with unnecessary information.

PULMONARY EMBOLISM

A thrombus, which has developed in the deep veins of the lower extremities, breaks loose from its attachment and travels through the venous circulation into the pulmonary circulation, where it will partially or completely occlude a pulmonary artery. A massive pulmonary embolism is one in which more than 50% of the pulmonary artery bed is occluded.

There are three conditions, referred to as Virchow's triad, that tend to precipitate thrombus formation: damaged endothelium of veins, venous stasis, and hypercoagulability of the blood.

With these three conditions present, a thrombus has a great chance of developing. Natural processes of clot dissolution may cause release of fragments, or external mechanisms such as direct trauma, muscle contraction, or changes in perfusion may contribute to the release of the thrombus. As the thrombus breaks loose, it flows through the venous circulation, entering the right ventricle and then lodging in small pulmonary arteries (Fig. 14-1). Compromise will occur more readily if there is underlying COPD, congestive heart failure, or other chronic conditions.

Pulmonary hypertension is due to pulmonary arterial obstruction. If the obstruction is partial or develops slowly, the patient may survive to be treated. However, if the obstruction is rapid and total, the patient may suffer sudden death. Chronic pulmonary hypertension does not usually occur with a single embolus. It usually results from multiple emboli of middle size vessels.

Etiology

Pulmonary emboli may develop in patients with no predisposing factor. Some predisposing factors include stasis of venous blood due to immobilization, varicose veins, obesity, pregnancy, and congestive heart failure. Aging, vasculitis, and trauma to the vessel wall during

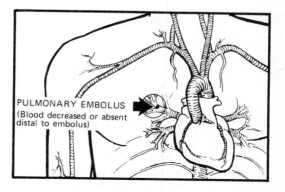

PULMONARY EMBOLUS
(Blood decreased or absent distal to embolus)

Figure 14-1. Pulmonary embolism.

venipuncture or prolonged intravenous therapy, venous wall damage due to soft tissue trauma, fractures, or infiltration by malignant cells may cause thrombi. Hypercoagulability is related to thrombocytosis, increased platelet activity following surgery, trauma, parturition, polycythemia, and hemoconcentration. All of these may be factors, and patients with any of these conditions or diagnoses should be considered at high risk for developing pulmonary emboli. Rare causes of thrombus formation include thrombus formation in the heart secondary to acute myocardial infarction, atrial fibrillation, subacute bacterial endocarditis, and cardioversion.

Clinical Presentation

Increased respiratory rate (due to increased dead space) and tachycardia are the most common signs of pulmonary embolism. The signs and symptoms of pulmonary emboli must be divided into the clinical pictures of a massive embolism and a submassive embolism. Massive embolism occurs suddenly. The patient may have crushing, substernal chest pain and appear to be in shock. The patient may be hypotensive, dyspneic, cyanotic, apprehensive, or comatose. Respirations are rapid, shallow, and gasping. Arterial pulse is rapid, and the volume is diminished. If awake, the patient may express feelings of impending doom.

Submassive embolism may present only fleeting minimal symptoms. If the submassive embolism has occluded a medium-size artery, tachypnea, dyspnea, tachycardia, generalized chest discomfort, and pleuritic-type chest pain may develop within a few hours. Fever, cough, and hemoptysis may occur over several hours (or days). A pleural friction rub and a pleural effusion may develop.

Diagnosis

Routine chest x-ray may be normal or in about 20% of such cases may show some consolidation. ECG may be normal but most often shows sinus tachycardia, or it may show right ventricular strain. Blood chemistries are nonspecific and the arterial blood gases are unreliable indicators of pulmonary embolism. If the PaO_2 is above 80 mm Hg on room air, a pulmonary embolism is less likely, although one may exist and not occlude major arteries.

The most useful tests are nuclear studies and pulmonary angiography. A lung scan that is normal usually rules out a pulmonary embolism. If a lung scan shows perfusion defects on segments that appear normal on chest x-ray, then pulmonary embolism is likely. A lung scan may be abnormal due simply to COPD.

Pulmonary angiography is the most accurate way to diagnose pulmonary embolism. An angiogram is the standard by which other tests are compared. An angiogram should be obtained before surgical therapy is instituted.

Complications

Complications of pulmonary embolism may be pulmonary infarction due to extension of emboli. Any embolus that is large enough to alter hemodynamics can result in complications such as stroke, myocardial infarction, cardiac dysrhythmias that are not amenable to therapy, liver failure and necrosis secondary to congestion, pneumonia, pulmonary abscesses, ARDS, shock and death.

Treatment

Heparin is the immediate drug of choice. Within 30 minutes of a bolus, anticoagulation should be documented. A partial thromboplastin time of 55 to 85 seconds is adequate anticoagulation. Heparin impedes clotting by preventing fibrin formation.

Anticoagulation is continued by a heparin bolus every four to six hours or a continuous intravenous heparin drip. Continuous intravenous heparin is preferred for patients at high risk or with a massive embolus. A continuous infusion maintains a steady therapeutic blood level. In contrast, the heparin bolus every four to six hours causes peak levels for short times and subtherapeutic levels for the remaining time before another bolus is due. Heparin is usually continued for several days or when oral anticoagulation can become effective.

Oral anticoagulants are often started three to four days before the heparin is stopped to avoid a period of no anticoagulant therapy. Oral anticoagulants are usually given for six to eight weeks if the patient is asymptomatic. They may be given indefinitely or for the remainder of the patient's life for multiple reasons.

Streptokinase, urokinase, and tissue plasminogen activation are thrombolytic enzymes being used to dissolve or lyse the emboli. These three thrombolytic agents are administered only by intravenous infusion. Therapeutic action begins immediately and ceases with the interruption of the intravenous administration. However, residual effects may last for as long as 12 to 24 hours.

Surgery is reserved for those patients who do not

respond to anticoagulants, who have rebound effects to heparin, or who have recurrent emboli. Procedures may include ligation or clipping of the inferior vena cava, filter placement in the vena cava, and embolectomy. Embolectomy is a serious operation and is usually reserved for the massive emboli or for the decompensating patient who cannot be stabilized. The vena caval umbrella inserted in the inferior vena cava may filter emboli and eliminate the necessity of major surgery in some patients.

Nursing Intervention

These measures will help prevent emboli in potential patients. Ambulate patients as much as their clinical condition allows. Nonambulating patients may have regular active and passive exercises assisted by the nurse or physical therapist. Elevation of the legs, use of pneumatic devices, and use of an antiembolic hose will help prevent stasis of venous blood. Deep breathing exercises and adequate fluid intake will help to maintain adequate ventilation, circulation, and expectoration of pulmonary secretions. Education of the patient and family about risk factors of embolism development and prevention measurements is important.

CHEST TRAUMA

Chest injuries are common in multiple trauma. The more systems involved in the trauma, the more critical each injury becomes. Chest injuries are especially serious in the elderly, the obese, and patients with cardiac or pulmonary disease. The older the patient, the more likely the presence of underlying health problems, and physiologic reserve is diminished. Statistically, if there is a chest injury alone, there is a 5 to 10% mortality rate. If there is a chest injury and another injury, the mortality rate is 30%. Chest trauma occurs in six out of ten motor vehicle accidents.

Classification

Chest trauma can be classified into one of three categories: closed chest injury, open chest injury, and visceral injury. Any chest injury interrupts the normal thoracic pressures and movements. Treatment of all chest injuries is to reestablish normal and adequate hemodynamic and ventilatory function. The type and location of the trauma determine the presentation, diagnosis, treatment, and complications of chest trauma. Diagnosis and treatment of chest trauma are delayed until it is certain that an adequate and patent airway exists. If the airway is not patent and multiple trauma exists, insertion of a large 14-gauge needle into the cricothyroid membrane will suffice until cervical spine injuries have been ruled out and endotracheal intubation or tracheostomy may be performed. The most common injuries in chest trauma are fractured ribs and pneumothoraces.

Closed Chest Injuries

These are usually the result of a blunt force that does not penetrate the chest wall. Motor vehicle accidents, falls, and violent assaults are the common causes of closed chest injury.

Among the most common closed chest injuries are rib fractures. Symptoms will be pain, dyspnea, ecchymosis, and splinting on movement. It is not common to have a fracture of the first rib. When a very strong force is applied to the upper thoracic cage, the result is a "starburst" fracture, that is, pieces of bone going in all directions. Examination for neck injuries, brachial plexus injury, pneumothorax, aortic rupture or tear, and very often thoracic outlet syndrome is a must. Fracture of the first rib is life threatening and indicates severe underlying thoracic and/or abdominal injuries.

Fracture of the second rib is commonly termed "the hangman's fracture." Ribs 3 to 8 are the most commonly fractured. If a single rib is fractured, pain relief is usually the only treatment necessary. The intact rib on each side of the fractured rib stabilizes the fracture and keeps it in alignment for healing. Fractures of ribs 9 to 12 arouse suspicion of the possibility of laceration and/or rupture of the spleen and liver.

Treatment and Nursing Intervention. The objective is to relieve the pain of fractured ribs without compromising ventilatory efficiency. Intercostal nerve block is most efficient in relieving pain without interfering with coughing, sighing, and deep breathing. Bronchial hygiene and physical therapy are used to prevent development of atelectasis. Binders are not recommended because they decrease excursion over a wide area of the chest, predisposing the patient to hypoxemia and atelectasis.

Flail Chest

A flail chest is two or more adjacent ribs with two or more fractures. The involved portion of the chest wall may be so unstable that it will move paradoxically or opposite the rest of the chest wall when the patient breathes (Fig. 14-2). The flail chest may be especially

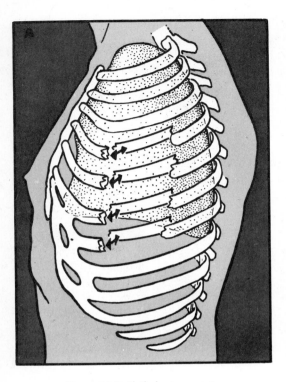

Figure 14-2. Flail chest segment.

severe if it is associated with a transverse fracture of the sternum. Symptoms of flail chest include rapid, shallow respirations, cyanosis, severe chest wall pain, shock, bony crepitation at the site of fracture, and paradoxical chest movement. There may be signs of pulmonary contusion.

Treatment and Nursing Intervention. Specific treatment is to stabilize the flail segment and to restore normal breathing. In an emergency, anything (e.g., sandbags or hands) can be used to stabilize the chest wall and help immobilize the segment. Critical care may include intubation, positive pressure ventilation, and PEEP. The current treatment emphasizes the alleviation of pain as the top priority, even over stabilization measures such as mechanical ventilation.

Fracture of the Sternum
Sternal fracture is suspected when there is paradoxical movement of the anterior chest wall. It may be stabilized with traction or with endotracheal intubation, mechanical ventilation, and PEEP. Sternal fractures may

be associated with myocardial injuries. Cardiac contusion should be ruled out.

Simple Closed Pneumothorax
This can be a result of blunt penetrating trauma resulting in air buildup in the pleural cavity, decreasing vital capacity. The closed pneumothorax is potentially dangerous because air cannot escape the chest. If air continues to enter the pleural space and intrapleural pressure increases, pressure on the other lung and heart will continue. Tension pneumothorax is a possibility.

Diagnosis is by physical exam and chest x-ray. Symptoms include dyspnea and restlessness, cardiac pain radiating throughout the chest, diminished or absent breath sounds on the affected side, decreased chest wall movement, signs of increasing respiratory distress, and tracheal shift toward the unaffected side.

If the patient is symptomatic, a chest tube is inserted in the second or third intercostal space (ICS) at the midclavicular line to drain the air. Chest tubes are sutured in place and connected to an underwater seal. Daily x-rays monitor the reexpansion of the lung. If the pneumothorax is small enough, needle aspiration or thoracentesis may be sufficient treatment.

Tension Pneumothorax
Tension pneumothorax may be caused by blunt trauma tearing the pleura or by iatrogenic causes. This condition is potentially life threatening, since air can accumulate in the pleural space but cannot escape. As the patient inhales, air is sucked into the pleura through the tear. As the patient begins to exhale, the torn pleura is "sucked back" against the parenchyma, creating a one-way valve system that prevents the air from being exhaled (Fig. 14-3). On inspiration, more air is drawn in through the tear. The accumulation of air in the thorax results in severe hemodynamic imbalances.

General symptoms include dyspnea, progressive cyanosis and chest pain. On the affected side, symptoms include diminished or absent breath sounds and hyperresonant percussion sounds. The mediastinum, the trachea, and the point of maximum intensity all shift away from the affected side.

Air under tension in the pleural cavity is immediately removed. A large 14-gauge needle is inserted in the second or third ICS at the midclavicular line and aimed toward the shoulder (Fig. 14-4), or a chest tube is placed. The chest tube is usually connected to a water seal or suction drainage. The insertion site of the tube is covered with a sterile dressing. Once the imme-

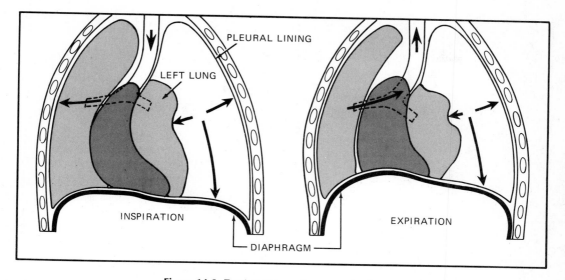

Figure 14-3. Tension pneumothorax mechanics.

diate crisis is over, X rays are used to determine whether the chest tube is properly positioned and whether additional tubes are indicated.

Open Pneumothorax

An open pneumothorax is caused by a penetrating injury that allows air to enter and exit the pleural space. An open pneumothorax is less dangerous than a closed pneumothorax because there is less likelihood of developing a tension pneumothorax. Treatment is the same as for a closed pneumothorax.

Hemothorax

Hemothorax may develop from blunt or penetrating chest trauma or from iatrogenic causes. The two major effects of a hemothorax are the accumulation of blood in the lungs, collapsing alveoli, and systemic hypovolemia.

The symptoms of a hemothorax depend upon the size of the blood accumulation. Small amounts of blood (400 mL or less) will causes minimal symptoms and minimal chest x-ray changes. Larger amounts of blood usually present signs of shock inducing tachycardia, tachypnea, hypotension, and nervousness. Breath sounds may be diminished or absent, and there is dullness to percussion.

Small hemothoraxes may resolve spontaneously because of low pulmonary system pressure and the presence of thromboplastin in the lungs. Large hemo-

thoraxes are treated with the insertion of one or more chest tubes in the fifth or sixth ICS in the midaxillary line (Fig. 14-5). The chest tube is sutured in place and covered with a sterile dressing after connection to an underwater seal with suction. Severe or uncontrollable

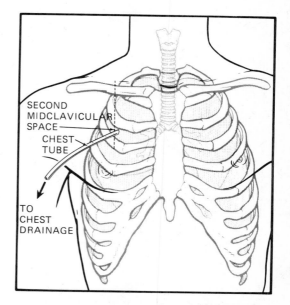

Figure 14-4. Insertion of chest tube for tension pneumothorax.

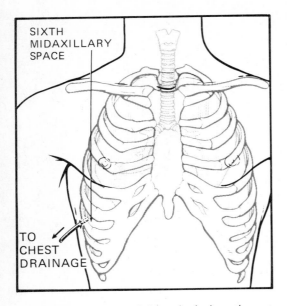

SIXTH
MIDAXILLARY
SPACE

TO
CHEST
DRAINAGE

Figure 14-5. Insertion of chest tube for hemothorax.

hemothoraces may require a thoracotomy to arrest the bleeding.

It is controversial to "milk" chest tubes every hour to prevent occlusion due to the presence of fibrin, since doing so may increase intrathoracic pressures. Monitoring the patient's ability to expel secretions and suc-

tioning when necessary are important in preventing hypoxia and atelectasis. Bronchial hygiene and aggressive chest physical therapy will help avoid infection. Analgesic medications will make these nursing procedures more tolerable for the patient. Sputum cultures should be performed if fever develops. Psychological support of the patient and reassurances that the tubes are only temporary will help decrease the patient's anxiety.

Open Chest Injury

Open Sucking Chest Injuries. These occur as the result of blunt, penetrating, or deceleration forces. As the chest wall is opened, air rushes in and collapses the exposed lung. The mediastinum is pushed toward the opposite lung, preventing it from functioning normally. Unless the condition is rapidly corrected, severe hemodynamic compromise occurs (Fig. 14-6). Immediate treatment consists of covering the wound. Vaseline gauze is the covering of choice. Bear in mind that the patient generally will not have severe symptoms unless the pneumothorax is >20% or preexisting lung disease exists.

The symptoms of open tension pneumothorax are obviously the appearance of the chest wall and the distinctive sound of air being sucked into the chest. The chest wall appears to cave in or to have been pushed in at the injury site. The patient may have

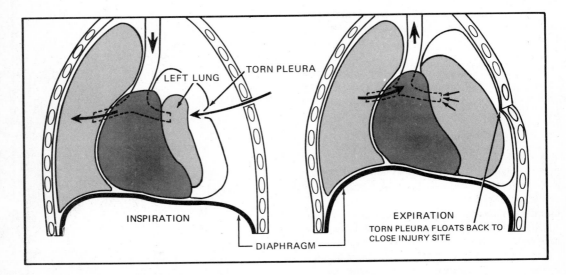

TORN PLEURA

LEFT LUNG

INSPIRATION

DIAPHRAGM

EXPIRATION
TORN PLEURA FLOATS BACK TO
CLOSE INJURY SITE

Figure 14-6. Open tension pneumothorax ("sucking chest wound").

dyspnea, tachycardia, or hypoxia and is usually hyperventilating. Subcutaneous emphysema may be present.

Treatment is to stop the in-rushing air. Chest tubes are inserted to drain the air if the wound is small. If the wound is large, thoracotomy will be required to debride the wound and repair the damage from the injury.

Nursing interventions include close monitoring for signs of increasing respiratory distress, extension of the pneumothorax, and possible cardiac involvement previously undetected. Suctioning may be required to prevent atelectasis and hypoxemia and to decrease the chance of infection from retained secretions. In addition to the pneumothorax, a hemothorax may develop, requiring immediate treatment if the patient is deteriorating or going into shock. Nursing care of the chest tubes and psychological support are the same as for patients with closed pneumothoraces.

Subcutaneous Emphysema

Subcutaneous emphysema occurs when a communication exists between the pleural space and subcutaneous tissue. By itself, it is not dangerous and does not require treatment. The familiar crunching or popping that occurs on palpation is the clue to a diagnosis of subcutaneous emphysema. Finding the cause of the subcutaneous emphysema is the focus of treatment. Subcutaneous emphysema is the clue to bronchial or tracheal injuries. If the major airways are lacerated, death usually results from loss of ventilation.

Visceral Injuries

Pulmonary Contusion. The most common visceral injury is pulmonary contusion. Contusions may occur as the result of blunt chest trauma or penetrating lung trauma. Pulmonary contusion is damage to the lung parenchyma, resulting in localized edema and hemorrhage. Motor vehicle accidents are the most common cause of lung contusion, since the chest hits the steering wheel during an accident, which compresses the lung against the thoracic cage, the sternum, and/or the vertebrae. It is assumed that the pressure of striking the steering wheel compresses the thoracic cage, diminishing its size and compressing the lungs due to the increased intrathoracic pressure. As the pressure from hitting the steering wheel decreases, the thoracic cage increases in size, decreasing the intrathoracic pressure and the pressure on the lung parenchyma. This allows expansion of the lung parenchyma (under pressure), rupturing capillaries and resulting in hemorrhage.

Figure 14-7 shows the mechanics of pulmonary contusion and the consequences.

The diagnosis of pulmonary contusion due to blunt trauma is difficult, since symptoms may not occur for 4 to 72 hours posttrauma. X-rays may be normal or may reveal localized opacification in the injured area. The affected area may be larger than revealed by the chest x-ray.

Depending upon the severity of the trauma, symptoms may include tachypnea, tachycardia, and blood-tinged secretions. Crackles may be heard throughout all lung fields due to retained secretions. Arterial blood gases reveal a decreased $Paco_2$ and Pao_2 and a worsening of the Pao_2/Fio_2 ratio or a/A ratio, indicating increasing Qs/Qt.

Treatment and Nursing Intervention. The objectives of treating lung contusion are a patent airway, adequate oxygenation, and restoration of normal lung function. If the contusion is mild, monitoring and supplemental oxygen by mask may be sufficient. If deterioration occurs with this conservative treatment, many physicians prefer to treat the lung contusion as ARDS to arrest the progressive deterioration.

Controversy exists over the use of steroids and crystalloid (Ringer's lactate) versus colloid (dextran, Plasmanate, etc.) fluid replacement. Since moderate to severe pulmonary contusions are often accompanied by multisystem injuries, the fluid administration must be balanced against hemodynamic and pulmonary function. Nasotracheal suctioning, aggressive chest physiotherapy, and humidification may help the patient expel secretions and allow more accurate assessment of the situation. The onset of agitation and anxiety may indicate the presence of hypoxia and may be a first sign of impending deterioration. A fever may be the first sign of infection.

Pulmonary Laceration. The next most common visceral injury is pulmonary laceration, which results in pneumothorax. If the force of the injury is sufficient to lacerate the lungs, cardiac injury is quite likely to have occurred. Bleeding following pulmonary laceration is a common and potentially dangerous occurrence. Laceration may occur from tearing due to rib fractures or direct puncture. If bleeding is active, a hemopneumothorax may result.

Cardiac Contusion. This is the most common blunt injury to the heart. It is only rarely fatal. Signs and

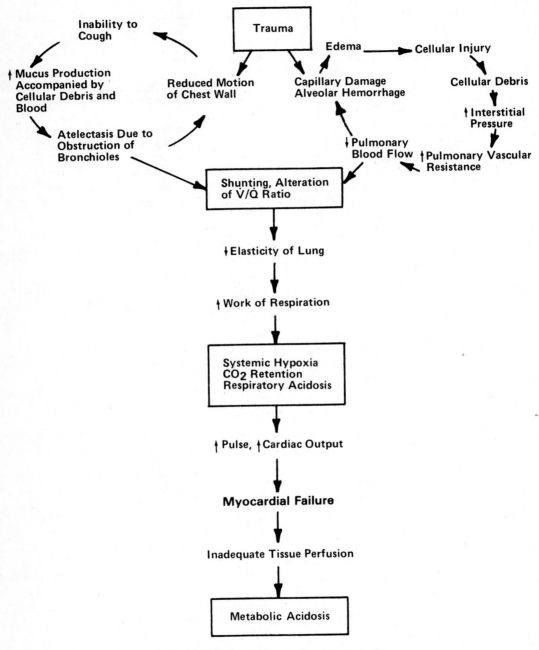

Figure 14-7. Mechanics of pulmonary contusion.

symptoms are the same as for myocardial ischemia and/or infarction. Specific treatment is to monitor cardiac status with daily ECGs, since some ST- and T-wave changes may not become apparent for up to 48 hours, and to treat dysrhythmias as they occur. Isoenzymes, specifically CK-MB band, are perhaps the most accurate indicators of myocardial injury. Severe visceral injury may result in delayed cardiac rupture, ventricular septal defect, and ventricular aneurysm, all of which would receive conventional treatment. Symptoms include angina-like chest pain, unexplained tachycardia, and after some time elapse, a pericardial friction rub.

Cardiac Rupture

This is a blunt trauma injury and is the most common cause of death. In sequence of frequency of rupture, it is right ventricle, left ventricle, right atrium, and left atrium. There is no treatment for cardiac rupture other than surgical intervention.

Valvular Injury

This is a blunt trauma injury. The aortic valve is the most commonly injured valve. Signs and symptoms are valve regurgitation and congestive heart failure. Specific treatment could include valve replacement or the normal medical treatment for congestive heart failure.

Cardiac Tamponade

This may result from blunt or penetrating trauma. Blood gets into the pericardial sac but cannot get out. As more blood enters the sac, more pressure is placed against the heart, decreasing venous return and cardiac output (Fig. 14-8).

Cardiac tamponade presents with hypotension, muffled or distant heart sounds, and distended neck veins. Additional clues are a falling systolic blood pressure, narrow pulse pressure, pulsus paradoxus (more than a 10-degree drop in systolic blood pressure during inspiration and expiration), elevated central venous pressure, and various degrees of shock.

Treatment and Nursing Intervention. The objective of treatment is to confirm the diagnosis and relieve the tamponade. This is best accomplished by a pericardiocentesis. Anesthesia is achieved with xylocaine, and then a 3-inch spinal or cardiac needle is introduced at a 35° angle in the right paraxiphoid space (Fig. 14-9). An ECG lead may be attached to the nee-

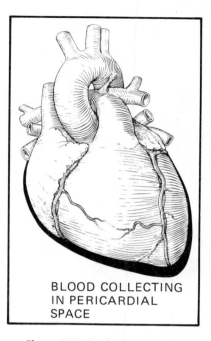

BLOOD COLLECTING
IN PERICARDIAL
SPACE

Figure 14-8. Cardiac tamponade.

dle. This will show by cardiac monitoring if the needle tip enters the myocardium (ST segment elevation). The needle can be withdrawn slightly and the diagnosis confirmed by aspiration of pericardial fluid (pericardiocentesis). This also relieves symptoms if it is a slowly developing tamponade. If pericardiocentesis does not relieve the tamponade, thoracotomy for direct repair of the pericardial wound is indicated.

Nursing interventions include monitoring of the respiratory and cardiovascular systems especially closely for early signs of deterioration, assisting with preparations for the pericardiocentesis and with the procedure itself, providing emotional support for the patient, and continuing close monitoring after the procedure for recurring signs of tamponade.

Diaphragmatic Rupture and/or Herniation

This is associated with both blunt and penetrating trauma. It is almost always accompanied by multisystem injuries. In the majority of cases, the left hemidiaphragm is the part of the diaphragm that is injured. (Perhaps the more solid liver protects the right hemidiaphragm.)

Primary symptoms include marked or increasing respiratory distress, severe shoulder pain on the same

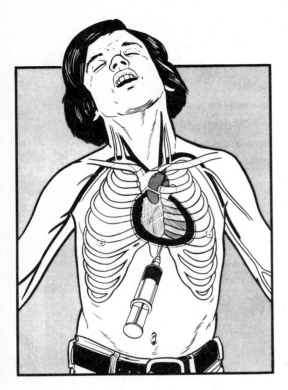

Figure 14-9. Paraxiphoid approach to pericardiocentesis.

side as the tear (due to air entering the thoracic cavity), an inability to insert a nasogastric tube (it cannot pass the kinked esophagus), and increasing signs of cardiopulmonary collapse. The immediate result of a significant tear in the diaphragm is the herniation of the abdominal contents into the thoracic cavity. Bowel sounds heard in the chest are pathognomonic of diaphragmatic rupture and herniation.

The diagnosis is established if bowel sounds are heard in the chest. X-ray may reveal an elevated, arched shadow of a high left hemidiaphragm, a shift of the heart and mediastinum to the right, shadows appearing above the diaphragm, and abnormal air/fluid levels. Diagnosis is aided by water-soluble contrast studies and fiberoptic endoscopy.

Treatment and Nursing Intervention. Immediate treatment is to establish adequate respiratory function. This is most frequently accomplished by endotracheal intubation and mechanical respiration. Stabilizing a patient in shock prior to surgery may or may not be

possible, depending upon the severity of the rupture. Definitive therapy consists of surgical repair of the torn diaphragm and replacement of the abdominal organs in the abdominal cavity. Gastrointestinal obstruction or bleeding is treated by conventional methods.

The nursing intervention of the highest priority is to monitor the patient's respiration status to ensure adequate oxygenation. Cardiovascular monitoring is the next priority, since the increased pressure and contents of the thoracic cavity will usually cause marked hemodynamic compromise, and cardiovascular collapse is not uncommon.

Esophageal Perforation

Esophageal perforation is due to penetrating injuries or iatrogenic causes. Perforation is suspected when there is posterior injury to the mediastinum or an unexplainable pneumothorax. Early diagnosis and treatment may be life saving, while a delayed or missed diagnosis may cause permanent disability or death. The possibility of severe morbidity and mortality is related to the degree of contamination, the site of the perforation, and the delay in diagnosis and initiation of treatment.

A definitive diagnosis is made by having the patient swallow a water solution contrast medium under fluoroscopy, which will reveal any esophageal tear or leak. Chest x-ray may reveal a widening mediastinum, rib fractures, pleural effusions, pulmonary contusion, and/or hydropneumothorax, among other things. Symptoms include pain, choking, hoarseness, dysphagia, dyspnea, and upper abdominal pain. Stridor, decreased breath sounds, cyanosis, or shock not consistent with the apparent degree of injury suggests an esophageal tear.

Treatment and Nursing Intervention. Specific treatment includes insertion of a nasogastric tube, endotracheal intubation, and surgical repair of the tear if diagnosis is made within 6 to 12 hours. After that time lapse, edema, necrosis of tissue, and infection will probably prevent primary healing, since suturing of the tear may well not hold. In these instances, the esophagus may be ligated above the tear and oral secretion drainage achieved with a cervical esophagostomy. The esophagus is also ligated below the tear, and stomach drainage is achieved by a gastrostomy. The tear then heals by secondary intention, and at a later date, the esophagus may be reopened and reconstructed if necessary. Massive broad-spectrum antibiotic therapy is maintained until the situation has resolved.

Nursing interventions include close monitoring of

the respiratory system, since it is frequently damaged and usually infected from the esophageal contents. Secretions must be continuously drained both from the mouth and the endotracheal tube. Infection is monitored by the administration of antibiotics and the nurse's report of the patient's response to them. Nutritionally, it is important to maintain a positive nitrogen balance to promote healing. This may be accomplished by gastrostomy feedings or hyperalimentation. Physical therapy, as soon as tolerated by the patient, will help avoid musculoskeletal problems. Passive range of motion progressing to active and resistive exercise is the usually sequence of physical therapy. Psychological support of the patient and reassurances that the situation will be temporary will help alleviate the patient's fears and anxieties.

Tracheobronchial Injuries

This type of injury may be the result of blunt or penetrating trauma. Shearing forces are the cause of these injuries, since the trachea is attached in the cervical outlet and the thoracic inlet. The remainder of the airways are not as fixed in the chest, and significant movement is likely. The movement of nonfixed airways results in a shearing effect on the portion of the airways that is fixed and secured to other tissues. Diagnosis of a tracheal or bronchus tear is made by careful bronchoscopy, which allows the physician to identify the source of the tear, and to rule out abnormalities in the trachea and bronchus, and plan the best surgical approach for repairing the tear. Symptoms include failure of a lung to reexpand after proper treatment of pneumothorax, increasing subcutaneous emphysema, occasionally hemoptysis, the development of a pneumomediastinum, and a deterioration of the patient's condition that is out of proportion to the known injuries.

Treatment and Nursing Intervention. Treatment consists of intubation, ventilatory support, and surgical repair of the injury. Nursing interventions include close monitoring of the respiratory and cardiovascular systems. Control of respiratory secretions to prevent hypoxia, atelectasis, and infection is of paramount importance. Alterations in the cardiovascular status may indicate fresh bleeding and impending shock.

Aortic Rupture

Aortic rupture is the result of blunt trauma deceleration injury. Although most patients die immediately, 10 to 20% survive to reach a hospital when a tamponade

occurs around the rupture. This allows some blood to leave the left ventricle and pass beyond the distal end of the rupture.

Aortic rupture is diagnosed by aortogram. X ray may reveal a widened mediastinum, which is suggestive of aortic rupture. The aortogram will identify the area of rupture. Figure 14-10 identifies the most common sites of aortic rupture.

Symptoms may include an increased blood pressure and pulse in the upper extremities, a decreased blood pressure and pulse in the lower extremities, and the X-ray picture of a widened mediastinum. Shortness of breath, weakness, chest or back pain, and varied abnormalities involving the lower extremities may be present.

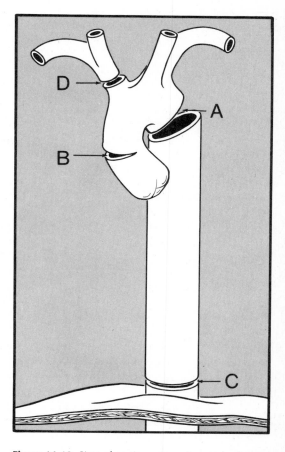

Figure 14-10. Sites of aortic rupture. A = arch of aorta; B = area just above aortic valve; C = end of thoracic aorta; D = subclavian vein. A is the most common; D is the least common.

Treatment and Nursing Intervention. Treatment consists of thoracotomy to repair the rupture. If the thoractomy cannot be performed immediately, the patient is medically treated as a patient with dissecting aortic aneurysm until surgery.

Nursing interventions include monitoring the respiratory, cardiovascular, neurologic, and renal systems, since these suffer first due to the decreased blood flow. Sodium nitroprusside is usually administered until the patient can be taken to surgery. Nursing care of the patient on ventilatory support and in need of close monitoring before and after surgery applies to the patient with a ruptured aorta.

PLEURAL DRAINAGE

Design of Systems

Drainage of air and fluid from the pleural space requires an evacuation system that allows air and fluids to exit but not reenter. This is accomplished by placing the pleural chest tube into a water seal chamber a few centimeters below water, which allows air to exit the pleural space but not to reenter. Several variations of the water seal valve are now in existence, but the principle of drainage remains the same.

Some pleural units place a collection chamber before the water seal chamber to avoid the effect of increasing resistance to air evacuation. As fluid accumulates in the water seal, the hydrostatic resistance to air leaving the pleural space increases. The collection chamber before the water seal chamber reduces this problem. The water seal is situated at the end of the pleural tube to provide minimal resistance to pressure changes in the pleural space. Suction chambers have been developed to accelerate reexpansion of the pleural space. While the value of suction is controversial, many physicians routinely order low suction levels between 10 and 40 cm H_2O. Low levels are employed to avoid injury to pulmonary parenchymal tissue.

Air leaving the pleural space is readily seen by the bubbling in the water seal chamber. When air has ceased leaking from the pleural space, bubbling in the water seal chamber ceases. Evacuation of fluid is noted by measuring the amount of fluid in the collection chamber.

Placement of Chest Tubes

For evacuation of air, chest tubes are placed in locations where air will migrate, i.e., superiorly and ante-riorly in a patient lying flat. Air evacuation chest tubes are placed near the second ICS in the midclavicular line. Chest tubes are placed in gravity-dependent positions to facilitate fluid evacuation. Fluid drainage tubes are placed near the fifth ICS in the midaxillary line. Placement lower than the fifth ICS increases the risk of puncturing abdominal viscera.

Clamping Chest Tubes

Chest tubes should not be clamped if bubbling is present in the water seal chamber. The potential for a tension pneumothorax exists if a tube is clamped while air is still exiting the pleural space. If no air is leaking from the pleural space, the clamping of a chest is generally not a problem, provided no major blood accumulation is also present.

BIBLIOGRAPHY

Ahrens, T.S. (1987). Concepts in the assessment of oxygenation. *Focus Crit Care, 14*, 1, 36–44.

Ahrens, T.S. (1989). Intrapulmonary shunting and deadspace analysis. *Crit Care Nurs Clin, 1*, 3.

Ahrens, T.S., & Rutherford, K.P. (1987). The new pulmonary math: Applying the a/A ratio. *AJN, 87*, 337–340.

Berte, J.B. (1986). *Critical Care—The Lung.* Norwalk: Appleton-Century-Crofts.

Bostick, J., & Wendelgass, S.T. (1987). Normal saline instillation as part of the suctioning procedure: Effects on PaO2 and amount of secretions. *Heart Lung, 16*, 5, 532–537.

Bradley, R.B. (1987). Adult respiratory distress syndrome. *Focus Crit Care, 14*, 5, 48–59.

Burrows, B., et al. (1983). *Respiratory Disorders: A Pathophysiologic Approach.* Chicago: Yearbook Medical Publishers.

Chulay, M. (1988). Arterial blood gas changes with a hyperinflation and hyperoxygenation suctioning intervention in critically ill patients. *Heart Lung, 17*, 6, 654–616.

Civetta, J.M., Taylor, R.W., & Kirby, R.R. (1989). *Introduction to Critical Care.* Philadelphia: J.B. Lippincott.

Eisenberg, P.R., Hansbrough, J.R., Anderson, D., & Schuster, D.P. (1987).A prospective study of lung water measurement during patient management in an intensive care unit. *Am Rev Respir Dis, 136*, 662–668.

Hasegawa, E.A.J. (1986). The endotracheal use of emergency drugs. *Heart Lung, 15*, 1, 60–63.

Kirby, R.R., Smith, R.A., & Desautels, D.A. (1985). *Mechanical Ventilation.* New York: Churchill Livingstone.

Roberts, S.L. (1987). Pulmonary tissue perfusion altered: Emboli. *Heart Lung, 16*, 2, 128–137.

Rudy, E.B., Baun, M., Stone, K., & Turner, B. (1986). The relationship between endotracheal suctioning and changes in intracranial pressure: A review of the literature. *Heart Lung, 15,* 5, 488–494.

Schuch, C.S., & Prince, J.G. (1987). Determination of time required for blood gas homeostasis in the intubated post-open heart surgery adult after a ventilator change. *Heart Lung, 16,* 4, 364–370.

Shapiro, B.A. (1985). *Clinical Application of Respiratory Care.* Chicago: Yearbook Medical Publishers.

Slonim, M., & Hamilton, L.H. (1987). *Respiratory Physiology.* St. Louis: C.V. Mosby.

Stone, K.S., Vorst, E.C., Lanham, B., & Zahn, S. (1989). Effects of lung hyperinflation on mean arterial pressure and postsuctioning hypoxemia. *Heart Lung, 18,* 4, 377–385.

Stratton, C.W. (1986). Bacterial pneumonias—An overview with emphasis on pathogenesis, diagnosis and treatment. *Heart Lung, 15,* 3, 226–244.

von Hippel, A. (1986). *A Manual of Thoracic Surgery.* Anchorage: Stone Age Co.

Weilitz, P.B. (1989). New modes of mechanical ventilation. *Crit Care Nurs Clin 1*(4), 689–695.

Weilitz, P.B. (1991). *Pocket Guide to Respiratory Care.* St. Louis: Mosby-Yearbook, Inc.

Weilitz, P.B. (1991). Weaning from mechanical ventilation: old and new strategies. *Crit Care Clin 3*(4), 585–590.

West, J.B. (1990). *Respiratory Physiology—The Essentials.* Baltimore: Williams & Wilkins.

White, K.M. (1985). Completing the hemodynamic picture: SvO2. *Heart Lung, 14,* 272–280.

PART 3

Neurology

Teresa Halloran, RN, MSN, CCRN

Anatomy of the Nervous System

Perhaps the area of the CCRN exam that is most difficult is the section on principles of neurology. The difficulty in neurology can be traced to the complexity of understanding central and autonomic nervous system dysfunction. The focus of the CCRN exam, however, is not on all potential disturbances of the nervous system. The primary focus is on problems that are common in general critical nursing practice. This focus makes understanding the neurological aspect of the CCRN test more manageable.

In its present format, the CCRN exam devotes 8% (about 16 questions) to neurological concepts. If you are not comfortable with neurological concepts, review the following chapters carefully. The key aspects covered in the CCRN exam include encephalopathies, head trauma, cerebral bleeding/emboli, aneurysms, space-occupying lesions (brain tumors), neurological infectious diseases, seizure disorders, and acute spinal cord injury, all of which are discussed in the following seven chapters. Study the chapters, seek patients with neurological conditions representing the key concepts, and practice neurological assessments and neurological tests during your clinical practice. These guidelines will help provide an understanding of neurology for both your practice and the CCRN exam.

It is customary to divide the nervous system into three segments to facilitate comprehension of the system and its dysfunctions. The three segments are the central nervous system (CNS) (composed of the brain and spinal cord), the peripheral nervous system (composed of the cranial, spinal, and peripheral nerves), and the autonomic nervous system (composed of the sympathetic and parasympathetic systems).

EXTRACEREBRAL STRUCTURES

Extracerebral structures include the scalp, skull, and meninges. These structures provide protection to the brain.

Scalp

The letters in the word "scalp" form a mnemonic for remembering the cranial coverings (Fig. 15-1). "Sca" represents a single layer of skin, cutaneous, and adipose tissue. This layer contains blood vessels, but these cannot contract. Consequently, when the scalp is lacerated, it bleeds more than an identical cut else-

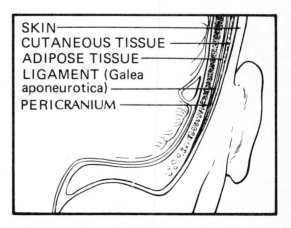

Figure 15-1. Layers of the scalp.

where on the body. The "l" is the dense, fibrous ligament-like layer called the galea aponeurotica. This layer helps to absorb the forces of external trauma. The "p" represents the pericranium, which contains fewer bone-forming elements than does the periosteum.

Skull

The bony calvarium (skull) is composed of several bones fused to form a solid, nondistensible unit. The cranium is hollow and very rigid. The skull has a volume of 1400 to 1500 mL. It provides strong protection to the head without being heavy. To achieve this, there is an outer and an inner layer of regular bone structure. The middle layer is called the diploë (or diploic space), which is spongy and lightweight.

Eight bones comprise the cranium (Fig. 15-2): the frontal and occipital bones (both single) and pairs of parietal, temporal, sphenoid, and ethmoid bones. The main function of the bony calvarium is to protect the brain from external forces. The bones formed during fetal life do not completely fuse until the infant is about 18 to 24 months of age. The fusion of these bones forms three landmarks. The coronal suture is the fusion of the frontal and parietal bones. The sagittal suture is the fusion of the two parietal bones. The lamboidal suture is the fusion of the parietal bones and the occipital bone.

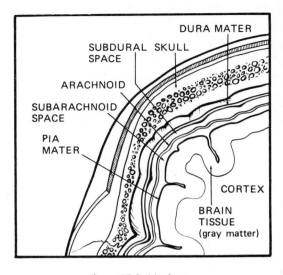

Figure 15-3. Meninges.

Fossae

The internal surface of the cranium has three distinct ridges that serve to divide the brain area into anterior, middle, and posterior segments called fossae (singular, fossa).

Meninges

The three membranes covering the entire brain surface, the spinal cord, and the spinal canal below the cord are the meninges (Fig. 15-3). A mnemonic ("pad") may help distinguish the meningeal coverings: the pia mater, arachnoid layer, and dura mater. The meningeal layers absorb shocks from sudden movements or trauma. The meninges literally "pad" the brain. Between each layer of the meninges is a space containing certain structures.

Starting from the brain per se, the first meningeal layer is the pia mater. The pia mater is contiguous with the brain surface and its convolutions.

The "a" of "pad" represents the arachnoid layer of the meninges. The arachnoid is a delicate, avascular membrane between the dura mater and pia mater. It looks much like a lacy spiderweb with projections onto the pia mater, forming a space. This space between the arachnoid layer and pia mater, the subarachnoid space, contains many cerebral arteries and veins that are bathed by cerebrospinal fluid (CSF). The arachnoid membrane also has projections, called arachnoid villi,

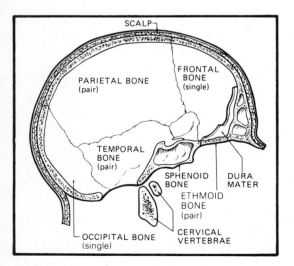

Figure 15-2. Cranium.

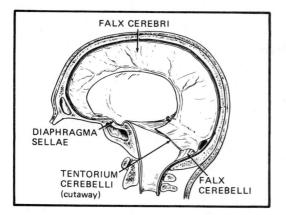

Figure 15-4. Sagittal section showing processes formed by the inner layer of the dura mater.

that absorb CSF. The subarachnoid space enlarges at the base of the brain to form the subarachnoid cisterns.

The most exterior layer of the meninges is the dura mater. The dura mater is actually two layers of tough fibrous membrane that protects the underlying cortical matter. The outermost layer forms the periosteum of the cranial cavity. The inner layer, which is lined with flat cells, contains arteries and veins. Between the two layers are clefts, which form the dural venous sinuses. The inner layer also gives rise to several folds that divide the cranial cavity into compartments. Three important folds are the falx cerebri (separating the cerebral hemispheres), the falx cerebelli (separating the right and left cerebellar hemispheres), and the tentorium cerebelli (separating the cerebral hemispheres from the cerebellum) (Fig. 15-4). These compartmental dividers are significant anatomical landmarks in the brain. The extradural space, also called the epidural space, is a potential space between the inner table of the skull and the outermost meningeal layer, the dura mater. This potential space becomes real when an individual experiencing a blow to the head develops an epidural hematoma. Epidural hematomas commonly result from a laceration of the middle meningeal artery in association with a skull fracture at the parietotemporal junction.

Another potential space, the subdural space, lies between the dura mater and the arachnoid. This is the site of subdural hematomas. This type of hematoma is most often venous in origin, resulting from tearing of the dural veins.

CENTRAL NERVOUS SYSTEM

The brain is nervous tissue that fills up the cranial vault. It weighs about 3 pounds in the adult male. Although it is an integrated unit, for study purposes, it can be divided into six major parts (Fig. 15-5): cerebrum (telencephalon), diencephalon, midbrain (mesencephalon), pons, cerebellum, and medulla oblongata.

Cerebrum

The cerebrum is contained in the anterior and middle fossae of the cranium. The left and right cerebral hemispheres are incompletely separated by a deep medial longitudinal fissure. This fissure, called the falx cerebri, is formed by the sagittal folds of the dura mater. The two cerebral hemispheres are joined by the corpus callosum (Fig. 15-6).

In addition to this function, the corpus callosum provides a path for fibers to cross from one hemisphere to the other. Each hemisphere has a lateral ventricle. These two hemispheres are sometimes referred to as the telencephalon.

The cerebral surface is covered with convolutions that give rise to gyri (raised portions) and sulci or fissures (depressions in the surface). The cerebral surface is about six cells deep and is called the cerebral cortex. Because the area normally appears gray, these six layers (Fig. 15-7) are called gray matter. This cortex is estimated to contain 14 billion nerve cells.

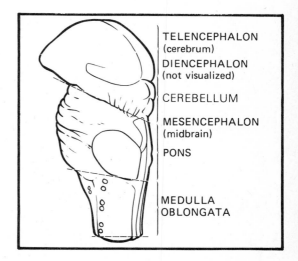

Figure 15-5. Gross anatomical sections of the brain.

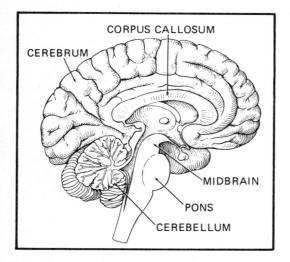

Figure 15-6. Midsagittal section showing the corpus callosum.

A lateral view of the cerebral hemispheres shows two fissures dividing the hemisphere (Fig. 15-8). The lateral fissure (also called the fissure of Sylvius) divides the frontal lobe and the temporal lobe (named for

the overlying bones). This area contains the primary auditory center. The central sulcus, also known as the fissure of Rolando, divides the frontal lobe from the parietal lobe. Immediately in front of the central sulcus is the precentral gyrus, which is the primary motor area. Immediately posterior to the central sulcus is the postcentral gyrus, which is the primary sensory cortical area.

In looking at pictures of the brain surface that do not show the cerebellum, imagine the brain as a boxing glove. The thumb of the boxing glove always points toward the frontal area of the brain. For descriptive purposes, the lateral surface of the hemisphere is divided into four lobes. The frontal lobe (approximately the anterior one-third of the hemisphere) is the portion that is anterior to the central sulcus and above the lateral fissure. The frontal lobe is responsible for voluntary motor function and higher mental functions such as judgment, foresight, affect, and personality. The parietal lobe extends from the central sulcus to the parieto-occipital fissure. This lobe is responsible for sensory function, sensory association, and higher-level processing of general sensory modalities. The occipital lobe is that part lying behind, or caudal to, an arbitrary line drawn from the parieto-occipital fissure to the pre-

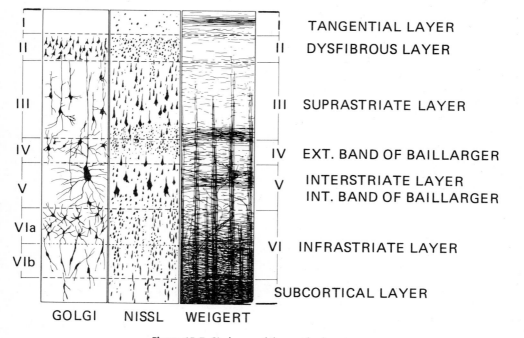

Figure 15-7. Six layers of the cerebral cortex.

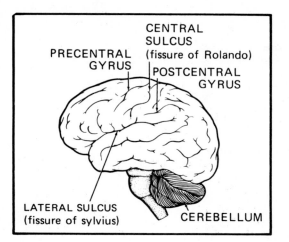

Figure 15-8 Fissures, sulci, and gyri dividing the cerebral hemisphere.

occipital notch. The function of the occipital lobe is visual reception and visual association.

The temporal lobes are located under the lateral fissures of Sylvius. The temporal lobes are each divided into primary auditory receptive, secondary auditory association, and tertiary visual association areas.

The basal ganglia, or basal nuclei, are also part of the telencephalon. The basal ganglia include the caudate nucleus, putamen, globus pallidus, claustrum, subthalamic nucleus, and substantia nigra (Fig. 15-9). Specific functions of the brain segments are listed in Table 15-1.

Diencephalon

The diencephalon, the most superior portion of the brain stem, is covered by the cerebrum (Fig. 15-10). It is a paired structure with a thin fluid space between the two sides. The diencephalon is composed of the thalamus, the hypothalamus, and the limbic system. The thalamus, the largest structure in the diencephalon, integrates all body sensations except smell. It is also the major relay area for all neuronal impulses. The hypothalamus connects with the limbic system, thalamus, mesencephalon, and hypophysis (pituitary gland).

Mesencephalon

The mesencephalon, or midbrain, is located between the diencephalon and the pons. It contains the major motor nerves for eye movement, carries impulses down from the cerebrum, and controls the wakefulness of the brain through the reticular activating system (RAS) (Fig. 15-11). RAS fibers connect with the thala-

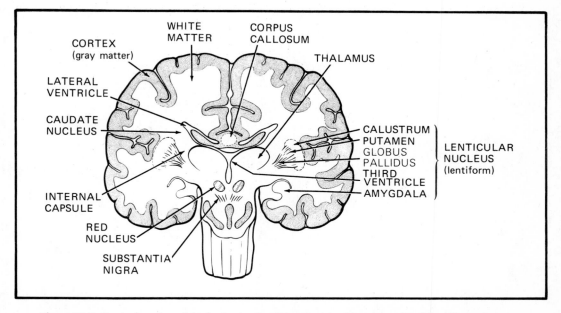

Figure 15-9. Coronal section of the brain showing internal parts of basal ganglia of the telencephalon.

TABLE 15-1. FUNCTIONS OF SPECIFIC BRAIN STRUCTURES

Structure	Function
Cerebrum (divided into cerebral hemispheres)	Governs all sensory and motor thought and learning; analyzes, associates, integrates, and stores information
Cerebral cortex (4 lobes)	
1. Frontal lobe	Motor function; motor speech area; controls morals, values, emotions, and judgment
2. Parietal lobe	Integrates general sensation; governs discrimination; interprets pain, touch, temperature, and pressure
3. Temporal lobe	Auditory center; sensory speech center
4. Occipital lobe	Visual area
Basal ganglia	Central motor movement
Thalamus (diencephalon)	Screens and relays sensory impulses to cortex; lowest level of crude conscious awareness
Hypothalamus (diencephalon)	Regulates autonomic nervous system, stress response, sleep, appetite, body temperature, water balance, and emotions
Midbrain (mesencephalon)	Motor condition, conjugate eye movements
Pons	Contains projection tracts between spinal cord, medulla, and brain
Medulla oblongata	Contains all afferent and efferent tracts, most pyramidal tracts, and cardiac, respiratory, vasomotor, and vomiting centers
Cerebellum	Connected by cerebellar peduncles to other parts of CNS; coordinates muscle movement, posture, equilibrium, and muscle tone
Limbic system	Regulation of some visceral activities; some function in emotional personality

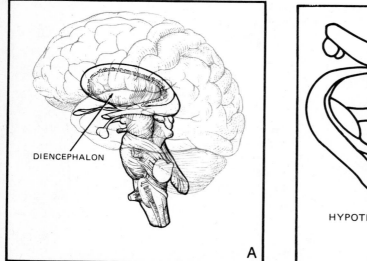

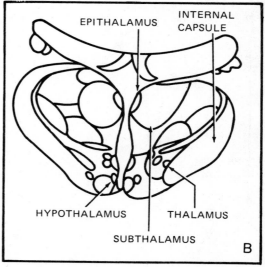

Figure 15-10. Position of the diencephalon (**A**) and the internal components of the diencephalon (**B**).

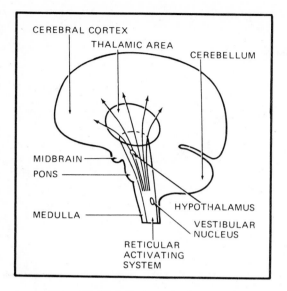

Figure 15-11. Reticular activating system.

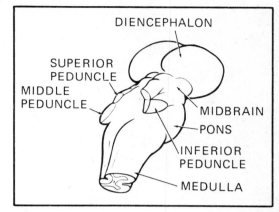

Figure 15-12. Cerebellar peduncles.

mus, cerebral cortex, cerebellum, and spinal cord. This area contains nuclei of the third and fourth cranial nerves.

Pons

The pons is situated between the midbrain and the medulla oblongata. The pons forms a bridge (thus its name, from the Latin word for bridge) between the cerebellar hemispheres and contains the neurons for sensory input and motor output for the face. This area contains nuclei of the fifth, sixth, and seventh cranial nerves.

Medulla Oblongata

Located between the pons and the spinal cord, the medulla oblongata is the structure that marks the change between the spinal cord and the brain per se. The corticospinal tracts, which mediate voluntary motor function, descend through the medulla, where they decussate in the lower medulla. This structure is responsible for specific symptoms of dysfunction that occur ipsilaterally (same side as the lesion or injury) or contralaterally (opposite side). Collectively, the mesencephalon, pons, and medulla oblongata are termed the brain stem.

Cerebellum

The cerebellum is situated in the posterior fossa of the cranial cavity, separated from the cerebrum by dura mater folds forming the tentorium cerebelli. The cerebral hemispheres are above the tentorium cerebelli and are thus supratentorial structures. The two cerebellar hemispheres are connected to each other by a structure called the vermis. They are connected to the brain stem by cerebellar peduncles. There are three cerebellar peduncles (Fig. 15-12). The superior cerebellar peduncles send impulses from the cerebellum to the thalamus. The middle cerebellar peduncles receive cerebral cortex information from nuclei in the pons. The inferior cerebellar peduncles receive impulses that reveal body and extremity positions.

Gray and white matter compose the cerebellum. The cerebellum receives input from the brain stem and spinal cord nuclei, whose axons project to the cerebellar cortex. These tracts carry excitatory impulses to the cerebellar cortex.

Equilibrium, posture, muscle tone, and ultimately muscle coordination are mediated by the cerebellum.

CIRCULATION AND FORMATION OF CEREBROSPINAL FLUID

There are four ventricles (cavities) involved in the CSF system (Fig. 15-13). The largest two are the lateral ventricles, which are located in the cerebral hemispheres. The lateral ventricles are connected to the third ventricle via the interventricular foramen (the foramen of Monro). The cerebral aqueduct of Sylvius arises from the floor of the third ventricle. This channel passes down through the brain stem to the fourth ventricle. The fourth ventricle is continuous with the

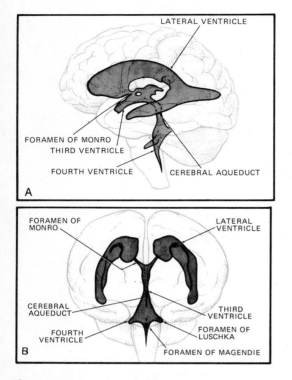

Figure 15-13. Lateral view of the ventricular system of the brain (**A**) and anterior view of the ventricular system of the brain (**B**).

protect them from colliding with the cranium and vertebrae in response to moving forces. The CSF also reduces the gravitational weight of the brain. To a limited extent, the CSF adjusts to changes in the intracranial vault's pressure and volume. If the pressure or volume increases in the vault, more CSF will be absorbed and/or pushed into the spinal canal in an attempt to maintain normal pressure. Normally, 125 to 150 mL of CSF is in the ventricles and the subarachnoid space. An average of 500 to 800 mL (or approximately 25 to 35 mL/hour) of CSF is produced in 24 hours. The CSF also participates in the exchange of nutrients and waste material between the blood and the CNS cells.

Cerebral Blood Supply

The brain is supplied with oxygenated blood from two arterial systems: the internal carotid arteries and the vertebral arteries. As a reserve for these two systems, the circle of Willis helps provide adequate circulation through its anastomoses. The circle of Willis anastomoses are between the two vertebral arteries and the two carotid arteries (Fig. 15-14).

central canal of the spinal cord. CSF is synthesized by the choroid plexus. This is an area of modified epithelial cells covering tufts of capillaries found in all ventricles but predominating in the anterior segment of the lateral ventricles. CSF is a clear, colorless liquid having a few cells, some protein, glucose, and a large amount of sodium chloride.

The foramen of Monro allows the CSF to leave the lateral ventricles and flow into the third ventricle. From the third ventricle, CSF flows through the aqueduct of Sylvius into the fourth ventricle. Foramina of Luschka and Magendie direct the CSF from the fourth ventricle into the cisterns and subarachnoid space.

After circulating (in the subarachnoid space) over the entire brain and spinal cord, the CSF is reabsorbed by the arachnoid villi in dural sinuses and by pacchionian bodies found in the superior sagittal sinus.

The CSF cushions the brain and spinal cord to

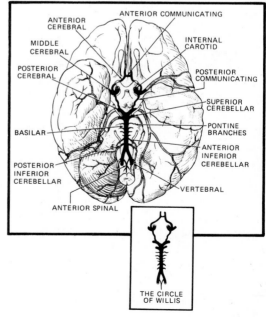

Figure 15-14. Circle of Willis.

External Cerebral Blood Supply

The external carotid arteries bifurcate and form the occipital, temporal, and maxillary arteries. The occipital arteries supply the posterior fossa. The temporal arteries supply the temporal region. The maxillary arteries form the middle meningeal arteries, which supply the anterior, middle, and posterior portions of the meninges and the fossae. While not a part of cerebral circulation, the external carotid artery and its branches have been used to supplement cerebral circulation in patients with cerebrovascular disease.

Internal Cerebral Blood Supply

On entering the skull, the internal carotid artery follows the carotid groove upward through the cavernous sinus and the sphenoid bone and into the circle of Willis at the base of the brain. Before this, smaller vessels originate, one of which is the ophthalmic artery to the retina. Temporary blockage of this vessel by microemboli may cause fleeting monocular blindness (amaurosis fugax).

The internal carotid arteries bifurcate to form the anterior cerebral arteries, the anterior communicating arteries, the middle cerebral arteries, the posterior communicating arteries, and the anterior choroidal arteries. The anterior communicating artery connects the left and right anterior cerebral arteries. The posterior communicating artery connects the internal carotid arteries to the basilar artery. These communicating arteries do not supply any part of the brain directly, but some are collateral channels helping to form the circle in the circle of Willis.

The vertebral arteries enter the posterior fossa and join to form the basilar artery. The basilar artery bifurcates to form the superior cerebellar arteries and the posterior cerebral arteries. The superior cerebellar arteries supply the pons and the cerebellum. Posterior cerebral arteries supply the posterior one-third of the cerebrum.

The anterior cerebral, anterior communicating, posterior communicating, and posterior cerebral arteries anastomose with each other to form the circle of Willis. All of these arteries are involved in supplying blood to the anterior two-thirds of the cerebrum.

Only about 50% of all people have a "classic" circle of Willis. The most common difference is that the posterior communicating artery is not present and the posterior cerebral artery comes directly from the internal carotid artery.

Veins run parallel with many of the arteries. The middle meningeal arteries are special in that the veins that accompany these arteries are positioned between the arteries and the bones of the cranium. This helps protect the middle meningeal artery, which is frequently torn in skull fractures of the temporal bones.

As there is an internal and external arterial blood

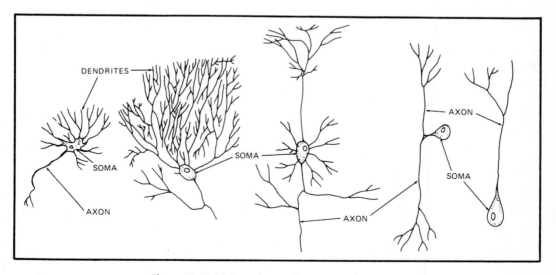

Figure 15-15. Various shapes of neurons and neuroglia.

supply, there is a corresponding internal and external venous return system. Many of the veins are important in aneurysms and as surgical landmarks. The veins that drain the dura mater and diploë of the skull (external) empty into the venous sinuses, which are located between the layers of the dura mater. Internal cerebral veins also empty into venous sinuses.

Venous sinuses are lined with epithelium; they have no valves and no muscle in the walls. The sinuses connect with emissary veins, which in turn connect with external cranial veins that empty into the internal jugular veins. The superior sagittal sinus receives venous blood from the superior cerebral veins. The inferior sagittal sinus receives venous blood from the middle cerebral hemisphere veins. The straight sinus receives venous blood from the internal cerebral veins. There are many other sinuses that receive venous blood from other areas of the brain.

Components of Nervous Tissue

There are two main types of cells in the brain: neurons (Fig. 15-15) and neuroglia (glial cells). The neuron is the functioning unit of the nervous system; its function is to transmit impulses. There are more than 10 billion neurons in the CNS, and three-fourths of them are in

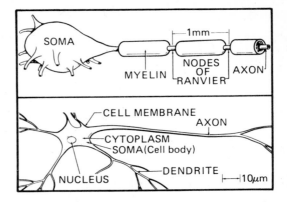

Figure 15-16. Schematic diagram of the structures of the neuron.

the cerebral cortex. Neurons are categorized in two ways: by the direction of impulse flow and/or by the number of processes emanating from the neuron cell body.

Neurons that transmit impulses to the spinal cord or brain are afferent sensory neurons. Those transmitting impulses away from the brain or spinal cord are called efferent motor neurons. Interneurons transmit

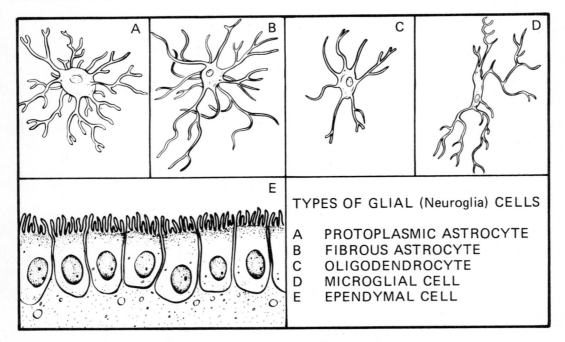

Figure 15-17. Types of glial cells (neuroglia).

impulses from sensory neurons to motor neurons. The mnemonic "same" can be used to remember the direction and type of neuron: "sa" for sensory afferent and "me" for motor efferent.

Neurons are one of three types, according to the number of processes that exist. Unipolar neurons have one process coming from the cell body. After a short distance, this one process splits to form one axon and one dendrite. Bipolar neurons have one axon and one dendrite coming from the cell body. Multipolar neurons have one axon and multiple dendrites.

Upper motor neurons originate above the brainstem, enter the spinal column and stop in the anterior horn of the spinal cord. Injury to upper motor neuron lesions will produce a type of spastic paralysis since spinal reflexes are still intact below the injury. This is unlike lower motor neuron lesions which originate in the anterior horn of the spinal column and end in skeletal muscles. Injury to lower motor neurons will be associated with flaccid paralysis of the affected muscles.

All neurons, regardless of the category, have certain unique structures (Fig. 15-16): axons, dendrites, neurofibrils, Nissl bodies, myelin, neurilemma, and nodes of Ranvier.

The cell body of a neuron is called a soma or perikaryon. It contains a nucleus and many cytoplasmic organelles. The axon transmits impulses away from the soma. There is one axon per neuron. Dendrites are short processes that transmit impulses to the soma. Neurofibrils are thin, threadlike fibers forming a network in the cytoplasm. Nissl bodies specialize in protein synthesis with RNA to maintain and regenerate the neuronal processes.

Myelin is a protein-lipid compound that covers some axons. In the CNS, myelin is reduced to oligodendrocytes. In the peripheral nervous system, myelin is produced by Schwann cells. Myelin covers axons of nerve cells between the nodes of Ranvier. The nodes of Ranvier are bare spots at regular intervals that speed the conduction of impulses.

The neurilemma is an outer coating of the neurons outside the CNS. The neurilemma encompasses all structures, even myelin. It is the neurilemma that provides for peripheral nerve regeneration. Since the neurilemma is not found on neurons of the brain and spinal cord, these neurons cannot regenerate.

Neurons require an extensive support system to maintain optimal function. The neuroglia are responsible for this support system (Fig. 15-17). Neuroglia are composed of glial cells, and they outnumber the neu-

rons by ten to one. Four types of specific cells comprise the glial support system.

1. Astrocytes are star-shaped cells that form the actual tissue support system.
2. Microglia are tiny cells that lie quiescent until nervous tissue is damaged. Because of their origin, microglia are part of the reticuloendothelial cell system. They wander in and out of the CNS in response to need. When damage occurs, the microglia become mobile and travel to the damaged tissue. They enlarge and phagocytize the debris.
3. Oligodendroglia help support the nervous tissue, but their primary function is the original

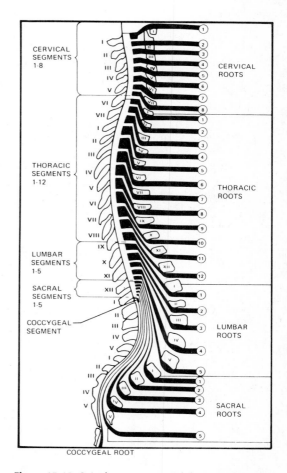

Figure 15-18. Spinal nerve roots and their attachment to the spinal cord.

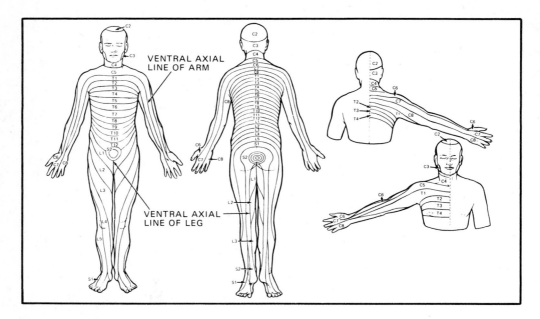

Figure 15-19. Dermatomes.

formation of myelin in the CNS during fetal, neonatal, and early years. Once the myelin has been formed, the oligodendroglia cannot form it again.

4. Ependyma are special glial cells that are found lining the ventricles of the brain and the central canal in the spinal cord.

The spinal cord is the second part of the central nervous system. It is examined in Chapter 17.

PERIPHERAL NERVOUS SYSTEM

The peripheral nerves, the spinal nerves, and the cranial nerves form the peripheral nervous system. There are 31 pairs of spinal nerves and 12 pairs of cranial nerves.

The 31 pairs of spinal nerves are numbered in relation to the vertebral level at which they emerge from the spinal cord. Spinal nerves do not attach directly to the spinal cord. Instead, the spinal nerves attach to a shorter anterior (ventral, motor) root and a short posterior (dorsal, sensory) root (Fig. 15-18). The posterior root has a bulge consisting of neuron cell bodies. This bulge is called a spinal ganglia. There are 8 cervical, 12 thoracic, 5 lumbar, 5 sacral, and 1 coccygeal spinal pair of ganglia.

Peripheral nerves often encompass more than one spinal nerve root. A good example is the sciatic nerve, which includes all of the spinal nerve roots in the sacrum.

Spinal Nerve Fibers

There are four types of nerve fibers comprising the spinal nerves.

1. Motor fibers originate in the ventral (anterior) horn of the spinal cord, with efferent fibers relaying motor impulses from the CNS to peripheral skeletal muscles.
2. Sensory fibers originate in the dorsal (posterior) horn of the spinal cord, with afferent fibers relaying sensory impulses from organs and muscles to the CNS.
3. Meningeal fibers transmit sensory and vasomotor innervation to the spinal meninges.
4. Autonomic fibers will be considered separately.

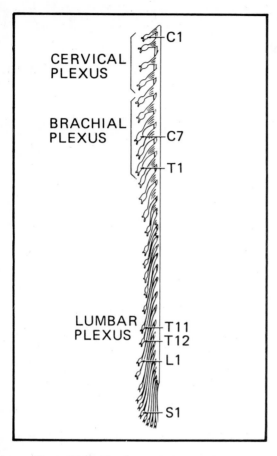

Figure 15-20. The three spinal nerve plexuses.

Dermatomes

Each spinal nerve dorsal root innervates a specific portion of skin. These skin regions, called dermatomes (Fig. 15-19), are clinically important in identifying areas of spinal cord injury.

Plexuses

The spinal nerves interweave in three areas that are termed the cervical, brachial, and lumbosacral plexuses (Fig. 15-20). The cervical plexus involves spinal nerves C-1 to C-4. It sends motor impulses to neck muscles and the diaphragm. It receives sensory impulses from the neck and head. The brachial plexus is composed of spinal nerves C-4 to C-8 and T-1. It inner-

vates the arms. The lumbosacral plexus is formed by spinal nerves L-1 to L-5 and S-1 to S-3. This plexus innervates the legs.

Cranial Nerves

Twelve pairs of cranial nerves complete the peripheral nervous system. Three pairs of cranial nerves are totally sensory, five pairs are totally motor, and four pairs are combined sensorimotor. Origin of the nerves is seen in Fig. 15-21. By convention, the cranial nerves are numbered by roman numerals as well as named. The cranial nerves are summarized in Table 15-2. The standard mnemonic may help keep them in order: On Old Olympus's Towering Top A Finn And German Viewed Some Hops.

AUTONOMIC NERVOUS SYSTEM

The sympathetic nervous system and the parasympathetic nervous system together form the autonomic nervous system. Technically, the autonomic nervous system is part of the peripheral nervous system. Sympathetic stimulation, e.g. epinephrine administration or parasympathetic inhibition, e.g. atropine, cause similar responses such as papillary dilation.

The sympathetic nervous system releases norepinephrine, which stimulates and prepares our bodies for "fight or flight." Norepinephrine is categorized as an adrenergic chemical (hormone). Fibers originating in the thoracic and lumbar areas form the peripheral sympathetic nervous system division.

The parasympathetic nervous system releases acetylcholine, which is categorized as a cholinergic chemical (hormone). In reality, the parasympathetic system is an antagonist to the sympathetic system and mediates or slows body responses when the "fight, fright, or flight" situation no longer exists. Fibers originating in the cranial and sacral areas form the peripheral parasympathetic nervous system division.

Nerve Structures of the Autonomic Nervous System

The sympathetic nervous system has a chain of ganglia situated on both sides of the vertebrae (Fig. 15-22). Nerve fibers between the spinal cord and the ganglia are termed preganglionic fibers (or axons). The nerve fibers between the ganglia and visceral end organ are called postganglionic fibers (or axons). The norepinephrine that is released to maintain body function

TABLE 15-2. SUMMARY OF CRANIAL NERVES

Number	Name	Major Functions
I	Olfactory	Sense of smell
II	Optic	Central and peripheral vision
III	Oculomotor	Eye movement; elevation of upper eyelid; pupil constriction
IV	Trochlear	Downward and inward eye movement
V	Trigeminal	Touch, pain, temperature; jaw and eye muscle proprioception; mastication
VI	Abducens	Abduction of the eye
VII	Facial	Close eyelid, muscles of facial expression; secretion by glands of mouth and eyes; taste (anterior two-thirds of tongue)
VIII	Acoustic Vestibular branch	Equilibrium
	Cochlear branch	Hearing
IX	Glossopharyngeal	Movement of pharyngeal muscles; secretion by parotid glands; pharyngeal and posterior tongue sensation
X	Vagus	Pharyngeal and laryngeal movement; visceral activities; pharyngeal and laryngeal sensation; taste
XI	Spinal accessory	Pharyngeal, sternocleidomastoid, and trapezius movement
XII	Hypoglossal	Tongue movement

is not easily or rapidly neutralized, so the effect is sustained for a period of time. The sympathetic system may be referred to as the thoracolumbar system, since major ganglia arise in the thoracic and lumbar regions.

The parasympathetic nervous system does not have a chain of ganglia next to the vertebral column. The preganglionic fibers (or axons) originate in the brain and sacrum (Fig. 15-23). These axons are long to allow them to reach specific organs. Ganglia are found adjacent to or within specific organs, so postganglionic fibers (or axons) are short. The chemical released by the parasympathetic system, acetylcholine, is rapidly neutralized by cholinesterase. Because of this, the parasympathetic effect is brief and must be renewed fairly regularly to counter the sympathetic stimulation. This system may be referred to as the craniosacral system, since the preganglionic fibers arise from certain cranial nerves and in the sacral spinal cord.

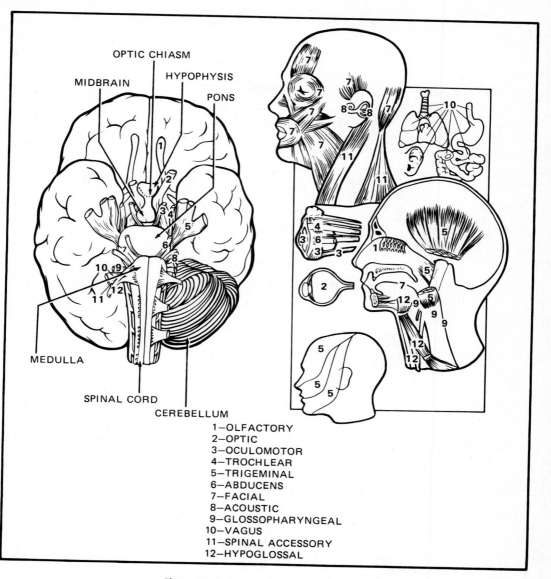

Figure 15-21. Origin of the cranial nerves.

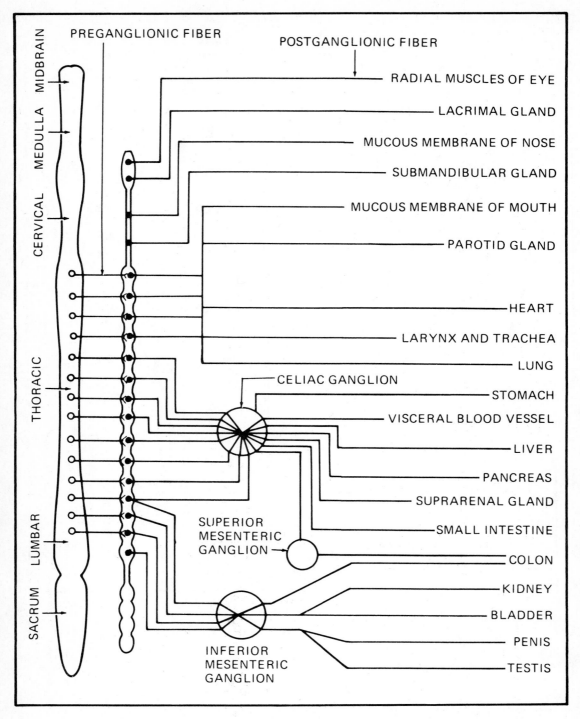

Figure 15-22. Sympathetic nervous system ganglia.

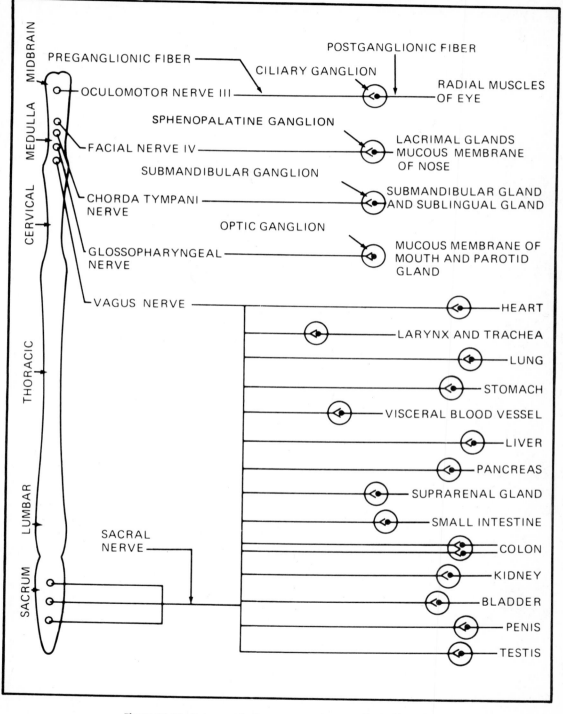

Figure 15-23. Parasympathetic nervous system ganglionic fibers.

CHAPTER 16

Physiology of the Nervous System

Editor's Note

Like the previous chapter on anatomy of the nervous system, this chapter on physiology is designed to acquaint you with the key functions of the nervous system. The CCRN exam will not likely test directly on this area. However, understanding the physiology of the nervous system is crucial to understanding clinical disorders. Use this chapter as an aid to improve your general understanding of neurological function, an understanding that can be used to better assess clinical conditions presented in subsequent chapters.

NEURAL CELL DEPOLARIZATION AND REPOLARIZATION

Depolarization and repolarization of the nerve cell follow the same principles as depolarization and repolarization of the cardiac cell.

Depolarization

The neuron in a resting state (resting membrane potential) is positively charged outside the cell membrane and negatively charged on the inner surface of the cell membrane. When the cell is stimulated, sodium rapidly enters the cell and potassium leaves the cell. This produces a positive ionic charge at the entry site and decreases the resting membrane potential. This positive ionic charge is transmitted along the length of the neuron and is termed a wave of depolarization.

Repolarization

As soon as potassium reenters the cell and sodium leaves the cell, the resting state of the cell is reestablished. This is called repolarization. A specific

mechanism exists to force the sodium ions that entered the cell's cytoplasm back into the extracellular fluid. The mechanism is termed the sodium pump. Without the sodium pump, ion homeostasis could not be preserved. At the same time, a potassium pump exists to maintain potassium ion homeostasis by forcing potassium ions back into the cell.

An action potential exists when an ionic charge on one side of the membrane is different from an ionic charge on the other. Depolarization occurs when a stimulus is strong enough (threshold) to alter the cell membrane permeability to sodium, allowing a change in the ionic charge. (Sodium ions enter and potassium ions leave the cell interior.) Once an action potential exists and a stimulus of threshold-level magnitude occurs, the neuron totally depolarizes. The neuron depolarizes following the all-or-none principle: it depolarizes in its entirety or else it does not depolarize at all. As with the cardiac cell, the neuron has a complete refractory period during which it is repolarizing and cannot be stimulated. Also like the cardiac cell, the neuron has a relative refractory period. During this period, the neuron can be stimulated (or excited), but only when the stimulus is at a threshold level.

Two terms are important in relation to action potentials. Summation refers to repetitive, accumulated discharges that eventually reach threshold level (much like building blocks placed one on top of the other until the top is reached). Facilitation is an increase in every subsequent neuron stimulus even though the stimulus remains below threshold levels. No action potential occurs in facilitation. Action potential does occur in summation.

The rapid velocity of conduction of the impulse is due in part to the neuron structure (Fig. 16-1) and the size of the nerve fiber. Myelin is a protective, lipid insulation of the neuron that is nonconductive, thus preventing an easy flow of ions into the nerve fiber. The myelin sheath is segmented. At specified inter-

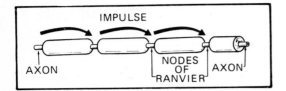

Figure 16-1. Nodes of Ranvier providing saltatory conduction.

vals, the myelin sheath is totally absent. These noninsulated points are called nodes of Ranvier. Ions flow easily around the nerve fiber at the nodes of Ranvier. The action potential on myelinated nerve fibers jumps from one node of Ranvier to the next node of Ranvier. This process, called saltatory conduction, is far faster than conduction in an unmyelinated fiber. In unmyelinated fibers, the impulse must travel the entire length of the neuron.

CHEMICAL SYNAPSES

A synapse is a point of junction, but not of contact, between one neuron and another neuron, a muscle cell, or a gland cell. Synapses differ in shape and size but function similarly in transmitting impulses.

The neuron's axon enlarges at its end, forming a synaptic knob (also called a terminal button or a presynaptic terminal) (Fig. 16-2). The synaptic knob con-

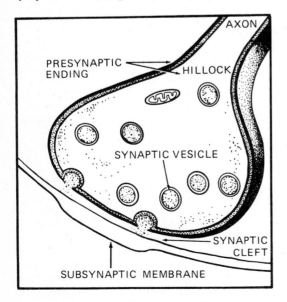

Figure 16-2. Chemical synapse.

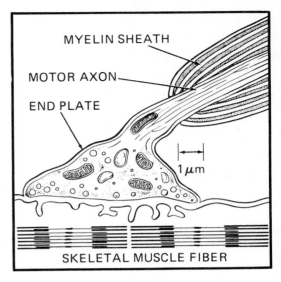

Figure 16-3. Neuromuscular junction or neuromuscular end plate.

tains vesicles that are filled with specific neurotransmitter chemicals. When the axonal knob is stimulated, these chemicals are released from the vesicles. The presynaptic terminal is separated from the postsynaptic side by a minute space termed the synaptic cleft. The postsynaptic membrane is slightly thicker at the synaptic cleft than elsewhere and is termed the subsynaptic membrane. The extra thickness is thought to be due to an increased number of receptor sites for the neurotransmitter.

When the axons of a motor neuron synapse with skeletal muscle, the presynaptic terminal (synaptic knob) is called a neuromuscular junction or a neuromuscular end plate (Fig. 16-3). At this specific synapse, the presynaptic terminal looks like a plate. The neuromuscular junction is the only synapse specifically named.

NEUROTRANSMITTERS

Acetylcholine

Acetylcholine is the neurotransmitter chemical found in the vesicles of neuromuscular junctions and in the parasympathetic system. Acetylcholine is the primary neurotransmitter of the peripheral nervous system. As the action potential in the axon reaches the neuromuscular junction, the neuromuscular junction is stimulated to release the chemical in its vesicles. The chemical diffuses across the synaptic cleft, coming in contact with receptors on the postsynaptic membrane.

Acetylcholine acts on the postsynaptic membrane briefly before it is neutralized by the enzyme acetylcholinesterase. The milliseconds during which acetylcholine is in contact with the postsynaptic membrane are enough to propagate conduction of an impulse. Acetylcholinesterase is found in abundance in skeletal muscles and blood, so it very rapidly breaks down acetylcholine into acetic acid and choline. This rapid degradation of acetylcholine ensures that only one action potential occurs at a time at the receptor sites on the postsynaptic membrane. The end products (acetic acid and choline) are resynthesized in the synaptic vesicles for use again.

The end result of the release of acetylcholine at many peripheral synapses is muscular contraction. The amount of acetylcholine released is determined in part by calcium ion diffusion into the presynaptic terminal. Calcium ions are necessary for depolarization at other peripheral synapses; therefore, it is assumed that calcium plays a similar role at all chemical synapses.

Acetylcholine is a cholinergic neurotransmitter. It is felt that more cholinergic synapses exist in the central nervous system (CNS), but they have not been positively identified.

Monoamines

The monoamines that have been identified as neurotransmitters in the CNS include the catecholamines dopamine, norepinephrine, and epinephrine and the indolamine serotonin. Catecholamines are produced in the brain and in the sympathetic ganglia from their amino acid precursor tyrosine. Serotonin is produced in the brain and other tissues from the amino acid tryptophan. The activity of the monoamine neurotransmitters in the synaptic cleft is limited by their reuptake into the presynaptic ending, where they are recycled into vesicles for future release.

Dopamine is a precursor to epinephrine and norepinephrine. Dopamine acts as an inhibitory chemical transmitter and is one of the most important chemicals involved in basal ganglionic functions (acetylcholine is the other important transmitter in basal ganglionic functions). Dopamine is decreased in the brains of patients with parkinsonism. It may play a role in eating, drinking, and sexual behavior.

Epinephrine and norepinephrine are found in adrenergic fibers of the sympathetic nervous system. In the CNS, norepinephrine cell bodies are confined to the brain stem, but their axons extend to all parts of the CNS. Epinephrine neurons are restricted to the lower brain stem.

Like dopamine, norepinephrine has been found to have inhibitory influences on postsynaptic neurons. Little is known of the action of epinephrine as a central neurotransmitter. Within the sympathetic nervous system, epinephrine and norepinephrine are found in adrenergic fibers. They exert a generalized "fight, flight, or fright" response in the body.

Serotonin is also a monoamine chemical. It is an inhibitory transmitter and is linked to slow-wave sleep patterns. Although serotonin has been implicated in a physiological role with sleep, psychotic states, pain transmission, and response to hallucinogenic drugs, little is known about its specific function.

GABA (gamma-aminobutyric acid) is a neutral amino acid that has an inhibitory effect on synaptic function. It is found in the CNS.

REFLEXES

A reflex is a stereotypical reaction of the CNS to specific sensory stimuli. Some reflexes, such as brainstem reflexes (subtentorial), are usually associated with abnormalities in pupillary and oculocephalic responses. Injury to the brainstem will produce changes in the above reflexes as well as basic physiologic functions such as respiration, blood pressure, and heart rate. There are two major types of reflexes, monosynaptic and polysynaptic.

Monosynaptic Reflex Arc

This constitutes the simplest reflex in the body (Fig. 16-4). Inside every group of muscles is a structure called a muscle spindle. The muscle spindle is made of small fibers that are bound together by afferent sensory fibers (Fig. 16-5). As a muscle spindle is stretched, an action potential develops and a sensory impulse travels to the dorsal root ganglion. From the ganglion, the impulse enters the spinal cord. In the gray matter (unmyelinated) of the spinal cord, the impulse synapses with interneurons in the anterior portion of the cord. These interneurons have efferent (motor) fibers that leave the spinal cord through the anterior (ventral) root. The efferent fibers carry an impulse back to the original muscle. The muscle contracts upon receiving this impulse.

The monosynaptic reflex arc is more important in research than in practice. The muscle stretch reflex (knee jerk) is the most commonly tested reflex.

Polysynaptic Reflex Arc

The withdrawal reflex is a common example of the polysynaptic reflex (Fig. 16-6). Afferent nerve fibers in the peripheral muscles are excited, producing an

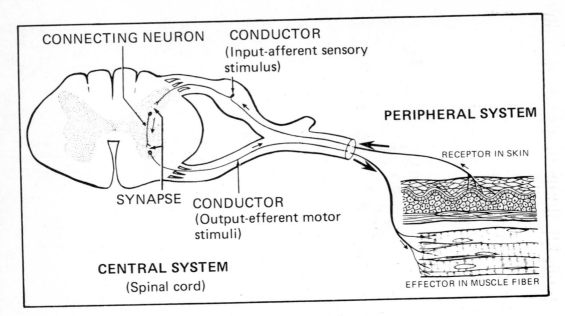

Figure 16-4. Monosynaptic reflex arc.

impulse. This impulse enters the spinal cord via a dorsal root ganglion. This excited neuron will synapse with appropriate interneurons within the gray matter of the spinal cord.

The interneurons in the anterior (ventral) horn emerge from the spinal cord through efferent (motor) fibers. These fibers transmit the motor impulse to the original muscle that produced the sensory impulse.

The muscle then contracts. There are literally hundreds of interneurons with which the impulse could and does synapse, thus the name polysynaptic reflex arc.

When impulses effect a muscular contraction, other impulses must negate the function of opposing muscle groups. For the knee to bend, extensor muscles are inhibited and concurrently flexor muscles are excited. This is termed the law of reciprocal innervation.

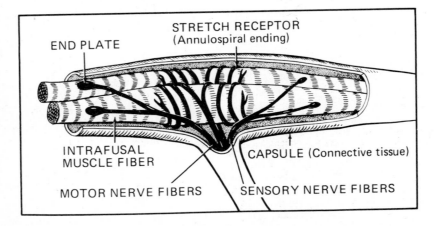

Figure 16-5. Muscle spindle.

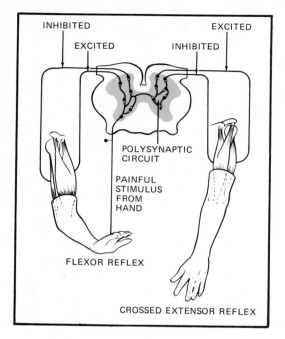

INHIBITED   EXCITED
   EXCITED   INHIBITED

POLYSYNAPTIC
CIRCUIT

PAINFUL
STIMULUS
FROM
HAND

FLEXOR REFLEX

CROSSED EXTENSOR REFLEX

Figure 16-6. Polysynaptic reflex arc.

METABOLISM IN THE BRAIN

White matter (myelinated) and gray matter (unmyelinated) have the same metabolic needs.

The cerebral need for oxygen does not decrease in a resting state. Even though it weighs only about 3 pounds (2% of body weight), brain tissue requires about 20% of the body's oxygen supply. The brain needs a constant supply of oxygen and is unable to store oxygen for future use. Energy is necessary for metabolic functions of the brain, and this energy is obtained from the oxidation of glucose. All oxidative reactions require oxygen. Hypoxia may occur without irreversible anoxic injury to brain cells. If the anoxic state lasts four or more minutes at normal body temperature, cerebral neurons are destroyed. Once destroyed, cerebral neurons cannot regenerate. The areas of the brain most sensitive to hypoxia are the cerebral hemispheres, particularly the hippocampus, which is most likely to be damaged by small amounts of decreased oxygen. Since the cerebral cortex is only six layers (cells) deep (see Fig. 15–7), the entire cerebral cortex, especially layer four, is very sensitive to de-

creases in oxygen. Damage here results in the so-called laminar cortical necrosis.

The brain stem is the area most resistant to hypoxic damage. If hypoxia occurs in this area beyond the four- or five-minute limit, irreversible coma or a persistent vegetative state usually develops.

NUTRITIONAL NEEDS

The extensive, continuous activity of the brain results in very high metabolic energy needs. Glucose, a carbohydrate, is the main source of energy (ATP) for cellular activity. Glucose and oxygen are essential for reestablishing electrochemical gradients for impulse transmission, for the synthesis of neurotransmitters, and for maintaining cellular integrity. If the cerebral glucose level is less than 70 mg/100 mL, confusion results. With a glucose level of less than 20 mg/100 mL, coma develops, followed by death (without treatment). Whereas hypoglycemia causes confusion, coma, and death, hyperglycemia does not appear to have a direct influence on nervous system functions. Certain vitamins are essential in adequate amounts to ensure normal CNS functions.

Vitamin B_1 (thiamine) is important in the Krebs cycle of energy production. Insufficient B_1, common in alcoholics, causes the Wernicke-Korsakoff syndrome, which in late stages causes cerebellar degeneration.

Vitamin B_{12} function is not understood. However, insufficient B_{12} results in a gradual degeneration of the brain, optic nerves, spinal cord (especially posterior and lateral columns), and the dorsal root entry zone of the peripheral nerves. Degeneration often starts with the spinal cord. Pernicious anemia is the dominant systemic disease with vitamin B_{12} deficiency. A deficiency is also present in alcoholism and other malnutritional states.

Pyridoxine is a coenzyme that participates in many enzymatic reactions in the CNS. Pyridoxine deficiencies produce polyneuropathies, seborrheic dermatitis, glossitis, and conjunctivitis.

Nicotinic acid is needed for synthesis of coenzymes. Insufficient nicotinic acid results in altered mentation leading to coma, extrapyramidal rigidity, and tremors of the extremities. This form of encephalopathy seems to be becoming nonexistent in the United States. There may be a relationship between inadequate nicotinic acid and pellagra.

CIRCULATORY NEEDS

The brain needs a more continuous supply of oxygenated blood, even during sleep, than any other organ, since the brain's needs are never decreased. The cerebral blood flow is determined in part by the cerebral perfusion pressure. This pressure is the difference between mean arterial (systemic) pressure and intracranial pressure (CPP = MAP − ICP). The size of the cerebrovascular system, activity, disease, fever, injury, and other factors determine the actual amount of blood needed at any given time.

Hypercapnia ($Paco_2$ > 45 mm Hg) and to a lesser extent hypoxia (Pao_2 < 60 mm Hg) will cause an arteriolar dilatation of the cerebral arteries, which increases the amount of blood flowing into the brain regardless of the actual amount needed. This may cause an increased intracranial pressure that the healthy brain can accommodate but an injured or diseased brain cannot.

Increases in intracranial pressure will result in a decrease in blood perfusion to the brain due to compression of the arteries, veins, and brain mass as a whole. The brain has its own autoregulatory mechanism that functions mainly by increasing (constriction of arteries) or decreasing (dilatation of arteries) resistance to blood flow, thus altering the diameter of the vessels. Autoregulation maintains constant blood flow over a range of perfusion pressures. The limits of autoregulation are generally thought to be a mean arterial pressure of between 50 and 150 mm Hg. This system works well until the intracranial pressure increases beyond a certain unknown point, after which compensatory mechanisms fail.

BLOOD-BRAIN BARRIER

Between the blood and brain is a barrier that controls the diffusion of substances from the blood into the extracellular fluid or the cerebrospinal fluid of the brain. The location and structure of this barrier are thought to be related to the "tight junctions" of cerebral endothelial cells. The permeability of cerebral capillaries and the choroid plexus controls the movement of specific substances.

Water, oxygen, glucose, and carbon dioxide move quickly through the blood-brain barrier. Other substances move either slowly or not at all across the barrier. This control determines the level of metabolism, the ionic composition, and the homeostasis of cerebral tissue.

In addition to a blood-brain barrier, there is a blood-cerebrospinal fluid barrier. This barrier functions like the blood-brain barrier in controlling the composition of the cerebrospinal fluid. This is a vitally important function because substances in the cerebrospinal fluid are rapidly absorbed into the interstitial brain fluid.

CHAPTER 17

The Vertebrae and the Spinal Cord: Function and Dysfunction

Editor's Note

In this chapter, the anatomy, physiology, and concepts of spinal cord dysfunction are reviewed. The CCRN exam usually has one to three questions on dysfunction or trauma associated with the spinal cord. This chapter should provide you with the information necessary to address questions about the spinal cord. Again, keep in mind that anatomy and physiology questions are usually not directly asked on the CCRN exam. For example, the number of vertebrae would not be asked. Focus your studying on the function of the cord and clinical conditions that are altered by cord injury and dysfunction.

VERTEBRAL COLUMN

The spinal cord is protected by and housed by the vertebrae. There are a total of 33 vertebrae.

Divisions of the Vertebral Column
There are eight cervical vertebrae. Some texts state that there are seven cervical vertebrae. These texts apparently count the atlas and axis as one, since they articulate directly with each other. There are 12 thoracic vertebrae, 5 lumbar and 5 sacral vertebrae, and 3 to 5 vertebrae fused as the coccygeal segment.

Typical Vertebra
The body of a typical vertebra (Fig. 17-1) is the solid portion that lies anteriorly. Opposite the vertebral body is the spinous process (the bony segment that one can feel down the back). Projecting laterally from each side of the vertebra are the transverse processes. The lamina is the curved portion of bone joining the transverse processes to the spinous process. The lamina is the most frequently fractured portion of the vertebra. The vertebrae may sustain any fracture of any type in ways that other bones in the body can. Between the vertebral body and the spinous process is the spinal foramen, the cavity through which the spinal cord passes.

Cervical Vertebrae
The cervical vertebrae are the smallest. Figure 17-2 shows the atlas vertebra (C-1), which articulates with the occipital bone and the axis vertebrae (C-2). The axis has an odontoid process (the only one) that permits C-1 to articulate directly and to provide rotation of the head. Trauma to the odontoid process is sometimes called the hangman's fracture when this process is broken and the head is no longer stabilized by C-1's articulation. If C-2 is fractured, the required force is so great that the vertebra bursts like a star. This causes multiple bone fragments that may penetrate the spinal cord nerves as well as vascular structures.

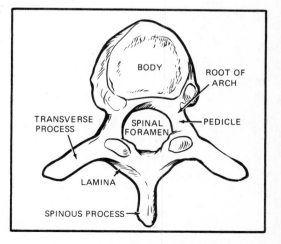

Figure 17-1. Typical vertebra.

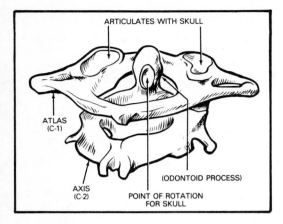

Figure 17-2. Articulation of C-1 and C-2 vertebrae.

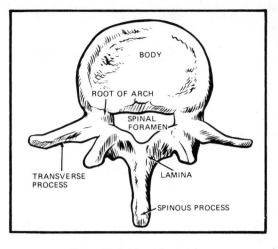

Figure 17-3. Thoracic vertebra.

Thoracic Vertebrae
The 12 thoracic vertebrae (Fig. 17-3) have points of attachment for the ribs to help support the chest musculature.

Lumbar Vertebrae
The five lumbar vertebrae (Fig. 17-4) are the largest. They support the back muscles. These vertebral discs are the most frequently herniated.

Sacral Vertebrae
The five sacral vertebrae (Fig. 17-5) are fused to form the sacrum, a frequent point of low back pain.

Coccyx Vertebrae
Depending upon the individual, three to five vertebrae are fused to form the coccyx (Fig. 17-5).

Intervertebral Discs
Between each of the lumbar, thoracic, and cervical vertebrae, excluding the atlas and axis, is an interver-

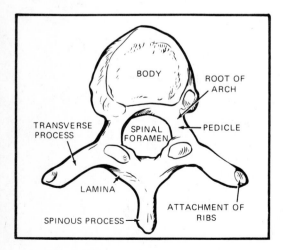

Figure 17-4. Lumbar vertebra.

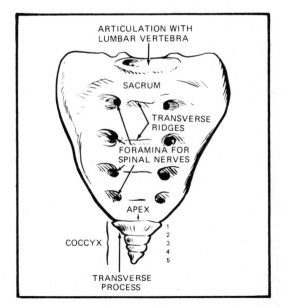

Figure 17-5. Sacral vertebrae and coccyx.

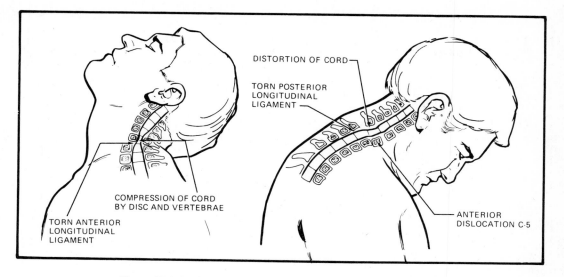

DISTORTION OF CORD

TORN POSTERIOR
LONGITUDINAL
LIGAMENT

COMPRESSION OF CORD
BY DISC AND VERTEBRAE

TORN ANTERIOR
LONGITUDINAL
LIGAMENT

ANTERIOR
DISLOCATION C-5

Figure 17-6. Hyperextension and hyperflexion of the spinal cord.

tebral disc. The disc is a fibrocartilaginous material designed to absorb the shocks or pressure between one vertebra and another. The center portion of the disc is a gelatinous layer called the nucleus pulposus. Unexpected movement or force may rupture the disc, forcing the nucleus pulposus out of position—the so-called slipped disc. When out of position, the disc may impinge upon the spinal canal, the spinal cord, or the emerging spinal nerves.

Unfortunately, it is very common for the spinal cord to be damaged by extreme hyperextension or hyperflexion forces (Fig. 17-6). Damage may occur with or without fracture of the vertebrae.

SPINAL CORD

The spinal cord is the second major component of the central nervous system (the brain is the other). The spinal cord is vital for life and is protected by vertebrae.

Location

The spinal cord (Fig. 17-7) is continuous with the medulla oblongata in the brain stem. It is located in the spinal canal of the vertebrae. The vertebrae extend from the foramen magnum to the coccyx. Within the vertebrae, the spinal cord extends from the foramen magnum to the first lumbar vertebra. The spinal cord does not extend to the lower end of the vertebral col-

umn. Its tapered end is called the conus medullaris. The cord is some 25 cm shorter than the vertebral column. The filium terminale is a group of fibers extending from the conus medullaris at the L-1 vertebral level to the first coccygeal vertebra.

Structure

The spinal cord is oval and is surrounded by the meninges that also encase the brain. Between the first lumbar and second sacral vertebrae, the arachnoid membrane enlarges somewhat to form the space known as the lumbar cistern, which is used for lumbar punctures. The spinal cord has a minute cavity in its center, the central canal. This canal is an extension of the fourth ventricle and contains cerebrospinal fluid.

The spinal cord is composed of both white (myelinated) and gray (unmyelinated) tissue. The gray matter appears (with a little imagination) to be shaped like an H that is surrounded by white matter (Fig. 17-8). The amount of gray matter varies with its location in the vertebral column. A mnemonic may help distinguish white from gray matter and myelinated from unmyelinated fibers. The fourth letter of gray is "y," as is the fourth letter of unmyelinated; thus, gray matter is unmyelinated fibers.

Gray matter is composed of nerve cells and unmyelinated fibers arranged in three columns (Fig. 17-9). The anterior gray columns are also known as the anterior horns. They contain cell bodies of efferent

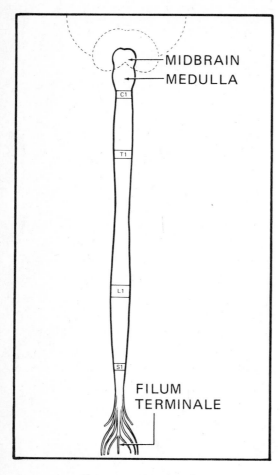

Figure 17-7. Spinal cord.

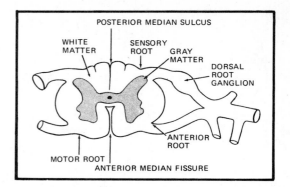

Figure 17-8. Gray and white matter of the spinal cord (cross section).

sal and ventral spinocerebellar tracts, and spinotectal tract. These tracts carry sensory impulses and are identified in Fig. 17-11.

The significant descending tracts (Fig. 17-11) are the rubrospinal tract, ventral and lateral corticospinal tracts, and tectospinal tract. These carry motor impulses and are identified in Fig. 17-11.

Lower motor neurons are spinal and cranial motor neurons that directly innervate muscles. Lesions cause flaccid paralysis, muscular atrophy, and absence of reflex responses. Upper motor neurons in the brain and spinal cord activate lower motor neurons. Lesions cause spastic paralysis and hyperactive reflexes.

Spinal Cord Injuries

Spinal cord injuries are more and more common and are a result mainly of auto accidents, diving accidents, athletic accidents, falls, and gunshot wounds. Spinal injuries may be classified by many criteria.

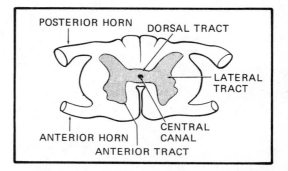

Figure 17-9. Columns (tracts) of gray matter in the spinal cord (cross section).

(motor) fibers. The middle gray columns, known as the lateral columns, contain preganglionic fibers of the autonomic nervous system. The lateral columns are largest in the upper cervical, thoracic, and midsacral regions. The posterior columns, also known as the posterior horns, contain cell bodies of afferent (sensory) fibers.

The white matter (myelinated) is arranged in three columns called the anterior, lateral, and posterior funiculi (singular, funiculus) (Fig. 17-10). Within these columns or funiculi are ascending (sensory) and descending (motor) tracts termed fasciculi.

The significant ascending tracts (Fig. 17-11) are the fasciculus gracilis, fasciculus cuneatus, lateral spinothalamic tract, anterior spinothalamic tract, dor-

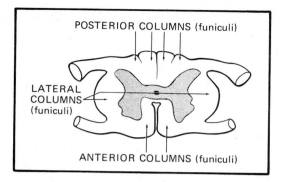

Figure 17-10. Funiculi of white matter in the spinal cord.

Classification

1. The injury may be at the cervical, thoracic, or lumbar level. Cervical injury is the most common.
2. The degree of spinal cord involvement may be either complete or incomplete. Complete cord involvement by lesion (or transection) results in total loss of sensory and motor function below the level of the lesion. This loss is a result of irreversible damage to the spinal cord. If the cervical cord is involved, quadriplegia is the common result. If the thoracic or lumbar cord is involved, paraplegia is the common result. Incomplete cord lesion involvement (or partial transection) leaves some tracts intact. The degree of sensory/motor loss varies according to the level of lesion. Three syndromes are commonly the result of incomplete lesions.

   a. The central cord syndrome is characterized by microscopic hemorrhage and edema to the central cord (Fig. 17-12). When the damage is in the cervical central cord, it is termed central cord syndrome. There is motor weakness in both the upper and lower extremities, but the weakness is much greater in the upper extremities.

   Sensory dysfunction varies according to the site of injury or lesion, generally being more pronounced in the upper extremities. Reflexes in the lower extremities may be hyperactive temporarily. Bladder dysfunction is common. This syndrome is frequently due to hyperextension of an osteoarthritic spine. It is the most common type of cord injury when there is no overt fracture or dislocation. The extent of recovery depends upon the resolution of edema

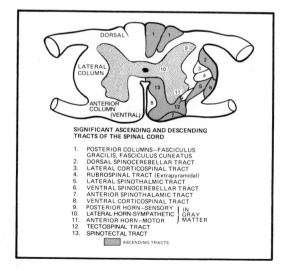

SIGNIFICANT ASCENDING AND DESCENDING TRACTS OF THE SPINAL CORD

1. POSTERIOR COLUMNS—FASCICULUS GRACILIS, FASCICULUS CUNEATUS
2. DORSAL SPINOCEREBELLAR TRACT
3. LATERAL CORTICOSPINAL TRACT
4. RUBROSPINAL TRACT (Extrapyramidal)
5. LATERAL SPINOTHALMIC TRACT
6. VENTRAL SPINOCEREBELLAR TRACT
7. ANTERIOR SPINOTHALAMIC TRACT
8. VENTRAL CORTICOSPINAL TRACT
9. POSTERIOR HORN—SENSORY } IN
10. LATERAL HORN—SYMPATHETIC } GRAY
11. ANTERIOR HORN—MOTOR } MATTER
12. TECTOSPINAL TRACT
13. SPINOTECTAL TRACT

ASCENDING TRACTS

Figure 17-11. Significant ascending and descending tracts of the spinal cord. The left half of the picture is a mirror image of the right half.

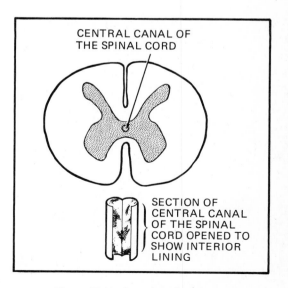

Figure 17-12. Central cord syndrome.

and the intactness of the spinal cord tracts. As improvement occurs, it proceeds from proximal to distal parts.

b. Anterior cord syndrome is characterized by injury resulting in an acute compression of the anterior portion of the spinal cord, often a flexion injury (Fig. 17-13). Compression is usually caused by a disc or bony fragment. It may also be caused by an actual destruction of the anterior cord by an anterior spinal artery occlusion caused by a thrombus. Symptoms include immediate anterior paralysis that is complete from the injury or compression down. Hypesthesia (decreased sensation) and hypalgesia (decreased pain sensation) occur below the level of injury. Since the posterior cord tracts are not injured, there are sensations of touch, position vibration, and motion. If the syndrome is caused by compression of the anterior cord from bony fragments, surgical decompression is indicated.

c. Brown-Séquard's syndrome is due to transection or lesion of one-half of the spinal cord (Fig. 17-14). There is a loss of motor function (paralysis) and position and vibratory sense, as well as vasomotor paralysis on the same (ipsilateral) side and below the hemisection. On the opposite (contralateral) side of the hemisection, there is loss of pain and temperature sensation below the level of the lesion or hemisection.

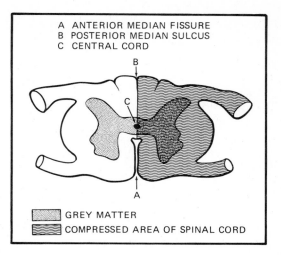

Figure 17-14. Brown-Séquard's syndrome.

3. Spinal cord injuries may be categorized as stable (vertebral column is aligned) or unstable (vertebral column is not aligned).
4. Injuries may be classified according to the injury to the vertebral column. Such types include dislocation, subluxation, compression fracture, and hangman's fracture (C-2).
5. Injuries may be classified in relation to the specific level of injury. These injuries are summarized in Table 17-1.
6. The final classification of spinal cord injuries is in relation to the mechanism involved, i.e., either hyperextension or hyperflexion. Rarely, rotational injuries occur.

Spinal cord injuries are frequently associated with head or other systems trauma.

Treatment of spinal cord injuries involves initial stabilization of the spinal column and eventual immobilization. The spinal column can be immobilized by cervical traction (such as with cervical tongs) or halo devices anchored to upper body casts. Many experimental therapies, such as early administration of high dose methyprednisolone, are being developed for the treatment of spinal injuries although it is unlikely these would be addressed on the CCRN exam.

Spinal Shock. Spinal shock is a state that exists when irreversible damage has occurred to the spinal cord, resulting in areflexia and flaccid paralysis below the level of injury.

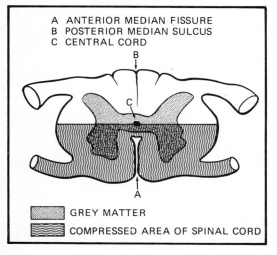

Figure 17-13. Anterior cord syndrome.

TABLE 17-1. CLASSIFICATION OF INJURY ACCORDING TO SPECIFIC VERTEBRAL LEVEL

Injury Level	Intact Function	Lost Function
Below L-2	Mixed motor/sensory, depending on intact nerve fibers	Mixed motor/sensory; possibly bladder, bowels, and sexual functioning
T-1 to L-1 or L-2	Arm function	Leg functions; bladder, bowels, and sexual functioning
C-7, C-8	Triceps muscle, head rotation, respiration	No intrinsic muscles of hand; no other function retained
C-6, C-7	Biceps muscle, head rotation, respiration	No triceps; no other function retained
C-5, C-6	Gross arm movement, head rotation, diaphragmatic respiration	No other function retained
C-4, C-5	Head rotation, diaphragmatic respiration	No other function intact
C-3, C-4	Head rotation	No other function intact (many die)
C-1, C-2	None	Most die

Spinal shock may affect any and all body systems and is more severe in cervical vertebral injuries than other vertebral injuries. The duration of spinal shock is two days to several months. One knows that spinal shock is resolving when flaccid paralysis becomes a spastic paralysis and reflexes return.

Complications. Immediate postinjury problems are (1) maintaining a patent airway, (2) maintaining adequate ventilation, (3) maintaining an adequate circulating blood volume, and (4) preventing an extension of cord damage.

Respiratory System. Cervical injury or fracture above C-4 presents problems in that total respiratory function is lost. Artificial ventilation will be required to keep the patient alive; however, most of these patients will die. Injury or fracture of C-4 or the lower cervical vertebrae will result in diaphragmatic breathing if the phrenic nerve is functioning. Hypoventilation almost always occurs with diaphragmatic respirations because there is a decrease in vital capacity and tidal volume.

Since cervical fractures or severe injuries cause a paralysis of abdominal musculature and frequently intercostal musculature, the patient is unable to cough effectively enough to remove secretions; this leads to atelectasis and pneumonia. Artificial airways provide direct access for pathogens, so bronchial hygiene and chest physiotherapy become extremely important. If

multiple trauma is involved, a neurogenic pulmonary edema may result from the sudden changes in thoracic pressures at the time of the injury. The occurrence of pulmonary edema (as opposed to neurogenic pulmonary edema) is probably due to fluid overload.

Cardiovascular System. Any cord transection above the level of T-5 abolishes the influence of the sympathetic nervous system. Consequently, immediate problems are bradycardia and hypotension. If the bradycardia is only slight, close cardiac monitoring may reveal a stable cardiac condition. Junctional escape beats may be observed, and a junctional rhythm may become established. If the bradycardia is marked, appropriate medications to increase the heart rate and avoid hypoxia will be necessary.

With the abolition of the influences of the sympathetic nervous system, vasodilatation occurs, decreasing venous return of blood to the heart. This decreases cardiac output, and hypotension results. Intravenous fluids may resolve the problem, or vasopressor drugs may be required.

Renal System. Urinary retention is a common development in acute spinal injuries and spinal shock. The bladder is hyperirritable. There is a loss of inhibition of reflex from the brain. Consequently, the patient will void small amounts of urine frequently. In spite of this, the bladder becomes distended since this phenomenon is actually urinary retention with overflow. Urinary retention increases the chance of infection. In addition, urinary calculi are likely to develop in a distended bladder retaining urine. Catheterization is indicated.

Gastrointestinal System. If the cord transection has occurred above T-5, the loss of sympathetic innervation may lead to the development of an ileus or gastric distension. A nasogastric tube to intermittent suction may relieve the gastric distension, and standard treatment will be used for an ileus. A common occurrence in the past has been the development of biochemical stress ulcers due to excessive release of hydrochloric acid in the stomach. An H_2 antagonist is frequently used to prevent the occurrence of these ulcers during the initial extreme body stress. Because of the absence of clinical signs, intra-abdominal bleeding may occur and be difficult to diagnose. There will be no pain, tenderness, guarding, or such. Continued hypotension despite vigorous treatment is suspicious. Ex-

panding girth of the abdomen may sometimes, but not always, be ascertainable. If the rectum is not emptied on a regular basis, the patient may develop a fecal impaction.

Musculoskeletal System. The integrity of the patient's skin is of primary importance. The deterioration of denervated skin can occur very quickly, leading to major, life-threatening infection. The use of Roto-Beds (Fig. 17-15) and their variations helps to prevent breakdown of the skin. A certain degree of muscle atrophy will occur during the flaccid paralysis state, while contractures tend to occur during the spastic paralysis stage.

Poikilothermism is the adjustment of the body temperature toward the room temperature. This adaptation occurs in these injuries because the interruption of the sympathetic nervous system prevents its temperature-controlling fibers to send impulses that will reach the hypothalamus.

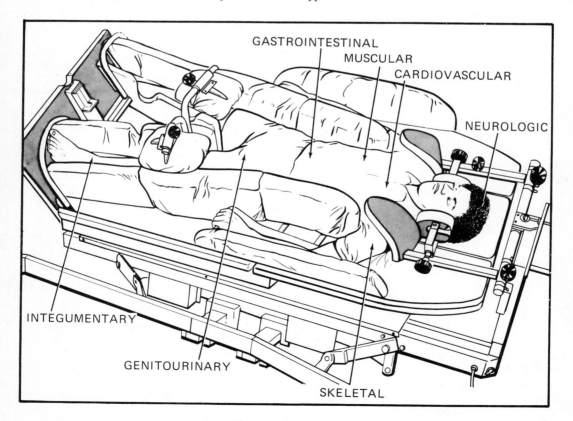

Figure 17-15. Roto-Bed.

Metabolic Needs. Correcting an existing acid-base disturbance and maintaining acid-base balance will promote the function of other body systems. Recall that nasogastric suctioning may lead to alkalosis, and decreased perfusion may lead to acidosis. Electrolytes must be monitored until a normal diet is resumed and suctioning has been discontinued. A positive nitrogen balance and a high-protein diet will help prevent skin breakdown and infections and will help decrease the rate of muscle atrophy.

Nursing Intervention. The primary nursing intervention is ensuring a patent airway at all times to provide for adequate ventilation. Most patients with cervical fractures will have an endotracheal tube or a tracheostomy. Frequent, gentle suctioning of the nasopharynx, oropharynx, and endotracheal tube or tracheostomy is imperative to help prevent hypoxia secondary to retained secretions. However, suctioning must not exceed 10 to 15 seconds, and the patient should be hyperventilated before and after the procedure to prevent a cardiac arrest, which may occur if hypoxia develops and the patient has a bradycardia or junctional rhythm. Chest physiotherapy protocols should be followed according to neurological and cardiovascular parameters. The patient's vital capacity, tidal volume, and arterial blood gases should be carefully and frequently monitored until the patient is stable and ventilatory support is no longer needed.

Cardiovascular monitoring of dysrhythmias and hypotension is essential. Dysrhythmias may require standard treatment or only continued close monitoring. Hypotension is often controlled with fluids intravenously, which requires that the nurse monitor the patient for the development of pulmonary edema.

The prevention of extension of cord injury is the next major nursing responsibility. If traction is employed, the rope knots should be taped, weights hanging freely, and traction lines should be kept straight or as positioned by the physician.

Renal status is usually monitored hourly in the first few days following injury. The amount of intravenous fluids necessary to prevent hypotension is usually sufficient to prevent renal complications of oliguria or anuria unless there is multiple trauma involving the kidneys. The common renal problem after vertebral and cord injury above the sacral level is urinary retention. A Foley catheter is often used in the early stages of the injury. If a Foley catheter is not inserted, intermittent catheterization is needed to ensure that an excessive urinary volume is not retained in the bladder, leading to further problems.

Gastrointestinal interventions include initial drainage of the stomach contents, after which the nasogastric tube is usually connected to intermittent suction since gastric distension occurs and acid secretions are increased in the first few days. Contents suctioned should be routinely tested for blood since biochemical stress ulcers may occur.

Musculoskeletal needs of the patient include proper body alignment, support of bony prominences to prevent skin breakdown, and frequent turning (unless the patient is on a Roto-Bed) to promote circulation and induce comfort. During the flaccid paralysis stage, extremities should be maintained in a functional position. During the spastic stage of the paralysis, medications and some physical therapy may help control the spasms.

Metabolic needs of the patient are initially met with intravenous fluids. As soon as the patient is stabilized, tube feedings are often started. Depending upon the site of the injury and the residual deficits, the patient may be able to start oral feedings relatively soon after the injury. Rarely is hyperalimentation used unless there are protracted multiple trauma injuries.

AUTONOMIC DYSREFLEXIA

Autonomic dysreflexia, also called autonomic hyperreflexia, is a life-threatening condition requiring immediate resolution.

The most common precipitating etiology is a distended bladder or rectum. Contraction of the bladder or rectum, stimulation of the skin, or stimulation of the pain receptors may also cause autonomic hyperreflexia.

Symptoms include hypertension, blurred vision, throbbing headache, marked diaphoresis above the level of the lesion, bradycardia, piloerection (body hair erect) due to pilomotor spasm, nasal congestion, and nausea.

Pathophysiology of this condition involves the stimulation of sensory receptors below the level of cord lesion. The intact autonomic system reacts with a reflex arteriolar spasm that increases blood pressure. Baroreceptors in cerebral vessels, the carotid sinus, and the aorta sense the hypertension and stimulate the parasympathetic system. The heart rate is decreased, but the visceral and peripheral vessels do not dilate because efferent impulses cannot pass through the cord lesion.

Nursing interventions in this very serious emergency are notification of the physician, assessment to determine the cause, and elevation of the head of the bed or placement of the patient into a sitting position if possible. Blood pressure should be monitored every three to five minutes. Abdominal palpation for a distended bladder is done very gently to avoid increasing the stimulus. Catheter irrigation performed very slowly and gently may open a plugged catheter. A digital rectal exam should be done only after application of a Nupercainal-type ointment to decrease rectal stimulation and to prevent an increase of symptoms. If signs and symptoms persist after the bladder and bowel have been thoroughly checked, the next step is to check the skin for irritation.

CHAPTER 18

Acute Head Injuries and Craniotomies

Editor's Note

The CCRN exam may have one to three questions on the material covered in this chapter. The primary focus of this chapter is content from the exam such as head injury and space-occupying lesions (brain tumors).

ACUTE HEAD INJURIES

Acute head injuries are almost always the result of violence or automobile accidents. A history is often very difficult to obtain, but it can be vital in establishing potential damage done by acceleration/deceleration forces. Acceleration injuries may be called coup (pronounced coo), and deceleration forces may be called contracoup.

Examination of the Patient

Airway. Always establish a patent airway. Use only an oral or nasopharyngeal airway, not an endotracheal tube, until the cross-table lateral x rays confirm that there is no neck fracture. If the oral airway does not provide a patent airway, an emergency tracheostomy or cricoidotomy is preferable to manipulating the neck for insertion of an endotracheal tube if an x-ray examination has not been done.

Cardiac and Respiratory Function. Continually monitor these systems to ensure early intervention in cases of dysfunction. Inadequate function of either system may result in extension of neurological impairment.

Shock. Monitor for signs of impending shock. Be prepared to intervene by establishing an intravenous line while awaiting specific instructions from the physician. If shock occurs, it is not due to intracranial bleeding if the cranium is intact. There is insufficient room in the cranium to contain the volume of blood necessary to cause hypovolemic shock.

Abdomen. Palpate for involuntary guarding and increasing girth, which may indicate an intra-abdominal hemorrhage leading to shock.

Long Bones. Long bones such as the femur and other extremity bones need to be checked for fractures. Such fractures may lead to fat emboli, shock, and other complications.

Neurological Examination

Scalp. Check for tears and/or swelling, which may indicate a subgaleal hematoma.

Face. Palpate eye orbits, nose, teeth, maxilla, and mandible for facial fractures. Some facial fractures may provide for leakage of cerebrospinal fluid (CSF), and this would be an entry port for infection.

Ears. Blood in the external canal usually indicates a basal skull fracture.

Carotid Arteries. Palpate each carotid artery by itself to check for cerebral hemorrhage. If the carotids cannot be palpated, check for palpation of the superficial temporal arteries, which are a branch of the external carotids.

Mentation. There are five possible states or levels of consciousness. The definition and/or progression may differ in various institutions.

1. Alert—The patient is oriented to person, place, and time.

2. Lethargic—The patient prefers to sleep; when the patient is aroused, the degree of alertness or confusion is variable.
3. Obtunded—The patient can be aroused with minimal stimulation but will drift off to sleep quickly.
4. Stuporous—The patient is aroused only by constant, deep, and usually painful stimuli. The patient may respond by some attempt to withdraw, moan, or exhibit decerebrate or decorticate positioning.
5. Coma—The patient cannot be aroused.

The Glasgow Coma Scale (Table 18-1) is one of the standards for use in identifying levels of consciousness (mentation) and for prognosis of the outcome of the injury. Level of consciousness is the first neurological test performed in head injuries.

Cranial Nerves. Some of the 12 cranial nerves can be checked during routine patent care and during neurological checks.

II. Optic nerve (this will be covered in detail at the end of the chapter). The most common result of injury to the optic tract is homonymous hemianopsia. When looking at the optic disc, one usually sees a sharp, clear outline. If pulsations in the veins of the optic disc are visible, there is usually no increased intracranial pressure. Papilledema is present when the head of the optic nerve appears raised or increased (bulging) instead of flat.

III. Oculomotor nerve. This controls four of the six eye muscles (exceptions are the lateral rectus and superior oblique). The parasympathetic nerves cause pupil constriction. The sympathetic nerves cause pupil dilatation.

IV. Trochlear nerve. This controls the superior oblique muscle. It turns the eye down and out.

V. Trigeminal nerve. Cornea sensation provides the sensory side of arc for corneal reflex. The seventh nerve (facial) provides the motor side of arc.

VI. Abducens nerve. This controls the lateral rectus muscle. It turns the eye out.

VII. Facial nerve. It exits the skull through the bone in the mastoid area. It controls the muscles of facial expression and plays a part in the production of tears.

X. Vagus nerve. This controls palate deviation. If the nerve is damaged, the uvula deviates away from the side of the paralysis. In vagal nerve paralysis, there is ipsilateral paralysis of the palate, pharynx, and larynx muscles. The soft palate at rest is usually lower on the affected side, and if the patient says "ah," it elevates on the intact side.

XI. (Spinal) accessory nerve. It turns the head by use of sternocleidomastoid muscles.

XII. Hypoglossal nerve. This controls tongue movement. If this nerve is damaged, the patient cannot move the tongue from side to side, and tongue protrusion results in deviation toward the side of nerve damage.

TABLE 18-1. GLASGOW COMA SCALE

Eye Opening (E)	Best Motor Response (M)	Verbal Response (V)
Spontaneous = 4	Obeys = 6	Oriented = 5
To speech = 3	Localizes = 5	Confused conversation = 4
To pain = 2	Withdraws = 4	Inappropriate words = 3
No response = 1	Abnormal Flexion = 3	Incomprehensible sounds = 2
	Extension = 2	No response = 1
	No response = 1	

Motor Function. Check whether the patient moves all extremities voluntarily and equally. Note a one-sided weakness. If muscle weakness is suspected, have the patient close the eyes and extend the arms directly in front. If there is a muscle weakness, there will be a drifting downward of the weakened extremity. Usually, there is no spasticity immediately after an injury. Flaccidity is usually present for about ten days.

Sensation. In trauma, patients usually respond only to pain. The response to sensation may include decorticate or decerebrate positioning in the unconscious patient.

Classification of Injury

Closed Head Injuries. The scalp is intact. The injury can be concussion, contusion, and/or skull fracture.

Concussion. There is an elimination of consciousness due to blunt trauma to the head by an accelerative or decelerative force. Some authorities place artificial time limits on unconsciousness to differentiate concussion from contusion or coma. Clinically, duration of unconsciousness may alter the classification of the injury, but the primary consideration is that of neurological deficits. Concussions usually clear spontaneously after varying time intervals, with the patient having no residual neurological deficit other than total amnesia for the time of unconsciousness. The patient with a mild to moderate concussion will have recovered consciousness within about 12 hours (as the accepted standard). It may be two or three days before the patient can recall correctly all factors leading to the concussion.

Contusion. As with concussion, there is an immediate elimination of consciousness due to accelerative or decelerative blunt trauma forces to the head. These forces propel the brain against the rigid cranium (the coup force). With initial impact, the brain is then rotated or thrown back in the opposite direction (the contracoup force) (Fig. 18-1). This trauma invariably results in cerebral bruising and edema. If the forces are strong enough, lacerations and scattered intracerebral hemorrhages may occur. These usually occur along the axis line of the coup and contracoup forces. In severe contusion, subarachnoid hemorrhage may occur, resulting in coma. Mild contusions will clear as the bruising and edema resolve, leaving no neurological deficit. Severe contusions that do not resolve, as indicated by the patient remaining comatose, indicate that the original bruising or lacerations caused a necrosis of brain tissue (possibly secondary to prolonged cerebral hypoxia at the injury sites).

Skull Fractures. Skull fractures are usually classified as linear, depressed, or basilar. A linear skull fracture that does not tear the dura mater will heal without treatment. If the linear fracture occurs over the temporal lobe and tears the dura mater (Fig. 18-2), there is a chance that the middle meningeal artery will also be

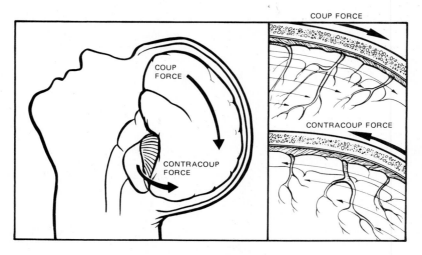

Figure 18-1. Coup and contracoup forces.

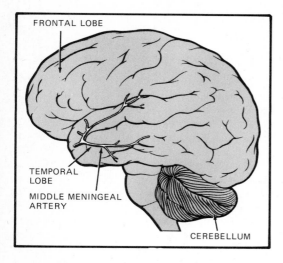

FRONTAL LOBE

TEMPORAL LOBE

MIDDLE MENINGEAL ARTERY

CEREBELLUM

Figure 18-2. Linear skull fracture over the middle meningeal artery.

torn. This constitutes a medical emergency, since the bleeding is arterial (commonly known as an acute epidural hematoma). The fracture may tear the dura mater over a venous sinus, resulting in a slow bleeding causing a chronic (nonacute) epidural hematoma. A depressed skull fracture that is not depressed more than the thickness of the skull is usually just monitored. However, a depressed skull fracture greater than the thickness of the skull (usually more than 5 to 7 mm) requires surgery to relieve the compression. If the dura is torn, bone fragments may have entered brain tissue, requiring removal, and the chance of infection is greatly increased.

With a basilar skull fracture, there is a high risk of injury to cranial nerves, infections, and residual neurological deficits due to coup and contracoup forces (Fig. 18-3). Basilar fractures may occur in the anterior or posterior fossa. CSF draining from the nose (rhinorrhea) or the ear canal (otorrhea) is a sign of basilar fracture. The "battle sign" is an area of ecchymosis over the mastoid projection and indicates either a temporal or basilar fracture in the posterior fossa. "Raccoon eyes" are a sign of bleeding into the paranasal sinuses, with ecchymosis developing around the eyes. This indicates a basilar fracture in the anterior fossa. Other symptoms of basilar fracture include tinnitus, facial paralysis, hearing difficulty, nystagmus, and conjugate deviation gaze. Patients with rhinorrhea will

complain of a salty taste as the CSF drains into the pharynx. Otorrhea can be tested with Tes-tape for glucose. If glucose is present, the drainage is CSF. Severe neurological deficits are common with basilar fractures.

Compound Injuries. Compound injuries include a laceration of the scalp with a head injury or skull fracture. If there is a laceration with a head injury (depressed fracture), surgery is usually performed immediately because of the threat of infection.

Intracranial Mass Lesions

Acute Epidural Hematoma. Epidural hematomas are a true neurosurgical emergency. They occur at the time of the injury (Fig. 18-4) and are usually associated with a temporal or parietal skull fracture with laceration of the middle meningeal artery (and often vein). There is usually a loss of consciousness, which may be followed by a brief period (up to four to six hours) of lucidity and then coma. During the lucid period, nausea and vomiting often occur. Other signs include ipsilateral oculomotor paralysis, contralateral hemiparesis/hemiplegia, and positive Babinski reflexes.

In one type of epidural hematoma, the linear fracture occurs across the sagittal sinus or the transverse sinus. In this instance, venous blood oozes into the area above the dura mater, producing a chronic epidural hematoma. Symptoms may be delayed for several days.

Subdural Hematomas. There are two types of subdural hematomas, acute and chronic. In the acute subdural hematoma (Fig. 18-5), symptoms may occur from the first two or three days up to two weeks (subacute subdural hematoma). The hematoma consists of some gel and some xanthochromic liquid. Symptoms include headaches, slowness in thinking, confusion, and sometimes agitation. These symptoms progressively worsen. Acute subdural hematomas usually present with signs of increasing intracranial pressure, decreasing level of consciousness, and ipsilateral oculomotor paralysis with contralateral hemiparesis.

In the chronic subdural hematoma, a period of weeks may follow the injury before symptoms occur. These symptoms include giddiness, exaggeration of certain personality traits, confusion, occasionally headaches, and rarely a seizure. The CSF may be clear, bloody, or xanthochromic. Intracranial pressure may be normal, elevated, or decreased. If symptoms do not

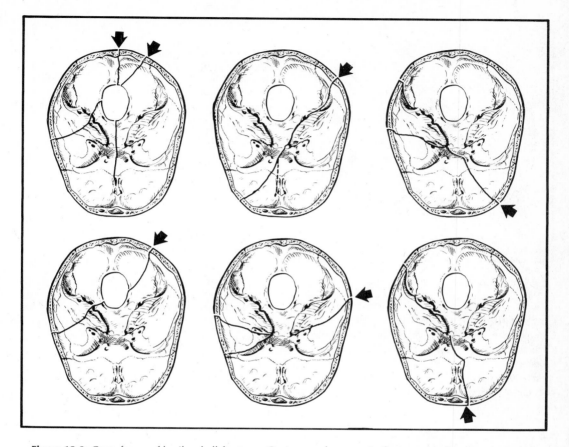

Figure 18-3. Coup forces of basilar skull fractures. Contracoup forces go in the opposite direction along similar paths.

occur for several weeks, a membrane forms around the subdural hematoma, walling it off from the rest of the brain. (In some cases, this walled-off section will calcify.)

Subdural hematoma may occur spontaneously without any form of injury in patients on anticoagulant therapy or in those with clotting dysfunction. A CAT scan will provide a diagnosis. Surgery is the treatment of choice in both forms of subdural hematomas.

Intracerebral Hemorrhage. Many intracerebral hemorrhages occur as hypertensive strokes (Fig. 18-6). Other causes include skull fracture, penetrating trauma (bullets), contracoup decelerative forces, and systemic diseases, such as leukemias and aplastic anemias. If the hemorrhage occurs in the internal capsule of the brain, paralysis results. If the hemorrhage occurs in the

dominant hemisphere, dysfunction is variable, dependent upon the location of hemorrhage. Signs and symptoms include nausea, vomiting, dizziness, headache, signs of increasing intracranial pressure, and a contralateral hemiplegia. A delayed intracerebral hemorrhage may occur hours to days after a closed head injury.

Subarachnoid Hemorrhage. This may occur after trauma due to hypertension with atherosclerosis or due to a congenital aneurysm or arteriovenous malformation. Symptoms usually include headache, dizziness, tinnitus, facial pain (pressure on the fifth cranial nerve), ptosis, a unilaterally dilated pupil, nuchal rigidity, and hemiparesis or hemiplegia. Areas and function affected by a subarachnoid hemorrhage on the dominant hemisphere are shown in Fig. 18-7.

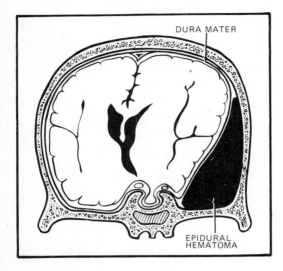

Figure 18-4. Epidural hematoma.

Complications of Closed Head Injuries

Complications include cerebral edema, hydrocephalus, seizures, increased intracranial pressure, diabetes insipidus, and residual neurologic deficits. Metabolic complications include respiratory insufficiency, infection, and systemic dysfunction as a result of associated trauma.

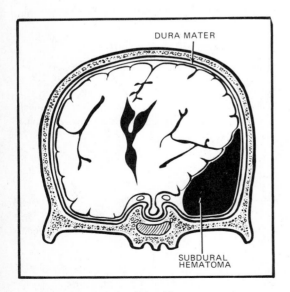

Figure 18-5. Subdural hematoma.

Complications of Intracranial Hemorrhage

Respiratory hypoxia, secondary to the intracranial hemorrhage, causes hypoxemia and hypercapnia. This results in an increased cerebral blood flow, which increases intracranial pressure. The increased pressure results in neurologic dysfunctions. Subarachnoid hemorrhage may occur because of the increased pressure or trauma, and a hydrocephalus may result. If the hypothalamus or pituitary gland is affected, diabetes insipidus will most likely occur. Biochemical stress ulcers are common and are frequently associated with electrolyte disturbances. Dependent upon the site and degree of injury, seizures may develop. Infections, both cerebrospinal and respiratory, are continuous threats.

Complications of Intraventricular Hemorrhage

These patients usually die. A frequent complication is acute hydrocephalus with increased intracranial pressure. A long-term complication is a communicating hydrocephalus. A drain may be placed. A rising Pco_2 will dilate cerebral vessels, increasing blood flow and pressure. For these reasons, the Pco_2 is maintained at between 25 and 30 mm Hg.

Nursing Intervention

The primary nursing intervention after assurance of a patent airway and the prevention of hypoxia is the frequent neurological assessment. Signs of increasing intracranial pressure may be treated with osmotic diuretics, hyperventilation, diuretics, or drainage of CSF via intraventricular cannulas. Nursing interventions include facilitating venous drainage by elevating the head of the bed 15 to 30 degrees and maintaining the patient's head in a neutral position, avoiding hypoxemia or hypercarpea with suctioning procedures, preventing hyperthermia and shivering, and avoiding Valsalva maneuvers. Intracranial pressure monitoring may be instituted. In some centers, barbiturate coma therapy may be utilized.

Monitoring vital signs and maintaining fluid balance and accurate intake and output records will help in evaluating treatment modalities aimed at stabilizing the patient. Standard procedures to prevent infections are employed.

Diagnostic Tests and Findings

Computerized axial tomography (CAT scan or CT) is the premier diagnostic test for head injuries. It will

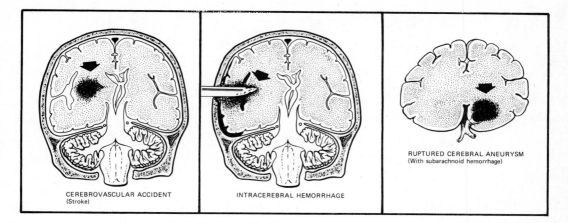

Figure 18-6. Examples of intracerebral hemorrhages.

reveal whether, (1) air has entered the brain from fractures of the eye, mastoid, or sinuses, (2) blood is present in brain tissue or in the ventricular system, (3) blood is on the surface of the brain or in the basal cisterns, (4) ventricles are of normal size and in normal position, and (5) the pineal gland has calcified and is in normal position.

Lumbar puncture is contraindicated by increased intracranial pressure and is rarely done in the diagnosis of head injuries.

Arterial blood gases in intracranial hematoma reveal respiratory alkalosis (due to hyperventilation). Metabolic acidosis may occur if the patient is in shock, is hypoxic, or has a high level of physical activity (combativeness will produce lactic acidosis, as does decerebrate posturing).

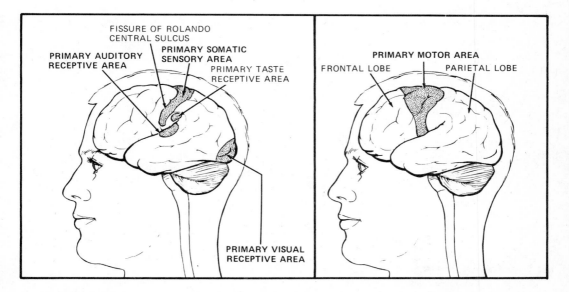

Figure 18-7. Areas and functions affected by subarachnoid hemorrhage. (**A**) Somatic sensory areas. (**B**) Primary motor area (strip). Because of rapidly increased intracranial pressures of the subarachnoid hemorrhage, the entire brain can be affected.

In closed head injuries, skull x-ray, brain scan, and angiogram studies may be essentially normal. A CAT scan may show cerebral edema and areas of petechial hemorrhage in severe contusions. Hydrocephalus may be present. The echoencephalogram has a high percentage of false results.

In intracranial hematomas, a CAT scan will show increased density that indicates the presence, location, and extent of the hematoma. Skull films may show fractures or increased intracranial pressure, a calcified pineal gland, or a choroid plexus shifted from midline. Cerebral angiography may reveal an avascular mantle with displacement or stretching of vessels. Cervical spine x rays may show injury. A brain scan may show increased uptake of isotope in the area of hematoma or tumor. An echoencephalogram may reveal a shift of midline structures and is reserved for use in diagnosing the cause of coma in patients for whom other tests have failed to reveal the cause.

VISUAL PATHWAY DEFECTS

Visual field defects may occur due to cranial trauma, various other pathologies, or craniotomies. Figure 18-8 demonstrates the most common visual field defects. The key to interpreting visual defects seen in Fig. 20-8 is that the left eye is on the left and the right eye is on the right in the figure. The image is not reversed as with heart drawings.

Visual images from the peripheral field (temporal) hit on the nasal side of each retina. Fibers from the nasal side of each retina carry the visual impulses along the optic nerve toward the optic tract. Just prior to the optic tract, these fibers cross (at the optic chiasm). They then continue on the inside of the optic tract through the optic radiation to the end of the optic tract.

Visual images from the central (nasal) field of vision hit on the outer, temporal side of each retina. Fibers from the outer side of the each retina carry the impulses to the optic nerve and follow the optic nerve tract on the outside, through the optic radiation to the end of the tract. Lesions between the eye and the point where nerve fibers cross cause a blind eye. Lesions of the eye itself will also cause unilateral blindness.

A lesion at the point where the optic nerve fibers cross (the optic chiasm) will result in bitemporal blindness. Images from the periphery of both eyes are blocked, resulting in bitemporal blindness.

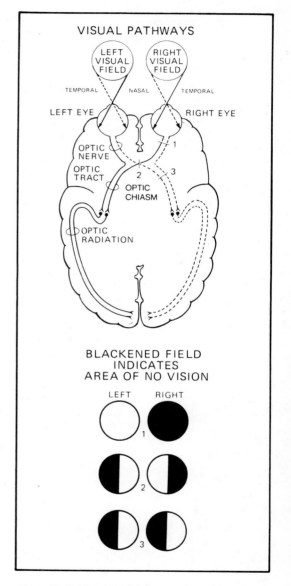

Figure 18-8. Visual field defects. (Adapted from B. Bates, *A Guide to Physical Examination*, Philadelphia: J. B. Lippincott, p. 49, 1974. Reprinted with permission of J. B. Lippincott.)

A lesion of the fibers of the right optic tract blocks visual images on the same side of each eye. This is a left homonymous (same side) hemianopsia (one-half the visual field).

In the same way, a lesion of fibers of the left optic tract blocks visual images on the same side of each eye. In this case, a right homonymous (same side) hemianopsia (one-half the visual field) exists. These are the two most common visual defects found associated with optic tract injuries.

A lesion may occur in the optic radiation. If the lesion is completely across the optic radiation, a homonymous hemianopsia develops. However, if the lesion affects only the outer fibers, a homonymous quadrantic defect occurs.

CRANIOTOMIES

Craniotomies are performed for many reasons. Postoperative care includes routine postoperative care plus:

1. Neurological monitoring compares pre- and postoperative functions, right side-to-left side function, and hour-to-hour functions.
2. Pain control may be achieved with codeine and or other narcotic analgesics. Careful neurological monitoring is necessary.
3. Intracranial pressure must be maintained within the normal range. This is achieved by the administration of glucocorticoids (however controversial), by diuretic therapy, by elevating the head of the bed 15 to 30°, and by keeping Pco_2 between 25 and 35 mm Hg.
4. Patent drainage tubes, which may be used for 24 to 48 hours, help control intracranial pressure and help monitor the type and amount of drainage.
5. A clear drainage through dressings may be CSF and should be reported to the physician immediately.
6. Stress ulcers (also known as Cushing's ulcers) are a common occurrence. They may be treated and/or prevented with use of H_2 antagonists and/or antacids.
7. Cardiovascular status is monitored, since certain head injuries cause a bradycardia. Bradycardia may be a precursor to other dysrhythmias and cardiac failure. Intravenous fluid needs are calculated daily to prevent fluid overload and to maintain electrolyte balance.

Diabetes insipidus occurs with some head injuries and with other cerebral pathologies. This condition is covered in Chapter 34.

CHAPTER 19

Meningitis, Guillain-Barré Syndrome, and Myasthenia Gravis

Editor's Note

With respect to infectious diseases of the neurologic system, the CCRN exam is more likely to address meningitis than myasthenia gravis and Guillain-Barré syndrome. As you read this chapter, focus on the infectious process of the neurologic system. It will help to have a fundamental understanding of the other conditions discussed, although they are unlikely to be included in the CCRN exam. Expect one to three questions on the test from content in this chapter.

MENINGITIS

Definition

Meningitis is an acute infection of the pia and arachnoid membrane surrounding the brain and the spinal cord. Therefore, meningitis is always a cerebrospinal infection.

Pathophysiology

A pathogenic organism gains access to the pia-arachnoid space and causes an inflammatory reaction in the pia and arachnoid, in the cerebrospinal fluid (CSF), and in the ventricles of the brain, since these are all communicating structures. The first response is a hyperemia of the meningeal vessels, followed by the infiltration of neutrophils into the subarachnoid space. An exudate forms and very quickly enlarges, covering the base of the brain and extending through the subarachnoid space and into the sheaths of cranial and spinal nerves. Polymorphonuclear leukocytes attempt to control the invading pathogen. Within a few days, leukocytes and histiocytes increase in number in an attempt to "wall off" the exudate from the pathogen or

its toxins. Toward the end of the second week, the cellular exudate has formed two layers. The outer layer is composed of polymorphonuclear leukocytes and fibrin directly under the arachnoid membrane. The inner layer is composed of lymphocytes, plasma cells, and macrophages and is next to the pia.

With appropriate drug therapy destroying the pathogen, these two layers begin to resolve. The outer cellular layer against the arachnoid disappears. If the infection was arrested quickly enough, the inner layer will also disappear. However, if the infection lasts for several weeks, the inner layer, which contains fibrin, forms a permanent fibrous structure over the meninges. This produces a thickened, often cloudy arachnoid membrane and causes adhesions between the pia and arachnoid membranes.

The adhesions and prior inflammation result in congestion of tissues and blood vessels. A degeneration of nerve cells follows, eventually resulting in congestion of adjacent brain tissue. This congestion causes cortical irritation and increased intracranial pressure. Cerebral edema may lead to hydrocephalus. If uninterrupted, a progression of vasculitis with cortical necrosis, petechial hemorrhage within the brain, hydrocephalus, and cranial nerve damage occurs.

Etiology

Organisms obtain access to the subarachnoid space through penetrating head injuries, basal skull fractures with a torn dura mater, intracranial pressure monitoring, cranial surgery, mastoiditis, acute otitis media, lumbar punctures, injury to the paranasal sinuses, and sepsis. The organism may be viral or bacterial. The most common bacterium is the meningococcus. After neurological surgery, *Staphylococcus aureus* or *S. epidermidis* is a common bacterial contaminant. In children, the bacterium is *Haemophilus influenzae*. Other bacteria include streptococci, pneumococci, and occasionally the tuberculous organism.

Clinical Presentation

Suspect meningitis if a fever, severe headache, and nuchal rigidity (resistance to flexion of the neck) exist. Positive Kernig's and Brudzinski's signs, photophobia, decreased sensorium, and signs of increased intracranial pressure are common. Kernig's sign is the inability to fully extend the leg when the thigh is flexed to the abdomen. Brudzinski's sign is the involuntary adduction and flexion of the legs with attempts to flex the neck. With meningitis, a headache becomes progressively worse and is accompanied by nausea, vomiting, irritability, confusion, and seizures. If the causative organism is meningococcus, a skin rash is common.

Diagnosis

A major diagnostic tool is examination of the CSF. Variations of the CSF depend upon the causative organism. CSF protein levels are usually elevated and higher in bacterial than in viral cases. A decreased CSF sugar is common in bacterial meningitis and may be normal in viral meningitis. The CSF appears purulent and turbid in bacterial meningitis. It may be the same or clear in viral meningitis. The most predominant cell in the CSF is the polymorphonuclear leukocyte.

Cultures of blood, sputum, and nasopharyngeal secretions are performed to identify the causative organism.

X-rays of the skull may demonstrate infected sinuses. CAT scans are usually normal in uncomplicated meningitis. In other cases, CAT scans may reveal evidence of increased intracranial pressure.

Complications

The most common complication of meningitis is residual neurological dysfunction. Cranial nerve dysfunction often occurs with cranial nerve III, IV, VI, or VII in bacterial meningitis. Usually the dysfunction disappears within a few weeks. Hearing loss may be permanent after bacterial meningitis but is not a complication of viral meningitis.

Cranial nerve irritation can have serious sequelae. Cranial nerve II is compressed by increased intracranial pressure. Papilledema is often present, and blindness may occur. When cranial nerves III, IV, and VI are irritated, ocular movements are affected. Ptosis, unequal pupils, and diplopia are common. Irritation of cranial nerve V is evidenced by sensory and corneal changes, and irritation of cranial nerve VII results in facial paresis. Irritation of cranial nerve VIII causes tinnitus, vertigo, and deafness.

Hemiparesis, dysphasia, and hemianopsia may occur. These signs usually resolve within several hours. Failure of resolution to occur suggests a cerebral abscess, subdural empyema, subdural effusion, or cortical venous thrombophlebitis.

Acute cerebral edema may occur with bacterial meningitis, causing seizures, third-nerve palsy, bradycardia, hypertension, coma, and death.

A noncommunicating hydrocephalus may occur if the inner layer of the exudate has caused adhesions that prevent the normal flow of CSF from the ventricles. Surgical implantation of a shunt is the only treatment.

Nursing Intervention

Administration of antibiotics at scheduled times maintains a therapeutic blood level. Isolation precautions will protect the staff and visitors but need not be continued past 48 hours after the institution of antibiotic therapy.

Body temperature can be controlled by use of antipyretic drugs as indicated and a hypothermia blanket.

Headache is usually treated with analgesics. A darkened, quiet room will help both the headache and photophobia.

If seizures occur, anticonvulsant medication is indicated. Documentation, progression, limb involvement, and duration of the seizures will help determine an effective medication regimen.

Dyspnea and respiratory distress require standard treatment. A central venous pressure line or a pulmonary artery catheter may be inserted to monitor fluid balance and the cardiovascular status. Standard nursing procedures for these types of complications are followed.

Editor's Note

It is possible to have a question or two addressing Guillain-Barré syndrome, primarily from the perspective of the acute respiratory failure that develops in advanced states of this condition. Review the content in this section with an understanding of the critical implications for this condition.

GUILLAIN-BARRÉ SYNDROME

Definition

Guillain-Barré syndrome is an acute inflammatory disease, thought to be autoimmune or viral, that affects peripheral nerves, spinal nerves, and sometimes cranial nerves, first with edema and then with demyelination. Synonyms for Guillain-Barré syndrome include Landry-Guillain-Barré disease, acute inflammatory polyradiculoneuropathy, and infectious polyneuritis.

Pathophysiology

In the normal course of the disease, the patient usually has an upper respiratory or gastrointestinal infection one to two weeks prior to the development of Guillain-Barré syndrome. The predominant pattern is weakness starting in the lower extremities and advancing (often very rapidly) to motor paralysis and progressing up the body. The progression may stop at any point. The first pathological sign of the syndrome is a perivascular lymphocytic infiltration. Following this, characteristic infiltration occurs in the myelin, breaking it down but not damaging the axon. This is called segmental demyelination. If the syndrome progresses, the infiltration becomes more intense and affects the axon, resulting in muscle denervation and atrophy. If the infiltration occurs in the distal segment of the axon, regeneration will occur because the nerve cell body has been spared. If the infiltration occurs at the proximal end of the axon, the nerve cell body may die and regeneration cannot occur. This is known as Wallerian degeneration. Collateral motor fibers may reinnervate the destroyed muscle, restoring the lost function partially or completely. As the infiltration process ends, recovery of motor function begins proximally and progresses distally.

Etiology

Specific etiologic agents are unknown. The most popular theory currently is that a slow-acting measles virus is the causative agent. Guillain-Barré syndrome occurs at any age, with a peak incidence between 30 and 40 years of age. Males and females are affected equally.

Clinical Presentation

Symptoms usually develop one to three weeks after an upper respiratory infection and occasionally after a gastrointestinal infection. Infrequently, polyneuritis may occur after surgery or after immunization against a lymphomatous disease such as rabies or swine flu.

Weakness of the lower extremities evolving more or less symmetrically occurs over a period of hours to days to weeks, usually peaking by the 14th day. Distal muscles are the more severely affected. Paresthesia (numbness and tingling) is frequent, but pain is rare. Paralysis usually follows paresthesia in the extremities.

Hypotonia and areflexia are common, persistent symptoms. Objective sensory loss is variable, with deep sensibility more affected than superficial sensations.

Autonomic nervous function is rarely altered. Sinus tachycardia, hypertension, and anhydrosis (absence of sweating) are uncommon findings. Urinary retention occurs occasionally, but catheterization is seldom needed for more than a few days.

If cranial nerve involvement occurs, it is most frequent in cranial nerve VII, and then in cranial nerves VI, III, XII, V, and X (most to least frequent). Consequently, dysphasia is common if the paresthesia and paralysis extend to the cranial nerves.

Variations in Clinical Presentation. Ascending paralysis moves from legs to trunk to arms to head. It usually peaks in 10 to 14 days. Fisher's variant is complete ophthalmoplegia (paralysis of the eye muscles), ataxia, and areflexia.

Cases with a steady or stepwise progression over weeks or months may be asymmetrical. Some body parts will be recovering while others are getting worse. There may be relapses, but these are uncommon.

Diagnosis

Examination of the CSF is done to determine whether the CSF protein is elevated (up to 700 mg%) with only a few cells present. This condition represents albuminocytologic dissociation (high protein/few cells), which is specific for Guillain-Barré syndrome.

Complications

The most serious complication is respiratory failure as the paralysis advances upward. Constant monitoring will provide for immediate intervention if failure occurs. Respiratory monitoring is typically provided by measuring forced vital capacities and peak (or negative) inspiratory efforts. Arterial blood gases (ABGs) may be monitored to detect the development of a respiratory acidosis.

Infection, either respiratory or urinary, may occur, and intervention begun if fever develops. Due to muscle atony and immobility, ileus development, venous thrombophlebitis, and pulmonary emboli may occur.

Treatment and Nursing Intervention

The objective of therapy is to support body systems until recovery occurs. Respiratory failure and infection are serious threats to recovery. Monitoring the vital capacity and ABGs is essential. If the vital capacity drops to less than 800 cc, the peak negative pressure drops to below -20 cm H_2O, or the ABGs reflect development of a respiratory acidosis, intubation or tracheostomy may be done so that the patient can be mechanically ventilated. Strict sterile suctioning is needed to prevent infection whether the patient has an endotracheal tube or a tracheostomy. Excellent bronchial hygiene and chest physiotherapy will help clear secretions and prevent respiratory deterioration. If fever develops, sputum cultures should be obtained to identify a specific pathogen (if one is present in the respiratory tract) so that appropriate antibiotic therapy may be instituted.

A communication system must be established with the patient, using whatever muscle action is possible. This is extremely difficult if the disease progresses to involvement of the cranial nerves. At the peak of a severe syndrome, communication from the patient may be impossible. The nurse must explain all procedures before doing them and reassure the patient that muscle function will soon return to some part of the body so that the patient can then communicate needs and desires.

Monitoring of blood pressure, cardiac rate, and cardiac rhythm is important, since some transient cardiac dysrhythmias have been reported. Hypotension, secondary to the muscular atony, may occur in severe cases or at the peak of the attack. Vasopressor agents may be required. Otherwise, vasoactive drugs are seldom used because the patient's sensitivity to drugs is altered.

Urinary retention for a few days is not uncommon. Intermittent catheterization may be preferred to use of a Foley catheter in an effort to avoid urinary tract infection.

Physiotherapy is indicated very early to help counter the hazards of immobility. Passive range of motion and attention to body extremity position help maintain function and prevent contractures.

Nutritional needs must be met with consideration of gastric dilatation, ileus development, and aspiration potential if the gag reflex is lost. Initially, tube feedings may be used to ensure adequate caloric intake; in some centers, hyperalimentation may be started.

Fluid and electrolytes are monitored carefully to prevent electrolyte imbalances and possible occurrence of ADH secretion dysfunction.

Steroid therapy is controversial, as is anticoagulant therapy unless signs of a phlebitis or pulmonary embolism develop.

Plasmapheresis

This is the general process of separating blood components in order to remove specific portions of the blood. Lymphoresis removes lymphocytes and so forth; plasmapheresis removes specific components in the plasma. In myasthenic patients, the plan is to remove autoantibodies that are believed to cause the disease. While the role of plasmapheresis is unclear in certain diseases, there is an apparent benefit to its use in diseases such as myasthenia gravis and Guillain-Barré syndrome.

Prognosis

Provided complications from respiratory failure can be avoided, good recovery with minimal permanent neurological dysfunction can be expected. Without critical-care medical treatment and nursing, morbidity and mortality will increase due to respiratory failure.

Editor's Note

Remember, it is unlikely that the CCRN will cover myasthenia in any detail if at all. Focus on the critical-care aspects of this condition and do not try to remember all components of the disease.

MYASTHENIA GRAVIS AND CRISIS

Definition

Myasthenia gravis is considered an autoimmune disease affecting postsynaptic receptor sites. It is a chronic disorder of neuromuscular transmission resulting in weakness with exercise and improving strength with rest.

Pathophysiology

Three theories have been proposed as the pathophysiology of myasthenia gravis. Acetylcholine is released at nerve terminals and combines at the postsynaptic muscle membrane to produce an electrochemical reaction. The electrochemical reaction results in muscle contraction. In myasthenia gravis, there are too few postsynaptic receptor sites for the amount of acetylcholine released to bind with to provide for a full muscular contraction, not enough acetylcholine is released to cause full muscle contraction, or acetylcholinesterase degrades the acetylcholine before sufficient amounts can cause a full muscle contraction.

Etiology

The most prevalent hypothesis is that myasthenia gravis is an autoimmune process damaging the postsynaptic membrane. A statistically significant number of cases are associated with thymoma and thymic hyperplasia. This view is substantiated by the detection of serum antibodies, produced by sensitized lymphocytes or thymocytes that block the action of acetylcholine and the production of immune bodies by the thymus, that are capable of reproducing the disease in experimental animal models.

Occurrence

Myasthenia gravis occurs in from 1 in 10,000 to 1 in 50,000 people. It may occur at any age, but it rarely occurs in those under 10 or over 70 years old. Peak occurrence is between 20 and 30 years of age. Under the age of 40, the ratio of occurrence in women to men is 3:1, after 40, it is 1:1.

Clinical Presentation

The clinical presentation of myasthenia gravis is characterized by easy fatigability of voluntary muscle groups with repeated use. Pathognomonic signs of myasthenia gravis include uneven drooping of the eyelids, a smile that resembles a snarl, a drooping lower jaw that must be supported by the hand, and a partially immobile mouth with the corners turned downward. However, few patients are first seen with these signs. In more than 90% of cases, eyebrow and extraocular muscles are involved, accompanied by weakness in eye closure. Ptosis and diplopia are common. The next most commonly affected muscles exhibiting symptoms are those of facial expression, mastication, swallowing, and speaking (dysarthria). Hoarseness occurs after only a few minutes of talking. Neck flexor and extensor muscles, the shoulder girdle, and hip flexors are less frequently involved. There usually is no sensory disturbance.

The course of myasthenia gravis is variable. Remission may occur for no discernible reason in less than half the cases and usually does not last longer than one to two months. The disease then becomes progressive. Frequently, the disease is slow but progressive from onset. The greatest danger of death is during the first year and again during years four through seven in progressive cases. Stabilization of the disease occurs after this time, and severe recurrence is rare. Infection of any kind, but especially respiratory, trauma of any kind, and emotional stress make the disease worse.

Associated Conditions

Approximately 15% of patients have a tumor of the thymus. There is an increasing incidence of tumors in older males. Thyroiditis, thyrotoxicosis, lupus erythematosus, and rheumatoid arthritis occur more often than statistically expected. A pregnancy may make the disease worse or better or may have no effect. Close to 15% of babies born to myasthenic mothers exhibit symptoms of the disease. The symptoms are usually transient and resolve within 1 to 12 weeks.

Diagnosis

A history of an increasing muscular fatigability that improves with rest is a common characteristic of myasthenia gravis. Various laboratory tests can be used to aid in a diagnosis. However, anticholinesterase tests are considered conclusive.

Edrophonium chloride (Tensilon) is injected intravenously after the patient's muscle strength has been assessed. Ten milligrams of Tensilon, given in 2 to 5 mg doses, is the limit used to test for myasthenia gravis. The duration of action for Tensilon is about five minutes.

Tensilon is an anticholinesterase agent. When injected, it increases the level of acetylcholine at the myoneural junction by blocking cholinesterase (which breaks down acetylcholine). A clinical increase in muscle strength is positive for myasthenia gravis. No improvement or a deterioration in muscle strength is negative for myasthenia gravis.

If use of Tensilon is not conclusive, neostigmine bromide, 0.5 mg intravenously or 1.5 mg intramuscularly, may be used. Atropine sulfate (0.6 mg) should be given prior to intravenous neostigmine and may be needed with intramuscular injection of neostigmine to counter nausea, vomiting, increased salivation, and sweating. Intravenous neostigmine may cause ventricular fibrillation or cardiac arrest. After intramuscular injection, maximum effect will be apparent within 30 minutes, but effects may last two to three hours. Curare is seldom used because of its paralytic action, but it serves as a definitive test if properly administered.

Treatment

The major objectives of therapy are to improve neuromuscular transmission and prevent complications. Early thymectomy may be employed.

Neuromuscular transmission is improved by administration of anticholinesterase drugs. Pyridostigmine bromide (Mestinon) is a popular choice. If Mestinon is not adequate to establish control of neuromuscular transmission, neostigmine (Prostigmin) is used. Prednisone has become an adjunctive drug of choice. It is extremely important to medicate the patient on schedule and to document carefully the patient's muscular response. The major difference between Mestinon and neostigmine is their duration of action. Mestinon has a four-hour effect; neostigmine, two hours. Steroids may decrease the amount of anticholinesterase drug required to control myasthenic symptoms. The use of steroids results in suppression of immune responses and the resultant problem of infection and biochemical stress.

Thymectomy produces an improvement in or remission of symptoms in many patients. An improvement may be gradual over several years (up to ten). Frequently, steroid and anticholinesterase drugs are needed in smaller dosages after thymectomy. New treatments include thoracic duct drainage and plasmapheresis.

Nursing Intervention

A major nursing intervention is to maintain adequate ventilation in spite of a weak cough, an inability to clear secretions, and an increased likelihood of aspiration. Vital capacity is checked every two to four hours. Ventilators often are set up and kept available.

Prevention of aspiration, prevention of infection from any source, and emotional support of the patient are very important. If the patient is on a respirator, a communication system should be established. If the patient has had a thymectomy, monitoring and nursing treatment as provided for any patient with a thoracotomy must be followed.

Specific drugs that impair neuromuscular transmission must be avoided. The aminoglycoside antibiotics and true mycin drugs are contraindicated. Such drugs include aureomycin, kanamycin, polymyxin, neomycin, streptomycin, and gentamicin. Quinidine, procainamide, morphine sulfate, and sedatives will aggravate muscle weakness.

Nursing education as to the importance of taking prescribed medications on schedule is extremely important, since an early or late dose may immediately affect muscle strength. Regulation of daily living habits to avoid fatigue and provide rest must be

planned according to the patient's life style as much as possible. The patient should know that minor infection or illness may precipitate an acute attack.

Postthymectomy Nursing Interventions

Routine postsurgical care is needed plus:

1. Post–thoracic surgery procedures (e.g., chest tubes)
2. Ventilatory support with frequent suctioning
3. Anticholinesterase and steroid drugs started slowly
4. Reassurance that positive effects of a thymectomy occur over long periods (even years)
5. Protection from infections (e.g., sterile technique for suctioning, intermittent urinary catheterization rather than an indwelling catheter)

Complications: Myasthenic or Cholinergic Crisis?

Myasthenic and cholinergic crises both have extreme weakness as the predominant symptom. Myasthenic crisis is caused by insufficient drug dose. Cholinergic crisis is due to an overdose of drugs, and the patient has increased salivation and sweating. An impending cholinergic crisis can be detected by constricting pupils. Two millimeters is the maximum constriction that should be allowed before intervention. To distinguish between these crises, a Tensilon test is used, with a ventilator on standby. If the patient becomes weaker, a cholinergic (overdose) crisis exists. Treatment is to discontinue anticholinesterase drugs. After 72 hours, drug therapy is usually restarted in small increments. Atropine (an anticholinergic drug) may control symptoms but may also block important symptoms of anticholinesterase overdose. Monitoring ventilatory function with arterial blood gases is imperative.

Myasthenic crisis is established by muscular improvement with the Tensilon test. Anticholinesterase drugs are given and repeated as needed. Steroids are usually avoided during a crisis. Monitoring, assessing, and documenting muscular strength and ABGs are continued throughout the crisis. Identification of the precipitating etiology is important to treat and/or correct the cause. Communication with the patient throughout treatment, by whatever means possible, facilitates rest and enhances trust in the nurse.

CHAPTER 20

Seizures, Status Epilepticus, Cerebrovascular Accidents

Editor's Note

In this chapter, concepts are covered that address the CCRN exam items of intracranial hemorrhage and seizures. You can expect one to three exam questions on this content.

SEIZURES

Seizures are a manifestation of excessive neuronal discharge in the brain. They may be associated with infection, trauma, tumor, cerebrovascular disease, or genetic, congenital, or metabolic dysfunction. A convulsion is musculoskeletal contractions accompanying a seizure.

Definition

A seizure is a symptom of paroxysmal electrical discharges in the brain resulting in autonomic, sensory, and/or motor dysfunction. If seizures are recurrent and transient, the condition is classified as epilepsy.

Classification of seizure disorders is summarized in Table 20-1.

Types of Seizures

Grand mal seizures may also be termed convulsive or tonic-clonic seizures. These are characterized by a loss of consciousness. Myoclonic seizures are characterized by violent contraction of muscle groups, usually without a loss of consciousness. Petit mal seizures are common only in the 4- to 12-year-old range. They are called absences rather than seizures, since loss of consciousness is for a period of seconds, with no generalized motor activity. Focal (partial) seizures have a lesion in an identifiable area of the brain. Focal seizures are of two types: simple (no loss of consciousness) and complex (with loss of consciousness). Focal motor seizures are also called Jacksonian seizures. Focal sensory seizures may involve somatosensory, visual, auditory, olfactory, or vertiginous components. Psychomotor seizures are also termed temporal lobe seizures and limbic seizures. They are characterized by an exaggerated emotional component and a bizarre behavioral component.

Pathophysiology

It is not known whether seizures occur because of an increased neuronal excitability or a decreased neuronal inhibitory force. Focal neurons appear to be unusually sensitive to acetylcholine and possibly a deficit in specific neurotransmitters. Altered cell permeability and/

TABLE 20-1. CLASSIFICATION OF SEIZURES

A. Generalized Children and infants	1. Tonic-clonic	2. Absence	3. Bilateral myoclonus
	4. Infantile spasm	5. Atonic seizures	6. Tonic seizures
B. Partial seizures	1. Simple; motor, sensory, affective	2. Complex; temporal lobe or psychomotor seizures	
C. Partial (focal) seizures with secondary generalization			

or alteration in electrolytes may have a role in seizure activity. It is logical to assume that an electrical threshold for seizures exists in all persons. Factors thought to lower electrical threshold of neurons include fever, fatigue, altered electrolyte and water balance, stress, emotional distress, and/or pregnancy. Regardless of these factors, hyperexcited neurons become hyperactive. As these localized neuronal discharges become intense, the hyperirritability spreads synaptically to adjacent neurons. In many instances, the entire brain is involved. When only one hemisphere is involved, consciousness is preserved. When both cerebral hemispheres are involved, there is usually a loss of consciousness. An exception is a bilateral simple partial seizure. Also, in a complex partial seizure, consciousness may be altered but not lost, since the seizure is in the limbic system (even though it is bilateral).

Etiology

Multiple etiologies of epilepsy are known. The most common is the abrupt cessation of antileptic drugs or other chronic sedative medications. Other causes include trauma, tumor, injuries (both perinatal and postnatal), CNS infections, and cerebral vascular disease, including arteriovenous malformations. Metabolic and toxic disorders may cause seizures. The role of genetics and heredity is controversial at this time. In a large number of cases, the cause is unknown. These cases are termed idiopathic epilepsy.

Clinical Presentation

Tonic-Clonic (Grand Mal Seizures). A peculiar sensation or feeling known as an aura (prodroma) may occur at the beginning of a seizure. An aura also accompanies complex partial seizures. For those who do experience an aura, it is almost always the same sensation or feeling. As consciousness is lost, the patient falls (if he or she is upright). The body becomes rigid. Air is forced from the lungs and may result in a high-pitched, loud cry. The jaws become locked, and the tongue is often caught between clenched teeth. Pupils dilate and are nonreactive. Apnea results in cyanosis. Bladder incontinence is common. This is the tonic phase of the grand mal seizure and lasts 10 to 20 seconds.

The clonic phase of the grand mal seizure is a period of violent, rhythmic, symmetric, alternating contraction and relaxation involving the entire body. Increased salivation, mixed with blood if the tongue

has been bitten, results in frothing at the mouth. The patient has a tachycardia, is profusely diaphoretic, and remains apneic. The tonic and clonic phases last one to five minutes.

In the postictal phase, the seizure subsides, the patient resumes breathing, cyanosis clears, and the pupils react. The patient should be bagged with a high volume of oxygen during this stage to help compensate for the period of apnea. The patient is fatigued, has a headache, is sleepy and confused, and may have amnesia of the entire seizure excepting the aura. A residual neurologic deficit may continue for several hours (Todd's paralysis).

Absences (Petit Mal Seizures). These are generalized seizures consisting of frequent episodes of loss of consciousness termed absences. The absences last from two to ten seconds and are characterized by ceasing motor activity, stopping speech in midsentence, and/or staring into space. During the seizure, the child (it is rarely seen after age 12) may twitch the lips or the lips may droop. The eyes may roll upward. There is no change in muscle tone. The patient may stagger or stumble, but rarely falls. Petit mal is benign neurologically. It may interfere with classroom learning.

Bilateral Myoclonus (Myoclonic Seizures). These seizures are characterized by sudden, violent contractions of muscle groups. They may be generalized or focal, symmetrical (both sides) or asymmetrical (one side). Loss of consciousness is unusual in certain types of myoclonic seizure activity. The seizures may be a single jerking movement, intermittent periods of active seizure, or present in varying degree all of the waking time. The seizures are absent during sleep, being precipitated by stimulation and intensified with intentional movement.

Atonic Seizures (Akinetic Seizures). These may occur by themselves or in cases of petit mal epilepsy. There is a sudden, brief loss of muscle tone with or without a loss of consciousness. The child falls often and may be labeled clumsy or awkward. Akinetic seizures may cloud the picture of petit mal epilepsy. These seizures often result from serious neurological disease which cannot be treated.

Simple Partial (Focal) Motor Seizures. These seizures are also known as Jacksonian seizures. The focal point is in the motor strip area (the prerolandic

gyrus). The typical seizure starts with a twitching of the fingers or toes or around the lips on one side of the body. The muscle movement becomes more severe and spreads (marches) by involving more muscle groups until one side of the body is totally involved. Consciousness is maintained unless the Jacksonian seizure becomes generalized and spreads to the remainder of the body.

Simple Partial (Focal) Sensory Seizures. These seizures may be described by the patient as a numbness, tingling, or "pins and needles" sensation. If the causative lesion is in the postrolandic gyrus (the sensory strip between the frontal and parietal lobes), the seizure may progress like the Jacksonian seizure. Visual sensations usually indicate an occipital lobe lesion. Auditory sensations are most commonly a buzzing or ringing of the ears, often accompanied by olfactory symptoms and dizziness. This indicates a temporal lobe lesion.

Complex Partial Psychomotor Seizures. An aura often precedes a seizure. The aura includes complex visceral and/or perceptual hallucinations. The patient appears to be in an awake but nonresponsive state. Simple or elaborate behavior patterns may be carried out during the seizure. The behavior patterns are automatisms; that is, the patient performs the behavioral pattern like a robot. The average seizure lasts about five minutes. Attempts to interrupt the behavior pattern often precipitate violence. The seizure may end abruptly with the patient having complete amnesia, or the patient may have a period of headache, confusion, or sleepiness.

Diagnosis

The patient's history of seizure activity (duration, frequency, intensity, and progression) is one of the most useful tools in establishing a diagnosis. Physical examination, laboratory studies, radiologic studies, and electroencephalograms may reveal factors supporting a diagnosis of epilepsy, or the studies may all be within normal limits.

Treatment

If seizures are the result of tumor, infection, or metabolic dysfunction, correcting the underlying cause is the goal of therapy. In a majority of cases, an underlying cause may not be identifiable or amenable to curative therapy. These cases are treated with anticonvul-

sive drugs. It is common to use combinations of drugs to achieve control of seizure activity. The most common drugs include phenytoin sodium (Dilantin), phenobarbital, primidone (Mysoline), ethosuximide (Zarontin), clonazepam (Clonopin), and carbamazepine (Tegretol). A recently introduced drug is valproic acid (Depakene). For the therapeutic serum levels of these drugs, their affinities for specific types of seizures, and their side effects, the reader is referred to any standard pharmacology text.

If drug therapy is ineffective, if seizures are intractable, and if the seizures prohibit a normal semblance of life, surgery may be performed. After identification of the specific epileptic focus and the patient's dominant hemisphere, a cerebral lobectomy or hemispherectomy may be done. Seizures may continue for a period after the surgery.

Nursing Intervention and Complications

There are five major areas of nursing interventions for the patient having seizures.

1. Protect the patient from injury. Remove objects that might cause injury from the immediate environment. Stay with the patient during the seizure. Bedrails should be padded. The patient should not be restrained, but efforts to keep the patient's head from injury are appropriate (e.g., if a seizure occurs when the patient is out of bed, a pillow may be placed under the head or a nurse may cradle, *not* restrain, the patient's head to protect it). *Nothing* should ever be used to pry open the mouth or be forced into the mouth during a seizure. Damage to the mouth and tongue occurs at the start of a seizure, and only more damage will occur if objects are forced into the mouth.
2. Observing (and recording) seizure patterns may help identify the seizure focus. Data include precipitating factors, presence and type of aura, duration of unconsciousness, pattern and progression of seizure activity, body parts involved (generalized or one-sided), incontinence, and postictal activity.
3. Assessment of the respiratory system is extremely important. The danger of a grand mal seizure is that the patient is apneic during the seizure. The respiratory status may be further compromised by aspiration. Oxygen should be at the bedside.

4. Administration of medication on a regularly timed basis and evaluation of the effects of the medication on controlling seizures as well as the psychological effects on the patient are important actions and assessments. Teaching the patient the beneficial effects of following the prescribed medication regimen and identifying patient objections will allow teaching that may result in better patient compliance in the future.

5. Promoting physical and mental health may sharply curtail the number of seizures. Regular routines for eating, sleeping, and physical activity should be established. Activity tends to decrease the occurrence of seizures. Alcohol, stress, and fatigue tend to precipitate seizures. Modifying these factors will alter the seizure pattern.

STATUS EPILEPTICUS

Definition

Status epilepticus is present when seizures follow each other so closely that a state of consciousness is not recovered between seizures. Status epilepticus usually refers to grand mal seizures, but any form of seizures may evolve into status epilepticus.

Pathophysiology

Pathophysiology is the same as for epilepsy except that the seizures are almost continuous. The rapidly repeating grand mal seizures lead to hypoxemia (patients are apneic during grand mal seizures) and cerebral anoxia. The increased metabolic activity of the brain causes a hypoglycemic and hyperthermic state. Hypoxemia, hypoglycemia, and hyperthermia may themselves precipitate seizure activity, resulting in a vicious cycle.

Etiology

Inadequate dosage of antileptic medication in a known epileptic is a common precipitating factor. Other factors include sudden withdrawal of antileptic drugs and other sedative drugs, intercurrent infection (commonly in the CNS), cerebral vascular disease, and cerebral hypoxia, anoxia, and edema. Progressive neurological diseases such as brain tumor and subdural hematoma may cause status epilepticus. A common triad of causes consists of alcohol abuse, drug abuse, and sleep deprivation. Head trauma or pregnancy (pre-eclamptic state) may precipitate status epilepticus. Metabolic disorders as a cause include hypoglycemia, uremia, and electrolyte imbalances.

Incidence and Prognosis

Approximately 6% of known epileptics will develop status epilepticus. Almost 50% of the cases of status epilepticus occur in known epileptics. From 10 to 30% of patients with status epilepticus will die. Death is commonly due to respiratory and metabolic acidosis, hypoxemia, hypoglycemia, hyperthermia, electrolyte disturbances, and/or renal failure.

Clinical Presentation

There are three variants in the clinical picture of status epilepticus.

1. Grand mal status is a life-threatening emergency. Seizures are of the tonic-clonic type without a period of consciousness between seizures.
2. Petit mal status may exhibit as many as 200 to 300 absences per day.
3. Partial or focal status is termed epilepsia continua. Focal seizures occur continuously or regularly. Consciousness is usually maintained unless generalization occurs.

Electrical status occurs in every type of status epilepticus and is not a distinct type. It is always associated with some clinical abnormality. An electroencephalogram shows continuous epileptic activity. There is also a complex partial status.

Treatment

The goal of therapy is to restore physiologic homeostasis and to stop the seizures. The first step in treatment is to ensure a patent airway. The second step is to draw blood (for glucose, electrolytes, BUN, ABGs, and CPK) and establish an intravenous line. (This is often achieved as a one-step process with jelcos or angiocaths.) If there is the slightest possibility of hypoglycemia, 50% glucose is given intravenously. The third step is administering medications to stop seizure activity.

Diazepam (Valium) intravenously is often the drug of choice in spite of its potential for suppressing respirations. It very quickly enters the brain and quickly leaves the brain. But these very properties often make diazepam a poor drug for status epilepticus. After intravenous injection, diazepam will be completely out of brain tissue in 30 minutes.

Phenytoin is given intravenously. It must be injected slowly (50 mg/minute), and cardiac monitoring is essential for early intervention in dysrhythmias. Bradycardia and hypotension are especially common in patients over 40. Phenytoin requires 15 to 20 minutes to peak in brain tissue, and it remains in brain tissue over a long period.

If seizures persist after 30 minutes, there is a high probability that acute CNS disease caused the seizures. Phenobarbital may be tried. A slow intravenous injection is recommended. Respiratory depression and hypotension may develop. Phenobarbital and diazepam should not be administered concurrently. If diazepam is used to stop seizures, phenytoin is given simultaneously to block recurrence of the seizures.

Lidocaine as a 20% solution in normal saline may be tried. Some medical centers use general anesthesia (barbiturate coma) to a depth of electroencephalogram silence when other drugs have failed.

Paraldehyde may be used intramuscularly or rectally. Intravenous administration is hazardous. It must be diluted and given very slowly.

Nursing Intervention

Maintaining a patent airway is extremely important. An intravenous line should be maintained. Cardiac drugs should be available, as cardiac monitoring may reveal dysrhythmias. Hyperthermia is treated frequently with a hypothermia blanket. Fluid and electrolyte balance is monitored. Neurologic status is monitored continuously.

CEREBROVASCULAR ACCIDENT

Definition

A cerebrovascular accident (CVA) is a sudden focal neurologic deficit due to cerebrovascular disease. A CVA is the most common cause of cerebral dysfunction in this country.

Etiology

The end result of any interruption of oxygen to brain tissue for more than a few minutes is the death of those neurons not being oxygenated. The decrease in oxygen may be partial or complete. It is caused by thrombi, emboli, tumor, hemorrhage, hypertension, and compression or spasm of cerebral arteries.

Clinical Presentation

The common symptom in CVAs regardless of the etiology is the sudden onset of symptoms. Specific symptoms depend upon the location of the injury and the hemispheric dominance of the patient. Homonymous hemianopsia, hemiparesis, and/or hemiplegia are common symptoms.

If the right cerebral hemisphere is involved, there are spatial-perceptual deficits resulting in apraxia. Apraxia may be constructional or dressing. Constructional apraxia is the inability to complete the left half of figures one is drawing or arranging words in an incorrect manner, superimposing words, and such. A constructional apraxia usually includes an inability to complete the drawing of a picture (e.g., a clock). Dressing apraxia is the inability to dress oneself properly. Both constructional apraxia and dressing apraxia are common in right cerebral CVAs. Neglect of the paralyzed side, impulsive quick behavior, and poor judgment of abilities and limitations occur with right cerebral CVAs.

Left cerebral hemispheric CVAs have astereognosis and autotopagnosia. Astereognosis is an inability to identify a common object placed in the hand with one's eyes closed. Autotopagnosia is an inability to determine the position of parts of the body in relation to the rest of the body.

In addition, these CVAs tend to cause a finger agnosia (inability to identify a finger being touched) and a right-left disorientation. Behavior is slow, cautious, and disorganized. Aphasia, both expressive and receptive, is common. Expressive aphasia is the inability to express oneself verbally and understandably. Receptive aphasia is loss of the ability to understand the spoken or written word.

Regardless of which hemisphere is involved in a CVA, the patients tend to have a reduced memory span, are emotionally labile, and have spasticity of the affected extremities. Some patients will have an anosognosia, which is the denial of a neurological deficit such as hemiplegia. Anosognosia is different from a psychological denial stage. Deviation of the head and eyes is toward the cerebral hemisphere involved in the CVA of pontine lesions. Frontal lobe lesions produce the opposite signs.

Diagnosis of CVA

The diagnosis of CVA is usually made on the basis of history and clinical symptoms. The history frequently reveals transient ischemic attacks, reversible ischemic neurologic deficits, and possibly "small" strokes in the past. A CAT scan will reveal decreased density in ischemic and infarcted areas. It will reveal increased density in hemorrhage areas. Angiography may show spasms, arteriovenous malformations, and aneurysms.

Treatment

In most centers, treatment is supportive. Anticoagulant therapy may be considered if embolic etiology is suspected. Research is continuing and looks promising for extracranial and intracranial bypass anastomoses in reversible ischemic neurological deficits. Carotid endarterectomy and bypass patients are seen in critical-care areas more than the uncomplicated CVA patient.

Nursing Intervention

To some extent, nursing interventions (and patient complications) depend upon the site of a CVA as well as the patient's age, general health, and extent of neurologic deficit.

Communication with the patient is achieved in any way possible—through writing, pictures, gestures, and so on. Different aphasias make this task difficult.

Monitoring and assessing neurologic status will identify extensions of deficit that may be treatable.

Supportive comfort measures are important; these include training, positioning, skin care, fluid and nutritional intake, emotional support, and early implementation of rehabilitation.

CHAPTER 21

Intracranial Pressure, Aneurysm, Coma, and Brain Herniation

Editor's Note

This chapter covers concepts that address CCRN test areas of aneurysm and encephalopathies. Expect one to three exam questions on the contents of this chapter.

INTRACRANIAL PRESSURE

Within a very narrow range, the contents of the cranial vault can adjust to increases in intracranial pressure (ICP). When the limits of the range and time are exceeded, the ICP rises precipitously.

Components of the Cranial Vault

There are three components that almost completely fill the cranial vault: brain tissue (about 88% of the volume), cerebrospinal fluid (CSF) (about 9 to 10% of the volume), and intravascular fluid (2 to 11% of the volume).

Munro-Kellie Hypothesis

This hypothesis is the basis for ICP monitoring. The hypothesis states that in the adult, the cranial vault is nondistensible (it is bone) and the components of the vault are essentially incompressible. Based on these tenets, a relationship between the vault and its contents can be construed.

An increase in one component of the vault contents necessitates a reciprocal decrease in either or both of the other components. If the reciprocal decrease does not occur, there is a rise in intracranial pressure. This pressure increase is termed intracranial hypertension. Normal ICP is less than 10 mm Hg. Most practitioners treat a sustained ICP of above 15 to 20 mm Hg.

Compensatory Mechanisms for Increasing ICP

Initial increases in the volume of the cranium are compensated for by two mechanisms.

1. A decrease in intravascular fluid (blood) occurs by compression of the low-pressure venous system. Intravascular volume is the most alterable component of the three in the cranium (brain tissue, CSF, and blood). There is a specific limit to the extent of compressibility. When this limit is exceeded, ICP rises.
2. The CSF is the second compensatory mechanism for increasing ICP. As the ICP rises, CSF is displaced from the cranial vault into the spinal canal. When maximum displacement of CSF has occurred, there is probably an increase in CSF absorption, which aids compensatory mechanisms.

These mechanisms function to keep the ICP constant. They function well when the ICP increases slowly. Even then, the mechanisms will lose their compensatory function at a certain point (variable with the individual). If the ICP rises rapidly, the compensatory mechanisms are unable to function.

Intracranial Compliance

The relationship of change in pressure to change in volume is termed compliance. When intracranial compliance is low, a small increase in volume causes a large rise in pressure. The ICP provides information about intracranial compliance. Cerebral perfusion pressure (CPP) is as important as compliance or more so. CPP can be calculated from ICP, being the difference between mean arterial pressure (MAP) and mean ICP.

$$CPP = MAP - ICP$$

CPP is the pressure in the cerebral vascular system. This pressure approximates cerebral blood flow

(CBF). Decreases in CPP reduce CBF. CBF affects delivery of both oxygen and glucose to the brain tissue. The normal brain has an extremely good autoregulatory system that maintains normal blood flow with CPP as low as 50 mm Hg. In the injured brain, activity of the autoregulatory system is not known. Thus, many authorities consider a CPP of 60 mm Hg to be the least acceptable pressure. If the patient is neurologically unstable, CPP is extremely important when mean arterial pressure (MAP or SAP) is low or when ICP is high. If MAP is low or ICP is high, the brain is not being adequately perfused with oxygenated blood.

Indicators for ICP Monitoring

The outcome of many neurological conditions can be mediated by early recognition and intervention of increasing ICP. Six areas are identified:

1. Head injuries. A Glasgow Coma Score of 8 or less indicates significant neurological impairment. The parameters and scoring for the Glasgow Coma Score are shown in Table 18-1. With ICP monitoring, early signs of intracranial problems can be identified and treatment initiated before clinical signs and symptoms develop.
2. Evaluation of an increasing ICP for effectiveness. This includes fluid balance, osmotic diuretics, possibly glucocorticoids, therapy, and hyperventilation.
3. Postoperative cerebral edema. Certain brain tumors grow slowly, allowing the cranial contents to compensate for the increasing mass volume. After the tumor is removed, cerebral edema may be severe and life threatening. ICP monitoring will allow early intervention.
4. Reye-Johnson syndrome. The mortality of the Reye-Johnson syndrome may be due to cerebral hypoglycemia and ischemia. This could be the result of poor cerebral perfusion and increasing ICP. By monitoring the ICP, therapies can be used to maintain a good CPP.
5. Infections and edema. Infections are not usually associated with increasing ICP. If coma (and/or brain stem involvement) is present, cerebral edema is a potential problem.
6. Monitoring. Preoperative and postoperative monitoring is common in intracerebral hemorrhage. The evacuation of a tumor, treatment of an underlying lesion, and evacuation of the

hemorrhagic hematoma may result in cerebral edema and increasing ICP.

Sites for Measurement of ICP

ICP can be measured in many areas: the lumbar sac, cisterna magna, fontanels in newborns, cerebral ventricles, cranial subdural space, and cranial epidural space. ICP values will depend upon (1) the site selected for monitoring and (2) the patient's position. The ICP is usually measured supratentorially by an intraventricular cannula or by a subdural catheter or bolt or epidural sensor.

Monitoring Systems

The monitoring system has three parts: a sensor, a transducer, and a recording instrument. It is like an arterial pressure monitoring system except that the ICP monitoring system is closed, with no heparinized continuous flush system and no interflow.

The sensor is a fluid-filled catheter, a cannula, or a bolt that communicates between the epidural, subdural, or intraventricular space and the transducer (Fig. 21-1).

The transducer converts the pressure signal to an electrical signal that can be recorded.

The recorder is usually a bedside monitor with or without a digital readout and with a waveform display.

Monitoring Techniques

Three common techniques being used are epidural, subarachnoid, and intraventricular monitoring.

In epidural monitoring, the sensor is placed between the skull and dura, with the pressure-sensitive membrane toward the dura (Fig. 21-2). The advantage of this device is that it leaves the dura intact. Techni-

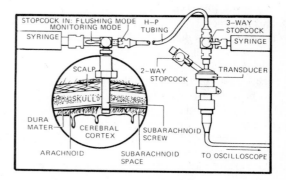

Figure 21-1. An ICP system.

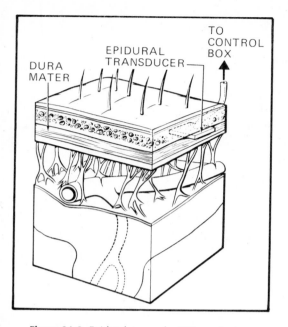

Figure 21-2. Epidural sensor for ICP monitoring.

cally, this may protect the patient from intracerebral infection. Disadvantages are summarized in Table 21-1. The subarachnoid screw may be the most commonly used method of ICP monitoring (Fig. 21-3). A hollow screw is inserted into the subarachnoid space and is connected by fluid-filled tubing to the transducer. Advantages of the screw include direct measurement of the CSF and the ability to drain or sample the CSF. Disadvantages are summarized in Table 21-1.

Intraventricular monitoring is the most difficult form of monitoring because it involves the insertion of a cannula into one of the lateral ventricles (Fig. 21-4). Insertion is usually into the nondominant cerebral hemisphere, since brain tissue must be penetrated. The cannula is usually connected to a stopcock or pressure tubing (fluid filled) to a transducer. The transducer is positioned at a level of the foramen of Monro. The major advantages of the intraventricular cannula are the ability to measure the CSF directly and to drain or sample the CSF as desired. Disadvantages are summarized in Table 21-1.

ICP Waveforms

There are three waveforms (A, B, and C) seen in ICP monitoring (Fig. 21-5). The shape of the waves is af-

fected by both cardiac pulsations and the respiratory cycle.

"A" waves, or plateau waves, occur when there is a sudden, sustained rise in ICP. "A" waves may be present for 5 to 20 minutes. "A" waves are not normally present if the ICP is less than 50 mm Hg.

"B" waves are evident when the ICP rises to approximately 50 mm Hg. These waves are variable in shape and size and usually last for one-half to three minutes. They can occur with changes in the cardiac status.

"C" waves have been identified in ICP monitoring. Their significance has not been established.

With intraventricular monitoring, sharp peaked waveforms occur. Systolic and diastolic portions of the wave cycle are "dampened." A dampened waveform is acceptable in ICP monitoring because the ICP mean is the measurement of significance. *Caution:* Do not confuse this with the waveforms of pulmonary ar-

TABLE 21-1. SOME DISADVANTAGES OF ICP MONITORING

All ICP monitoring has an inherently high risk of infection, some routes more than others.

Intraventricular

May cause increased damage during insertion, especially with cerebral trauma, edema, and/or increased ICP.

Increased chance of damage also to misshapen, tortuous, small, or displaced ventricles.

Statistical increase of infection with this form of monitoring.

Epidural

Wound, bone, or epidural infection may occur and progress to an intracerebral infection and/or a generalized sepsis.

May be plugged by brain tissue.

Waveforms are dampened and may give faulty tracing.

Insertion must be in operating room.

Transducer and unit expensive.

Subarachnoid

Plugging often occurs, giving false tracing.

May be flushed away from patient.

Recalibration of transducer with every plugging. This increases chance of infection and chance of false readings.

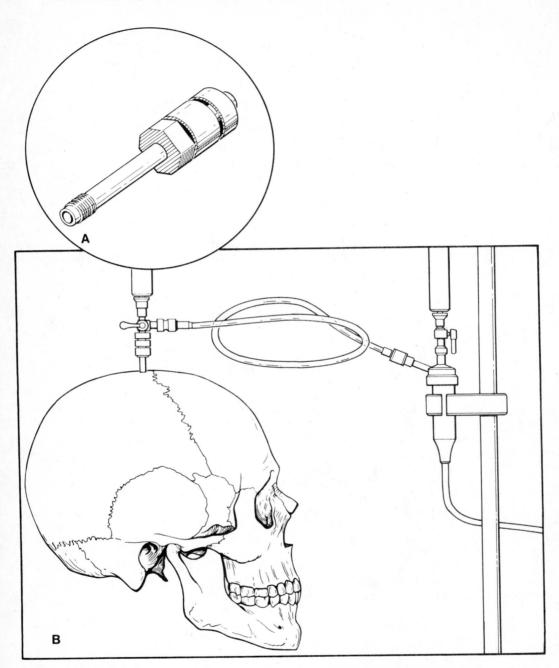

Figure 21-3. Subarachnoid screw for ICP monitoring (**A**) and subarachnoid screw and monitoring transducer in place (**B**).

tery monitoring, where dampened waveforms are *not* acceptable.

Flat line tracings are unacceptable. The flat line may be high or low. It indicates occlusion of the monitoring tip. As long as a tracing is scalloped in phase with arterial pulsation, the readings are acceptable.

Implications and Interventions

ICP monitoring is useful in early interventions (stages 1 and 2) to control the ICP.

1. Cellular hypoxia is most likely to occur during the "A" waves (plateau waves). "A" waves indicate sustained pressure peaks up to 100 mm Hg (roughly 136 cm H_2O). These waves frequently coincide with headache, decreasing level of consciousness (LOC), and a generalized neurological deterioration. If the patient is on a respirator, hyperventilation is utilized to maintain the $Paco_2$ between 25 and 35. This will cause a vasoconstriction that may help control ICP.
2. With increasing ICP, the LOC decreases and the reticular activating system, or "alerting system," fails. Medications such as mannitol, steroids, and diuretics may help decrease the ICP.

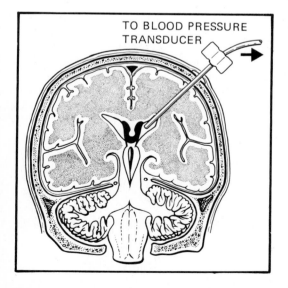

Figure 21-4. Intraventricular cannula for ICP monitoring.

3. Motor responses such as hemiparesis or decorticate or decerebrate positioning occur as a result of cortical and midbrain compression of motor tracts. In some centers, barbiturate coma therapy may be tried. Some centers will only continue treatments if the aforementioned conditions 1 and 2 exist.
4. Changes in vital signs and the respiratory pattern are late changes indicating brain stem compression (the pons and medulla oblongata). Interventions will include those listed in conditions 1, 2, and 3. Prognosis is poor.

Nursing Intervention

Most nursing procedures have an effect on the ICP. Turning the patient may increase the ICP. If the patient can cooperate, having him or her exhale while turning prevents a Valsalva maneuver (Valsalva maneuvers increase ICP). If two nursing actions both increase ICP, space the nursing care to allow the ICP to diminish after the first action before starting the second action.

Suctioning is imperative if the patient cannot clear secretions. Suctioning increases ICP and decreases oxygen availability during the procedure. Limiting suctioning to a maximum of ten seconds, hyperventilating the patient before and after the procedure.

Dehydration and electrolyte imbalances may occur rapidly in conditions precipitating increased ICP. Careful monitoring of the electrolytes and serum osmolality will allow early interventions to regulate ICP responses.

Infections are a major threat in intraventricular and subdural monitoring. If irrigation is performed by the physician, an antibiotic solution may be used. Fever increases cerebral metabolism and may compromise the ICP. Hypothermia blankets may be used to help control febrile states. The most important step in preventing infection is maintaining a closed system.

Glucocorticoids may be used to decrease cerebral edema. Maintaining an elevated head (15 to 30 degrees) is thought to help cerebral edema by promoting venous return from the cranium.

Physical signs of an increased ICP, such as hypertension and bradycardia, should be monitored consistently. It has become obvious through ICP monitoring that the physical signs of decreasing LOC, Cushing's triad, and pupillary changes occur late in the course of an increasing ICP. Reliance on only these physical parameters may result in irreversible brain damage and/or death.

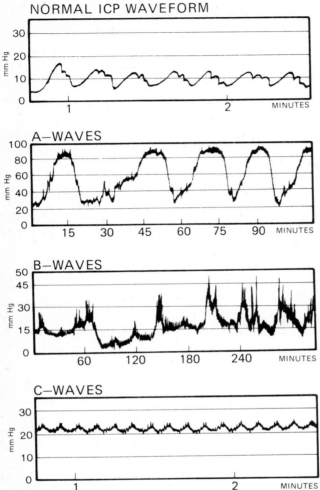

NORMAL ICP WAVEFORM

1. Normal waveform has steep upward systolic slope, followed by downward diastolic slope with dicrotic notch. Ordinarily, this waveform occurs continuously and indicates an ICP measurement between 4 and 15 mm Hg.

A—WAVES

2. The A—waves (sometimes called plateau waves) typically reach elevations of 50 to 100 mm Hg and then drop sharply. If they're recurring or are sustained for several minutes, A—waves indicate a rapid, dangerous rise in ICP and a decreased ability to compensate. Consider such waves ominous. Sustained A—waves may indicate irreversible brain damage.

B—WAVES

3. The B—waves are sharp and rhythmic, with a sawtooth pattern. They occur every 1½ to 2 minutes and may reach elevations of 50 mm Hg. But high elevations aren't sustained. They seem to occur more frequently with decreasing compensation. Sometimes they precede A-waves. Watch them closely.

C—WAVES

4. C—waves are rapid and rhythmic, less sharp in appearance than B—waves, and may fluctuate with respirations or changing systemic blood pressure. C—waves aren't clinically significant.

Figure 21-5. ICP waveforms. (Adapted from *Coping with Neurologic Disorders,* Nursing Photobook series, Springhouse, PA: Intermed Communications, Inc., p. 87, 1981.)

INTRACRANIAL ANEURYSMS

Definition

An aneurysm is considered to be a congenital developmental defect in the muscle layer of arteries, normally occurring at points of bifurcation. (Recall that there are three layers in the arterial wall: the inner endothelial layer [the intima, a middle smooth muscle layer], the media, and an outer layer of connective tissue [the adventitia].)

Pathophysiology

The congenital weakness of the arterial wall results in a gradual "ballooning out" of that segment of the artery over a period of years. When an increase in vascular pressure rises to a sufficient (unknown) pressure, the weakened ballooning segment of the artery bursts.

Location, Incidence, and Etiology

Most cerebral aneurysms develop in the anterior arteries of the circle of Willis. Aneurysms are the fourth leading cause of cerebrovascular problems. Aneurysms are rare in children and teenagers and most common in the middle age group. Slightly more females than males have aneurysms. Some 10 to 20% of patients with aneurysms have more than one (may be found on the same or opposite side).

Etiological factors may include hypertension (in a majority of cases). No specific precipitating factors are present in all patients. Congenital anomalies account for some aneurysms, and others occur for unknown reasons.

Clinical Presentation

Aneurysms are commonly asymptomatic until a bleed occurs. The exception is a very large aneurysm, which may cause symptoms related to pressure against surrounding tissues. Severe headache (unlike any other headache) occurs as the aneurysm starts to bleed. Unconsciousness may occur and be transient or sustained secondary to ischemia and/or necrosis of brain tissue. Nausea and vomiting are common. Transient neurological deficits include numbness, aphasias, and paresis.

Nuchal rigidity, photophobia, diplopia, Kernig's sign (inability to fully extend leg when thigh is flexed to the abdomen), Brudzinski's sign (involuntary adduction and flexion of legs when neck is flexed), and headache are common because of meningeal irritation. All of these signs except diplopia are sometimes grouped together under the term meningismus.

Diagnosis

A lumbar puncture is usually performed. Elevated CSF pressure, elevated protein levels, elevated red blood cells, and grossly bloody spinal fluid indicate hemorrhage in the subarachnoid space.

CAT scanning will reveal areas of intracerebral

bleed. *Note:* In the adult, an intracerebral bleed is never the cause of a hypovolemic shock state if the cranium is intact. The intact cranium does not have sufficient space to accommodate the quantity of blood required to cause a hypovolemic shock state.

Carotid and vertebral angiography may reveal the presence of other small aneurysms. Angiography may determine the patient's suitability for preventative measures such as hypotensive drugs or intracranial-extracranial bypass anastomosis, clipping/ligating, or reinforcing the artery.

Classification of Clinical State Postaneurysmal Rupture

Aneurysms may be placed in one of five categories (grades). These grades are summarized in Table 21-2. If patients can be stabilized in grade I or II, they may be candidates for surgical intervention.

Prognosis

The prognosis depends upon the site and severity of the bleed. Persistent coma beyond two days is a poor sign. Rebleeds may occur as the original clot that formed around the bleed is absorbed (or lysed). This usually occurs between the seventh and eleventh days after the original bleed and carries a poor prognosis. Increasing and/or persistent vasospasm results in increasing cerebral ischemia. Vasospasm is commonly seen about the third day postbleed. Marked cerebral edema and/or the development of hydrocephalus indicates a poor prognosis.

Nursing Intervention

Stabilization of the patient is the primary objective of treatment. Once the patient is stabilized and the condi-

TABLE 21-2. GRADES OF ANEURYSMS

Symptom	Grade I	Grade II	Grade III	Grade IV	Grade V
LOC	Alert	Decreased	Confused	Unresponsive	Moribund
Headache	Slight	Mild to severe	—	—	—
Nuchal rigidity	Slight	×	×	×	—
Vasospasm	—	—	—	May be present	May be present
Decerebrate posturing	—	—	—	—	×

× = present; dash = absent.

tion approaches grade I or II, surgical intervention is usually successful.

1. Complete bed rest with a quiet, dark environment promotes stabilization.
2. Although the procedure is controversial, the head of the bed may be elevated in an attempt to promote cerebral venous return by gravity. It is usually elevated 15 to 30 degrees.
3. Dehydrating the patient is avoided, but fluid intake is limited to decrease the possibility of rebleed from hypervolemia or increase ICP. If vasospasm occurs and is not controlled by other means, short periods of hypervolemia may be tried.
4. If alert, the patient should avoid Valsalva maneuvers and any other action that produces straining, such as forced cough to clear secretions and such. These actions will increase ICP and may start a rebleed.
5. Sedating drugs may be used to decrease stress, anxiety, or restlessness and may have the additional side effect of lowering the blood pressure in a hypertensive patient. Antihypertensive drugs may be used to prevent increases in pressure rather than to bring hypertension down to normal levels.
6. Antifibrinolytic drugs, usually epsilon-aminocaproic acid (Amicar), may be given by mouth, if the patient is alert, or intravenously. This drug may delay lysis of the aneurysmal clot. If the drug is given intravenously, a continuous infusion should be used to ensure a continuous therapeutic blood level (130 mg/mL). Efficacy of this treatment modality is controversial.
7. Antispasmodic drugs (e.g., reserpine) and/or anticonvulsants (e.g., phenytoin) may be used if conditions indicate the need.
8. Calcium channel blockers that cross the blood-brain barrier may be used to treat vasospasm.

Surgical Intervention and Nursing Implications

If an aneurysm is diagnosed prior to a bleed, surgery may be performed to prevent a bleed, depending upon the size and location of the aneurysm. If an aneurysmal bleed has occurred and the patient has stabilized in grade I or II, surgery may be performed.

Surgery may consist of one of several procedures:

1. Clipping the aneurysm is probably the oldest and the most frequent surgical treatment (Fig. 21-6). If the aneurysm is extremely large, clipping may not be possible.
2. Reinforcing the aneurysm by wrapping some of the new mesh materials around it and the artery may prevent further enlargement or rupture (Fig. 21-6). Caution must be taken not to decrease the arterial lumen, especially if atherosclerotic disease is present.
3. Trapping the aneurysm by ligating proximal and distal to the aneurysm may be the procedure of choice if the aneurysm is large (Fig. 21-6).
4. Embolization of the aneurysmal clot may be performed once the patient is stabilized, especially if the aneurysmal clot is impinging upon important structures (Fig. 21-6).

If the aneurysm cannot be reached and/or surgical risk of one of the above procedures is extremely high, the common carotid artery may be clamped. Prior to this procedure, angiography must demonstrate that vascular perfusion of the involved hemisphere is adequate from the opposite side.

The major nursing responsibilities are assessment of the neurological status for signs of increasing intracranial pressure, observing for signs of impending seizures, and performing the routine postoperative and postcraniotomy care.

ENCEPHALOPATHIES, COMA, AND BRAIN HERNIATION

Encephalopathies

The primary change produced in the critical care area by encephalopathies is either a behavior change or an alteration in LOC. Three common reasons for a change in LOC are reduction in oxygen delivery, reduction in blood glucose, and reduction in CPP. In addition, the accumulation of various metabolites of renal and hepatic failure can cause a change in LOC and behavior.

In any situation where a patient does not respond appropriately, the aforementioned considerations should be assessed for their impact. The specific alterations in behavior and LOC from renal and hepatic failure are addressed in later chapters.

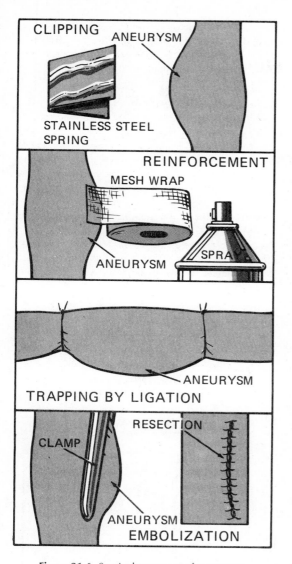

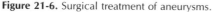

Figure 21-6. Surgical treatment of aneurysms.

Coma

Two general types of pathological processes lead to coma: (1) conditions that widely and directly depress function of the cerebral hemispheres and (2) conditions that depress or destroy brain stem-activating mechanisms.

Three categories of disease are important in the aforementioned pathological processes leading to coma.

1. A supratentorial mass lesion will encroach on deep diencephalic structures, compressing or destroying the ascending reticular activating system.
2. A subtentorial mass or destructive lesion may directly damage the brain stem central core.
3. Metabolic disorders may result in generalized interruption of brain function.

Coma does not occur as a result of focal injury or ischemia in a specific lobe. Coma occurs only when both cerebral hemispheres or brain stem divisions are dysfunctional. The major catastrophe of coma is death due to brain herniation.

Routes of Herniation

There are two main paths of herniation. Brain tissue can herniate through the tentorial notch and/or through the foramen magnum. Herniation through the tentorial notch will be central herniation or uncal herniation. The symptoms differ markedly with each.

Central herniation occurs when the cerebral hemisphere is compressed against the incisura (the opening in the tentorium cerebelli). This compresses the midbrain.

Uncal herniation occurs when the uncus (medial part of the temporal lobe) impacts upon the tentorial notch. This compresses the upper brain stem, especially the cerebral peduncles, and also traps the ipsilateral third cranial nerve.

Pathophysiology of Central Herniation

The tentorium cerebelli divides the supratentorial structures from the infratentorial structures. The tentorium cerebelli actually separates the cerebral hemispheres from the cerebellum. The tentorium cerebelli has an opening, the incisura (also called the tentorial notch). The midbrain passes through this opening. Increasing ICP forces the cerebral hemispheres and the basal nuclei through the tentorial notch. This displacement compresses the diencephalon, midbrain, and pons. Divisions of the basilar artery are also displaced, causing ischemia and brain stem deterioration.

The displacement also blocks the aqueduct of Sylvius, effectively preventing the downward displacement of CSF (a compensatory mechanism of increasing ICP). This further increases ICP. Central herniation usually progresses in a head-to-tail direction. Thus, an alteration in LOC is often a subtle first sign of impending herniation.

Pathophysiology of Uncal Herniation

The uncus is the median portion of the temporal lobe that hangs on the edge of the incisura (tentorial notch). An expanding temporal lobe lesion or increasing middle fossa pressure may force the uncus over the edge of the incisura. The movement of the uncus compresses the mesencephalon (midbrain) against the opposite edge of the incisura. Uncal herniation often presses the oculomotor nerve and posterior cerebral artery against the incisura. The earliest consistent sign in uncal herniation along with a change in LOC is a unilaterally dilating pupil.

Etiology

Herniation is the result of increased ICP beyond compensatory levels. Papilledema (edema of the optic disc) is a positive sign of increased ICP. However, in acute intracranial hypertension, papilledema may not occur immediately. In acute cases, elevated ICP may result in herniation before sufficient time has elapsed to allow for the development of papilledema.

Stages of Herniation

There are four distinct stages as central herniation progresses: early diencephalic, late diencephalic, midbrain–upper pons, and lower pons–upper medulla.

There are three stages in uncal herniation. The first stage is the uncal syndrome–early III nerve. The second stage is the uncal syndrome–late III nerve. The third stage is the same lower pons–upper medulla stage as in central herniation.

Monitoring Parameters in Herniation

Specific parameters can be monitored to indicate impending or active herniation.

In central herniation, the parameters are LOC, pupillary function (size and reaction to light), respiratory pattern, oculocephalic responses (doll's eyes) and oculovestibular responses (ice water caloric test), motor response, and ciliospinal reflex.

In uncal herniation, pupillary response and third-nerve palsy are early important signs. Then LOC (both content and degree of alertness), delirium, or lethargy suggests impending herniation. Respiratory, oculocephalic, and oculovestibular responses do not come into play until LOC has declined.

Parameter Norms and Testing Methods

1. LOC. LOC was discussed in Chapter 18 and will not be addressed again.
2. Pupils. Pupillary reaction is controlled by both sympathetic and parasympathetic tracts. These

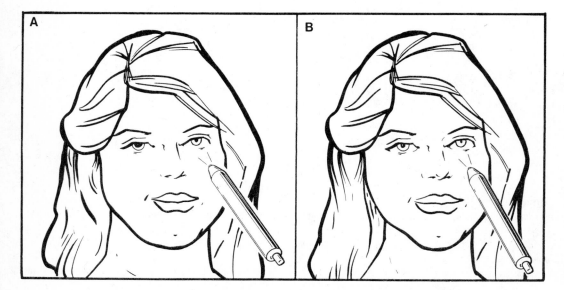

Figure 21-7. Pupillary light reflex (**A**) and consensual light reflex (**B**).

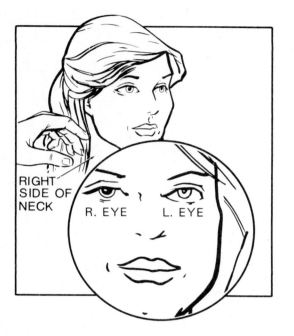

RIGHT
SIDE OF
NECK   R. EYE   L. EYE

Figure 21-8. Pupil response in the ciliospinal reflex (depicted in inset).

tracts are not easily affected by metabolic states. Therefore, the pupil light reflex is the single most important indicator in differentiating metabolic or structural (neurological) coma.

The pupil light reflex (Fig. 21-7) is best tested in a darkened room (although this is not always possible). In a normal state, a pupil will constrict when a light is directed into it. Normally, there is also a consensual response; that is, the eye not having a light beam directed into it constricts with the eye being tested.

3. Ciliospinal reflex. This is tested by pinching the skin on the back edge of the neck (Fig. 21-8). Normally, this action causes ipsilateral pupil dilatation.

4. Eye movements. The key eye movements observed in the comatose patient are the spontaneous motion of each eye, the resting position of each eye, and responses of the eyes to the oculocephalic and oculovestibular tests.

The resting position of the eyes may be conjugate, disconjugate, or skewed. Conju-

gate position is any resting position with both eyes in the same position. Disconjugate position is a resting position with the eyes in different positions. Right eye midline midposition and left eye midline, fixed to the right side, is an example of disconjugate eyes. Skewed eyes are any vertical disconjugate positioning. Skewing indicates a brain stem lesion.

The oculocephalic response (Fig. 21-9) is often called doll's eyes. Doll's eyes can be tested only in the unconscious patient and is normally recorded as present or absent. To test the oculocephalic response, hold the patient's eyelids open and quickly but gently turn the head to one side. The normal response is for the eyes to conjugately deviate in the contraversive direction of the head turning. Repeat by flexing and extending the head. Again, the normal response is conjugate (parallel) contraversive movement of the eyes in the direction of head movement. This is referred to as doll's eyes present. Abnormal responses are referred to as doll's eyes absent. If the eyes move in the same direction of head position (i.e., flex head and eyes go down, or turn head to right and eyes go right or no further than midline), the test is abnormal (doll's eyes absent). Cranial nerves III, IV, and VI, which are responsible for ocular movements, are not intact. Turning the head to both the right and the left will test each pair of these nerves. Doll's eyes must *never* be tested unless cervical spinal cord or vertebral injuries have been ruled out.

The oculovestibular reflex (the ice water caloric test) is more powerful in eliciting eye movements. An intact tympanic membrane is essential. The head of the bed is elevated about 30 degrees. The physician slowly injects ice water until nystagmus or eye deviation occurs (or until 200 cc of ice water has been used). In the unconscious patient, the eyes move slowly toward the irrigated ear and remain there two to three minutes (Fig. 21-10). This indicates a supratentorial lesion or a metabolic condition. An extremely abnormal movement (skewing, jerky rotation) usually indicates a cerebellar or brain stem lesion.

5. Motor responses. Motor responses are not dependent on LOC, but they may and usually do correlate with LOC. These are important

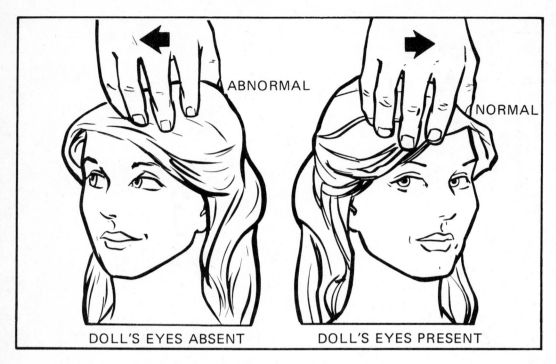

ABNORMAL

NORMAL

DOLL'S EYES ABSENT

DOLL'S EYES PRESENT

Figure 21-9. Oculocephalic response (doll's eyes phenomenon).

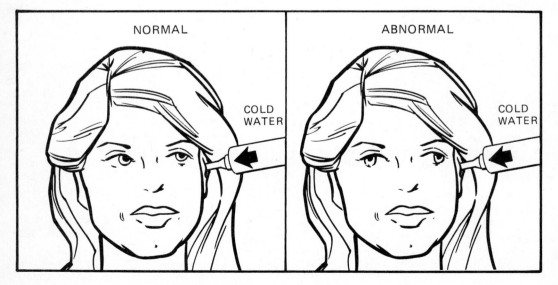

NORMAL

ABNORMAL

COLD WATER

COLD WATER

Figure 21-10. Pupil response in the oculovestibular reflex.

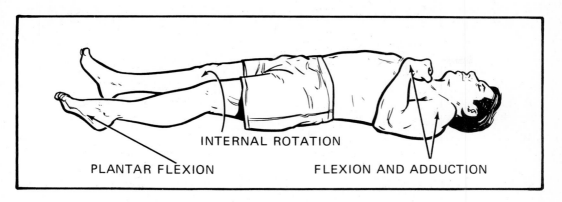

Figure 21-11. Decorticate posture (abnormal flexion response).

sources of information concerning the geographical spread of neurological dysfunction.

A cerebral hemisphere frontal lobe dysfunction is characterized by paraplegia in flexion, tonic grasping, and exaggerated snout reflexes. Decorticate posture (Fig. 21-11) is characterized by flexion of the arm, wrist, and fingers. Adduction of arms along with extension and internal rotation with plantar flexion of the lower extremities complete the motor responses. Decorticate posturing is synonymous with abnormal flexion response. Decerebrate posture is characterized by opisthotonos (arching of the back so that the head and heels remain on the surface and the remainder of the back is raised), with arms slightly extended, adducted, and hyperpronated (Fig. 21-12).

The legs are stiffly extended, and the feet are flexed in a plantar position. Abnormal extension response is synonymous with decerebrate posture.

6. Respiratory patterns. These patterns were discussed in Part 2 and will not be addressed again here.

Table 21-3 identifies the stages and parameter responses in central herniation. Table 21-4 identifies the stages and parameter responses in uncal herniation.

Herniation Through the Foramen Magnum

If the ICP rises precipitously, the pressure may be of sufficient force to compress the cerebellum and medulla oblongata through the foramen magnum. A lumbar puncture performed in the presence of high ICP

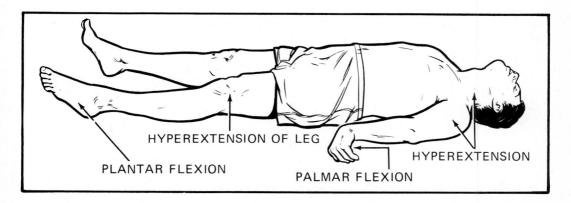

Figure 21-12. Decerebrate posture (abnormal extension response).

TABLE 21-3. STAGES AND PARAMETERS OF CENTRAL HERNIATION

	Central—Early Diencephalic	Central—Late Diencephalic	Midbrain—Upper Pons	Lower Pons—Upper Medulla
Respirations				
Pupillary response				
Consensual light response				
Ciliospinal reflex				
Oculovestibular response				
Doll's eye response				
Babinski response				
Body position response	Rest / Stimulus			

TABLE 21-4. STAGES AND PARAMETERS OF UNCAL HERNIATION

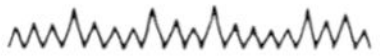

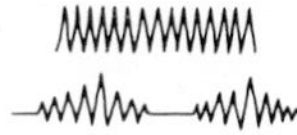

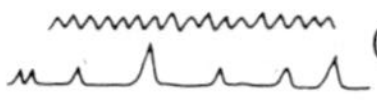

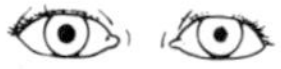

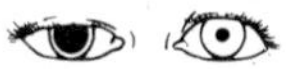

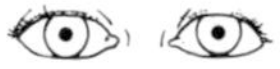

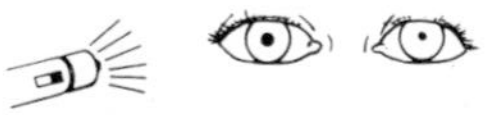

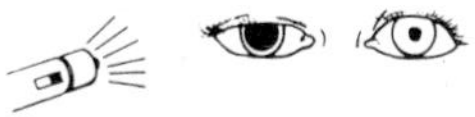

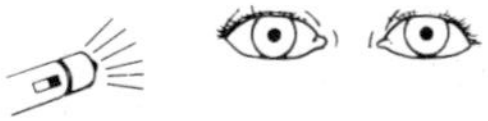

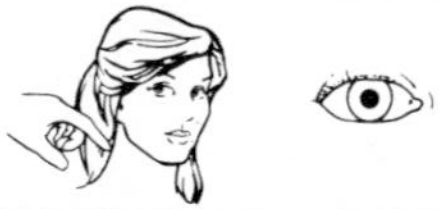

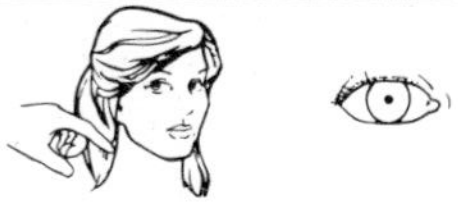

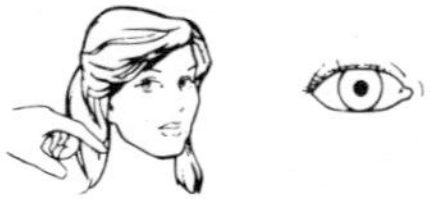

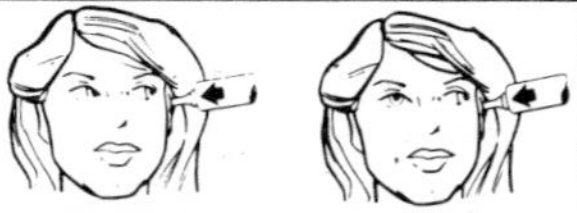

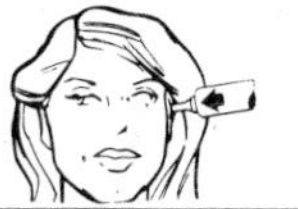

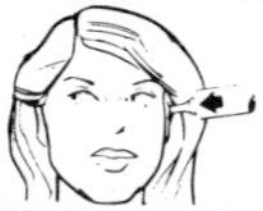

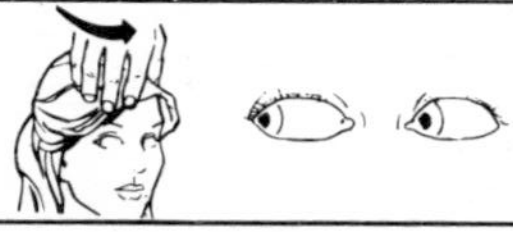

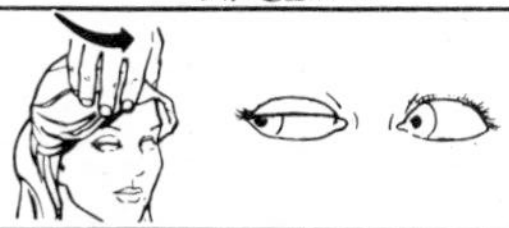

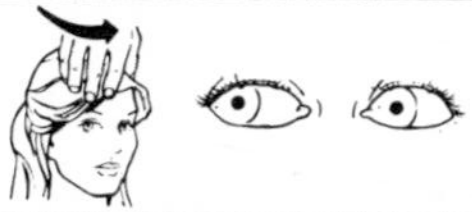

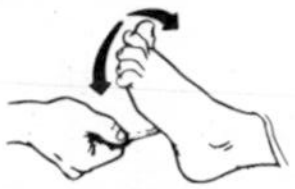

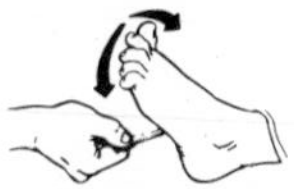

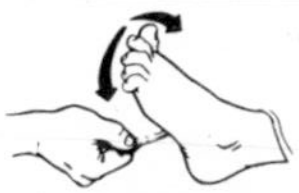

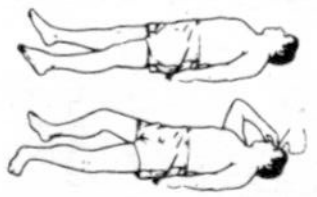

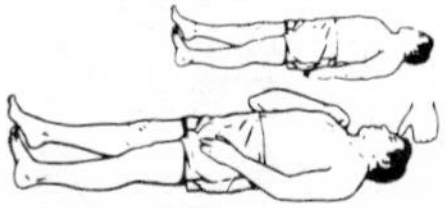

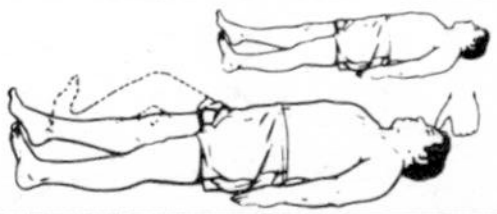

may result in brain stem herniation through the foramen magnum as the counterpressure in the spinal canal is lost. Herniation through the foramen magnum results in death secondary to cardiopulmonary arrest. This form of herniation is not clinically separable from central and uncal herniation.

BIBLIOGRAPHY

Adelstein, W., & Watson, P. (1983). Cervical cord injuries. *J Neurosurg Nurs, 15,* 65–71.

Bastnagel-Mason, P.J. (1992). Neurodiagnostic testing in critically injured adults. *Crit Care Nurse, 12,* 64–75.

Bell, J., and Hannon, K. (1986). Pathophysiology involved in autonomic dysreflexia. *J Neurosurg Nurs, 16,* 86–88.

Brucia, J. A., Owen, D.C., & Rudy, E.B. (1992). The effects of lidocaine on intracranial hypertension. *J Neurosci Nurs, 24,* 4, 205–214.

Butterworth, J.F., & DeWitt, D.S. (1989). Severe head trauma: Pathophysiology and management. *Crit Care Clin, 5,* 4, 807–820.

Chipps, E. (1992). Transphenoidal surgery for pituitary tumors. *Crit Care Nurs, 12,* 1, 30–39.

Cummings, R. (1992). Understanding external ventricular drainage. *J Neurosci Nurs, 24,* 2, 84–87.

Dudas, S., & Stevens, K. (1984). Central cord injury: Implications for nursing. *J Neurosurg Nurs, 16,* 2, 84–88.

Franco, L.M. (1984). Cerebral contusion, a prototype for head injury. *J Neurosurg Nurs, 16,* 1, 45–49.

Gilman, S., & Newman, S.W. (1987). *Manter and Gatz's Essentials of Clinical Neuroanatomy and Neurophysiology,* 7th ed. Philadelphia: F.A. Davis Co.

Giubilato, R. (1982). Acute care of the high level quadriplegic patient. *J Neurosurg Nurs, 14,* 3, 128–132.

Gruppi, L.A. (1987). Acoustic neuromas: Nursing management during the acute postoperative period. *Crit Care Nurse, 7,* 5, 16–25.

Harper, J. (1989). Use of steroids in cerebral edema: Therapeutic implications. *Heart Lung, 17,* 1, 70–75.

Hickey, J. (1986). *The Clinical Practice of Neurological and Neurosurgical Nursing,* 2nd ed. Philadelphia: J.B. Lippincott.

Hudak, C.M., Lohr, T.S., & Gallo, B.M. (eds.). (1986). *Critical Care Nursing,* 4th ed. Philadelphia: J.B. Lippincott.

Ingersoll, G.L., & Leyden, D.B. (1987). The Glasgow coma scale for patients with head injuries. *Crit Care Nurse, 7,* 5, 26–32.

Lindamann, C. (1992). S.I.A.D.H.: Is your patient at risk? *Nursing, 22,* 6, 60–63.

Manifold, S.L. (1986). Craniocerebral trauma. *Focus Crit Care, 13,* 2, 22–35.

Mathewson, M. (1985). Ascending and descending spinal cord tracts. *Crit Care Nurse, 5,* 10–14.

Morrison, C.A. (1987). Brain herniation syndromes. *Crit Care Nurse, 7,* 5, 34–38.

Nikas, D.L. (1987). Critical aspects of head trauma. *Crit Care Nurs Q, 10,* 1, 19–44.

Pollack-Latham, C. (1987). Intracranial pressure monitoring: Physiologic principles. *Crit Care Nurse, 7,* 5, 40–52.

Pryden, M. (1983). Guillain-Barré syndrome: Disease process. *J Neurosurg Nurs, 15,* 1.

Ross, A.M., Pitts, L.H., & Kobayashi, S. (1992). Prognosticators of outcome after major head injury in the elderly. *J Neurosci Nurs, 24,* 2, 88–93.

Rudy, E., Turner, B., Baum, M., et al. (1991). Endotracheal suctioning in adults with head injury. *Heart Lung, 20,* 667–674.

Segatore, M. (1992). Fever after traumatic brain injury. *J Neurosci Nurs, 24,* 2, 104–109.

Tikkanen, P.L. (1984). Landry Guillain-Barré syndrome. *J Neurosci Nurs, 16,* 6.

Vulcan, B.M. (1987). Acute bacterial meningitis in infancy and childhood. *Crit Care Nurse, 7,* 5, 53–65.

Young, W.L., & McCormick, P.C. (1989). Perioperative management of intracranial catastrophes. *Crit Care Clin, 5,* 4, 821–841.

PART 4

Gastroenterology

Lori Geisman, RN, MSN, CCRN

Anatomy and Physiology of the Gastrointestinal System

Editor's Note

This chapter provides a good review of the general anatomy and physiology of gastrointestinal function. Few if any questions from this chapter will be included on the CCRN exam. Use this chapter to strengthen your overall understanding of gastrointestinal anatomy and physiology.

The process of digestion and absorption of nutrients requires an intact and healthy gastrointestinal tract epithelial lining that is able to resist the effects of its own digestive secretions. It involves the movement of materials through the gastrointestinal tract at a rate that facilitates absorption, and it requires the presence of enzymes that are needed for digestion and absorption of nutrients.

In this system, enzymes and hormones are produced, vitamins are synthesized and stored, and food is dismantled and then reassembled. Nutrients, vitamins, minerals, electrolytes, and water enter the body through the gastrointestinal tract. Catalysts and reactants play a role, and some are recycled and used again. Finally, wastes are collected and eliminated.

UPPER GASTROINTESTINAL SYSTEM

Oral Cavity (Mouth)

The oral cavity consists of the lips, cheeks, teeth, gums, tongue, palate, and salivary glands. Its main functions include ingestion, mastication, salivation, and the first phase of swallowing (deglutition).

The salivary glands' total daily secretion is between 1 and 1.5 liters of saliva. Saliva is secreted in the mouth. The salivary glands consist of the parotid,

submaxillary, sublingual, and buccal glands. Saliva has three functions. The first of these is protection and lubrication. Saliva is rich in mucus, which serves to protect the oral mucosa and to coat the food as it passes through the mouth, pharynx, and esophagus. The sublingual and buccal glands produce only mucous types of secretions. The second function is its protective antimicrobial action. The saliva not only cleanses the mouth but contains the enzyme lysosome, which has an antibacterial action. Third, saliva contains ptyalin and amylase, which initiates the digestion of dietary starches.

Secretions from the salivary glands are primarily regulated by the autonomic nervous system. Parasympathetic stimulation decreases flow. These nuclei are controlled mainly by taste impulses and tactile sensory impulses from the mouth.

Tongue

The tongue is a mass of striated and skeletal muscles that is covered by a mucous membrane. It is a highly mobile, muscular, and tactile organ, and it plays an important part in articulate speech. It is also necessary to the digestive tract, being involved in mastication and swallowing as well as being the chief organ of taste. The surface of the tongue and its side edges are covered with papillae. The papillae contain the taste buds, which are highly specialized nerve endings. A perfectly dry tongue cannot taste, and the sense itself is limited to four discriminations: bitter, sweet, salty, and sour. Many of the finer sensations attributed to taste are actually received by the organ of smell.

Swallowing is initiated when a bolus of food is pushed backward by the tongue into the pharynx, a voluntary act. The bolus stimulates swallowing receptor areas located in the pharynx, transmitting impulses to the medulla oblongata via the trigeminal nerve. The autonomic nervous system is activated, and a series of pharyngeal, laryngeal, and esophageal contractions result from transmission via the glossopharyngeal and vagus nerves.

Pharynx

The pharynx connects the oral cavity to the esophagus. The pharyngeal walls are composed of longitudinal and circular striated muscle fibers that surround the fibrous tissues involved in deglutition. The pharynx is divided into three sections: nasopharynx, oropharynx, and laryngeal pharynx.

Esophagus

The pharynx ends at the level of the sixth cervical vertebra to become the esophagus. The total length of the esophagus is about 25 cm (10 inches). The upper one-fifth lies in the neck; the lower four-fifths lie in the thorax. It is located posterior to the trachea and is capable of altering its own size.

Three cellular layers comprise the wall of the esophagus. The innermost layer of cells is the mucosal layer made up of squamous epithelium. The middle layer is muscle arranged circularly around the lumen. The upper one-third of this middle layer is skeletal (striated) muscle controlled directly by nerves from the brain; the remainder is smooth muscle that is only indirectly controlled by the central nervous system through the effects of the autonomic nervous system on the intramural plexus. The outermost layer of cells is longitudinal muscle fibers.

When food is pushed from the pharynx through the hypopharyngeal sphincter into the esophagus, the propulsion continues throughout the length of the esophagus and is known as peristaltic waves controlled by vagal response. These peristaltic waves often exert as much as 50 to 70 cm of water pressure. The peristaltic waves move the food bolus down the esophagus, through the gastroesophageal sphincter, and into the stomach. Food normally passes from the mouth through the esophagus and into the stomach in about seven seconds.

Two sphincters control food boluses from moving in and out of the esophagus. The hypopharyngeal sphincter, the superior end of the esophagus, opens to allow food to enter the esophagus from the pharynx. When the hypopharyngeal sphincter is relaxed, it is closed due to a passive elastic tension. When the skeletal muscles contract, the sphincter opens and a bolus of food may enter the esophagus, creating a peristaltic wave that advances the food through the esophagus.

The sphincter may also open during vomiting to allow the food to be regurgitated.

The gastroesophageal sphincter, also known as the cardiac sphincter, functions in the same way as the hypopharyngeal sphincter. The gastroesophageal sphincter controls food boluses leaving the esophagus into the stomach. It opens as peristaltic waves travel along the esophagus to allow the bolus of food to enter and closes to prevent a reflux of food and acid. If the sphincter cannot close, a condition known as achalasia exists. Achalasia is damage of the myenteric level of nerves that innervate the sphincter and prevent it from closing.

A condition known as reflux may occur as a result of inappropriate relaxation of the gastroesophageal sphincter. It may occur in a variety of conditions such as pregnancy, obesity, excess caffeine and tobacco intake, hiatal hernia, and some medication ingestions. Treatment of the problem may help relieve the sensation of chest pain. Diet change may also relieve discomfort.

The opening in the diaphragm that allows passage of the esophagus is the esophageal hiatus. As soon as the esophagus passes through the opening, it almost immediately enters the stomach. If this opening becomes enlarged, the stomach usually bulges into the opening. This condition is termed a hiatal hernia.

No enzymes are secreted in the esophagus. The esophagus secretes only mucus. The mucus protects the mucosa from excoriation from food that is in its most abrasive form.

Stomach

The stomach is the most dilated portion of the digestive tract and has an average capacity of about 1 liter. It is located in the epigastric, umbilical, and left hypochondriac regions of the abdomen. It is subject to considerable variation in shape and size, but an average stomach is J shaped in general outline and has a maximum length of about 25 cm (10 inches) and a maximum breadth of about 14 cm.

The stomach is generally described as having three sections: the fundus, the body, and the pylorus (Fig. 22-1). The upper lateral border of the stomach is called the lesser curvature. The lesser curvature carries downward the line of the right border of the esophagus and throughout most of its extent is nearly vertical. The lower lateral border is called the greater curvature. The greater curvature is subject to considerable variation in length and position, depending on the condition of the stomach at the time of examination.

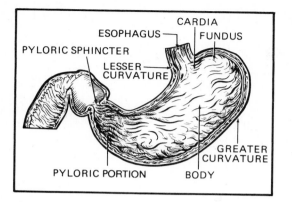

Figure 22-1. Divisions and curvatures of the stomach.

Openings of the Stomach. The esophagus has thickened, circular muscles at the distal end just as it passes into the stomach. These thickened circular muscles form the cardiac sphincter.

The pyloric sphincter has the same anatomical structure and the same physiologic function as the cardiac sphincter. The pyloric sphincter controls the opening at the distal end of the stomach into the duodenum. It lies 3 cm to the right of the midline and about 5 cm below the tip of the sternum. The sphincter is slightly open most of the time, permitting fluids to be squirted out but preventing escape of solids.

Layers. The stomach wall is composed of three muscular layers. The outer layer consists of longitudinal muscle fibers. The middle layer consists of circular fibers. The innermost third layer consists of transverse (oblique) fibers (Fig. 22-2).

The gastric mucosa lines the interior of the stomach. The mucous membrane is thick and velvety, with the appearance of a honeycomb. In the body and the pyloric end, the muscularis mucosa is thrown into folds or ridges called rugae. These rugae allow for distension.

The interior mucosa of the stomach has a layer called the submucosa. The layer is composed of blood and lymph vessels and connective and fibrous tissue.

Visceral peritoneum covers the exterior of the stomach and consists of tissue which "hangs" in a double layer from the greater curvature of the stomach to cover the anterior side of abdominal viscera. This is the greater omentum (Fig. 22-3).

Gastric Glands. Glands are present throughout the gastrointestinal tract to secrete chemicals that mix with the food and digest it. These secretions are of two types: (1) mucus, which protects the wall of the gastrointestinal tract and liquefies the stomach contents, and (2) enzymes and allied substances that break the large chemical compounds of the food into simple compounds.

Mucus is secreted by every portion of the gastrointestinal tract. It contains a large amount of mucoprotein that is resistant to almost all digestive juices. Mucus also lubricates the passage of food along the mucosa, and it forms a thin film everywhere to prevent the food and hydrochloric acid from excoriating the mucosa. It is amphoteric, which means that it is capable of neutralizing either acids or bases. All of these properties make mucus an excellent substance for protecting the mucosa from physical damage and preventing digestion of the wall of the gut by the digestive juices.

A number of substances, such as aspirin, bile salts, ethyl alcohol, and acetic acid, have been shown to alter ion influxes and potential differences across

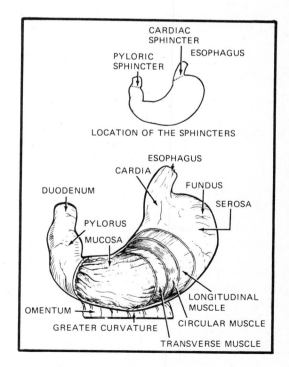

Figure 22-2. Layers of the stomach wall.

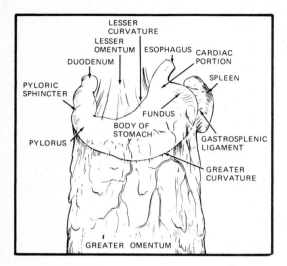

Figure 22-3. Greater omentum.

gastric mucosa, and these changes have been interpreted as a reflection of damage to the gastric mucosa. How these substances disrupt the gastric mucosa is not known. Possibly, active ion transport is inhibited or metabolic processes are altered, thus leading to changes in the permeability of the mucosa, predisposing a person to destruction of mucosa cells (ulcer formation).

The proximal portion of the stomach, the cardia, receives the bolus of food from the esophagus. This stimulates gastric glands to secrete lipase, pepsin, the intrinsic factor, mucus, hydrochloric acid, and gastrone (inhibits secretion of the acids), collectively known as gastric juice. The mucosa of the stomach contains few gastric glands at the fundus, many glands in the body, and fewer glands at the antral (pyloric) portion of the body.

Gastric glands are tubular. The narrow neck of each gland opens into the stomach. Chief cells in the gastric gland's neck have two functions: to secrete mucus and to regenerate cells both for the glands themselves and for the intestinal surface epithelial tissue. Argentaffin cells are present in the tissues of the gastric glands. These cells contain granules which are thought to be the origin of serotonin.

The fundus (blind end of the gland) has parietal (oxyntic) cells that secrete hydrochloric acid, water, and the intrinsic factor. Hydrochloric acid is an enzyme involved in the digestion of proteins. It also acti-

vates other enzymes in the stomach for digestion and kills bacteria. Hydrochloric acid secretion may be increased by four endogenous substances: histamine, gastrin, calcium, and acetylcholine. Atropine, a muscarinic antagonist, may block hydrochloric acid secretion caused by acetylcholine. Cimetidine, ranitidine, nizatidime, and famotidine, which are histamine H2 receptor antagonists, block histamine-induced hydrochloric acid secretion.

The intrinsic factor from the parietal cell is a mucoprotein that is essential for absorption of vitamin B_{12}. Once released from the parietal cells, the intrinsic factor adheres to epithelial cells in the ileum. If the ileum is surgically resected, exogenous B_{12} must be taken for life.

Zymogenic (chief) cells found in the body of a gastric gland secrete pepsinogen, an inactive proteolytic enzyme. The hydrochloric acid activates the pepsinogen to form pepsin, which is an enzyme that begins the digestion of proteins by splitting amino acid bonds.

The pyloric (antral) portion of the stomach has increased depth, size, and muscle and secretes mucus and pepsinogen. The hormone gastrin, a large polypeptide, is secreted from G cells in the antral mucosa and is absorbed into the bloodstream. This hormone then passes by way of the blood to the fundic glands of the stomach and causes them to secrete a strongly acidic gastric juice. The acid, in turn, greatly aids in the digestion of the meats that first initiated the gastrin mechanism. In this way, the stomach helps to tailor-make the secretion to fit the particular type of food eaten.

Gastric Motility. The rugae allow for a great distention of the stomach without increasing pressure (Laplace's law), which may be termed a receptive relaxation phenomenon. This may allow for stomach contents to approach 6 to 7 liters before peristaltic contractions are initiated.

Factors affecting gastric motility include quantity of contents, pH of contents, degree of mixing and peristalsis that has occurred, and the capacity of the duodenum to accept chyme from the stomach.

Usually, the fundus of the stomach is stimulated to initiate oscillations (mild "mixing waves") when about 1 liter of food is in the stomach, but there may be considerably more food present. These mixing waves occur approximately once every 20 seconds. When the food (bolus) is digested to the chyme state, it is ready for passage into the duodenum.

However, mixing waves alone are unable to achieve this. If no other influences are functional, malabsorption states will occur. To help the conversion of food boluses to chyme, the mixing waves assist the hormones and acids to mix with the food. As the peristaltic contractions move toward the antral (pyloric) portion of the stomach, they become very strong in order to force the chyme into the duodenum. A pH of 1 to 3 is obtained by the hormone gastrin stimulating the release of hydrochloric acid into the chyme and also stimulating peristaltic contractions, which will occur at a rate of about three per minute.

The enterogastric reflex (which causes lower gastrin and acid secretion) will delay the progression of chyme. This reflex is under vagal influence. It is stimulated by the degree of distension of the duodenum, by the presence of any degree of irritation of the duodenal mucosa, by the osmolality, acidity, and degree of emulsification of the chyme.

Chyme must be of the proper consistency and acidity, and the duodenum must be receptive for the strong antral peristaltic contractions to force the chyme through the pyloric valve. The small size of the pyloric sphincter opening results in little chyme entering the duodenum. Most of the chyme is squirted back toward the body of the stomach as the pyloric valve relaxes and closes. This is an important action in the mixing of the chyme.

Gastric Emptying. The stomach empties at a rate proportional to the volume of its contents. Chemical composition of the chyme in the duodenum determines the rate and quantity of additional chyme entering the duodenum. The duodenum contains osmoreceptors, chemoreceptors, and baroreceptors (stretch receptors for volume distension) that influence duodenal activity. If the chyme has a high fat content upon entering the duodenum, a release of cholecystokinin occurs, inhibiting further release of chyme. High fat content is the factor most known for inhibiting gastric emptying. Secretin may also be released to inhibit gastric emptying by inhibiting the gastrin mechanism.

Other factors such as emotional depression, sadness, and pain (both physical and psychological) inhibit emptying of the stomach. An inadequate fluid intake will retard emptying of the stomach because a large quantity of liquid is necessary to turn fat, protein, and carbohydrates into chyme.

Normally about 2 liters of gastric juices (primarily hydrochloric acid) are secreted per day. The pH is 1 to 3. This acidity and its resultant irritation affect gastric emptying by decreasing it. Inadequate protein breakdown and hypertonicity of the chyme will also slow gastric emptying.

Factors increasing gastric motility include aggression, increased volume of chyme, and fluids. The more liquid the stomach chyme is, the greater will be the ease of emptying.

Control of Gastric Secretions

Gastric secretions may be controlled through autonomic nervous system functions, by hormonal alterations, and/or through baroreceptors.

The control of the gastric secretions, specifically hydrochloric acid, may be broken down into three phases: the cephalic, the gastric, and the intestinal phases. These three phases follow the path of food and then chyme through the alimentary tract. When the stomach is at rest, normal secretion occurs at a rate of about 0.5 mL/minute. This is known as the basal rate. With food in the stomach, the rate of secretion increases to about 3.0 mL/minute.

Cephalic Phase. The parasympathetic nervous system controls the first phase of regulation of gastric secretion via the vagus nerve. The sight, smell, taste, or thought of food is sufficient to stimulate the release of hydrochloric acid in preparation for the expected arrival of food boluses. In addition to pleasant thoughts of food, hunger, hypoglycemia, and anger will also stimulate secretion of hydrochloric acid.

Vagal control is decreased by certain drugs (especially the anticholinergic drugs), hyperglycemia, and duodenal distension. A vagotomy may eliminate the cephalic phase.

Gastric Phase. This second phase of control over gastric secretion begins when food actually enters the stomach. The predominant regulatory mechanism in this phase is hormonal. Gastrin is the major hormone and it increases acid secretion from the oxyntic cells. It is stimulated by antral distention, secretion of pepsinogen, and an alkaline pH in the stomach. This phase has a negative feedback effect—as hydrochloric acid is released in response to gastrin, the stomach contents eventually become acid. When the number of hydrogen ions (acidity; pH of 2) is adequately high, gastrin secretion decreases.

Intestinal Phase. This phase begins when chyme enters the duodenum. Chyme entering the duodenum is more acid than that in the body of the stomach because as polypeptide fragments move from the body of the stomach to the antrum, they stimulate acid secretion by an unknown mechanism (but to a lesser extent than in the stomach).

When the chyme has a pH below 2.5, it is accepted more slowly into the duodenum. In the gastric phase, the chyme becomes more alkaline so that it will move into the duodenum in the intestinal phase.

Fat in the duodenum stimulates the secretion of cholecystokinin, which directly decreases gastric motility. Of the food types leaving the stomach, carbohydrates are the most rapid, followed by protein and then fat.

Gastric Digestion. Gastric digestion includes carbohydrates, proteins, and fats. The stomach is a poor absorptive area of the gastrointestinal tract. Only a few highly lipid-soluble substances, such as alcohol, can be absorbed in small quantities.

Carbohydrates. Digestion of starches really begin in the mouth with action of ptyalin and continues in the stomach by hydrolyzing carbohydrates into oligosaccharides.

Protein. The first stage of protein breakdown by proteolytic enzymes occurs in the stomach.

Fats. Digestion of fats in the stomach is minimal. The only action the stomach has on fats is by gastric peristalsis, which reduces the size of triglyceride droplets and facilitates contact with a lipase secreted by von Ebner's glands.

LOWER GASTROINTESTINAL SYSTEM

The Small Intestine

The small intestine extends from the pyloric sphincter to the cecum. This 18- to 20-foot tube is divided into three segments. The first segment is the duodenum, which arises at the pyloric sphincter. It is a C-shaped segment about 10 inches long and ends at the ligament of Treitz. The middle segment, the jejunum, extends about 8 feet from the ligament of Treitz and has an alkaline pH (7.8). The third segment is the ileum, which is about 12 feet long. There is no distinct change from the jejunum to the ileum.

Layers of the Small Intestine Wall. The small intestinal wall has the same layering as does the stomach. The wall of the intestine consists of a secreting and absorbing mucous membrane called the mucosa. It is composed of epithelial and columnar cells, smaller blood vessels, nerve fibers, plasma, and blood cells. The next layer is the muscularis mucosa. The muscularis mucosa is lined with areolar tissue (the submucosa). The submucosa contains larger blood vessels, connective tissue, nerves, ganglia, and lymphoid elements. The submucosa is covered with two smooth muscular coats, an outer longitudinal one and an inner circular one. The intestine also possesses still another coat, since it is closely invested by peritoneum; this coat is the serous membrane (serosa) lining the walls of those cavities and reflected onto the walls of the tube.

The activity of gastrointestinal smooth muscle is controlled by local, humoral, and neural influences. The rhythmic movements are integrated by an intramural network that lies between the two muscular layers of the intestine. This network has two layers of nerve fibers, a submucosal network (Meissner's plexus) and a second layer that lies between the circular and longitudinal layers of smooth muscle (the myenteric or Auerbach's plexus). The intramural network is responsible for many of the locally controlled movements that occur in the digestive tract. The afferent fibers of this system are located largely within the submucosal network, and the motor fibers are within the myenteric plexus.

The intrinsic tone and rhythmic activity of the digestive tract can be modified by the autonomic nervous system. Generally, the parasympathetic nervous system increases gastrointestinal activity, while the sympathetic nervous system slows its activity.

Ileocecal Valve. At the junction of the ileum and the cecum is the ileocecal valve. This valve controls the flow of contents into the cecum and allows no regurgitation of cecal contents into the ileum.

Villi. Villi (singular villus) are the distinguishing characteristics of the small intestine (Fig. 22-4). These fingerlike projections into the lumen provide an extensive surface area. The villi and microvilli increase in absorptive capacity 600-fold for a total surface area of about 250 m^2. An extraordinary number of villi project from the mucosa into the lumen of the small intestine.

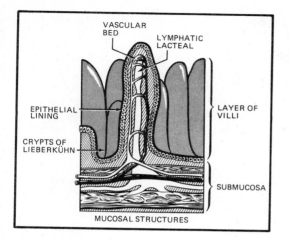

Figure 22-4. Structure of villi (a lacteal).

Each villus contains microvilli to actively absorb nutrients from the intestinal tract. Each villus contains a lymph vessel and a dense capillary bed to aid in the absorption process. This lymph vessel is called a lacteal. Carbohydrates, fats, proteins, vitamins, and minerals are absorbed into the small bowel through the villi.

Glands of the Small Intestine. The intestinal lumen is lined with simple, cuboidal, and columnar epithelial cells interspersed with goblet cells. The many goblet cells secrete mucus to protect the mucosa. The goblet cells decrease in numbers markedly toward the end of the ileum. Crypts of Lieberkühn (Fig. 22-5) are tubular glands found between the villi in the submucosa of the duodenum.

Absorptive and secreting cells have been identified but not differentiated in function. It is known that the crypts of Lieberkühn are extremely mitotic and replace villous cells. The entire intestinal epithelial surface is replaced every 32 hours.

Crypts of Lieberkühn are small pits found on the entire intestinal surface except in the area of Brunner's glands. The crypts of Lieberkühn secrete a watery fluid immediately absorbed by the villi. This supplies a carrier substance for absorption by villi as chyme contacts them. This secretion is controlled principally by local nervous reflexes.

Brunner's glands are mucus-secreting glands that are concentrated in the first portion of the duodenum, between the pylorus and the ampulla of Vater. The function of Brunner's glands is inhibited by the sympathetic nervous system. Lack of sufficient mucus may be related to the development site of peptic ulcers. Brunner's glands are thought to protect the duodenum from digestion by the gastric juices.

Peyer's patches are lymphoid follicles that lie in the mucosa and submucosa of the ileum. They participate in antibody synthesis and the body's immune responses.

The small bowel also secretes several hormones that enter the bloodstream and stimulate the pancreas to release its digestive secretions.

Movements of the Small Intestine. The presence of chyme in the small intestine stimulates baroreceptors that initiate a type of concentric contraction called segmentation. When the small intestine becomes distended, many constrictions occur either regularly or irregularly along the distended area. The constrictions then relax, but others occur at different points a few seconds later. Each contraction results in a segmentation of the chyme and moves the chyme forward about 1 to 2 cm. These segmenting contractions normally occur 7 to 12 times per minute. This helps to mix secretions of the small intestine with the chyme particles.

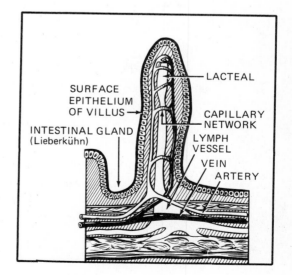

Figure 22-5. Crypts of Lieberkühn.

Propulsive contractions are called peristaltic contractions. They are elicited by distension of the intestine. Peristaltic contractions should be regularly spaced. The peristaltic waves (contractions) push the chyme slowly toward the colon. These waves are short and found predominantly in the first portions of the duodenum and jejunum.

Distension of the small intestine activates the nerves to continue the contraction sequence, known as the myenteric reflex. As the chyme nears the large intestine, contractions in the ileum increase. As chyme reaches the end of the ileum and is ready to enter the colon, a gastroileal reflex is stimulated. The gastroileal reflex regulates the movement of chyme from the small intestine into the large intestine. Between the ileum and the cecum is the ileocecal valve, which is normally closed. The tissue immediately before the ileocecal valve is highly muscular, forming the ileocecal sphincter, and the flaps of the ileocecal valve (Fig. 22-6) extend into the cecum. The sphincter is normally contracted except after a meal, when it relaxes and allows chyme to move from the ileum into the cecum. Chyme is prevented from returning to the ileum during colonic contraction due to the valve leaflets being floated out to close the ileocecal valve (in much the same way as the heart valves).

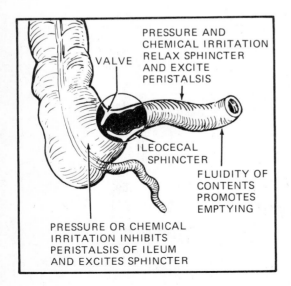

Figure 22-6. Gastroilial reflex.

Absorption Mechanisms in the Small Intestine.
Normally, absorption from the small intestine each day consists of several hundred grams of carbohydrates, 100 or more grams of fat, 50 to 100 grams of amino acids, 50 to 100 grams of ions, and 8 or 9 liters of water. Its absorptive capacity is much greater than this. There are five basic mechanisms for absorption in the small intestine: hydrolysis, nonionic movement, passive diffusion, facilitated diffusion, and active transport.

Hydrolysis. Hydrolysis is the chemical action of uniting compounds with water to split the compounds into simpler compounds. Enzymes and hormones act as catalysts in the process of hydrolysis. Catalysts speed up the process of hydrolysis. (Catalysts speed up a chemical reaction without entering into the reaction.)

Nonionic Movement. Nonionic transport allows substances to move freely in and out of cells with no energy or carrier substances needed. Such molecules include drugs and unconjugated bile salts.

Passive Diffusion. In passive diffusion, there is free movement of molecules based on a concentration gradient, primarily from an area of high concentration to an area of low concentration. Free fatty acids and water are molecules that move by passive diffusion.

Facilitated Diffusion. Facilitated diffusion may be defined as a process by which a carrier picks up an ion, crosses the cell membrane, liberates the ion inside the cell, and then returns outside to pick up another molecule (ion). This diffusion does not require energy, and ions cannot move alone against an electrochemical gradient.

Active Transport. For nutrients to be absorbed by active transport, energy (ATP) is required. Ions such as Na^+ and K^+ and molecules such as proteins and glucose require active transport.

Nutrient Digestion and Absorption.
Ninety percent of nutrients and 50% of water and electrolytes are absorbed in the jejunum. Meticulous nutritional counseling and follow-up are important for patients with small bowel resections.

Carbohydrates. Carbohydrates enter the duodenum in the forms of starch, polysaccharides (complex sugars), disaccharides, and monosaccharides. The starch and polysaccharides are hydrolyzed under the influence of amylase to form maltose. Maltose and directly ingested disaccharides such as sucrose, lactose, and maltose are hydrolyzed by intestinal enzymes into simple sugars of monosaccharides, which are then absorbed into the bloodstream via the intestinal mucosa.

Approximately 350 grams of carbohydrates are absorbed daily (60% starch, 30% sucrose, and 10% lactose). The three basic sugars are fructose, glucose, and galactose. Each of these basic sugars yields 4 kcal/gram. Glucose and galactose are actively transported across the small intestine wall into the blood. Fructose is transported by facilitated diffusion.

Proteins. Dietary proteins are first acted upon by enzymes called proteases. The principal proteases are pepsin (in the gastric secretion) and trypsin (in the pancreatic secretion). These enzymes catalyze the hydrolysis of the very large protein molecules into intermediate compounds (proteoses and peptones) and subsequently into amino acids. In the digestive sequence, protein is broken down into proteoses and peptones in the stomach. These simpler compounds are next broken down into polypeptides and thence into amino acids in the small intestine.

Approximately 70 to 90 grams of protein are absorbed daily, yielding 4 kcal/gram. Of the amino acids, eight (isoleucine, leucine, lysine, methionine, phenylalanine, threonine, tryptophan, and valine) are essential. Amino acids are absorbed (primarily from the duodenum and jejunum) by active transport into the blood of the intestinal villi. The transport is carrier mediated and requires an expenditure of energy.

Fats. Before fats can be digested, they must be emulsified. This function is performed in the small intestine by bile, which is secreted by the liver and stored in the gallbladder.

The bile salts aggregate to form micelles. These micelles have a fatty core but are still stable in the intestines because the surfaces of the micelles are ionized, which is a property that promotes water solubility. The fatty acids and the glycerides become absorbed in the fatty portions of these micelles as they are split away from fat globules and are then carried from the fat globules to the intestinal epithelium, where absorption occurs.

The emulsification of ingested fat globules provides a greater contact area between the fat molecules and pancreatic lipase, which is the principal fat-digestive enzyme. The end products of fat digestion are glycerides, fatty acids, and glycerol. Some fatty acids and glycerol may be absorbed into the blood via the blood vessels found in the villi of the intestinal mucosa. However, most fatty acids and glycerides are absorbed into the lymphatic system via the lacteals of the intestinal villi.

Approximately 60 to 100 grams of fat are absorbed daily, providing 9 kcal/gram.

Electrolytes. Electrolytes are absorbed in all parts of the intestine by active transport.

Water. Approximately 8 to 9 liters of water per day are absorbed from the intestine. Water is absorbed by diffusion and osmosis.

Water-Soluble Vitamins. The water-soluble vitamins, vitamin C and B complex, are absorbed in all parts of the intestine through passive diffusion directly into the blood.

Fat-Soluble Vitamins. The fat-soluble vitamins, A, D, E, and K, are absorbed from the gastrointestinal tract (mainly the jejunum) in the same way as lipids are. Once in the bloodstream, these vitamins are escorted by protein carriers because they are insoluble in water.

Calcium. The top portion of the duodenum is specialized for the absorption of calcium.

Iron. In the intestines, only about 10% of dietary iron is normally absorbed, but if the body's supply is diminished or if the need increases for any reason, absorption increases. This regulation is provided by a blood protein, transferrin, which captures iron from food and carries it to tissues throughout the body by active transport.

Large Intestine

The large intestine (colon) is 5 to 6 feet long and extends from the ileum to the anus. It is significantly different from the small intestine in that it contains no villi. The colon is 2.5 inches in diameter (larger than the small intestine) and has many sacculations (saclike segmentations) called haustra.

There are three segments of the colon: cecum, colon, and rectum. The colon is further subdivided into four sections: the ascending, transverse, descending, and sigmoid colons. The large intestine, or colon, is mainly responsible for the absorption of water and some electrolytes and the elimination of waste products.

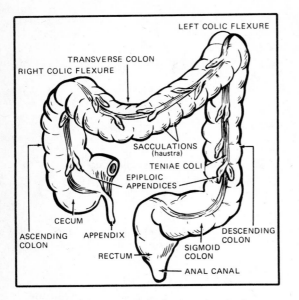

Figure 22-7. Large intestine (anterior view).

Cecum. The cecum is a blind-end sac (Fig. 22-7) into which the ileum empties its contents. The vermiform appendix is attached to the base of the cecum. The appendix has no known use and must be surgically removed if it becomes infected to prevent peritonitis.

Colon. Immediately above the cecum is the ascending colon, which passes upward to become the transverse colon at the right colic flexure (hepatic flexure). It then crosses the abdomen, now called the transverse colon, and becomes the descending colon at the left colic flexure (splenic flexure). At the iliac crest, the descending colon arches backward to form the sigmoid colon (Fig. 22-7). The sigmoid colon is the portion of the colon that crosses from the left side to the midline to become the rectum (Fig. 22-7), which follows the curvature of the lower sacrum and coccyx.

Rectum and Anus. The rectum is about 7 inches long. The distal 1 to 2 inches are the anal canal (Fig. 22-8). Mucous membrane lines the rectum and is arranged in vertical rows called rectal columns. Each rectal column contains an artery and a vein. These veins frequently enlarge to form hemorrhoids. Two sphincters control the anus (the exterior opening of the rectum). The internal sphincter is composed of invol-

untary smooth muscle. The external sphincter is voluntary striated muscle.

Layers of the Colon Wall. Epithelial cells form the mucosa of the colon, which is actively involved with absorption of water and some electrolytes. The muscle layers are different from those in the small intestine. The circular layer becomes somewhat spherical (Fig. 22-7), and the longitudinal layer fibers are evenly dispersed in three strips (called teniae coli) around the colon. This results in sacculation, and the resulting pouches are the haustra.

Colonic Motility. The colon moves its contents slowly through the colon system to allow for fluid absorption so that 800 to 900 mL of chyme liquid is absorbed along with nutrients. Thus, of the 1000 mL of chyme entering the colon, only 150 to 250 mL of fluid will be evacuated in the stool per day.

Mixing Movements in the Colon. Segmentation of chyme in the large intestine is caused by contraction of the inner muscle layer. There is a slow progress analward with segmentation in the colon. Mixing movements may also be called haustrations. As the circular segmenting contraction occurs, the teniae coli also contract. This provides for more surface contact of the contents to the lumen wall for absorption.

Propulsive Movements in the Colon. These are the result of the haustral contractions but are insufficient to provide for the necessary expulsion of waste products. A mass movement occurs due to an irritation

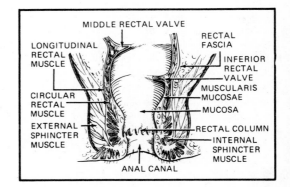

Figure 22-8. Section of the rectum.

or distension, usually in the transverse colon. These contractions, as a unit, force the entire mass of fecal material forward. A series of mass movements usually occur for up to 30 minutes and may then occur again in one-half to one full day.

Mass movements can cause increased colonic motility as a result of intense stimulation of the parasympathetic nervous system, irritation secondary to conditions such as ulcerative colitis, osmotic overload, or simply distension, use of drugs such as morphine sulfate or magnesium sulfate, an increase in bile salts, bacterial endotoxins, and high-residual diets. Hypermotility results in diarrhea and may cause severe fluid loss and electrolyte imbalance.

Mass movements are inhibited by all of the anticholinergic drugs and by diets deficient in bulk. This may result in constipation, since the extra length of time in the large intestine allows more fluid absorption.

Colonic Absorption. The colon may increase its absorption rate by threefold if threatened with large amounts of fluid. Most of the absorption in the colon occurs in its proximal half (the ascending and transverse colon). The distal colon functions principally for storage.

The mucosa of the large intestine has a very high capacity for active absorption of sodium, and the electrical potential created by the absorption of the sodium causes passive chloride absorption. The mucosa of the colon actively secretes bicarbonate and potassium as well.

Bacteria. Bacterial action in the colon causes the formation of gases, which provide bulk and help to propel the feces. They are capable of digesting small amounts of cellulose, in this way providing a few calories of nutrition to the body each day. These organisms also synthesize some important nutritional factors such as vitamin K, thiamin, riboflavin, vitamin B_{12}, folic acid, biotin, and nicotinic acid. The main anaerobic bacterium in the colon is *Bacteroides fragilis*. The main aerobic bacterium is *Escherichia coli*.

Defecation. The stimulus to defecate is the distension of the rectal wall resulting in the stimulation of the myenteric plexus. These nerves cause peristaltic waves in the rectum; the internal anal sphincter relaxes (receptive relaxation), and then the external anal sphincter relaxes so that defecation will occur.

Approximately 150 grams of feces are eliminated daily. Feces are three-fourths water and one-fourth solid matter. The organic constituents include undigested food residues, digestive secretions and enzymes, dead cells, bile pigments, and mucus. Thirty percent of the mass consists of bacteria, and another 30% is fat. The nature of the diet does not change the contents of the stool except for the amount of cellulose present. Stereobilinogen gives feces its brown color.

CHEMICAL MESSENGERS OF THE GASTROINTESTINAL SYSTEM

The gastrointestinal chemical messengers can act in one of three ways: under an endocrine stimulus, as a neurotransmitter, or as a neuroendocrine messenger.

An endocrine stimulus is a chemical substance formed in part of the body and carried to another part of the body to alter the functional activity or structure of that part. Examples are gastrin, secretion, gastric inhibitory hormone, insulin, and glucagon.

A neurotransmitter is any specific chemical agent released by a presynaptic cell, upon excitation, that crosses the synapse to stimulate or inhibit the postsynaptic cell. Examples are vasoactive intestinal peptide, acetylcholine, norepinephrine, and serotonin.

A neuroendocrine messenger consists of cells that release a hormone into the circulating blood in response to a neural stimulus. An example is cholecystokinin.

BLOOD SUPPLY OF THE GASTROINTESTINAL TRACT

Arterial Vascularization
The celiac artery, the superior mesenteric arteries, and the inferior mesenteric arteries all branch from the abdominal aorta. Figure 22-9 shows the arterial vascularization of the gastrointestinal tract.

Venous Blood Return
The venous circulation of the gastrointestinal system is unique in that the venous blood enters the portal vein system (Fig. 22-10). All blood from the gastrointestinal tract enters the portal vein system, which empties into the liver sinusoids. This makes the portal system extremely important for filtering microorganisms and

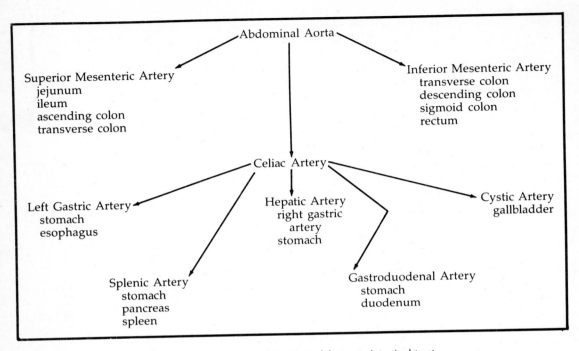

Figure 22-9. Arterial vascularization of the gastrointestinal tract.

for synthesizing many enzymes and clotting factors needed by the body. The liver also removes various absorbed nutrients, especially glucose and proteins, from the blood and stores them for later use by the body. Generally, the vein corresponding by name to the artery drains the same areas supplied by the artery.

The portal vein drains into the liver sinusoids. These sinusoids join branches of the hepatic artery to form the hepatic vein. In turn, the hepatic veins drain blood from the portal vein and hepatic artery into the inferior vena cava.

INNERVATION OF THE GASTROINTESTINAL SYSTEM

Compared with the other body systems, the gastrointestinal tract is unique in that it has its own separate intrinsic nervous system. The gastrointestinal tract can be influenced by the autonomic nervous system.

The intrinsic nervous system has two layers of neurons connected by specific fibers. The outer layer of neurons is called the myenteric plexus or Auer-

bach's plexus. It is located between the longitudinal and circular muscle layers. The inner layer of neurons, called the submucosal plexus or Meissner's plexus, is located in the submucosa.

Generally, the myenteric plexus controls movement of the gastrointestinal tract and the submucosal plexus (Meissner's plexus) controls the secretions of the gastrointestinal tract and sensory function through impulses received by stretch receptors in both the gastrointestinal wall and gastrointestinal epithelium.

Stimulation of the myenteric plexus results in increasing motor tone of the gastrointestinal wall and increasing intensity, rate, and speed of peristaltic waves. Increase in Meissner's plexus activity results in increasing secretions.

The extrinsic nerves of the autonomic nervous system can alter the effects of the gastrointestinal system at specific points or from the mouth to the stomach and then from the distal end of the colon to the anus. Parasympathetic supply for the gut is from the cranial X (vagus) and sacral nerves. Acetylcholine is the neurotransmitter from the postganglionic fiber. A few cranial parasympathetic fibers innervate the mouth and pharynx. Extensive parasympathetic innervation exists

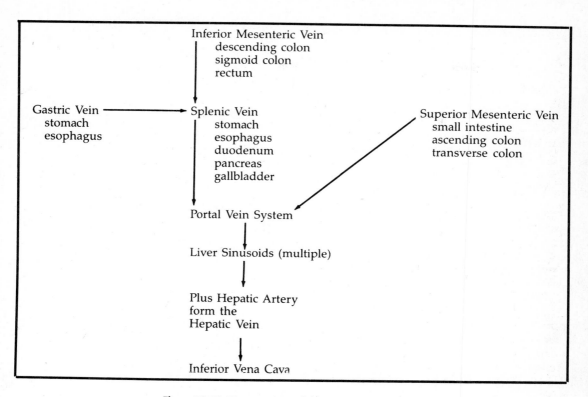

Figure 22-10. Venous return of the gastrointestinal tract.

in the esophagus, stomach, pancreas, and first half of the large intestine. The sacral parasympathetic fibers innervate the distal half of the large intestine, especially the sigmoidal, rectal, and anal portions.

The sympathetic nervous system fibers flow along blood vessels of the entire gut. The sympathetic fibers to the gastrointestinal tract originate in the spinal cord between segments T-8 and L-3. Its neurotransmitter, norepinephrine, inhibits gastrointestinal tract activity. This causes effects opposite those of the parasympathetic neurotransmitter, acetylcholine. If the effects are strong enough, the sympathetic system can virtually halt activity of the gastrointestinal tract.

ACCESSORY ORGANS OF DIGESTION

The accessory organs involved in making chyme suitable for nutrient absorption are the salivary glands, the pancreas, and the biliary system (liver and gallbladder).

Salivary Glands

There are three salivary glands: the parotid, the submandibular, and the sublingual (Fig. 22-11). All of the salivary glands are paired.

Hormones have no influence on the salivary glands. Salivary secretion is controlled by the superior and inferior salivatory nuclei located in the brain stem. Nervous stimuli of the glands occur from the thought, sight, and smell of food.

Pancreas

The pancreas is a soft, fish-shaped lobulated gland lying behind the stomach (Fig. 22-12). The gland is composed of three segments: the head, the body, and the tail.

The pancreas is both an endocrine and exocrine organ. The endocrine portion includes the secretion of insulin from the beta cells and the secretion of glucagon from the alpha cells (see above, "Chemical Messengers of the Gastrointestinal System"). The exocrine

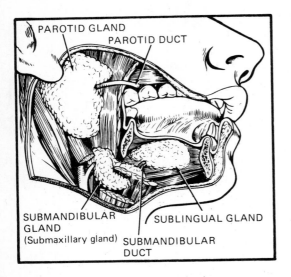

Figure 22-11. Salivary glands.

portion is related to the gastrointestinal system and produces three enzymes whose release is controlled by two hormones produced in the small intestine.

The main pancreatic duct is the duct of Wirsung, which runs the whole length of the pancreas from left to right and joins the common bile duct on the right.

The exocrine function of the pancreas is composed of acinar glands, which are little sacs called alveoli. These cells are arranged around a small central lumen into which the cells drain the exocrine enzymes

that they have synthesized. The central lumens drain into multiple ducts, which eventually drain into the main pancreatic duct. The ampulla of Vater (Fig. 22-13) is the short segment just before the common bile duct enters the duodenum.

The secretions of the acinar glands are digestive enzymes, water, and salts (sodium bicarbonate, sodium, and potassium). These colorless secretions total up to 1200 mL each day and are emptied into the upper portion of the small intestine 4 cm beyond the pylorus. They have a pH of 8.0 to 8.5. The pancreatic (acinar) fluid is composed of three major types of enzymes: amylytic, lipolytic, and proteolytic. At least 10% of the pancreatic enzymes must be present to prevent malabsorption states. During illness or injury the volume of pancreatic fluid usually decreases, and the composition may change.

The amylytic enzyme is predominantly alpha-amylase, first encountered in the saliva. The alpha-amylase is responsible for hydrolysis of carbohydrates. The end products of hydrolysis of carbohydrates are glucose and maltose (a disaccharide of two glucose molecules). The difference between salivary and pancreatic amylase is that the latter is able to digest raw starches as well as cooked starches. Amylase also contains calcium and is excreted in the urine.

The lipolytic enzymes are pancreatic lipase and phospholipase A, which are important in early stages of the digestion of fats. Lipase breaks down tri-

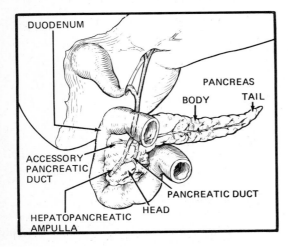

Figure 22-12. Pancreas.

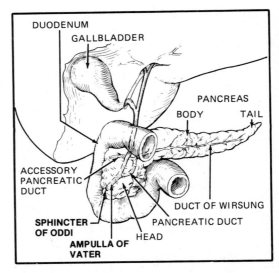

Figure 22-13. Ampulla of Vater and sphincter of Oddi.

glycerides to free fatty acids, glycerol, and mono-glycerides. Bile salts are essential for this function. Phospholipase A hydrolyzes lecithin (a complex lipid) to lysolecithin.

Proteolytic enzymes are actually proenzymes; that is, they must be altered to become biochemically active. The three most important proteolytic proenzymes are trypsinogen, chymotrypsinogen, and procarboxypeptidase.

Trypsin is involved in the activation of all three proenzymes to enzymes. The proteases are secreted in an inactive form; otherwise, they would act on pancreatic tissue and cause destruction. Once in the intestine, intestinal enterokinase acts on trypsinogen, converting it to trypsin. Trypsin then acts on the other proteases to convert them to active enzymes. These enzymes break amino acid bonds of protein chains, forming small polypeptides and single amino acids.

In addition to the digestive enzymes, pancreatic secretions contain large amounts of sodium bicarbonate, which reacts with the hydrochloric acid emptied into the duodenum in the chyme from the stomach to form sodium chloride and carbonic acid. The carbonic acid is absorbed into the blood and eliminated through the lungs as carbon dioxide. The net result is an increase in the quantity of sodium chloride, a neutral salt, in the intestine. Thus, pancreatic secretions neutralize the acidity of the chyme coming from the stomach. This is one of the most important functions of pancreatic secretion.

Two other important pancreatic enzymes are nuclease and deoxyribonuclease. These enzymes degrade nucleotides within DNA and RNA molecules into free mononucleotides.

Regulation of Pancreatic Secretions. The cells lining the acinar glands contain large amounts of carbonic anhydrase. The alkaline secretions (HCO_3-) of the duct cells (cells lining the acinar glands) mix with the amylytic, lipolytic, and proteolytic enzymes prior to reaching the major pancreatic duct, the duct of Wirsung.

Secretions of the pancreas are controlled by hormonal and neural factors. There are three phases of secretion: cephalic, gastric, and intestinal. The cephalic phase is activated by the same factors as in the cephalic state of the stomach and is mainly controlled by the vagus nerve (parasympathetic impulses). Stimulation of the vagus nerve (by thought, smell, taste, chewing, and swallowing of food) causes the secretory

cells of the pancreas to secrete highly concentrated enzymes with minimal amounts of HCO_3-. The quantity of fluid secreted, however, is usually so small that the enzymes remain in the ducts of the pancreas and later are floated into the intestinal tract by the copious secretion of fluid that follows secretin stimulation.

The gastric and intestinal phases are interrelated and controlled by two hormones, secretin and cholecystokinin. When the chyme is predominantly undigested proteins and fats, the pancreatic juice will be enzyme rich. When the chyme is mainly acidic (low pH), the pancreatic juice will be HCO_3- rich. The secretion of cholecystokinin stimulates the enzyme-rich secretion of pancreatic juices; secretin stimulates the release of HCO_3- and water-rich pancreatic juice. The pancreatic juices enter the duodenum along with the biliary system secretions at the sphincter of Oddi.

Biliary System
The biliary system is composed of the liver and gallbladder.

Liver. The liver is the single largest organ in the body, weighing 3 to 4 pounds. It is located in the right upper quadrant of the abdomen, lying up against the right inferior diaphragm.

Gross Structure. The liver is divided into a right and a left lobe by the falciform ligament (Fig. 22-14). The falciform ligament also attaches the liver to the abdominal wall and to the diaphragm. On the inferior liver surface is the quadrate lobe, and on the posterior liver surface is the caudate lobe. Both the quadrate and caudate lobes are small. Most of the liver is covered by peritoneum.

Functional Unit. Each of the hepatic lobes is further divided into numerous lobules. The hepatic lobule is the functioning unit of the liver (Fig. 22-15). Each lobule has a hepatic artery, a portal vein, and a bile duct known collectively as the portal triad. Between columns of epithelial cells are intralobular cavities called sinusoids. Each sinusoid is lined with Kupffer cells, which are phagocytic cells.

Blood Supply. Each sinusoid receives oxygenated blood from the hepatic arterioles and blood rich in metabolic precursors from the hepatic vein. The blood is filtered by the phagocytic Kupffer cells. Products removed from the blood include amino acids, nutrients, sugars, and bacterial debris. Blood leaves the

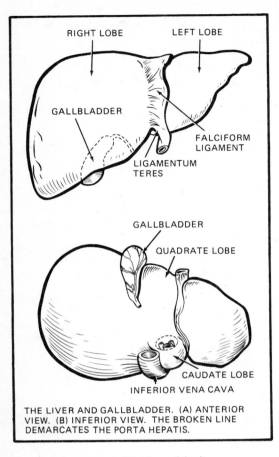

RIGHT LOBE   LEFT LOBE

GALLBLADDER

FALCIFORM
LIGAMENT

LIGAMENTUM
TERES

GALLBLADDER

QUADRATE LOBE

CAUDATE LOBE
INFERIOR VENA CAVA

THE LIVER AND GALLBLADDER. (A) ANTERIOR
VIEW. (B) INFERIOR VIEW. THE BROKEN LINE
DEMARCATES THE PORTA HEPATIS.

Figure 22-14. Divisions of the liver.

sinusoid by entering the central lobule vein. It then enters the hepatic veins and follows the normal venous circuit. Approximately 1500 mL of blood enters the liver each minute, making the liver one of the most vascular organs in the body.

Function. The role of the liver in digestion is to synthesize and transport bile pigments and bile salts for fat digestion. The liver cell, the hepatocyte, synthesizes bile (approximately 600 mL/day), which aids in the metabolism of carbohydrates, fats, and proteins. The bile is secreted into bile canaliculi (ducts), which branch and combine, eventually forming the right and left hepatic ducts. Immediately after leaving the liver, the right and left hepatic ducts merge to form the common hepatic duct. The hepatic ducts drain bile salts and the products of hemoglobin and drug metabolism.

The cystic duct of the gallbladder joins the common hepatic duct to form the common bile duct. The common bile duct joins the major pancreatic duct to form the ampulla of Vater just prior to entering the duodenum at the sphincter of Oddi.

The Kupffer cells of the liver sinusoids are typical reticuloendothelial cells. The Kupffer cells are tissue macrophages that are capable of removing and phagocytizing old and defective blood cells, bacteria, and other foreign material from the portal blood as it flows through the sinusoid. This phagocytic action removes the colon bacilli and detoxifies harmful substances that filter into the blood from the intestine.

The liver eliminates bilirubin (by-product of the breakdown of hemoglobin) from the blood through urine and feces. Failure to eliminate bilirubin causes jaundice.

The liver is involved in the metabolism of many hormones by virtue of its role in hormone biotransformation, activation, and excretion. It is particularly involved in the metabolism of steroid hormones such as the estrogens and progesterone, testosterone, glucocorticoids, and aldosterone. Steroid hormones are taken up from the circulation by the liver and then metabolized by hepatic enzymes. The steroid hormones directly influence many of the liver's biochemical and physiologic functions.

A major biochemical function of the liver is the detoxification and metabolism of drugs, vitamins, and hormones. Some compounds are metabolically converted to relatively inactive forms (steroid hormones),

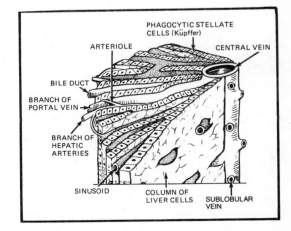

PHAGOCYTIC STELLATE
CELLS (Küpffer)

ARTERIOLE   CENTRAL VEIN

BILE DUCT

BRANCH OF
PORTAL VEIN

BRANCH OF
HEPATIC
ARTERIES

SINUSOID   COLUMN OF   SUBLOBULAR
                  LIVER CELLS   VEIN

Figure 22-15. Liver lobule.

whereas others become more biologically active (vitamin D). Of prime importance in maintaining homeostasis and protecting the body against ingested toxins is the ability of the liver to metabolize and detoxify a wide variety of absorbed substances that reach it directly in the portal blood.

The liver is essential in the regulation of carbohydrate metabolism, since it directly receives from the portal circulation most of the ingested carbohydrates and then, by hormonal regulation, controls the concentration of blood glucose in the fed and fasting states. The liver stores glycogen through glycogenesis (glucose to glycogen) and breaks it down in a process called glycogenolysis (glycogen to glucose) as needed. It also synthesizes glucose from amino acids (gluconeogenesis), lactic acid, and glycerol.

The liver is involved in many aspects of lipid synthesis and metabolism. It is a major site of triglyceride, cholesterol, and phospholipid synthesis. It is involved in the formation of lipoproteins, the conversion of carbohydrates and proteins to fats, and the formation of ketones from fatty acids.

The liver's role in protein metabolism includes the deamination of proteins for glucose availability, the formation of urea from ammonia so it may be eliminated from the blood, and the synthesis of plasma proteins such as albumin, haptoglobin, transferrin, and alpha and beta globulins.

The liver is the site of synthesis of the blood-clotting proteins fibrinogen (factor I), prothrombin (factor II), and factors V, VII, and X. It also stores the fat-soluble vitamins (A, D, and K), vitamin B_{12}, iron, and copper.

Gallbladder.

The gallbladder (Fig. 22-16) is a sac-like storage structure for bile.

Function. Bile is manufactured by the parenchymal cells (hepatocytes) of the liver and secreted by them into the bile canaliculi. The bile then travels to the hepatic duct, to the cystic duct, and then to the gallbladder for concentration (by as much as 12-fold) and storage. Upon stimulation, the gallbladder forces bile into the cystic duct, to the common bile duct, and into the duodenum. The adult gallbladder stores from 30 to 50 mL of bile. The major components of bile are bile acids, bile salts (sodium cholate and chenodenoxycholate), and pigments. The major pigment is mainly bilirubin. Other components include cholesterol, phos-

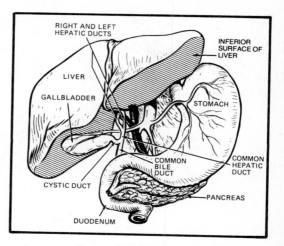

Figure 22-16. Location of the gallbladder.

pholipids (lecithin), alkaline phosphatase, electrolytes, and water.

Bile is responsible for the emulsification of fats and micelle formation. Inside the gallbladder, bile salts react with water, leaving a fat-soluble end to mix with cholesterol and/or lecithin. These formed particles are called micelles. Gallstones may form when the micelles become supersaturated with cholesterol. If bile salts are absent or diminished in the small intestine, normal fat digestion and absorption cannot occur. This results in fat malabsorption and steatorrhea (fatty stools). Most of the bile salts (approximately 80%) are reutilized by reabsorption in the ileum and enter the vascular system to be carried to the liver. The rest are excreted in the feces.

Bile pigments result from the degradation of hemoglobin. These pigments give the feces its brown color. Absence of bile pigments, as with obstructive jaundice, produces a whitish-gray feces.

Normally bile pigments do not form stones. However, in some diseases, there is an overconcentration of bile pigments, resulting in precipitation of bilirubinate stones. Most of gallstones (approximately 90%) are composed essentially of cholesterol.

Bilirubin is the main bile pigment. Once red blood cells have completed their 120-day sojourn through the circulatory system, they become fragile and rupture, releasing hemoglobin. The hemoglobin is phagocytized by cells of the reticuloendothelial system and thus split into heme and globin. It is from the heme ring that bile pigments are made. Bilirubin is the first pigment to be formed; however, it is soon reduced to free bilirubin and released into the plasma. Once in the plasma, free bilirubin combines quickly with plasma albumin and becomes protein-bound free (fat-soluble) bilirubin. It is now known as unconjugated or indirect bilirubin. Free bilirubin becomes conjugated (or direct) once it is absorbed into the hepatic ducts and combines with other substances. Conjugated bilirubin is now water soluble. Approximately 80% of protein becomes conjugated with glucuronide acid to form bilirubin glucuronide. Another 10% conjugates with sulfate to form bilirubin sulfate, and the remaining 10% conjugates with still other substances. In these three forms, bilirubin is excreted into the bile and passes through the bile ducts. From this point on, bilirubin is found in the plasma, intestinal contents, and urine.

A small amount of conjugated bilirubin formed by the hepatic cells escapes back into the plasma, creating a small portion of plasma bilirubin as conjugated rather than free. Most of the bilirubin passes into the intestines, where bacterial action produces urobilinogen. Some urobilinogen is reabsorbed by the portal blood and returned to the liver, which in turn reexcretes most of this urobilinogen back into the intestines. About 5% of this urobilinogen passes into the urine and is excreted as urobilin (oxidized urobilinogen). Urobilinogen oxidized in the feces becomes stereobilinogen.

Normally the total plasma concentration of both the free and conjugated forms of bilirubin is approximately 0.5 mg per 100 mL of plasma. In normal subjects, almost all of the bilirubin in the plasma appears to be in the unconjugated form. The concentration of bilirubin in the plasma represents a balance between the rate of entry of the pigment into the plasma and the hepatic clearance of bilirubin.

With jaundice, plasma levels of both unconjugated (indirect) and conjugated (direct) bilirubin are measured. If there is either a marked increase in the rate of formation of bilirubin or a defect in any of the processes underlying the hepatic clearance of unconjugated bilirubin (e.g., liver cell dysfunction), then conjugated bilirubin will accumulate in the plasma. In contrast, impairment to biliary flow either at a canalicular or bile ductular level (e.g., biliary tract obstruction) will cause reflux of conjugated bilirubin into the plasma.

Stimulation of the Gallbladder. The sphincter of Oddi opens upon vagal and hormonal stimulation. Vagal stimulation increases bile secretions through the sphincter of Oddi. The sphincter of Oddi in a normal state remains slightly opened, providing for a constant but minuscule amount of bile to enter the small intestine.

During normal digestion, the gallbladder contracts in response to the hormone cholecystokinin, pushing increased amounts of bile through the sphincter of Oddi into the duodenum. The gallbladder does not contract when there is no stimulation by cholecystokinin (e.g., between meals or during starvation diets).

GUIDE TO GASTROINTESTINAL ELEMENTS AND DIAGNOSTIC TESTS

Table 22-1 provides a quick reference to key chemical elements in the gastrointestinal system. Tables 22-2 to 22-5 provide quick references to common gastrointestinal diagnostic tests presented in the next several chapters.

NUTRITION

Under normal circumstances, human nutrition relies on a few key concepts. These concepts include minimal caloric needs (about 25 kcal/kg), minimal levels of substrate and vitamin ingestion, and ability of the gastrointestinal system to process the food. The CCRN exam traditionally has not focused heavily on nutritional concepts. This section is designed to provide enough information to cover the major current concepts of caloric need and substrate ingestion (gastrointestinal processing of food has been covered) in order to provide sufficient material for the exam. This section is not a comprehensive review of nutritional concepts. Controversial practices not supported by research (e.g., reducing diarrhea from tube feedings) are not addressed.

Caloric Needs

At rest, humans consume about 25 kcal/kg per day. A 70-kg man, for example, would consume 1750 kcal if he was on bedrest. During normal active states, the energy expended would increase to about 35 kcal/kg per day. Most critically ill patients are near the rest phase of about 25 kcal/kg/day. Many diseases do not markedly increase caloric need. Temperature elevations are the most common cause of increasing energy

TABLE 22-1. CHEMICAL ELEMENTS IN THE GI TRACT

Chemical Messenger	Origin	Stimulus	Inhibitors	Action
Gastrin (endocrine)	G cells of gastric antrum; duodenal mucosa	Distention of stomach from food. Presence of products from protein digestion; vagal stimulation; elevated blood levels of calcium and epinephrine	Acid in stomach	Stimulates secretion of HCl and pepsin; growth of gastric mucosa; relaxes ileocecal sphincter. Promotes antral activity. Stimulates parietal cells and chief cells
Secretin (endocrine)	Duodenal mucosa	Acid gastric contents entering the duodenum	Lack of acid gastric contents	Stimulates secretion of watery alkaline pancreatic fluid; stimulates pancreatic and hepatic HCO_3^-; augments action of cholecystokinin; decreases gastric acid secretion; stimulates secretion of pancreatic digestive enzymes; may inhibit gastric-emptying time
Cholecystokinin (neuroendocrine)	Duodenal mucosa	Products of protein and fat digestion entering the duodenum	Lack of stimulus	Stimulation of pancreatic enzyme secretion; stimulates gallbladder contraction caused by fat in the intestine; relaxation of the sphincter of Oddi; stimulation of pancreatic growth; inhibits gastric emptying; enhances insulin release; stimulates pepsin secretion; may weakly and selectively stimulate gastric acid secretion; stimulates motility of small bowel; augments secretion in stimulating secretion of alkaline pancreatic juice
Vasoactive intestinal peptide (neurotransmittor or neuropeptide)	Granules located in nerve terminals in the intestinal mucosa	Esophageal distention; intestinal distension; electrical vagal stimulation; intraduode-	None known	Relaxation of smooth muscle; vasodilation, and stimulation of pancreatic and intestinal secretion

(*continued*)

TABLE 22-1. (*Continued*)

Chemical Messenger	Origin	Stimulus	Inhibitors	Action
		nal fat or acid; serotonin; oxytocin; by intestinal ischemia		Stimulates insulin release; intestinal secretion of electrolytes and water; inhibits gastric acid secretion; dilates peripheral blood vessels and lowers blood pressure. Mediator of lower esophageal sphincter relaxation and of internal and sphincter relaxation
Gastric inhibitory hormone (endocrine)	Duodenal and jejunal mucosa	Presence of glucose and fat in the duodenum; not affected by acid. Released in response to bombesin and to beta-adrenergic stimulation	Lack of stimulus	Enhances insulin release; may inhibit gastric secretion
Insulin (endocrine)	Beta cells of the islets of Langerhans in the pancreas	Presence of glucose in the gut and blood	Low glucose levels	Controls glucose metabolism in the body by controlling the entry of glucose into the fat and muscle cells; increases the quantities of amino acids available in the cells for synthesizing proteins; stimulates the formation of proteins by ribosomes; stimulates the formation of RNA in cells; presence of insulin causes the body to use carbohydrates as fat; in the absence of insulin, fatty acids are mobilized and used in place of carbohydrates
Glucagon (endocrine)	Alpha cells of the islets of Langerhans in the pancreas	Low glucose concentrations (as low as 60 mg/100 mL of blood);	Normal-to-high glucose concentrations (greater than 60 mg/100	Regulates blood glucose level; mobilizes glucose from the liver by glycogenolysis (break-

(*continued*)

TABLE 22-1. (*Continued*)

Chemical Messenger	Origin	Stimulus	Inhibitors	Action
		severe exercise; and/or starvation	mL of blood)	down of the glycogen to glucose); increases gluconeogenesis (conversion of proteins to glucose) by the liver—does this by mobilizing proteins from the tissues of the body and then promotes the uptake of amino acids into the liver as well as conversion of the amino acids into glucose

expenditure (and caloric needs). Temperature elevations will increase energy needs by about 10% for each degree centigrade elevation.

Each patient should receive at least 25 kcal/kg per day for minimal nutritional support. There are many formulas to calculate (e.g., Harris-Benedict equation) or measure energy expenditure and caloric needs (indi-

TABLE 22-2. LIVER TESTS BASED ON DETOXIFICATION AND EXCRETORY FUNCTIONS

Type of Test	Associated Pathologies
Serum bilirubin (direct and indirect)	Increased indirect → hemolytic disorders Increased direct → liver or biliary tree disease; multiple blood transfusions; sepsis
Urine bilirubin	Indicates increased direct serum bilirubin and implies liver disease
Sodium sulfobromophthalein dye test	Indicates liver clearance function
Indocyanine green	Measures liver blood flow
Blood ammonia	Increased levels indicate hepatocellular disease and portal hypertension; detects hepatic encephalopathy
Serum bile acids	Sensitive to overall liver function

rect calorimetry), but for the purpose of the CCRN text, remember only the basic information on approximate caloric needs of the critically ill.

Substrates and nutrients are required in different degrees, depending on the condition of the person. For example, proteins are typically given in levels of about 1 gram/kg per day. Some patients may require more than this amount, and nitrogen balance studies should be performed to better determine specific protein needs. Protein deficits, such as albumin levels and total lymphocytes, are often used to assess the severity of malnutrition. Albumin levels less than 2.5 g/dLlymphocytes below 1000 mm_3 indicate potential malnutrition. The CCRN exam, however, currently does not require indepth knowledge regarding substrate, trace elements, or electrolyte concentrations as they relate to nutrition.

For the purpose of the test, information regarding basic nutritional support methods may be required. Enteral feedings, with the exception of solutions such as Pulmocare and Magnacal, usually have about 1 kcal/cc. Common formulas such as Osmolite, Ensure, and Jevity all have about 1 kcal/cc. Proper nutrition for a 70-kg man would require 1750 cc of full-strength enteral feeding (based on 25 kcal/kg and 1750 cc of enteral feeding = 1750 kcal).

Some enteral preparations have increased caloric values. Pulmocare and Magnacal, for example, have about 2 kcal/cc. In addition, some formulas, such as Pulmocare, have a potential advantage in the higher lipid concentration and subsequent reduced production of carbon dioxide. The reduced CO_2 production in theory reduces the stimulation to breathe. Patients with

TABLE 22-3. TESTS THAT MEASURE BIOSYNTHETIC FUNCTION OF THE LIVER—SERUM

Type of Test	Associated Pathologies
Albumin	Decreased levels may indicate chronic hepato-cellular disorders, malnutrition, protein-losing enteropathy, inflammatory bowel disease, and nephrotic syndrome.
Serum globulins (serum protein electrophoresis)	Increased levels indicate chronic liver disease.
Coagulation factors PT PTT Fibrinogen	Elevated in hepatitis, cirrhosis, vitamin K deficiencies, malabsorption, obstructive jaundice, and treatments with broad-spectrum antibiotics
Ceruloplasmin	Elevated values are seen with inflammatory diseases such as cholestatic disorders.
Ferritin	Low in iron deficiency; elevated in iron storage diseases such as hemochromatosis
Alpha-1-fetoprotein	Elevated in hepatocellular carcinoma

Serum enzymes

Aminotransferases SGPT SGOT	Elevated levels indicate acute hepatocellular disease.
Alkaline phosphatase 5'-Nucleotidase Gamma-Glutamyltranspeptidase	Elevated in inflammation of the biliary tree

TABLE 22-4. TESTS USEFUL IN THE DIAGNOSIS OF MALABSORPTION

Type of Test	Associated Pathologies
Stool fat	Steatorrhea
Xylose absorption	Disorders affecting the mucosa of the proximal small intestine
Small intestine biopsy	Value of the differential diagnosis of malabsorption
Schilling test for vitamin B_{12} absorption	Abnormal in disorders affecting the ileum such as regional enteritis and lymphomas
Secretin test	Used in a diagnosis of pancreatic insufficiency
Serum calcium, albumin, cholesterol, magnesium, and iron	Low level may be indicative of malabsorption.
Serum carotenes, vitamin A, and prothrombin time	May indicate malabsorption of the fat-soluble vitamins
Breath tests (hydrogen and bile acid)	Abnormal hydrogen breath test indicates lactase deficiency. Abnormal bile acid breath test indicates bacterial overgrowth syndromes.

Pancreatic function tests

Amylase	Increased levels are associated with pancreatitis.

TABLE 22-5. GASTROINTESTINAL AND RADIOLOGIC STUDIES

Upper gastrointestinal series	Barium and/or gas is taken orally to show structural or functional problems of the esophagus and stomach. Barium is usually followed through the small bowel with x rays to determine its rate of passage and to look for structural abnormalities.
Lower gastrointestinal series (barium enema)	The large colon is studied with barium and/or gas given per rectum. Sufficient barium and/or gas is given to distend the bowel and show any abnormalities in structure or a tumor.
Cholangiography	Oral cholangiography is based on the ability of the liver to extract from the blood a radiopaque dye that has been absorbed from the intestinal tract and then secrete it into bile. Indicates gallbladder disease. Intravenous cholangiography is based on the slow intravenous injection of a radiopaque dye, its extraction from blood by the liver, and then its rapid excretion into bile. Indicates cystic duct obstruction, most likely from gallstones.
Endoscopy (upper gastrointestinal endoscopy, colonoscopy, proctosigmoidoscopy, and fiberoptic sigmoidoscopy)	Endoscopy is the visualization of the inside of the body cavity by means of a lighted tube. Useful in diagnosing mass lesions, ulcers, strictures, dyspepsia, heartburn, bleeding, or cancers. Also used for biopsies and removal of foreign objects. Widely being used therapeutically sclerosing, polyp removal, heater probe therapy, and removal of gallstones from the common bile duct.
Percutaneous transhepatic cholangiography	Performed by inserting a long needle into the liver percutaneously, and injecting radiopaque dye into the bile duct. Useful in diagnosing obstructive jaundice.
Endoscopic retrograde cholangiopancreatography	The ampulla of Vater is cannulated through a side-viewing endoscope. A radiopaque dye is injected, and both the pancreatic and bile ducts can be visualized. Allows for diagnosing obstruction, malignancy, and inflammation. Endoscopic sphincterotomy and extraction of gallstones may also be performed.
Percutaneous liver biopsy	Puncture of the liver to diagnose hepatocellular disease, prolonged hepatitis, hepatomegaly, hepatic filling defects, fever, and staging of lymphoma
Angiography	The femoral artery is entered with a large needle that is then exchanged with a catheter that is passed into the celiac artery or one of its branches (superior mesenteric or hepatic). The contrast medium is injected, and films are taken. This procedure allows visualization of the visceral vessels to identify abnormalities of vascular structure and function, to visualize masses, and to note sites of bleeding.
CAT scan	Noninvasive procedure used in identifying masses. Provides a three-dimensional image.
Ultrasound	Noninvasive procedure using sound waves to outline the pancreas, liver, gallbladder, and spleen. It will distinguish fluid from solid structures and will show an abscess or the volume of fluid present in ascites.
Esophageal manometry	Contractions generated by the esophageal wall are measured as luminal pressures. Useful in the evaluation of achalasia, diffuse spasm, scleroderma, and other motility disorders.

difficulty weaning from mechanical ventilation may do better with a diet high in lipids due to a lessening of the drive to breathe.

Parenteral solutions have the ability to give higher levels of calories and substrates. Fifty percent dextrose (D_{50}) can give ten times the calories provided by D_5W. One liter of D_{50} can give about 1700 kcal, providing almost all caloric needs of the patient; 500 cc of a 20% lipid solution can give about 900 kcal (based on 9 kcal/gram of lipid and 20 grams/dL in the 500 cc of lipids).

Enteral solutions are preferred and should be started as soon as possible after entry into the unit. If the gastrointestinal system is unable to process food, parenteral solutions could be employed as a supplement or replacement for enteral feedings. Complications of enteral feedings, such as diarrhea, may require reduction in enteral volume with supplementation of parenteral solutions. Because of their high osmolality, parenteral solutions must usually be administered in a central vein. Some parenteral preparations, such as $D_{20}W$ or lipids, can be given peripherally. A common practice recently developed is the mixing of all parenteral solutions in a single intravenous bag.

CHAPTER 23

Gastrointestinal Hemorrhage and Esophageal Varices

Editor's note

The content of this chapter addresses the CCRN exam items of acute gastrointestinal hemorrhage and to some extent portal hypertension. Expect two to four questions on the exam regarding this content area.

Hematemesis is gross vomiting of blood. The blood may be fresh, indicated by a bright red color, or may be old, having the appearance of coffee grounds, with a black color. If the blood is excreted in the stool, fresh blood will be maroon and may have clots. Old blood turns feces black (called melena). Hematochezia is the passage of bright red blood through the rectum. Bleeding from the stomach or small intestine usually manifests as melena or maroon stools; bleeding from the colon manifests as maroon or bright red stools.

GASTROINTESTINAL HEMORRHAGE

Upper gastrointestinal (GI) hemorrhage is considered to be a bleed from the stomach or small intestine. Peptic disease, the most common cause of upper GI bleeding, refers to bleeding either from ulcers or from shallow erosions in the stomach, esophagus, or first part of the small intestine. Lower GI hemorrhage is from the colon.

Pathophysiology

Gastrointestinal bleeding occurs when a break in the lining of the GI tract erodes arteries, arterioles, or veins. The more serious bleeding usually occurs when arteries are eroded; however, some venous bleeding,

such as bleeding from esophageal varices associated with cirrhosis, can be just as catastrophic.

Etiology

Upper GI bleeding usually results from ulcers, erosions, acute mucosal tears, or esophageal varices. Ulcers are areas of breakdown in the wall of the GI tract that have significant depth. Erosions (e.g., gastritis, duodenitis, or esophagitis), also represent areas of breakdown in the wall, are much more superficial than ulcers. Approximately 80% of the ulcers are in the duodenum, with duodenal ulcers often causing bleeding.

There are multiple causes of ulcers or erosions, the most common being excessive acid production. Medications that work by decreasing acid production through H_2 inhibition, such as cimetidine (Tagamet) and ranitidine (Zantac), are effective in healing ulcers.

Other etiologies, such as side effects of medicines (e.g., arthritis medicines, aspirin, and prednisone), stress ulcers associated with surgery, severe burns, head trauma, sepsis, cardiac or respiratory failure, and alcohol use, also have been shown to cause ulcers and erosions. Stress ulcers are usually felt to be from ischemia, since acid production is usually not increased. Another type of ulcer may be due to infection caused by the bacterium *Helicobacter pylori.*

Lower GI bleeding usually results from colon tumors (e.g., cancer), diverticuli (which are outpouchings of the colon wall), or abnormal jumbles of arteries and veins (arteriovenous malformations [AVMs]).

Clinical Presentation

The great majority of ulcers and erosions do not cause bleeding. Usually the patient will present with recurring abdominal pain. The pain is usually burning or gnawing in character and is localized either below the xiphoid process, just inferior to the xiphoid in the epigastrium, or in the right upper quadrant of the abdomen. The pain is usually relieved by drinking milk or taking antacids and is usually worse between 30 minutes and 2 hours after eating. Alcohol, aspirin, caffeine, and spicy foods often worsen the pain.

When GI bleeding does occur, it usually manifests either as vomiting of fresh blood or old blood that has been acted on by gastric juices (coffee grounds) or as bloody bowel movements. A patient who has had a blood loss of less than 1 unit of blood, or 10% of the blood volume, usually will not have dizziness or orthostasis. A loss of more than 1 unit but less than 2 (10 to 20% of the blood volume) is associated with dizziness and orthostasis. Bleeding of more than 2 units (20% of blood volume) is often associated with shock (hypotension, cold, clammy skin, oliguria). Epigastric pain may or may not be present in GI bleeding. A slow bleed may produce only weakness, fatigue, and pallor.

Diagnosis

Diagnosis of the probable site of a bleed can usually be made from the history and physical examination. If coffee grounds or blood is vomited, the site of bleeding is the esophagus, stomach, or duodenum. Maroon or red blood with or without clots passed from the rectum is usually indicative of a bleed from the colon, but a severe upper GI bleed can sometimes manifest as passage of red blood through the rectum without vomiting of blood. Previous ulcer disease, alcohol, aspirin use, or liver disease can help determine the site of the bleed.

Passage of a nasogastric tube can sometimes be useful in assessing the site and severity of the bleed. Obtaining bright red blood indicates a more recent and usually a more severe bleed than the return of coffee grounds. However, for a variety of reasons, the nasogastric aspirate is far from perfect for assessing either the source or severity of the bleed.

Upper endoscopy is the best test for diagnosing and possibly treating an upper GI bleed. If done within 24 hours, it can detect the site of bleeding in a great majority of patients. Endoscopy involves passage of a long, flexible tube into the esophagus, stomach, and duodenum through which the physician can see the inside lining of the GI tract. Sometimes, however, bleeding is massive and a good examination with an endoscope is not possible. In such a case, a radiologic study called angiography is often used.

Bleeding from the colon is often diagnosed by a combination of colonoscopy and different radiologic studies, such as the tagged red blood cell or bleeding scan.

Complications

The major complications of GI bleeding are from the hemodynamic effects. Hypotension can cause serious organ damage, including cerebral infarction or myocardial infarction, renal failure, and intestinal infarction. All of these can be prevented if the patient has fluid and/or blood resuscitation given early enough after the onset of the bleed. Therefore, hemodynamic parameters need to be carefully monitored.

Also, aspiration of blood can cause severe respiratory difficulties, especially in unconscious or semiconscious patients. GI content aspiration predisposes patients to ARDS. Perforation and peritonitis occur very rarely.

Treatment

The most important aspect of treatment is the maintenance of blood pressure and circulating blood volume. This is accomplished by meticulous attention to pulse, blood pressure, and signs and symptoms of organ perfusion, such as urine output (at least 30 to 40 cc/hour) and mental status. Serial hemoglobin and hematocrit determinations are made to decide whether and when transfusion of blood is indicated. Large-bore intravenous access should be attained for possible blood product transfusions and also for intravenous fluids. The proper fluids to give to restore blood volume are isotonic solutions, such as normal saline or lactated Ringer's solution, or red blood cells, either as whole blood or as packed red blood cells. After multiple red cell transfusions, fresh frozen plasma or platelet transfusions may also be needed.

Iced saline lavage is controversial in the management of GI bleeds, and its use cannot be routinely recommended. Endoscopic therapy has become an important therapeutic modality. Laser, thermal, or electrical coagulation of the bleeding ulcer or erosion has become popular in the treatment of acutely bleeding upper GI tract lesions. Radiologic therapy, usually by angiography and infusion of vasopressin or clotting agents, and surgery are sometimes needed to manage GI bleeding.

Medical therapy with agents such as cimetidine (Tagamet), ranitidine (Zantac), famotidine (Pepcid), sucralfate (Carafate), and antacids has become the treatment of choice for ulcers and erosions. Although no studies have shown that these agents stop bleeding, they are very effective at healing such lesions. These agents decrease acid production and raise intragastric pH.

Fortunately, between 80 and 90% of GI hemorrhages cease spontaneously, with no more than medications such as cimetidine and ranitidine being used. Patients whose bleeding ceases spontaneously usually do very well, while those who need aggressive therapy are more prone to complications and risk of death.

Classic guidelines for considering surgery are transfusion requirement of greater than 4 units of blood in the first 24 hours, shock, or rebleeding. With the introduction of newer endoscopic therapies, these recommendations may change. Types of surgery may include vagotomy, pyloroplasty, and oversewing or resection of the ulcer. For stress ulcers, total gastrectomy may be needed.

Nursing Intervention

Fluid and electrolyte balance and adequate nutrition are key objectives of nursing treatment. Nursing interventions for hypovolemic shock should also be implemented.

Blood studies should include a complete blood count, type, and cross-match; electrolytes; blood urea nitrogen; and coagulation screen. One to two large-bore (14- to 16-gauge) intravenous lines should be started for rapid fluid and blood replacement.

Anticholinergic medications used to inhibit gastrointestinal action may have side effects such as dizziness, rash, mild diarrhea, leukopenia, blurred vision, headache, and urinary retention. These medications, in addition to the action of antacids, work to increase gastric pH. They will not stop bleeding.

The most important role for the nurse is to monitor the patient's hemodynamic status and observe for signs of continued bleeding. Careful attention to vital signs will guide fluid and blood replacement. Assessment of cardiac and pulmonary status will detect signs of possible fluid overload from too vigorous fluid and blood replacement, as pulmonary edema may develop.

If intra-arterial infusion of vasopressin is used, the patient must be monitored closely for bradycardia, hypotension, water intoxication, and postvasopressin diuresis. Renal status is measured by urinary output, which should be measured at least hourly and should be greater than 30 cc/hour. Tachydysrhythmias are a constant potential complication requiring monitoring and intervention as indicated.

The patency of the nasogastric tube should be maintained to monitor a recurrence of the bleed. Repeated blood from the rectum, return of red blood from a nasogastric tube, or recurrent hematemesis is an indication of continuing or recurrent hemorrhage.

Emotional support of the patient and family will help reduce stress and facilitate cooperation. As the bleeding is brought under control, reassurance will decrease the patient's fear.

ESOPHAGEAL VARICES

Esophageal varices are dilated, engorged, tortuous veins usually seen in the mid to distal esophagus. Varices are usually seen in patients with cirrhosis of the liver. Varices result from increased pressure in the portal veins (the veins that drain the stomach and the small and large intestines). With severe cirrhosis, the blood can no longer pass through the fibrotic liver and finds alternate pathways, through the veins in the distal esophagus. Being engorged, these veins are fragile and have a tendency to bleed, usually massively. Often they bleed within 12 months after they are discovered. Other causes of esophageal varices are splenic, portal, or hepatic vein thrombosis.

Clinical Presentation

Most patients with bleeding esophageal varices have signs of cirrhosis. Jaundice is often present. They usually have ascites, an abundance of intra-abdominal fluid causing abdominal distension. They often have elevated liver function tests, such as bilirubin, lactic dehydrogenase, AST (SGOT), ALT (SGPT), alkaline phosphatase, and prothrombin time.

Patients usually bleed massively and painlessly, with signs of shock present. They often become disoriented or lapse into coma as a complication of the bleeding and underlying cirrhosis.

Diagnosis

Diagnosis usually requires endoscopy since patients with cirrhosis often will not be bleeding from varices but rather from ulcerations in the esophagus, stomach, or duodenum. The history, physical examination, and laboratory blood studies are suggestive of cirrhosis.

Treatment

Treatment of esophageal varices is frustrating, as the bleeding is difficult to control and often recurs days to months later if initial control is achieved. Initially treatment includes control of shock and maintaining the patient's cardiopulmonary status. Endotracheal intubation may be necessary. Further treatment can be divided into five categories: medical, endoscopic, surgical, radiologic, and balloon tamponade.

Medical Therapy

Medical therapy of a continuous intravenous infusion of vasopressin (Pitressin) is often effective. Vasopressin often is the drug used first. Vasopressin works by reducing portal venous pressure. The dosage is 0.2 to 0.4 unit/minute. Vasopressin can cause serious cardiac ischemia and should be used with caution in patients with coronary artery disease. For patients who are receiving intra-arterial vasopressin, cardiac monitoring and frequent neurological assessments are performed because this drug is a very potent vasoconstrictor. Amyl nitrate, an antagonist vasodilator, should be at the bedside so that it is readily accessible if indications of angina pectoris, myocardial infarction, or encephalopathy occur. Patients with known coronary artery disease may be placed on nitroglycerin prophylactically.

Endoscopic Therapy

Endoscopic therapy consists of injecting a sclerosing, fibrosing agent, such as sodium tetradecyl sulfate, into the bleeding vein through the endoscope by a 23-gauge needle. Often effective, sclerotherapy requires considerable expertise in the actively bleeding patient.

Surgical Therapy

Portosystemic shunt surgery, aimed at bypassing the liver to lower pressure in the varices, is usually effective in stopping bleeding but can carry a 50% higher mortality in acutely bleeding patients.

Radiologic Therapy

Radiologic procedures, though available, are seldom used nowadays in the management of acute variceal hemorrhage.

Balloon Therapy

Balloon tamponade, using versions of the Sengstaken-Blakemore (SB) (Fig. 23-1) or Linton tube, is often effective in stopping acute bleeding. Unfortunately, there is a high incidence of rebleeding once these tubes are removed. These tubes are placed through the nose or mouth into the stomach. They utilize balloons in the early part of the stomach and/or esophagus to place pressure on the bleeding veins. These tubes, however, are fraught with dangers. Aspiration of blood, occlu-

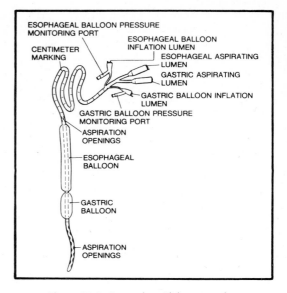

Figure 23-1. Sengstaken-Blakemore tube.

sion of the airway, esophageal necrosis, and esophageal rupture are all potential complications. Balloon pressures must be monitored carefully to prevent or recognize these complications early.

Nursing Intervention

A primary objective of nursing interventions is to control the bleeding to prevent or reverse hypovolemic shock. Attention to the patient's hemodynamic status is crucial. Monitoring electrolyte balance, fluid balance, and nutritional needs will enable early intervention if a problem appears imminent.

A patient with an SB or Linton tube to provide tamponade is continually observed for signs of asphyxiation or aspiration. These tubes can migrate and occlude the airway, or the patient may aspirate either blood or secretions into the lungs. Suctioning of pharyngeal secretion is required often. If suctioning does not improve the patient's respiratory status, check for breath sounds in the lungs. If no sounds are heard, most often the tube has slipped and is occluding the trachea. The nurse must immediately cut across all three tubes and remove the SB or Linton tube immediately. For this emergency, scissors are often taped to the head of the bed. Many patients with an SB or Linton tube will be prophylactically intubated to prevent airway occlusion. The mortality rate is high for this disease, approaching 33% for all patients with variceal bleeding, despite optimal medical and nursing therapy.

LOWER GASTROINTESTINAL BLEEDING

Etiology

The three major causes of lower GI bleeding are diverticulosis, AVMs, and colonic polyps or tumors.

Diverticulosis. Colonic diverticulosis is the presence of outpouchings, usually multiple and most often in the left side of the colon. Diverticulosis is felt partially to result from a relative deficiency of fiber in the American diet. It is very common in the United States, with approximately one-third of the population over the age of 60 affected. It usually is asymptomatic, but the diverticuli can become infected or bleed. The bleeding is usually painless and can be massive. The blood almost always appears red exiting the rectum. Therapy again consists of defense of hemodynamic status via fluids and often blood products, and most often bleeding ceases spontaneously. Diagnosis is usually made by colonoscopy or barium enema examination. Radiologic therapy by angiography and intra-arterial infusion of vasopressin to decrease blood flow to the affected bowel is often effective but rarely needed. Surgery in the form of partial colonic resection is also sometimes necessary to control diverticular hemorrhage. Presently, there is no effective endoscopic therapy.

Arteriovenous Malformations. AVMs, also called angiodysplasia, are closely packed tangles of arteries and veins that have a tendency to bleed. They are usually located on the right side of the colon but can be present anywhere in the colon, small intestine, or stomach. They are a very common cause of lower GI bleeding. Diagnosis is usually by colonoscopy, with bright red areas seen on the normally pink colon wall. They can also be noted by angiography, but not by barium enema examination. Therapy is possible with endoscopic laser, thermal, or electric coagulation using a small tube introduced through the colonoscope. Angiographic therapy with intra-arterial vasopressin infusion and surgical resection of the affected portion of the colon are also sometimes necessary. As with diverticulosis, bleeding usually ceases spontaneously. Initial therapy is aimed at stabilizing the patient's hemodynamic status.

Colon Polyps or Tumors. Colon tumors, such as cancer, or polyps, which are felt to be a premalignant growth, are usually asymptomatic. They often bleed, but usually very slowly. These lesions are slightly more likely than diverticuli or AVMs to produce pain with bleeding. Diagnosis is usually by colonoscopy or barium enema. Therapy is with either colonoscopic or surgical removal. As with any GI hemorrhage, initial therapy is aimed at stabilizing the patient hemodynamically.

Nursing Intervention

Nursing management of patients with lower GI bleeding is aimed at assessment of hemodynamic status. Careful assessment of vital signs, signs of hypovolemic shock, blood cell counts, coagulation studies, and electrolytes should be done frequently. Fluid and electrolyte losses should be replaced. Patients receiving intra-arterial vasopressin should be monitored for cardiac and neurological abnormalities.

CHAPTER 24

Viral Hepatitis

Editor's note

The content of this chapter addresses the CCRN exam test area including hepatic failure and coma. Expect one to three questions regarding this content area.

Viral hepatitis is hepatic inflammation caused by a variety of different viruses with a propensity to infect the liver. The major viruses have specific characteristics that help to differentiate the diseases that they cause. The four major groups of viruses causing viral hepatitis are hepatitis A, hepatitis B, hepatitis D (delta hepatitis), and hepatitis C viruses.

HEPATITIS A

Hepatitis A virus (HAV) is an RNA picornavirus that is excreted through the feces of infected individuals. It is spread through fecal-oral contact and is common in developing countries with poor sanitation. Ingestion of clams or oysters has been associated with occasional epidemics. It is a very common infection, with most infections in developing countries occurring early in life. Hepatitis A is often misdiagnosed as a gastroenteritis. Immunity after infection is lifelong. In adults with no prior immunization, the illness is more severe and usually icteric.

The incubation period is between 15 and 50 days. There are two phases of symptoms. The prodromal phase, occurring two to seven days before the icteric phase, consists of symptoms such as fatigue, nausea, vomiting, and low-grade fever. The icteric phase, usu-ally lasting between one and four weeks, follows. The icteric phase symptoms consist of darkened urine, light stools, and jaundice. Pruritis is not usually marked. Associated with symptoms are anorexia, nausea, vomiting, fever, and relatively mild abdominal pain. A diffuse rash may be present.

The most profound changes are in the liver function tests. Transaminases (SGOT, SGPT) rise dramatically, often into the thousands. Alkaline phosphatase also rises, but usually not to a similar degree. Bilirubin levels can range from normal to markedly elevated. Bilirubinuria is often present. Leukopenia is often seen, as is a mild anemia. Stools can be light colored, and steatorrhea may be present.

Patients are usually fully recovered within anywhere from six weeks to three months, but may have vague symptoms for up to a year. Rarely, fulminant hepatic failure and death occur. Mortality rates in large epidemics are approximately 19%. Hepatitis A has no progression to chronicity. The virus is excreted in the feces for up to two weeks before the icteric period and usually disappears prior to the resolution of the clinical hepatitis. Patients with acute hepatitis A should be placed on enteric precautions.

The antibody response to HAV is the key to diagnosis. The virus elicits both an IgM and an IgG antibody response. HAV-IgM appears in the acute infection and persists for two to six months. Detection of HAV-IgM is therefore indicative of infection within the last six months. IgG also appears in acute infection but persists for years. Therefore, the presence of IgG indicates a recent or past infection and probably ensures lifelong immunity.

Immune serum globulin is recommended for close personal contacts of an infected patient and in all those exposed to the food and water in an identified epidemic. This treatment has been shown to reduce the rate of infection in exposed subjects.

HEPATITIS B

Hepatitis B virus (HBV) is a DNA virus. It consists of a protein coat (known as the surface antigen [HbsAg]), and a core, which contains the double-stranded circular DNA, the e antigen (HbeAg), the core antigen (HbcAg), and the DNA polymerase. Each of these can be detected either in the liver itself or the circulating blood, and various antigens and antibodies have clinical relevance. HBsAg in the blood indicates either an acute or a chronic continuing infection. Surface antibody (HBsAb), however, indicates a resolved infection. HBeAg is associated with a high risk of infectivity and correlates with ongoing viral synthesis. It usually appears transiently during an acute attack. E antibody (HBeAb) is a marker of low infectivity and persists for a few months after the acute infection resolves. HBcAg is not currently detectable, but core antibody (HBcAb) is. IgM HBcAb indicates either acute or chronic infection, and IgG HBcAb is usually a marker for a past, nonactive infection.

Hepatitis B is usually transmitted through blood, but it can also be transmitted through saliva and sperm. It used to be a common cause of transfusion-associated hepatitis, but with present serologic screening of donors, hepatitis B is only rarely transmitted through blood transfusions. Major risk groups for hepatitis B are homosexuals, intravenous drug users, institutionalized persons, and health care professionals.

The incubation period for HBV infection is generally six to nine weeks. The patient usually is infectious both one to two weeks before and during the icteric phase. A serum sickness prodrome may occur, with symptoms such as rash and arthralgias. The clinical course can vary between mild and severe or can be asymptomatic. Fulminant hepatic failure and death can result. Symptoms and laboratory findings are similar to those for hepatitis A. The major difference between hepatitis A and hepatitis B is the 10% rate of chronicity in hepatitis B. While usually asymptomatic, this condition can lead to cirrhosis or hepatocellular carcinoma.

Therapy for acute hepatitis B is supportive once the infection is established. Prevention is the main focus, as no effective therapy to eradicate the infection exists. Presently there is a very effective vaccine to prevent hepatitis B infection that is composed of the surface antigen. Response to the vaccine and protection against infection are usually excellent. The vaccine is recommended for persons in the previously mentioned high-risk groups.

Persons exposed to hepatitis B, as in accidental needle sticks, should have hepatitis serologies checked. If they are HBsAg and HBsAb negative, then they should be given hepatitis B immune globulin (HBIG). In addition, the hepatitis B vaccine should be given. HBIG needs to be given only once, but the vaccine should be given again in one and six months. If the HBsAb is positive, the person exposed is already immune, and neither HBIG nor the vaccine need be given. If the HBsAg is positive, the individual is already infected and should be evaluated for acute or chronic hepatitis. Blood and body fluid precautions should be followed when dealing with infected individuals.

Health care workers in high-risk fields, such as intensive-care unit nurses and physicians, dialysis staff, and laboratory workers, should be given the hepatitis B vaccine even if no known exposure has occurred. No transmission of infections such as AIDS has been documented to occur from vaccination.

HEPATITIS D

Hepatitis D virus, also called delta hepatitis virus, is a viral particle. It is an RNA virus that infects only patients with coexistent hepatitis B infection. Therefore, a patient may have both hepatitis D and hepatitis B but cannot have hepatitis D alone. It can superinfect patients with either acute or chronic hepatitis B.

Delta hepatitis is uncommon. When present with acute hepatitis B, it usually causes a much more severe clinical hepatitis. Delta hepatitis infection of patients with chronic hepatitis B usually results in an acute exacerbation or worsening of symptoms, in addition to increases in liver function tests.

Because delta hepatitis requires infection with hepatitis B, the way to prevent infection is through immunization of groups at high risk of contracting hepatitis B. At present, there is no vaccine solely for hepatitis D and no satisfactory therapy.

HEPATITIS C

Hepatitis C virus, an RNA virus, is the major cause of transfusion-associated hepatitis today. The incubation period varies but is usually about seven weeks. Many of the infections are asymptomatic; when they are symptomatic, the disease is usually mild. Often the infection is diagnosed by screening liver function tests in an otherwise asymptomatic patient who has received a recent blood transfusion. The clinical manifestations are the same as for a mild case of hepatitis A or B.

Although usually spread through the blood by such means as blood transfusions, clotting factor transfusions, and sharing of needles by drug abusers, some cases have no such risk factors. Sexual transmission is also possible. Rare epidemics from food or water sources have also been described.

Although the initial clinical disease is usually mild, there is a high propensity for the infection to become chronic. It is estimated that up to 50% of acute infections, many of which are asymptomatic, lead to chronic hepatitis and sometimes to cirrhosis.

Hepatitis C antibody can detect chronic, but not acute, cases. Interferon therapy has been shown to be effective in some chronic hepatitis C infections.

NURSING INTERVENTIONS

Nursing priorities are aimed at reducing demands on the liver while promoting patient well-being, minimizing disturbance in self-concept due to communicability of disease, relieving symptoms and increasing patient comfort, promoting patient understanding of the disease process and rationale of treatment, and being aware of potential complications such as hemorrhage, hepatic coma, and permanent liver damage.

Placing the patient on bedrest with good skin care, providing a quiet environment by possibly limiting visitors, pacing activities, and increasing activity as tolerated can be interventions to prevent decreased mobility from decreased energy metabolism by the liver, activity restrictions, pain, and depression.

Nutritional monitoring is important due to an-orexia, nausea, and vomiting from visceral reflexes that may reduce peristalsis. Bile stasis as well as altered absorption and metabolism of ingested foods may also produce these symptoms. Diet is ordered according to the patient's need and tolerance. A low-fat, high-carbohydrate diet is most palatable to the anorexic patient. Protein should be given in low quantities. Counsel the patient to avoid alcoholic beverages. Accurate intake and outputs may be necessary due to severe continuing vomiting and diarrhea. Adequate hydration with intravenous fluids may be necessary. Serum electrolytes must also be monitored.

Particular attention must be paid to the patient's self-concept. Isolation measures are necessary to prevent cross-contamination. Annoying symptoms, confinement, isolation, and length of illness may lead to feelings of depression. Institute isolation procedures for all suspected cases of viral hepatitis. Patients with acute hepatitis A must be on enteric precautions. Patients with acute hepatitis B need to be on blood and body fluid precautions until the HBsAb appears or the HBsAg becomes negative. Isolation for acute hepatitis C includes blood and body fluid precautions. Explain all isolation procedures to the patient and family. Allow times with the patient for listening. Offer diversional activities based on energy levels.

Assess the patient's level of understanding of the disease process and provide specific information regarding prevention and transmission of the disease. Contacts may receive gamma globulin; personal items should not be shared; strict handwashing and sanitizing of clothes, dishes, and toilet facilities are necessary. While liver enzymes are elevated, avoid mucous membrane contact; blood donations should be discouraged. Discuss the side effects of and dangers of taking over-the-counter drugs and prescribed medications. Emphasis should be placed on the importance of follow-up physical examination and laboratory evaluation.

CHAPTER 25

Cirrhosis, Hepatic Failure, and Pancreatitis

Editor's note

This chapter addresses the CCRN exam areas of acute pancreatitis, hepatic failure and coma, and portal hypertension. This chapter overlaps slightly with the two previous chapters with regard to the content addressed by the exam. However, this format should make it easier to understand the major items addressed by each chapter and should reinforce understanding of earlier content.

CIRRHOSIS

Cirrhosis is the end stage of many types of liver disease. Basically, cirrhosis is defined as the abnormal fibrous regeneration of the liver, usually in response to chronic damage.

Types and Etiology

There are two major categories of cirrhosis, micronodular and macronodular. The distinction between the two is the size of the regenerating nodules. There are distinct causes under each category, but there can be overlap, with different diseases potentially causing either type. Cirrhosis usually results in increased resistance to blood flow through the liver and failure of the hepatic cells to function properly.

Micronodular cirrhosis is the most common type, and alcoholism is the most common cause of this type of cirrhosis in the United States. However, for unexplained reasons, only a minority of alcoholics develop cirrhosis. Cirrhosis is very unusual with less than five years of alcohol abuse, demonstrating that chronic injury is usually necessary for cirrhosis to develop. Alcohol itself directly injures liver cells, but other factors influence the development of cirrhosis.

Macronodular cirrhosis results from any of a variety of causes. Viral hepatitis B is the most common cause of this type of cirrhosis worldwide. Other causes include other types of infection, biliary cirrhosis, iron or copper overload, autoimmune diseases, and idiopathic or cryptogenic cirrhosis. Viral hepatitis A does not progress to cirrhosis.

All types of cirrhosis generally produce a firm, shrunken liver, although at times the liver can be enlarged. Fibrosis, or scarring, is prominent. Splenomegaly can also be present. The scarring provides resistance to normal blood flow through the liver. Loss of hepatocytes can result in hepatic failure.

Clinical Presentation

Usually patients present with gastrointestinal bleeding (often massive), ascites, jaundice, or abnormalities detected on routine blood testing. The patients may have weight loss, poor nutrition, and a history of alcohol abuse. Some patients may have no obvious signs of cirrhosis.

Ascites is usually present in moderate to advanced cirrhosis. The patient notes increased abdominal girth, a discomfort in the abdomen, and often pedal or ankle edema. Numerous factors are involved in ascites formation, including (1) low albumin level (the cirrhotic liver is often unable to make adequate albumin); (2) portal hypertension, resulting in leakage of fluid into the peritoneal cavity and poor fluid resorption; and (3) abnormal renal responses in cirrhosis, which lead to more fluid retention.

Endocrine changes can also be seen. Gynecomastia and testicular atrophy resulting from reduced testosterone levels are often seen in males, and menstrual irregularities are often seen in females.

Jaundice is also usually present in advanced cirrhosis. The eyes and skin generally assume a light to bright yellow discoloration as a consequence of elevated levels of bilirubin in the blood.

Other findings include a decreased or abnormal mentation, termed hepatic encephalopathy. This is often seen with an increased serum ammonia level and is caused by toxins usually filtered by the liver. Asterixis (an abnormal flapping of the hands), a hyperkinetic circulation, cyanosis, fetor hepaticus, renal failure, easy bruising, and low platelet, red, and white blood cell counts may be seen. Abnormal red clusters of blood vessels on the surface of the skin, termed spider angiomata, can also occur (Fig. 25-1).

Abnormalities in the serum concentrations of the hepatic transaminases and other enzymes (SGOT, SGPT, lactate dehydrogenase, alkaline phosphatase) are usually present. Abnormal coagulation tests (prothrombin and partial thromboplastin times) are often present, since the diseased liver frequently does not make sufficient clotting factors. Acidosis can occur either from shock or from the inability of the liver to clear lactate from the blood.

Diagnosis

Abnormalities in the patient's physical examination and laboratory data (Table 25-1) suggest the diagnosis. A liver biopsy is necessary to confirm the presence of cirrhosis and often determine the cause of the disease.

Treatment

At present, there is no satisfactory treatment to reverse cirrhosis. Treatment is aimed at decreasing any further damage, such as through the cessation of alcohol use. Different therapies, such as prednisone and interferon, are being studied. Protein restriction, fluid and salt restriction, diuretics, and vitamin K therapy are often necessary. Prevention of hepatitis B by immunizing high-risk population is probably the most important way to decrease the prevalence of cirrhosis worldwide.

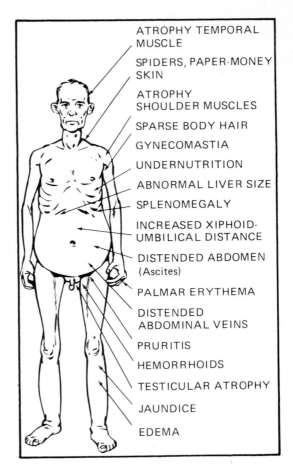

Figure 25-1. Advanced signs of cirrhosis.

ATROPHY TEMPORAL MUSCLE

SPIDERS, PAPER-MONEY SKIN

ATROPHY SHOULDER MUSCLES

SPARSE BODY HAIR

GYNECOMASTIA

UNDERNUTRITION

ABNORMAL LIVER SIZE

SPLENOMEGALY

INCREASED XIPHOID-UMBILICAL DISTANCE

DISTENDED ABDOMEN (Ascites)

PALMAR ERYTHEMA

DISTENDED ABDOMINAL VEINS

PRURITIS

HEMORRHOIDS

TESTICULAR ATROPHY

JAUNDICE

EDEMA

TABLE 25-1. LABORATORY TESTS FOR CIRRHOSIS

Decreased Levels	Increased Levels
WBC	Globulin
Hemoglobin	Total bilirubin
Hematocrit	Alkaline phosphatase
Albumin	Transaminase
Serum sodium	Lactate dehydrogenase
Serum potassium	Urine bilirubin
Serum chloride	Fecal urobilinogen
Serum magnesium	Urine urobilinogen
Folic acid	

Liver transplantation, although costly and necessarily involving lifelong intense medical care, is an option for highly selected patients with cirrhosis.

Nursing Intervention

Monitor the neurological status for behavior changes, increasing lethargy, and neuromuscular dysfunction such as asterixis. Provide a safe environment (siderails up, bed in low position, restraints as needed) for patients who are not completely lucid.

Nutritional intervention is mandatory since poor nutrition is influential in the development and progression of cirrhosis. Tube feedings or total parenteral nutrition (TPN) may be necessary. Increase protein (if there is no impending liver failure) to help regenerate liver tissue if the disease is not too far advanced. Carbohydrates should be increased (up to 2000–3000 kcal/day) to sustain weight and spare use of protein for healing. Vitamin supplements may be necessary.

Check the skin, gums, emesis, and stools often for bleeding and apply pressure at intramuscular sites. Notify the physician of the development of bleeding dyscrasias or an increase in bleeding. Assist patient to minimize trauma by avoiding the use of harsh toothbrushes, forceful nose blowing, and bodily injury.

Monitor fluid retention by weighing the patient daily. Check for dependent edema and maintain accurate intake and output records. Fluid and sodium restrictions may be necessary. Administer diuretics as required.

Paracentesis may be indicated in the patient with marked ascites. Paracentesis is generally not the initial treatment of ascites. If paracentesis is performed, note the amount of fluid removed and closely monitor the patient for signs of shock.

Monitor respiratory status for signs of ineffective breathing patterns. General debilitated states place patients at risk for acquired infections. Pressure on the diaphragm due to ascites causes reduced lung volumes, and hypoxemia may occur. Semi-Fowler's or high-Fowler's positions may be necessary. Auscultate lung sounds and turn, position, deep breathe, and position change every two hours. Additional laboratory tests to monitor include arterial blood gases (ABGs) and white blood cells (WBCs).

Skin breakdown, which is not uncommon, is due to edema and pruritus. Bathe the patient with moisturizing lotion, not soap. Turn the patient regularly (at least every two hours) and ensure rest to prevent an energy drain.

Educate the patient and family on the importance of proper diet, avoidance of alcohol, moderate exercise, and avoidance of any drugs (including over-the-counter medications), especially aspirin, unless the physician approves of their use.

HEPATIC FAILURE

Hepatic failure is the result of a very severe acute hepatitis or an advanced cirrhosis. It indicates failure of the liver to perform adequately either part or all of its functions.

Pathophysiology

Hepatocytes perform a variety of functions. The liver has a great deal of reserve, and it is estimated that 75 to 90% of normal liver cell function needs to be lost before liver failure results.

With hepatic failure, the liver is unable to adequately synthesize the plasma proteins. The most commonly deficient proteins are albumin and the coagulation factors. Inadequate albumin can lead to ascites and pedal edema. Deficient coagulation factors can lead to problems of easy bleeding or bruising.

Inability to metabolize substances that the liver normally breaks down leads to increased levels of potentially toxic chemicals in the blood. One of these potentially toxic agents is ammonia (NH_3). Increased levels are seen with mental status changes, i.e., hepatic encephalopathy. Hepatic encephalopathy may be mild or may lead to full coma.

Etiology

Hepatic failure occurs either with severe acute hepatitis or in the face of a chronic cirrhosis. Toxins such as acetaminophen may also cause hepatic failure.

Various factors precipitate hepatic failure in patients with cirrhosis. These include gastrointestinal bleeding, sedatives, chemical imbalances, dehydration, infections (especially spontaneous bacterial peritonitis), alcohol intake, and different anesthetics or surgeries, especially portacaval shunts.

Clinical Presentation

Patients usually present with gastrointestinal bleeding or mental status changes. Mental status changes can be subtle, such as a mild loss in short-term memory or mild confusion, or severe, resulting in coma. In mild changes, writing usually deteriorates (patient writes above and below the line), and the ability to concentrate diminishes. An abnormal flapping of the hands (asterixis) is usually present.

Hepatic encephalopathy can be divided into five stages. Stages 1 and 2 are the early stages, with slurred speech and mild confusion. Stage 3 has marked confusion, and the patient is in a precoma stage. Stage 4 is frank coma. Stage 5 is very deep coma without response to any stimuli.

Diagnosis

Diagnosis is made by recognizing the presence of underlying liver disease and noting the changes in mental status or laboratory values stated previously. Specifically, liver function tests such as SGOT, bilirubin, alkaline phosphatase, albumin, prothrombin time, and partial thromboplastin time are abnormal. Hepatitis A, B, and C studies should be checked to exclude these three infections. The hemoglobin should be checked for signs of gastrointestinal hemorrhage, and the WBC count should be checked as a clue to the presence of infection or sepsis.

Treatment

Hepatic encephalopathy is often amenable to therapy. The most important part of therapy is to reverse any precipitating factors. Treatment consists of changing the bacterial flora of the colon, thus decreasing the production of potentially toxic agents that are absorbed into the bloodstream. Lactulose, which is a poorly absorbed sugar, and neomycin, which is a poorly absorbed antibiotic, are the two most useful agents.

Correcting electrolyte disturbances such as hypokalemia, protein restriction, and therapy of gastrointestinal hemorrhage are also important factors of therapy. Intravascular volume should be maintained.

Nursing Intervention

Frequent assessment of the patient's neurological status is an index of the response to therapy. Administer medications as ordered, avoiding sedatives and hepatotoxic drugs (e.g., acetaminophen, amino acids). If the patient is comatose, initiate eye care to prevent corneal abrasions.

Monitor intake and output, fluid status, and electrolyte status. Signs of anemia, infection, alkalosis (increasing serum HCO_3-), melena, or hematemesis should be reported to the physician to provide an opportunity to prevent complications.

Replace dietary protein with calories from glucose. During recovery, introduce protein in very small increments (approximately 20 grams at a time). Administer nutrients through tube feedings or TPN.

Monitor respiratory status closely, especially during times of decreasing mental status. Maintain a patent airway and administer oxygen as needed.

Stop all nitrogen-containing drugs and administer neomycin (decreases gastric ammonia formation) and lactulose. Monitor all side effects of medications and decrease dosages as needed.

Emotional support of the patient (if alert) and the family with realistic responses to the patient's condition is appropriate and essential, since the expected outcome is poor.

ACUTE PANCREATITIS

Acute pancreatitis is an inflammatory disease of the pancreas resulting in enzymatic autodigestion of the pancreas.

Pathophysiology

Acute pancreatitis is felt to result from activation of pancreatic enzymes inside the pancreas itself. Normally, the enzymes are released from the pancreas in an inactive state and are then activated by fluids present in the duodenum. These enzymes normally digest food products, breaking down nutrients into substituents that can be absorbed by the intestinal cells.

In acute pancreatitis, the enzymes are activated before they leave the pancreatic duct and enter the duodenum. It is postulated that an obstruction, usually temporary, leads to activation of these enzymes. Once activated, they act on the pancreatic tissue, causing potentially severe damage to the pancreas. The enzyme trypsin is important mainly in the activation of other pancreatic enzymes. The enzymes phospholipase A_2 and elastase are probably the most important causes of pancreatic damage. Elastase damages blood vessel walls, and phospholipase A_2 acts on acinar cell and fat cell membranes.

Severe edema, necrosis, and hemorrhage can result in the pancreas and can spread to adjacent organs. Fat and pancreatic necrosis leads to an exudative phlegmon, or inflammatory mass, that induces hypoalbuminemia, and calcium sequestration can lead to a loss of ionized calcium.

Etiology

The two most common causes of pancreatitis are gallstones and alcohol, with alcohol the most common cause. Most alcohol-related pancreatitis occurs in heavy drinkers. Alcohol has been shown experimentally to increase the protein content of pancreatic juice, and intraductal protein plugs have been noted to form. This intraductal obstruction has been postulated to lead to activation of pancreatic enzymes. Likewise, gallstones in the distal common bile duct may block off the pancreatic duct, causing an obstruction that can lead to pancreatitis.

There are many other, less common causes of pancreatitis. Some examples are surgical or blunt trauma to the abdomen, hyperlipidemia (especially types I, IV, and V), hypercalcemia, certain drugs such as hydrochlorothiazide, ulcers in the stomach or duodenum, and certain infections. A considerable percentage of cases of acute pancreatitis do not have an identifiable cause and are known as idiopathic.

Clinical Presentation

Pain is the universal symptom. Usually the pain is in the epigastrium and radiates through to the back. The pain can be severe and is eased by sitting forward. Although intense abdominal tenderness may be present, guarding and rebound tenderness are usually not found. The abdomen may also be distended, and bowel sounds may be decreased or absent, as in an ileus pattern. Vomiting is often present, sometimes accompanied by fever, tachycardia, and hypotension. Pleural effusions, usually small, or atelectasis is sometimes present.

Four specific physical findings deserve mention. Grey-Turner's sign (ecchymoses in the flanks) and Cullen's sign (ecchymoses around the umbilicus) are due to hemorrhage and induration. Chvostek's sign (facial muscle twitching when the cheek is tapped) and Trousseau's sign (spasm of the hand with inflation of a blood pressure cuff over systolic blood pressure for greater than three minutes) are manifestations of hypocalcemia.

Diagnosis

Diagnosis is made by the clinical presentation discussed above and an elevated level of amylase or lipase, both pancreatic enzymes, on a serum sample (Table 25-2). Urinary amylase or a urinary amylase/creatinine ratio may also be elevated, but these measurements are rarely necessary. Liver function tests are often elevated, usually to a minor degree. Severe cases often have hypocalcemia, anemia, leukocytosis, hypoxemia, hypoalbuminemia, and hyperglycemia.

Other diseases that can be confused with pancreatitis include cholecystitis, ulcers, and myocardial infarction. Amylase measurement usually leads to the correct diagnosis.

Complications

Pancreatitis is a serious disease, and death can result in severe cases. Complications that can lead to major mor-

TABLE 25-2. LABORATORY TESTS TO DIAGNOSE PANCREATITIS

Markedly elevated serum amylase levels, often over 500 units.

Characteristically, amylase levels return to normal 48 hours after onset of pancreatitis.

Supportive laboratory values include:

1. Increased serum lipase levels
2. Low serum calcium (hypocalcemia)
3. WBC counts ranging from 8,000–20,000/mm^3, with increased polymorphonuclear cells
4. Elevated glucose levels as high as 500–900 mg/100 mL

bidity or mortality include hyperglycemia, hypocalcemia, renal failure, ARDS, infection, hypotension, blood coagulation disorders, abscess formation, fistula formation, and pancreatic pseudocyst formation.

Treatment

Treatment involves maintaining the cardiorespiratory status, placing the pancreas at rest, and careful observation and early treatment of any complications that may develop. Monitoring in an intensive-care unit may be needed for more serious cases, as well as pulmonary artery (Swan-Ganz) catheter insertion to maintain optimal intravascular blood volume.

The pancreas is placed at rest by strict adherence to an NPO (non per os, nothing by mouth) regime and often by nasogastric (NG) suction. Pain is treated by meperidine (Demerol) because morphine theoretically may worsen pancreatitis by raising the pressure in the pancreatic duct. Diazepam (Valium) or chlordiazepoxide (Librium) is often needed in alcoholics to prevent delirium tremens.

Surgery is infrequently needed, and only acutely in severe pancreatitis. Different techniques used are surgical drainage of abscesses, pancreatic lavage, and subtotal or total pancreatectomy. These procedures carry high morbidity and mortality.

Nursing Intervention

In acute cases, pancreatitis is life threatening and requires both vigorous treatment and nursing care. All vital signs are checked at least hourly. Intake and output should be documented carefully. Insensible losses should be taken into account. Monitor laboratory values such as hematocrit and hemoglobin, blood urea nitrogen, serum protein, creatinine, and electrolytes. Urine should be tested for glucose and acetone. If urine tests positive for glucose, serum glucose should be checked for hyperglycemia. Insulin should be used judiciously.

Observe for muscular twitching, jerking, or irritability. Frequent vomiting and/or gastric suctioning may cause loss of electrolytes, with the possible development of tetany. Calcium is lost because it binds to the fatty acids and is lost in the stool.

Respiratory status is monitored by ABGs and hourly auscultation of lungs for crackles, wheezing, and diminished breath sounds. Cardiac monitoring is essential to detect dysrhythmias, which are frequent with shock and/or electrolyte imbalances.

An NG tube is sometimes inserted and connected to suction to prevent a buildup of acid secretions in the stomach. Observe and record color, amount, and nature of NG drainage as well as pH and if blood is present. Mouth and nose care should be given hourly, especially if anticholinergic drugs are administered.

Nutritional support is very important. TPN should be administered in severe cases so as to not stimulate the gastrointestinal tract. Small amounts of clear liquids are allowed when the patient can tolerate the NG tube clamped. Eventually a bland high-protein, high-carbohydrate, low-fat diet with frequent small meals is recommended. Antacids and replacement enzymes should be given.

Medicate the patient to alleviate pain. Give meperidine rather than opiates because opiates produce spasms of the biliary and pancreatic ducts. Observe for side effects of all medications, especially antibiotics.

Emotional support is very important because the pain is severe, the NG tube is uncomfortable, and the monitoring equipment increases apprehension.

CHAPTER 26

Intestinal Infarction, Obstruction, and Perforation

Editor's note

This chapter addresses the areas of the CCRN exam on bowel infarction, obstruction, and perforation. Expect one to three questions on the exam regarding content addressed in this chapter.

INTESTINAL INFARCTION

The intestinal tract receives a rich blood supply. Three major vascular trunks from the aorta supply the intestinal tract: the celiac axis, superior, and inferior mesenteric arteries. Since there is much collateral flow, gradual occlusion of even two of these three major trunks usually does not cause clinical difficulties. Up to 20% of cardiac output after meals is delivered to the intestinal tract.

Because of this rich collateral circulation, mesenteric or intestinal infarction is unusual. Many patients have extensive atherosclerosis of the aorta and intestinal branches, but few have ischemia or infarction.

Pathophysiology and Etiology

Mesenteric ischemia usually results from one of two processes. In the first process, termed occlusive, cardiac output is usually adequate, but an embolus can dislodge from either the heart or aorta and flow into the superior mesenteric artery, lodging a short distance from the aorta and totally occluding blood flow in this area. Another etiology could be an acute thrombosis in a vessel with atherosclerosis, much as one sees with coronary occlusion. The result from this sudden occlusion is infarction of part or all of the small intestine and possibly some of the colon. With this sudden occlusion, the collateral circulation is unable to compensate by increasing blood flow to the ischemic bowel.

The second major type, termed nonocclusive, is related to atherosclerosis of the intestinal vasculature. Already there is narrowing of the blood vessels, but in the normal state these narrowings are not clinically significant. When cardiac output or blood pressure is compromised, such as in dehydration, myocardial infarction, atrial fibrillation, or shock from any cause, overall blood supply to the intestines may diminish below a critical level, at which point intestinal infarction can occur. In this type of infarction, the intestinal ischemia is secondary to an overall reduction in cardiac output.

Consequences of either type of ischemia in the intestines are similar. In milder cases, only the mucosa is affected, with sloughing of the mucosa, bleeding, and abdominal pain. With severe ischemia, the submucosal and muscular layers of the intestine can be involved. If the injury is severe, transmural bowel necrosis and perforation can occur. With transmural necrosis, peritonitis will result, and intestinal bacteria enter the bloodstream, causing sepsis. In these circumstances, the disease is usually fatal.

Clinical Presentation

Occlusive mesenteric ischemia usually presents dramatically. The patient often experiences the sudden onset of severe abdominal pain, usually located in the periumbilical area or the epigastrium. There is usually diaphoresis, and the patient prefers to sit up, being more uncomfortable when forced to lie still. The abdomen, in contrast to the impressive appearance of the patient, usually has little tenderness. Guarding, rigidity, and rebound tenderness are usually absent. If diagnosis and treatment are delayed, peritonitis and intestinal perforation result.

Nonocclusive mesenteric infarction, in contrast, does not present dramatically. Often the patient is hospitalized for other diseases. Intestinal infarction is usually preceded by a vague abdominal discomfort with few physical findings. Routine diagnostic studies undertaken for other causes of abdominal pain, such as ultrasound, upper GI series, and CAT scans, are usually negative in the course of the disease. With continuing ischemia, infarction and death usually result.

A milder form of nonocclusive ischemia can affect the colon without affecting the small bowel. In these patients, the clinical presentation is similar, but they experience bloody diarrhea and mild crampy pain. These patients usually do not go on to full-thickness infarction, perforation, and death, unlike those whose ischemia involves the small intestine as well.

Diagnosis

In occlusive disease, when the diagnosis is considered, and other causes such as perforated ulcer are excluded, the diagnosis can usually be confirmed at surgery or preoperatively by angiography. Angiography will reveal either an embolus or a thrombosis of the superior mesenteric artery, and surgery will reveal either ischemia or an infarcted small and possibly large intestine.

Nonocclusive disease is usually more difficult to diagnose. Symptoms are not as dramatic, and usually an acute surgical abdomen is not present. Blood analysis often reveals a leukocytosis, increased amylase and LDH, and decreased pH and bicarbonate, all of which are nonspecific abnormalities. A CAT scan may reveal air in the bowel wall or mesenteric vasculature but often is normal. Plain abdominal radiographs are usually of little help. Unfortunately, diagnosis is usually made at autopsy, at which time bowel infarction can readily be appreciated. Diagnosis can also be made during exploratory laparotomy, but at this point, chances of survival are slim.

Treatment

The treatment of occlusive disease has classically been surgical. Embolectomy or thrombectomy with or without bypass is usually performed. Surgical therapy also gives the opportunity to resect any questionable areas of intestine and to evaluate the extent of injury. There have been reports of angiographic management with infusion of thrombolytic (clot-dissolving) agents in patients considered to be poor surgical risks.

Therapy of nonocclusive disease is often also surgical. However, the underlying circulatory abnormality of poor cardiac output or hypotension should first be corrected. Early laparotomy and resection of infarcted intestine are necessary in patients whose pain

does not rapidly resolve with correction of the low-flow state.

Delay in diagnosis of either type is almost always associated with a fatal outcome. Even with the diagnosis made and surgical therapy performed in a timely manner, the mortality rate is high.

Nursing Intervention

Careful and astute assessment of patients with unexplained abdominal pain is the key to recognizing intestinal infarction. Monitor the type of pain and relieving factors.

Supportive management of patients with intestinal infarction includes nasogastric suction, appropriate fluid and electrolyte replacement, and administration of antibiotics after cultures have been obtained. Treatment of shock and metabolic acidosis should be managed with fluid therapy, since alpha-stimulating amines such as dopamine can have an adverse effect on intestinal perfusion, precipitating renal failure by reducing blood flow to the kidneys. Dopamine may be used in low doses if a pressor agent is necessary.

The primary objective of initial management should be to prepare the patient for possible surgery before these complications arise. Since most patients with intestinal infarction require surgery, once intestinal stabilization is present and the patient has gone to surgery, the nurse must redirect interventions to postoperative surgical care. Postoperative gastrointestinal surgery interventions will be covered later in this chapter.

INTESTINAL OBSTRUCTION

Intestinal obstruction is one of the most common indications for abdominal surgery. Obstruction is a common problem in the adult population; the patient usually presents with crampy abdominal pain, vomiting, and decreased passage of stool or flatus from the rectum. Intestinal obstruction is divided into gastroduodenal, proximal or distal small intestinal, and colonic.

Pathophysiology

Bowel obstruction often results in problems with fluid balance. Alteration in fluid balance is due to fluid trapped in the intestine and the reduced capacity to ingest and absorb fluids. Often patients have profound dehydration from decreased intake, vomiting, and fluid trapped in the intestinal loops. Serum chemical imbalances can occur specifically with sodium, potassium, chloride, and bicarbonate.

Etiology

In adults, the most common cause of intestinal obstruction is adhesions from previous surgery. When the peritoneal cavity is explored, as in a cholecystectomy or gastric surgery, fibrous bands often form between loops of intestine. Usually these fibrous bands, otherwise known as adhesions, are asymptomatic, but often they can obstruct different segments of the small intestine.

The other major causes of intestinal obstruction in adults are hernias, tumors, and ulcers. A loop of intestine can become incarcerated in a hernia, causing an obstruction. Tumors, usually of the colon, can grow so that they completely block off the lumen of the colon and thus produce obstruction. Ulcers, usually in the distal stomach or duodenum, can also cause a blockage from scarring and fibrosis.

Other, less common causes of obstruction include infections such as diverticulitis, abscesses, inflammation, ischemia, gallstones, or some congenital anomalies.

Clinical Presentation

The presentation depends on the location and etiology of the bowel obstruction. In patients with a gastro-duodenal or proximal small intestinal obstruction, vomiting and crampy epigastric pain are the major symptoms. The symptoms will occur early after the obstruction, usually within a few hours. However, if the obstruction is in the distal small intestine or colon, vague, crampy, periumbilical or diffuse abdominal pain is the initial symptom. Patients have vomiting usually hours to days after the start of the pain and may actually present for medical care before they have any vomiting at all. Commonly, tachycardia and dizziness due to dehydration are present. Later symptoms include decreased bowel movements and gas passage.

Examination often reveals a distended abdomen with hyperresonance or tympany on percussion, sounding like a kettle drum. Bowel sounds are usually increased and high pitched (tinkling), and the abdomen may be diffusely, though usually not severe, tender. There usually is no guarding or rebound tenderness. The fluid vomited may be yellow or green in proximal small bowel obstructions, or darker and feculent-smelling in distal small bowel or colonic obstructions.

Diagnosis

Diagnosis is made on the basis of history, a careful physical examination, and routine abdominal radiographs. The radiographs will usually show dilated small bowel loops with air-fluid levels, or a horizontal line on the radiograph above which air is seen. Surgery usually allows the diagnosis of the cause of the obstruction. Barium contrast, radiographic studies, either of the upper GI tract or via a barium enema, are sometimes used for diagnosis prior to surgical therapy.

Treatment

Treatment consists of correcting fluid and electrolyte imbalances. Intravenous fluids are given while carefully monitoring serum electrolyte concentrations, vital signs, and urine output. Passage of a nasogastric tube and applying suction to remove air and fluid can often reverse a small bowel obstruction from adhesions and should be used in virtually all cases of either proximal or distal bowel obstruction. Surgery is often necessary to break the bands of adhesions in obstructions and is almost always necessary in obstructions from tumors. If a hernia can be manually reduced, surgery may not be necessary. If bowel infarction or gangrene has occurred, intestinal resection and antibiotics are needed.

Nursing Intervention

Nursing interventions again are aimed at ensuring hemodynamic stability. Careful observation of fluid and electrolyte balances is of primary importance. Strict records of intake and output, daily weights, vital signs, and serum electrolyte concentrations are maintained.

Careful assessment of the patient's nutritional status must be done on a daily basis to prevent a catabolic state. Since the patient must be NPO, nutrition will need to be maintained by TPN if surgery is delayed or the obstruction does not resolve within a reasonable length of time.

Since nasogastric suction is very important in relieving a bowel obstruction, patency must always be maintained. Note consistency, type, color, amount, and pH of drainage.

As in intestinal infarction, the primary objective of initial management should be to prepare the patient for possible surgery to relieve the obstruction. Refer to gastrointestinal surgery nursing interventions for postoperative care of patients with bowel obstruction.

GASTROINTESTINAL PERFORATION

Perforation is usually a catastrophic event. The patient usually will have the sudden onset of abdominal pain and will appear very ill. Perforations occur in the stomach, duodenum, appendix, or colon. However, other areas of the GI tract can perforate at rare times.

Pathophysiology

Perforation of the intestinal tract results in leakage of intestinal contents into the peritoneal cavity. If the stomach or duodenum perforates, ingested foodstuffs, acids, and enzymes leak into the peritoneal cavity. If the appendix or colon perforates, feces, which contain large amounts of bacteria, are released into the peritoneal cavity. Any of these substances are irritating to the peritoneum and invoke an intense inflammatory reaction, with leakage of fluid and pus into the peritoneal cavity. Fever and leukocytosis result, and severe pain is usually present when the peritoneum becomes inflamed.

Etiology

The most common cause of intestinal perforation in the United States is appendicitis. If diagnosed early, appendicitis usually will not cause perforation. If diagnosis is delayed, the inflamed appendix may rupture, causing either a diffuse or localized peritonitis. Other major causes of colonic perforations are colonic diverticulitis, which represents infection of outpouchings from the colon, or colonic tumors, which can perforate through the bowel wall. The most common cause of gastric or duodenal perforations is ulcers. Small intestinal perforations rarely occur and are usually caused by tumors, congenital malformations, penetrating trauma, or ischemia.

Clinical Presentation

Patients usually present with the acute onset of abdominal pain. The pain is likely to begin in the periumbilical area and spread throughout the abdomen. The patient prefers to lie still, flat on the back, as movement usually accentuates the pain. Fever is often present, respirations are shallow, and a tachycardia may be present. Hypovolemia may be present and manifested as hypotension. Hypovolemia is secondary to fluid exudation into the peritoneal cavity and sequestration in the intestines from an ileus. The patient is often diaphoretic and looks moderately ill. Abdominal exam often reveals a boardlike abdomen with absent bowel sounds. Diffuse tenderness with muscle rigidity and rebound tenderness may be present. In the case of a local perforation that walls off, as occasionally occurs with a perforated appendix or gastric ulcer, the physical findings may be isolated to a certain area of the abdomen.

Diagnosis

Diagnosis usually is made by the history and physical examination. A leukocytosis with a left shift is usually present, and the hemoglobin may be falsely raised from intravascular volume depletion. Serum electrolytes may be abnormal. Plain radiographs of the abdomen often reveal free air underneath the diaphragm on an upright abdominal or chest film. An ileus pattern is often present. Diagnosis of the specific cause is usually made by exploratory laparotomy. In certain cases, either an upper GI series or colonic enema with a water-soluble contrast agent, such as gastrograffin, will show extravasation of the contrast agent, demonstrating an intestinal perforation.

Treatment

Therapy consists of surgical repair in the vast majority of cases. In some walled-off perforations in poor-risk patients, conservative management may be attempted, with nasogastric suction, intravenous fluids, and parenteral broad-spectrum antibiotics. Prior to surgical therapy, the hemodynamic status may need to be stabilized with intravenous fluids. Antibiotics should be given to treat the peritonitis. The overall prognosis depends upon the time from the perforation to definitive therapy, underlying medical disorders, and any complications resulting after the surgery. With prompt diagnosis and treatment, most patients will do well.

Nursing Intervention

Refer to the next chapter for intestinal infarction and intestinal obstruction nursing interventions.

CHAPTER 27

Gastrointestinal Surgery and Treatment

Editor's Note

This chapter addresses the CCRN exam areas of acute adominal trauma and, to some extent, all other GI concepts. Expect two to four questions on the exam in this content area.

GASTROINTESTINAL SURGERY

Esophagus

The most common surgical procedures related to the esophagus are those for the treatment of esophageal carcinoma. This disease usually occurs in males over the age of 60. Cigarette smoking and alcohol intake are the two major risk factors. The carcinoma is usually located in the mid-esophagus and is usually epidermoid. Patients usually have dysphagia as the main symptom and a recent unexplained weight loss. At the time of diagnosis, the great majority of tumors have spread beyond the esophagus to the mediastinum, lymph nodes, liver, or pulmonary system. Esophageal tumors frequently are not curable by either surgery, radiation therapy, or chemotherapy.

Surgery is undertaken to either cure the disease or palliate symptoms. Unfortunately, surgery is not always possible. The usual surgical procedure is esophagogastrectomy with primary esophageal-gastric anastomosis. The mortality rate associated with this procedure is anywhere from 2.8 to 17%. Another surgical procedure that was done more frequently in the past is primary esophagectomy with colonic interposition between the cervical esophagus and stomach. Radiation therapy is usually an effective palliation procedure for those who are not operable or have had a recurrence of their tumor. Current studies of chemotherapy do not show much benefit, but further studies of both chemotherapy and radiation therapy are in progress.

Stomach

Gastric surgery is generally performed for three diseases: ulcer disease, gastroesophageal reflux disease, and neoplastic disease.

Many different operations are performed for ulcer disease. One surgery is a vagotomy and pyloroplasty. The vagotomy (severing of the vagus nerve) results in decreased acid production because of the loss of vagally mediated gastric secretion. Pyloroplasty, or widening of the pyloric channel, is necessary to prevent gastric stasis. This surgery generally has a low rate of ulcer recurrence, but a combination of vagotomy and antrectomy has an even lower recurrence rate. In this more complicated surgery, the distal half of the stomach is removed to decrease gastrin production, another stimulus to acid production. The most recent development in ulcer surgery is the highly selective vagotomy, also called the parietal cell or proximal gastric vagotomy. In this operation, the vagal branches to the proximal stomach, the fundus, and body are severed. As this is where acid secretion occurs, this surgery decreases acid production without affecting the motor activity of the distal stomach. This surgery, however, is technically more difficult to perform than the other two.

Gastroesophageal reflux of acid results in problems with esophagitis and esophageal strictures. Usually these conditions can be treated medically, but some cases are refractory to conservative therapy. In such cases, surgery is necessary. One of the operations most commonly performed is the Nissen fundoplication. Fundoplication involves wrapping the fundus of the stomach around the lower esophagus and anchoring the distal esophagus in the abdominal cavity. This greatly reduces reflux of gastric juices into the esophagus, allowing the esophagitis to heal. Another procedure, done less commonly, involves the placement of a plastic ring around the distal esophagus to reduce reflux. This ring is called the Angelchick prosthesis.

Surgery for gastric neoplasms often takes many forms. Adenocarcinoma is the most common malignancy of the stomach. Symptoms often appear late, after spread has already occurred. In lesions that have not spread, the usual procedure is a subtotal gastrectomy, with removal of over half of the stomach. Some tumors are large enough to require a total gastrectomy. In patients with tumors that have already metastasized, gastric bypass in the form of gastrojejunostomy is often needed for palliation.

Small and Large Intestines

Surgery of the small intestine is usually performed for removal of tumors, treatment of hemorrhage, or correction of intestinal herniation. Tumors of the small intestine are rare, and therapy is usually with simple resection of the tumor itself plus a limited margin of normal intestine on either end. Hemorrhage is also uncommon and usually results from arteriovenous malformations, which in most cases form in the colon and not the small intestine. Small intestinal herniation can be either internal or external. Internal herniation is associated with trapping of intestinal loops by adhesive bands that form as a result of previous abdominal surgery. The herniation is referred to as internal because it is within the peritoneal cavity. External herniation involves trapping of an intestinal loop outside the peritoneal cavity, such as in inguinal, femoral, or ventral hernias. Surgical therapy of either type involves freeing the trapped loop of intestine and attempting to prevent its recurrence.

Surgery of the large intestine is usually for appendicitis, colonic carcinoma, diverticulitis, or lower gastrointestinal bleeding.

Appendicitis

Appendicitis is probably the major cause of an acute abdomen in Western civilization. The appendix arises from the cecum and varies in length. The appendix can become inflamed, distend, and perforate. Appendicitis is felt to arise from an obstruction in the more proximal part of the appendix, with stasis and bacterial proliferation distally. The visceral peritoneum initially gets inflamed, with resultant exudation of fluid and proteins. At this stage, pain is localized to the periumbilical area or right lower quadrant. As a response to the infection and inflammation, catecholamine is released, resulting in tachycardia and sweating. With further distension of the appendix and visceral peritoneal inflammation, inflammation of the adjacent parietal peritoneum results. This leads to the findings of localized involuntary abdominal musculature contractions, termed guarding. Rebound tenderness is often present in the right lower quadrant. With continuing obstruction and infection, the pus-filled appendix will perforate. Perforation results in release of pus and bacteria into the peritoneal cavity. An intense inflammation of the peritoneum results, with increased abdominal tenderness. If the infection is still isolated by loops of intestine to the right lower quadrant, the physical findings will be primarily in that site. If, however, the infected fluid spreads throughout the abdominal cavity, then diffuse direct tenderness, rigidity, and rebound tenderness of the abdomen result. At this stage, the intravascular blood volume will be low, the patient may be hypotensive, and urine output will fall. The patient prefers to lie quietly in bed without moving, and respirations are shallow. The temperature is usually elevated, the white blood cell (WBC) count is elevated with a shift to more immature forms of neutrophils, and the hemoglobin may be raised from hemoconcentration.

Therapy of appendicitis is surgical after fluid and electrolyte resuscitation is initiated. If there has been no perforation, an appendectomy is performed and recovery is usually rapid. If free perforation has occurred, copious irrigation of the peritoneal cavity with an antibiotic solution is required in addition to the appendectomy. Usually the surgical wound must be left open to protect against wound infection. Time to recovery and length of hospitalization are usually greater than in patients without perforation.

Colonic Carcinoma

Colonic carcinoma is presently the second leading cause of cancer death in the United States. Unfortunately, symptoms often appear late in the disease, after spread beyond the colon has occurred, or are ignored by the patient and attributed to other causes. One example of the latter is rectal bleeding, which is often perceived by patients as resulting from hemorrhoids. However, rectal bleeding can also be from a polyp or tumor in the rectum or sigmoid; it should be evaluated by sigmoidoscopy and possibly by barium enema examination. Other possible symptoms of colon cancer include constipation, diarrhea, and colonic obstruction. All of these are results of either a partial or complete mechanical colonic obstruction. Colon cancer may not produce early symptoms, but one early sign can often be found. Presence of microscopic amounts of blood (occult blood) not visible to the naked eye can be noted in many cases of colon cancer. Occult blood can be discovered by card tests, such as Hemoccult. Tests are recommended annually in all people over age 50 in the United States. If colon cancer is detected at an early stage, the likelihood of cure with surgical excision is excellent. However, if the tumor has spread, the chance of surgical cure is poor. Surgical excision involves removal of the tumor with wide margins of uninvolved intestine on either side, with resection of the areas of regional lymphatic drainage. Usually a permanent colostomy is not required, except in carcinoma of the distal rectum.

Diverticulitis

Diverticulitis is a common cause of abdominal pain in patients over the age of 50. It involves infection of one of the outpouchings of the colon prevalent in the older population. Patients may have anywhere from mild abdominal pain and tenderness to diffuse peritonitis from colonic perforation. Therapy is usually with antibiotics and bowel rest, but free perforation or abscess formation may mandate surgical exploration with performance of a temporary diverting colostomy.

Pancreas

Carcinoma of the pancreas is the fourth leading cause of cancer death in men and the fifth most common in women. It usually arises insidiously and is almost always incurable at the time of diagnosis. Risk factors for pancreatic cancer include cigarette smoking, certain dietary and environmental factors, and juvenile-onset diabetes mellitus.

Most patients with pancreatic cancer complain of a vague, dull epigastric discomfort that may radiate through to the back. Insidious weight loss and anorexia are also present. Approximately one-fourth of patients have a palpable abdominal mass. The tumor can spread to the duodenum, liver, lymph nodes, and lungs and can impinge on the stomach. Other symptoms vary with the sites of metastases. If the tumor is compressing on the stomach, gastric outlet obstruction and vomiting are common. If the bile duct is obstructed, jaundice, pruritis, and acholic stools can result. Diagnosis of pancreatic cancer is usually made by CAT scan of the abdomen, followed by either percutaneous needle biopsy or surgical exploration.

Most cases of pancreatic cancer are not surgically curable. Those that are resectable require extensive, complicated surgery for attempted cure. The two major procedures undertaken are pancreaticoduodenectomy (Whipple's procedure) and total pancreatectomy. Whipple's procedure involves resection of the head of the pancreas along with contiguous structures. The gastric antrum, duodenal C loop, gallbladder, and lymph nodes are removed. A loop of jejunum is anastomosed to the tail of the pancreas, the stomach, and the common bile duct. The procedure is difficult, and surgical mortality (death within 30 days of surgery) is 21%. Major complications of the procedure have been leakage or hemorrhage at the site of pancreaticojejunostomy. Five-year survival of one large series of patients treated by Whipple's procedure for pancreatic cancer was a disappointing 4%.

Total pancreatectomy is another option in pancreatic cancer. In this procedure, the same organs are removed as for Whipple's procedure, but a pancreaticojejunostomy is not necessary since the whole pancreas is removed. This procedure is technically simpler to perform than Whipple's procedure. Surgical mortality is decreased to 15%, but five-year survival is likely not improved.

Most surgical procedures for pancreatic cancer are palliative rather than curative. The aim is to treat or prevent common bile duct and gastric outlet obstruction. Therefore, anastomosis of the jejunum to either the gallbladder or common bile duct as well as gastrojejunostomy are most often done.

Nursing Intervention

Nursing priorities for patients undergoing gastrointestinal surgery should include promoting optimal physical conditions preoperatively, alleviating psychosocial concerns, meeting nutritional needs, promoting proper GI functioning postoperatively, and preventing complications.

Preoperatively, the patient must ideally be hemodynamically stable, have fluid and electrolyte balances in normal limits, be in a reasonable nutritional state (not catabolic), and be emotionally prepared for the impending surgery.

Postoperatively, the first goal of therapy is to ensure hemodynamic and respiratory stability. Maintain an airway by ventilation or oxygen therapy and assess the pulmonary effects of anesthesia. If the patient is not intubated, make sure the patient coughs and deep breathes every two hours (make sure you instruct on splinting the incision). Suction the endotracheal tube as needed and note the color, amount, and odor of the secretions. Monitor arterial blood gases on oximetry values if needed.

Assess vital signs at least every 30 to 60 minutes initially after surgery. Note urine output and maintain at least 30 cc/hour. If the patient has hemodynamic monitoring, note hemodynamic measurements every hour. Assess intake and output every hour, and monitor serum electrolytes as available. Assess the type and amount of drainage from the nasogastric tube and from incision and drainage tubes. Note any foul odor from any drainage. Assess for possible abdominal fluid accumulation or postoperative hemorrhage.

Maintain nutritional status by TPN if the patient will not tolerate oral or enteral intake within the first several days after surgery. The alimental route for nutrition is restricted due to cessation of peristalsis from intraoperative handling of intestines, anesthesia, and/or potassium loss with resultant decreased smooth muscle contractility. If the patient is not able to eat, maintain the patency of the nasogastric tube and record the characteristics of any drainage. Once bowel sounds are present, liquids, progressing to clear liquids and then to diets low in residue and high in protein, carbohydrates, and calories, may be initiated.

Maintain the integrity of the skin by monitoring for signs and symptoms of infection. Assess vital signs frequently, noting increased pulse, tachypnea, and apprehension. Check dressing and wound frequently during the first 24 hours for signs of bright blood or excessive incisional swelling. Note temperature elevations and elevated WBCs. Monitor for signs of peritonitis (rigidity, guarding, rebound tenderness, and the absence of bowel sounds).

Patients who have had pancreatic resections must have their blood glucose closely monitored.

Emotional support of the postoperative patient is important to both the patient and the family. This is extremely important for patients who have had ostomies placed. Maintain a reassuring, accepting environment and allow the patient time to vocalize fears and altered self-concept.

GASTROINTESTINAL TRAUMA

Blunt or Penetrating Abdominal Trauma

Since violence marks our present civilization, stab wounds and blunt injuries to the abdomen are increasingly seen in emergency rooms, operating rooms, and intensive-care units. Injury to the abdomen may occur from a blow to the abdomen in an automobile accident, altercation, or fall. These injuries may occur even though the abdominal wall is still intact. Other penetrating injuries, such as those from a stab wound, may appear superficial and unimportant, but they often are deep and may have lacerated several internal organs. Trauma of any kind is apt to cause bleeding or contusions and may open the bowel lumen to cause peritonitis. In closed abdominal wounds, the spleen, the kidneys, the duodenum (especially the third and fourth portions, which may be squeezed between the steering wheel and the spine), and the liver are injured in approximately that order of frequency; in stab wounds, the liver, stomach, and colon receive most of the injury because of their anterior location.

Diagnosis

Abdominal trauma may cause injury to the liver, spleen, pancreas, GI tract, spine, retroperitoneum, kidneys, and pelvic organs. Injuries to the spleen, liver, pancreas, and GI tract are the most difficult to diagnose by conventional radiologic methods. A CAT scan has been shown to be beneficial for the early diagnosis and accurate evaluation of the extent of internal injuries following abdominal trauma. A CAT scan is capable of detecting lacerations, subcapsular hematomas, and ruptures of all abdominal organs and therefore has advantages over organ-specific procedures. In addition, CAT scans directly image even small amounts of intra-abdominal hemorrhage, which cannot be identified by other conventional imaging techniques.

At some institutions, exploratory laparoscopy is done as an emergency procedure for the evaluation of patients who have suffered trauma to the abdomen. By this procedure, it can be determined which patients need laparotomy because of perforated viscera or lacerations of the liver or spleen.

Clinical Manifestations

If the injury is severe (especially with a significant blood loss), the patient may exhibit signs of hypovolemic shock (shallow respirations, weak rapid pulse, and decreased urine output). The patient may have pain, depending on the site and extent of injury. A physical insult to the abdomen is apt to cause cessation of bowel motility. If there is colonic injury, there may be blood in the stool and possible signs of intestinal perforation or obstruction.

In blunt trauma, the pancreas is particularly susceptible to rupture where it passes over the spine, and is often associated with duodenal rupture. With trauma to the pancreas, pancreatitis often follows but is usually asymptomatic. Elevation of serum amylase is not a dependable sign. Traumatic pancreatitis is often recognized only during exploratory laparotomy for gunshot or stab wounds. However, in the nonpenetrating, blunt abdominal trauma, traumatic pancreatitis often goes unnoticed because of the protected retroperitoneal location of the pancreas. This unnoticed pancreatitis may lead to the development of a pseudocyst, a subdiaphragmatic abscess, or massive GI hemorrhage. The disease, regardless of whether it is diagnosed during a laparotomy, carries a 14% mortality rate.

Symptoms of liver rupture are similar to those of splenic rupture, but they occur on the right side. There may be pain in the right upper quadrant, some tenderness, and if blood loss is great enough, signs of shock.

Treatment

Initial treatment is aimed at maintenance of the patient's hemodynamic status and prevention of shock. Rapid intravenous fluid and blood replacement may be necessary. Antibiotics may be necessary to prevent peritonitis, especially for open, penetrating wounds.

Surgical intervention must readily be instituted for those who are hemodynamically unstable. Most of these patients will undergo exploratory laparotomy to repair or remove injured organs and surrounding tissue. Vigorous rinsing of the abdominal cavity with an antimicrobial solution is necessary if bowel perforation has occurred. Patients with closed injuries require astute observation for organ failure or hemorrhage necessitating surgical intervention.

Nursing Intervention

Patients with abdominal injury must be carefully observed for coexisting cardiothoracic injury. Signs of pneumothorax, cardiac tamponade, cardiac rupture, and aortic or pulmonary vasculature injuries must be assessed.

Astute assessment of the patient's hemodynamic and respiratory status must be carried out continuously. Fluid and electrolyte replacements are given to counteract third spacing and hypovolemic shock. Anaerobic and aerobic coverage with antibiotics is immediately initiated. Ventilatory and oxygen support may be necessary.

A careful abdominal assessment is performed to evaluate injuries. The nurse must assess for rebound tenderness, muscle rigidity, anorexia, nausea, vomiting, abdominal distension, presence of bowel sounds, and pain. A nasogastric tube should be placed, and changes in drainage should be noticed.

Emotional support is important for the patient and family, since gastrointestinal trauma is usually quite unexpected and coping mechanisms are not readily available.

Other Trauma to the Gastrointestinal Tract

Caustic injury is usually produced by strong alkaline or acidic agents. The ingestion of caustic agents can initiate a progressive and devastating injury to the esophagus and stomach. Most caustic injuries are seen in patients who are very young, psychotic, alcoholic, or suicidal.

Acidic solutions usually cause immediate pain, and unless they are ingested intentionally, they are rapidly expelled. The alkali liquid solutions are often tasteless and odorless and thus are swallowed before protective reflexes can be invoked. Alkali solutions penetrate tissue more rapidly than acid solutions do and are more difficult to treat. Caustic injuries to the gastrointestinal mucosa are classified pathologically in the same manner as skin burns.

Symptoms may be present, especially early after the ingestion. Edema, ulceration, or a white membrane may be present over the palate, uvula, and pharynx. Hoarseness, stridor, dysphagia, epigastric pain, emesis of tissue or blood, tachypnea, and shock may be present. Late symptoms include perforation of the stomach or esophagus, mediastinitis, and peritonitis.

Early treatment includes neutralization of the caustic agent. Acid injuries should be neutralized with large volumes of water or milk. Alkali injuries occur so rapidly that even immediate attempts to neutralize them are probably unsuccessful and should not be undertaken because of the exothermic properties of dilution and neutralization.

Resuscitation should immediately be instituted. Establishment of an airway, fluid and blood resuscitation, and gastrointestinal rest (NPO) should be first priorities.

Endoscopic evaluation should be performed once the patient is stable to evaluate the extent of the damage. If there is perforation, a thoracotomy or laparotomy may be done to repair injured organs.

The morality rate after caustic ingestion is 1 to 3%. However, if the patient survives the acute effects of caustic ingestion, the reparative response can result in esophageal and gastric stenosis and an increased incidence of esophageal cancer.

Esophageal Perforation

The most common causes of esophageal perforation are medical tubes and instruments, forceful vomiting, and foreign bodies. Less frequent are perforations caused by gunshot wounds, necrotizing infections or tumors, and caustic agents.

Perforations are recognized by symptoms of respiratory distress, chest, neck, abdominal, and upper neck pain, and odynophagia. Subcutaneous crepitation, fever, shock, mediastinal crunching sound with the heartbeat, leukocytosis, and x-ray abnormalities may also occur.

The most important determinants of survival are the size and location of the perforation and whether gross contamination outside the esophagus has occurred. Most causes of esophageal perforation are surgically managed to repair the perforation.

GENERAL NURSING INTERVENTIONS FOR PATIENTS WITH GASTROINTESTINAL DISTURBANCE

Interventions to Maintain Fluid and Electrolyte Balance

1. Maintenance of accurate intake and output. Include number, character, amount, and site of GI fluid loss.
2. Monitoring of serum electrolytes per laboratory data. GI fluid losses through tube suction, ostomy drainage, diarrhea, and vomiting can cause losses of essential electrolytes, especially H^-, Cl^-, and K^+, and may produce alkalosis.
3. Correct use of GI tubes for decompression and diagnosis. Two types of tubes:
    a. Short tubes. These are used for the stomach and duodenum. Example: Nasogastric tubes.
       1. Levin (single lumen)
       2. Rehfuss (single lumen with metal tube)
       3. Salem sump (double lumen)
          The salem sump is most widely used because the second lumen, which is open to air, prevents the development of excessive negative pressure by bringing air into the cavity continuously. Low, intermittent levels of suction are used. The second port of the salem sump (pigtail) must be placed above the patient's midline to prevent reflux into the pigtail. Commercially made anti-reflux valves are available.
    b. Long tubes. These tubes are intended to extend the length of the small bowel. They can be 6 and 10 feet long.
       1. Miller-Abbott
       2. Cantor
       3. Harris
          The tube is threaded from the nose into the stomach and then through the pylorus, where peristaltic activity of the bowel carries it to the desired area. If peristalsis does not carry the tube to the appropriate place, gravity or guidance under fluoroscopy may be used. Once it is in the correct location, the tube is taped securely in place to prevent further migration.
          With all of the GI tubes, the material aspirated should be noted for color, odor, and quantity.
4. Maintenance of blood volume during GI hemorrhage.
    a. Blood volume replacement as needed.
    b. Monitor hematocrit/hemoglobin every day and prn during instability.
    c. Monitor amount, color, and area of bleeding.
    d. Oxygen therapy as needed.
    e. Monitor hemodynamic status.
5. Relief of nausea and vomiting.
    a. Monitor for distension; may place nasogastric tube to decompress stomach.
    b. Monitor emesis for amount, color, frequency, and presence of blood.
    c. Administer antiemetics.
    d. Place patient on side to prevent aspiration of vomitus.

Interventions to Maintain Nutritional Status

Patients in the intensive-care unit who are unable to eat must be fed enterally or parenterally. Normally, patients at rest require 25 kcal/kg/day. The nurse should assess the calories given versus what is needed.

1. Evaluation of the patient's nutritional status.
   a. History taking
      1. Medical history: Illness, surgery, GI disease, alcoholism, etc.
      2. Social history: Food storage and preparation facilities, money, and education.
      3. Drug history: Antibiotics, chemotherapy, anticonvulsants, etc.
      4. Diet history: 24-hour recall.
   b. Anthropometric measures. Physical measurements that reflect growth and development compared with standards specific for sex and age. Compares body fat and skeletal muscle obtained through triceps skinfold, midarm circumference, and midarm muscle circumference measurements.
   c. Types of proteins and biochemical tests
      1. Somatic protein (skeletal). Somatic protein is the protein of voluntary muscles. Indicators of somatic protein losses are low ideal body weight or usual body weight percentages, low fatfold thickness, negative nitrogen balance from nitrogen balance studies, and increased 24-hour urinary creatinine.
      2. Visceral protein. Visceral protein is the protein of the internal organs. Indicators of visceral protein losses are low total lymphocyte count (<1000), serum albumin (<3.5), and serum transferrin (<200 mg/dL).
   d. Measurements of immune function
      Various forms of protein malnutrition have been associated with depression of the immune system.
      1. Lymphocytes: White blood cells that defend against infection. Decrease in number as protein depletion occurs. Decrease for many other reasons also, so they are not nutrition specific.
      2. Antigen skin testing: A test of the immune system's competence, in which an antigen is injected just under the skin. A reaction means that the immune system is working normally.
2. Enteral feeding administration
   A person who has a functioning GI tract but is unable to eat enough food may be a candidate for a tube feeding.
   a. Types of tubes: Silicone or polyurethane (Silastic).
   b. Placement of tubes: Esophagostomy, gastrostomy, jejunostomy, transnasal, nasogastric, and nasoenteric (nasoduodenal or nasojejunal).
   c. Tube feeding formulas: Selected after the client's needs have been identified.
      1. Intact formulas. These contain protein, carbohydrates, and fats of higher molecular weights. A person must be able to digest and absorb nutrients without difficulty to use this type of formula.
      2. Hydrolyzed formulas. These contain smaller molecules of protein, fat, and carbohydrates. They are "predigested" and are recommended for those who lack digestive capabilities or who have a smaller than normal area for absorbing nutrients.
   d. Administration guidelines: Bolus feedings via gravity drip or continuous feedings via pump are used. It is controversial as to which method is preferred.
      Initial feedings:
      1. Check tube placement before feeding.
      2. Check residual amount in stomach. If greater than 100 to 150 cc, hold feeding.
      3. Diluting the feeding is controversial. Some institutions may prefer gradual progression to full-strength external feedings.
      4. Check drip rate every one to two hours.
      5. Feeding should be at or slightly below body temperature. Cold starts vasoconstriction, which reduces the flow of gastric digestive juices.
      6. Monitor intake and output.
      7. Changing feeding bag and tubing every day.
      8. Monitor laboratory data, especially serum electrolytes, two to three times weekly.
      9. Flush tube with 50 to 100 cc of water before and after each feeding to maintain patency.
   e. Complications
      1. Diarrhea: From bacterial contamination, lactose intolerance, hypertonic for-

mulas, low serum albumin, or drug therapy.
2. Dehydration: From excessive diarrhea, inadequate fluid intake, carbohydrate intolerance, or excessive protein intake.
3. Aspiration pneumonia: From regurgitation of formula that is subsequently inhaled into the lungs or from displacement of feeding tube.
4. Vomiting: From obstruction or stomach emptying very slowly.
5. Nausea, cramps, distension: From obstruction, stomach emptying very slowly, or intolerance to concentration or volume of formula.
6. Increased glucose levels: From excess glucose loads.

3. Total parental alimentation (hyperalimentation)
   If gastrointestinal absorption and delivery of nutrients are inadequate, impossible for prolonged periods of time, or contraindicated, nourishment should be provided parenterally.
   Total parental alimentation is done with a hypertonic mixture of dextrose, amino acids, electrolytes, vitamins, and trace minerals. It may be given peripherally or through central veins.
   a. Nutrient solutions
      The concentration and quantity of the solution are gradually increased until a desired state is reached.
      A typical TPN solution contains 25 to 75% dextrose and 3.5 to 8% amino acids. One liter of a D50 solution provides about 1700 kcal daily. Electrolytes, vitamins, and trace minerals are added. The fluid may be concentrated if it is infused through a central line.
   b. Lipid emulsions
      Lipids supply 9 kcal/gram, more than twice the energy supplied by a gram of glucose. They are isotonic. They prevent essential fatty acid deficiency.
   c. Administration guidelines
      1. Monitor serum electrolytes, albumin levels, and nitrogen balance studies. Increase TPN concentrations as nutritional status warrants.
      2. Monitor daily weight and daily intake and output.
      3. Monitor serum glucose and urine glucose every four to six hours. May need to administer insulin.
      4. Monitor infusion rate every one to two hours. If rate falls behind, monitor for hypoglycemia and spread whatever deficit has incurred over the next 24 hours.
   d. Complications
      1. Infection or sepsis: Stringent aseptic technique during catheter insertion and dressing changes.
      2. Thrombosis of great veins or embolism from the catheter: Remove catheter and start anticoagulation therapy if not contraindicated.
      3. Hyperosmolar nonketotic hyperglycemia: Discontinue TPN; give insulin, saline, and D5W to replace free water.
      4. Hyperglycemia: Insulin therapy, slow rate.
      5. Hypoglycemia: Check to make sure TPN has not been interrupted or the wrong concentration given.
      6. Electrolyte disturbances: Maintain appropriate concentrations.

Interventions to Maintain Bowel Elimination Status

1. Diarrhea
   a. Identify caustic factors.
   b. Record color, amount, and frequency of stools.
   c. Maintain intake and output to prevent dehydration.
   d. Monitor serum electrolytes.
   e. Check for blood in stools.
   f. Administer antidiarrheal medications to decrease intestinal motility if not contraindicated.
   g. Begin nutritional supplement.
2. Constipation
   a. Increase fluid intake if not concentrated.
   b. Monitor time and consistency of stools.
   c. Administer laxative or enema if not contraindicated. Needed after barium studies.

Interventions to Maintain Comfort Status

1. Pain
   a. Observe for signs and location of pain; determine type and severity.

b. Administer analgesics or sedatives; morphine sulfate is contraindicated in pancreatitis because it causes spasm of the sphincter of Oddi.

Interventions to Prevent Infection

1. Monitor temperature and WBCs.
2. Use strict aseptic technique when placing lines or changing dressings.
3. Use isolation techniques for specific diseases (e.g., hepatitis).
4. Assess sources of contamination. Culture infected drainage and blood.
5. Use good handwashing techniques to prevent cross-contamination.

Physical Assessment

Physical assessment of the GI system can be briefly summarized by following the steps listed below:

1. Begin the assessment with inspection of the abdomen. Do not begin palpation, particularly deep palpation until the last phase of assessment. This will avoid any stimulation of the GI system and avoid any initiation of painful stimuli.
2. Auscultation in the second phase of assessment. Bowel sounds are usually heard in all four abdominal quadrants. Observe for a change in sounds or bowel sound intensity and character. Bowel sounds are not always a reliable assessment tool due to the transmission of sound throughout the abdomen.
3. Percussion is the third step in assessment. Usually, the GI tract has air present and will result in hearing a resonant or hyperresonant sound. Tympanic sounds can be heard in the stomach although elsewhere this sound may indicate an obstruction.
4. Palpation, both superficial and deep, are the last phase of assessment. The goal is to detect abnormal organ size, such as liver or spleen enlargement, and to identify if pain is present in the abdomen.

BIBLIOGRAPHY

Achkar, E., Farmer, R.G., Fleshler B., Clinical gastroenterology. Philadelphia: Lea & Febiger. 1992. 2nd Ed.

Beal, J. (1982). *Critical Care for Surgical Patients.* New York: Macmillan Publishing Co., Inc.

Berk, E. (1985). *Gastroenterology,* 4th ed. Philadelphia: W.B. Saunders Co.

Bone, R. (1984). *Critical Care: A Comprehensive Approach.* Park Ridge: American College of Chest Physicians.

Cataldo, C., & Whitney, E. (1986). *Nutrition and Diet Therapy: Principles and Practice.* St. Paul: West Publishing Co.

Cello, J., et al. (1984). Endoscopic sclerotherapy versus portacaval shunt in patients with severe cirrhosis and variceal hemorrhage. *N Engl J Med, 311,* 25, 1589–1600.

Cello, J., et al. (1987). Endoscopic sclerotherapy versus portacaval shunt in patients with severe cirrhosis and variceal hemorrhage: Long-term follow-up. *N Engl J Med, 316,* 1, 11–15.

Cooke, M. & Sande, M. (1983). Diagnosis and outcome of bowel infarction on an acute medical service. *Am J Med, 75,* 984–992.

Cutter, J., & Mendeloff, A. (1981). Upper gastrointestinal bleeding: Nature and magnitude of the problem in the U.S. *Digest Dis Sci, 26,* 90.

Dalton-Loehner, D., & Connor, P. (1989). Beyond ileostomy: Surgery for a normal life. *RN,* July, 29–32.

Doenges, M., Jeffries, M., & Moorhouse, M. (1984). *Nursing Care Plans.* Philadelphia: F.A. Davis Co.

Gettrust, K., Ryan, S., & Engelman, D. (1985). *Applied Nursing Diagnosis.* New York: John Wiley & Sons.

Graham, D., & Lancellotti, F. (1987). Gastric ulcers: What to do for simple lesions and refractory disease. *J Crit Illness,* June, 82–86.

Green, P., et al. (1987). *Clinical Teaching Project: Acute Gastrointestinal Bleeding.* Thorofare, NJ: American Gastroenterological Association.

Griffiths, W., Neumann, D., & Welsh, J. (1979). The visible vessel as an indicator of uncontrolled or recurrent gastrointestinal hemorrhage. *N Engl J Med, 300,* 1411.

Hunt, P., Hansky, J., & Korman, M. (1979). Mortality in patients with hematemesis and melana: A prospective study. *Br Med J, 1,* 1238–1240.

Laine, L. (1987). Multipolar electrocoagulation in the treatment of active upper gastrointestinal tract hemorrhage. *N Eng J Med, 316,* 26, 1613–1617.

Larson, D., & Farnell, M. (1983). Upper gastrointestinal hemorrhage. *Mayo Clin Proc, 58,* 371–387.

Marta, M. (1987). Endoscopic retrograde cholangiopancreatography: Its role in diagnosis and treatment. *Focus Crit Care, 14,* 5, 62–63.

Miller, H. (1988). Liver transplanation: Postoperative ICU care. *Crit Care Nurse, 8,* 6, 19–31.

Ottinger, L. (1982). Mesenteric ischemia. *N Engl J Med, 307,* 9, 535–537.

Porth, C. (1982). *Pathophysiology: Concepts of Altered Health States.* Philadelphia: J.B. Lippincott Co.

Sabiston, D. (1986). *Textbook of Surgery,* 13th ed. Philadelphia: W.B. Saunders Co.

Sanowski, R. (1986). Thermal application for gastrointestinal bleeding. *J Clin Gastroenterol, 8,* 3, 239–243.

Schiff, L., & Schiff, E. (1987). *Diseases of the Liver,* 6th ed. Philadelphia: J.B. Lippincott Co.

Sherlock, D. (1985). *Diseases of the Liver and Biliary System,* 7th ed. Oxford: Blackwell Scientific Publications.

Shoemaker, W., et al. (1988). *Textbook of Critical Care.* Philadelphia: W.B. Saunders Co.

Sleisenger, M., & Fordtran, J. (1983). *Gastrointestinal Disease: Pathophysiology, Diagnosis, Management,* 3rd ed. Philadelphia: W.B. Saunders Co.

Sleisenger, M., & Fordtran, J. (1989). *Gastrointestinal Disease: Pathophysiology, Diagnosis, Management,* vol. 1, 4th ed. Philadelphia: W.B. Saunders Co.

Sleisenger, M., & Fordtran, J. (1989). *Gastrointestinal Disease: Pathophysiology, Diagnosis, Management,* vol. 1, 4th ed. Philadelphia: W.B. Saunders Co.

Stein, J. (1987). *Internal Medicine,* 2nd ed. Boston: Little, Brown & Co.

Sugawa, C., Schuman, B.M., Lucas, C.E. (1992). Gastrointestinal bleeding. New York: Igaku-Shoin.

Swain, C., et al. (1986). Controlled trial of Nd-YAG laser photocoagulation in bleeding peptic ulcers. *Lancet, i,* 1113.

Winawer, S.J. (1992). Management of gastrointestinal diseases. New York: Gower Medical Pub.

Zimmerman, T.A. (1986). Thinking critically about the Sengstaken-Blakemore tube. *Crit Care Nurse, 6,* 5, 72–75.

Zuckerman, G., et al. (1984). Controlled trial of medical therapy for active upper gastrointestinal bleeding and prevention of rebleeding. *Am J Med, 76,* 361–366.

PART 5

Renal

Deborah Klein, RN, MSN, CCRN

CHAPTER 28

Anatomy of the Renal System

Editor's Note

Renal patient care problems comprise approximately 5% (ten questions) of the CCRN exam. These ten questions are spread out over three major areas: acute renal failure, life-threatening electrolyte imbalances, and renal trauma. The following chapters contain information necessary to address each of these areas.

This chapter provides the essential concepts of renal anatomy, information that probably is not directly addressed on the CCRN exam. Understanding the contents of this chapter will, however, prepare you to better appreciate the clinical situations addressed by the CCRN exam. As you review this chapter, do not focus on minute concepts but rather concentrate on general anatomical features relevant to renal concepts that might be addressed in clinical practice.

KIDNEY

Location

The kidneys lie in the retroperitoneal space on each side of the vertebrae, with the upper border between T-11 on the right and T-12 on the left. This difference in position results from the natural displacement of the right kidney by the liver. The lower border is at approximately L-3. The posterior surfaces are protected by the last two ribs.

Protective Coverings

The kidneys are protected by coverings that prevent massive blood loss from trauma. The outermost protective covering is pararenal fat that completely surrounds the three coverings of the kidneys. The next layer is the renal fascia, a membrane sheet that surrounds a layer of perirenal fat. This perirenal fat is actually a very dense layer of adipose tissue. It is very compact and surrounds the innermost covering of the kidney, the fibrous renal capsule. The fibrous renal capsule is a thin, resistant membrane that is contiguous with the kidney tissue itself.

Shape and Size

The kidneys are bean-shaped organs with an indentation on their medial surfaces. The indented area is called the hilum. The hilum is the entrance site for the renal artery, lymphatics, and nerves and is also the exit site for the renal vein, ureters, lymphatics, and nerves. The average kidney is 10 to 12 cm long, 5 to 6 cm wide, and 3 to 4 cm thick. Its average weight is about 160 to 180 grams.

Gross Anatomy

The cortex is the outer one-third of the kidney tissue (Fig. 28-1). The cortex is composed of the glomeruli of all of the nephrons and the convoluted portions of the distal and proximal tubules. The cortex extends into the medulla between structures called pyramids. These extensions are the renal columns. The cortex itself extends inward from the renal capsule to the base of the pyramids.

The medulla is the inner portion of the kidney. The medulla contains the loops of Henle, the vasa recta, and the collecting ducts. These loops and ducts are arranged in triangles or pyramids. The tips of the pyramids are called papillae. Groups of papillae merge to form into a single papilla to enter the calyx, which collects urine flow from the collecting ducts. Calyces channel the urine into the renal pelvis. Eventually, the urine flows from the renal pelvis into the ureter.

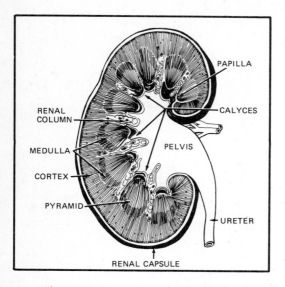

Figure 28-1. Gross anatomy of the kidney.

The number of calyces varies from 8 to 16 per kidney. Therefore, there is no symmetry in renal anatomy.

Nephron

The nephron is the functional unit of the kidney. Each kidney has more than one million nephrons. Up to 75% of the kidneys' nephrons can be destroyed before the remaining nephrons are unable to compensate. While compensation is occurring, the functioning nephrons filter a higher solute load. Because of this increased workload, the functioning nephrons hypertrophy. There are two types of nephrons, cortical and juxtamedullary.

Cortical nephrons (Fig. 28-2) have glomeruli that lie close to the cortical surface and have thin, short segments of the loops of Henle. The loops of Henle do enter the medulla but do not go past the outer medulla. Since the loops of Henle in the cortical nephrons are short and do not extend into the inner medulla, they do not participate in the concentration of urine. About 70% of the kidneys' nephrons are cortical nephrons with short or nonexistent loops of Henle.

The juxtamedullary nephrons (Fig. 28-3) are found in the inner one-third of the cortex. They have long loops of Henle that dip deep into the medulla and are surrounded by the peritubular network, the vasa

recta. These nephrons have a great capacity to retain sodium and concentrate urine due to the long loops of Henle.

In hypovolemic and hypotensive patients, a large portion of the renal blood flow is shunted from the cortical nephrons to the juxtamedullary nephrons to maintain urine formation.

Structural Anatomy. The nephron, as the functional unit of the kidney, is composed of the glomerulus, the proximal convoluted tubule, the loop of Henle, the distal convoluted tubule, and the collecting ducts.

The glomerulus is a network of capillaries (Fig. 28-4) that are spherical in shape and are formed by the afferent arterioles dividing into between two and eight subdivisions. These subdivisions branch to form as many as 50 capillary loops. The glomerulus is enclosed by an epithelial-lined membrane called Bowman's capsule. The efferent arteriole carries the blood out of the glomerulus.

The proximal convoluted tubule is about 14 mm in length. It receives the contents of the glomerulus. The lumen of the tubule contains tiny threadlike projections that help resorb the glomerular filtrate. The

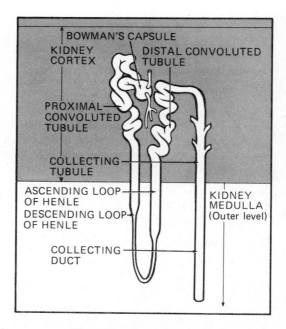

Figure 28-2. Cortical nephron.

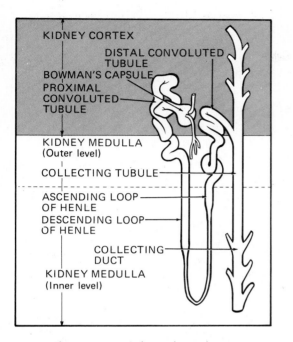

Figure 28-3. Juxtaglomerular nephron.

brush border increases the resorptive surface area per unit length of the tubule. The proximal convoluted tubule ends in the medulla of the kidney and becomes the descending limb of the loop of Henle.

The loop of Henle has three distinct portions (Fig. 28-5): a thick descending limb, a thin segment that is the actual loop, and a thick ascending limb. The loops of Henle in the cortical nephron reach just to the inside of the kidney medulla. The loops of Henle in the jux-tamedullary nephron reach almost to the tips of the pyramids (the papillae) and then start ascending to become the ascending limb of the loop of Henle. The peritubular capillary network surrounds the loop portion of the juxtamedullary nephron. As the long loop of Henle dips deep into the medulla, it is surrounded by the vasa recta. Thirty percent of the nephrons in each kidney are juxtamedullary nephrons.

The distal convoluted tubule begins where the ascending limb of the loop of Henle starts twisting. The distal convoluted tubule closely passes its own glomerulus and may even touch it. The distal convoluted tubule continues without convolutions to become the collecting tubule.

The collecting tubule extends to become the collecting duct, which empties into a common collecting duct that in turn empties into the renal pelvis.

Juxtaglomerular Apparatus. All nephrons have a juxtaglomerular apparatus (JGA) that contain three specific components. As the distal convoluted tubule passes between the afferent and efferent arterioles, there are specialized cells (Fig. 28-6) that are tightly packed together. These specialized cells are called the macula densa.

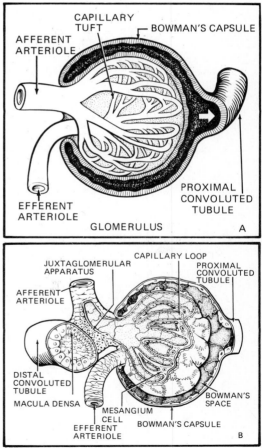

Figure 28-4. Schematic (**A**) and detailed (**B**) view of the glomerulus.

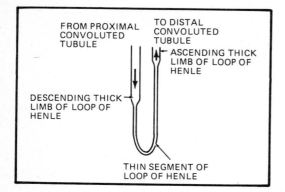

Figure 28-5. Loop of Henle.

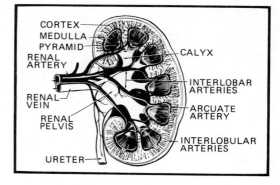

Figure 28-7. Vascular system of the kidney.

There are also specialized cells on the outside of the afferent and efferent arterioles near their entry point into the glomerulus that are referred to as polkissen cells or juxtaglomerular cells. These cells secrete granules of inactive renin.

The area where the distal convoluted tubule

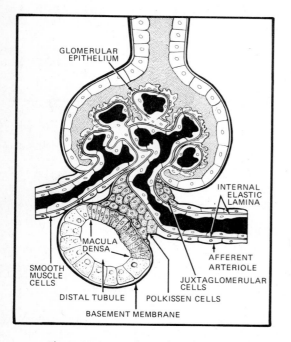

Figure 28-6. Juxtaglomerular apparatus.

passes by or touches the efferent arterioles is the third component of the JGA. The JGA and its actions are covered in Chapter 29.

Vascular System

One renal artery arises from the aorta and enters the kidney (Fig. 28-7). The renal artery enters in front of the midline of the kidney at the hilum and bifurcates immediately at the kidney pelvis.

After this first splitting at the kidney pelvis, the renal arteries develop many branches called interlobar arteries. These interlobar arteries, as their name implies, travel between lobes of the renal parenchyma inside the renal columns toward the point where the cortex and medulla meet.

At the interface of the cortex and medulla, the interlobar arteries branch to form the arcuate arteries. These arteries form arcs between the lobes of the parenchyma.

From each arcuate artery, multiple intralobular arteries spread into the cortex. These intralobular arteries form short muscular afferent arterioles that supply the glomeruli. Efferent arterioles drain the blood from the glomerulus and flow through the peritubular capillary network that surrounds the cortical portions of the tubules. The small amount of remaining arterial blood flows into straight capillary loops called vasa recta. These extend down into the medulla to provide arterial blood to the lower parts of the thin segments of the loop of Henle before looping upward to enter the intralobular veins. From the intralobular veins, the blood

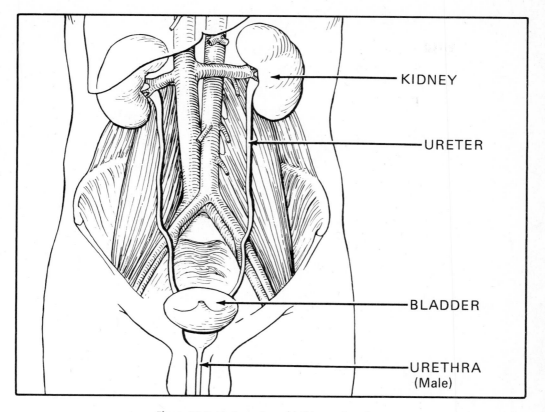

Figure 28-8. Ureter, urinary bladder, and urethra.

enters the arcuate veins, the interlobar veins, the renal veins, and the inferior vena cava.

Nerve Supply

The sympathetic nervous system controls constriction of renal arteries. These nerves follow the same course as the arterioles in order to maintain vasoactive tone of the arterioles.

The parasympathetic nervous system innervates the kidney through the vagus nerve fibers arising from the celiac plexus.

URETER, URINARY BLADDER, AND URETHRA

As the urine leaves the kidney pelvis, it enters the ureter. The ureter, approximately 10 inches in length, moves the urine along by peristaltic action to the urinary bladder, a hollow, muscular organ. It has a normal capacity of 250–500 ccs. At the bottom of the bladder is the urethra. It is about 6 to 8 inches long in males 1 to 1.25 inches in females (Fig. 28-8).

CHAPTER 29

Physiology of the Renal System

Editor's Note

The content in this chapter is designed to secure your understanding of the anatomy and physiology of the renal system. It is not likely that the CCRN exam will have questions taken directly from this section. However, a good understanding of the content in this chapter will assist you in answering questions relative to clinical situations that may appear on the exam.

Physiological processes of the kidney include the formation of urine, the regulation of body water and electrolytes, the excretion of metabolic waste products, the regulation of acid-base balance and blood pressure, and erythropoietin secretion.

FORMATION OF URINE

Three processes are involved in the formation of urine: glomerular filtration, tubular reabsorption, and tubular secretion.

Glomerular Filtration

The kidneys receive 20 to 25% of the cardiac output. Ninety-five percent of this quantity of blood will go through the glomerulus, where some solutes will be filtered out. An autoregulatory system exists to protect the glomerulus. The afferent and efferent renal arterioles constrict or dilate in response to systemic blood pressure. If systemic blood pressure increases, the afferent arteriole will constrict. This effectively reduces the pressure of the blood entering the glomerulus. In the same way, if systemic blood pressure decreases, the afferent arteriole will dilate to allow more blood to enter the glomerulus.

When the afferent arteriole constricts to reduce the pressure of blood in the glomerulus, the efferent arteriole relaxes (dilates) to allow the blood to leave more rapidly. This helps to control glomerular pressure. Conversely, when systemic pressure drops, the afferent arteriole dilates to let more blood into the glomerulus and the efferent arteriole constricts to help maintain the glomerular pressure. Below a mean blood pressure of about 60 mm Hg, this autoregulatory system fails and the glomerulus suffers the effects of hypotension.

Glomerular filtration is influenced by two factors, filtration pressure and glomerular permeability.

Filtration pressure is determined in part by the anatomical blood flow through the nephron. Each nephron is actually perfused by two capillary beds (Fig. 29-1). The glomerular capillary bed is perfused by the afferent arteriole with an average hydrostatic pressure of about 60 mm Hg. The peritubular capillary bed is perfused by the efferent arteriole, which resists blood flow. Because of this, the glomerular capillary bed has a high pressure (which may be termed glomerular hydrostatic pressure). The peritubular capillary bed has a low pressure of about 13 mm Hg.

The high pressure in the glomerulus tends to filter fluid out of the glomerulus and into Bowman's capsule. At the same time and following the same principles, the low pressure in the peritubular capillary bed tends to draw fluid from the interstitial spaces into the peritubular capillaries. The high pressures in the glomerulus cause a rapid filtration of fluid. The low pressure of the capillary bed of the peritubular system facilitates rapid uptake of the excreted tubular fluids by the peritubular capillaries. This diminishes backleak and increases net reabsorption.

Blood is brought into the glomerulus by the afferent arteriole. The pressure is close to 60 mm Hg, so

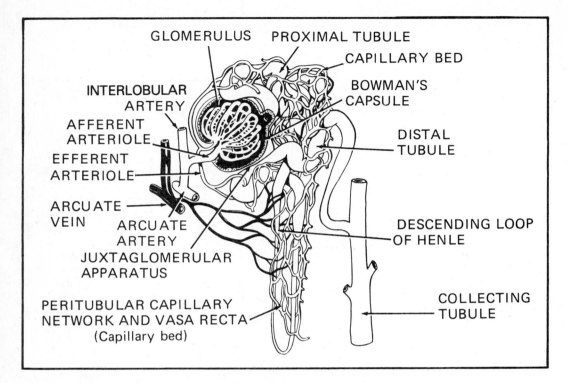

Figure 29-1. Capillary beds of a nephron.

fluid is forced from the glomerular capillaries into Bowman's capsule. This fluid is now called the glomerular ultrafiltrate. The fluid is called an ultrafiltrate because protein-size (and larger) molecules cannot filter out of the glomerular capillaries. Those proteins remain in the blood entering the peritubular capillaries from the efferent arteriole. The retained protein molecules cause an increase in the plasma osmotic pressure. The increased plasma osmotic pressure causes the rapid reabsorption of fluid from the peritubular interstitial spaces.

Glomerular permeability is the second influence on glomerular filtration. The glomerular membrane is different from other capillary membranes in the body. The glomerular membrane has three layers: the endothelial layer of the capillary, a basement membrane, and a layer of epithelial cells on the other surface of the capillary (Fig. 29-2). In spite of three layers, the glomerular membrane is 100 to 1000 times more permeable than the usual capillary. Obviously, it is not the three layers that increase the permeability. The endothelial cells lining the glomerular capillary are full of

thousands of tiny holes called fenestrae. Outside the capillary endothelium is a basement membrane similar to a mesh of fibers. The epithelial cells of the outer layer do not touch each other. The space between the cells is called a slit pore. Any particle greater than 7 millimicrons cannot penetrate the slit pore.

Composition of Glomerular Ultrafiltrate

Normally, the ultrafiltrate is free of protein and red blood cells since they are too large to pass through the slit pores. The semipermeable membrane of the glomerular capillary allows water, nutrients, electrolytes, and wastes to filter into Bowman's capsule.

Glomerular Filtration Rate

In the healthy kidney, the average glomerular filtration rate (GFR) is 125 mL/minute. The total quantity of glomerular filtrate per day is about 180 liters. More than 99% of this filtrate is reabsorbed in the tubules. The equation for calculating the GFR is the urine concentration of a substance times the urine flow rate divided by the plasma concentration of the same sub-

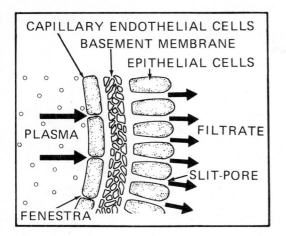

Figure 29-2. Three layers of the glomerular membrane.

stance. The substance must be freely filtered and not affected by the tubules (Fig. 29-3). The normal adult urine volume per 24 hours is about 1 to 1.5 liters.

Factors Affecting the Glomerular Filtration Rate

Any change in the glomerular hydrostatic pressure will alter the GFR. The most common cause of change in the hydrostatic pressure is a change in the systemic blood pressure. A change in systemic blood pressure changes the actual flow of blood into the glomerulus. Alterations in the afferent and efferent arteriole tone (constriction-dilatation) will also affect the glomerular pressure and hence the GFR.

Any alteration in the composition of the plasma, such as an increase in oncotic pressure (the osmotic pressure due to the presence of colloids in a solution), will alter the GFR. Such conditions as hyperproteinemia, hypoproteinemia, hypovolemia, or hyper-

volemia will also alter the composition of plasma due to alterations in the extracellular fluid (ECF) and intracellular fluid. Thus, these states will alter the GFR.

The GFR will automatically be altered by any abnormality of structure, presence of disease, or ingestion of nephrotoxic substances.

TUBULAR ABSORPTION AND SECRETION

The glomeruli filter a total of 180 liters per day, and normal urine output is 1 to 1.5 liters per day. The tubular function of the nephron is responsible (in part) for determining urinary output.

The nephron uses two processes, absorption and secretion, to convert this 180 liters of ultrafiltrate to just 1 to 1.5 liters of urine. These processes may be active or passive and are influenced by hormones, electrochemical gradients, and Starling's law. The following definitions may be useful in understanding renal function.

1. Diffusion is the movement of solutes from an area of high concentration to an area of low concentration.
2. Osmosis is the movement of water from an area of high water concentration to an area of low water concentration.
3. Absorption, as discussed here, is the movement of solutes and water from the tubule into the peritubular network (i.e., from the filtrate back into the bloodstream).
4. Secretion, as discussed here, is the movement of solutes and water from the peritubular network into the tubule (i.e., from the bloodstream back into the filtrate).
5. Passive transport is the movement of solutes by diffusion following concentration gradients and electrical gradients.
6. Active transport is the movement of any substance against an electrical or concentration gradient. Active transport requires energy, usually supplied by ATP.

A mnemonic may help unravel the maze of the movement of solutes in the various tubules. Cations are carried by active transport (CAT—carried active transport); anions are passively transported (ANI—a negative ion) Na^+, K^+ and H^+ are the most common cations in the body; Cl^- and HCO_3^- are the most common anions.

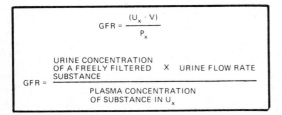

Figure 29-3. Equation for calculating the glomerular filtration rate.

As with most rules, there is always an exception. In the collecting duct, chloride (anion) is actively absorbed and the cations are passively absorbed. Table 29-1 traces the formation of urine, starting with the ultrafiltrate and ending with urine after passage through both convoluted tubules, the loop of Henle, and the collecting ducts.

The major function of the loop of Henle is to concentrate or dilute urine as necessary. This is accomplished by the countercurrent mechanism that maintains the hyperosmolar concentration in the renal medulla.

Body Water Regulation

Throughout the discussion of body regulation, the terms osmolarity and osmolality will be used interchangeably. Osmolarity is the concentration of particles in solution. Osmolality is the amount of solvent in relation to the particles.

The volume and concentration of body water content are maintained by the thirst-neurohypophyseal-renal axis. Approximately 60% of ideal body weight is water in males; in females, the proportion is 50 to 55%. Figure 29-4 shows the distribution of water throughout the body. There are three mechanisms that help regulate body fluid: thirst, antidiuretic hormone (ADH), and the countercurrent mechanism of the kidney.

Thirst. Thirst is the major force in our awareness of a need for water. The thirst center is located in the hypothalamus. Intracellular dehydration causes the sensation of thirst. The most common cause of intracellular dehydration is an increase in osmolar concentration of

TABLE 29-1. URINE FORMATION

Start	Proximal Convoluted Tubule	Loop of Henle (3 parts)	Distal Convoluted Tubule	Collecting Duct	Finish
Ultrafiltrate	60–80% of ultrafiltrate absorbed	**I. Descending limb** H_2O absorbed (highly permeable to H_2O)	**Absorbed** HCO_3^- H_2O if ADH is present	**Absorbed** Na^+ H_2O if ADH is present	Urine flows into renal pelvis, ureters, bladder
	Absorbed NA^+ Cl^- Glucose Amino acids All K^+ HCO_3^-	Fluid becomes increasingly hypertonic	Na^+ actively if aldosterone is adequate	**Secreted** H^+ K^+ NH_3	
		II. Thin segment loop Permeable to H_2O	**Secreted** K^+ H^+ Fluid is hypotonic		
	Secreted H^+ Urea Drugs Organic acids HCO_3^- and H^+ (regulates acid-base balance) H_2O passively absorbed Fluid isotonic to plasma	**III. Ascending limb** Cl^- absorbed actively; Na^+ absorbed Impermeable to H_2O			

Notes:
1. Sulfates, nitrates, and phosphates are absorbed only enough to maintain the ECF concentration.
2. All K^+ from the filtrate is absorbed in the proximal tubule.
3. The K^+ secreted in the distal convoluted tubule equals about 12% of the K^+ in the original filtrate. Under certain circumstances, secretion may exceed the original filtered load.

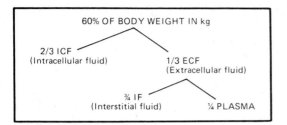

Figure 29-4. Distribution of water throughout the body.

the ECF. Increased sodium concentration of the ECF causes osmosis of fluid from the neuronal cells of the thirst center. Other important and frequent causes of thirst are excessive angiotensin II in the blood, hemorrhage, and low cardiac output.

The role of the thirst center is to maintain a conscious desire to drink the exact amount of fluid needed to maintain a normal body hydrated state or return a dehydrated state to the normal state of hydration.

Antidiuretic Hormone. ADH works closely with the thirst mechanism. The plasma protein and ECF sodium concentrations determine the osmolality of the ECF. Normal serum osmolality is 280 to 320 mosm/liter. Acid-base control mechanisms of the kidney adjust the negative ion in relation to the extracellular concentration (osmolality) to equal the positive ions in the body. ADH is synthesized in the supraoptic nuclei of the hypothalamus and then drips down the supraopticalhypophyseal tracts to the posterior pituitary (neurohyphosis), where it is stored. The supraoptic area of the hypothalamus is so close to the thirst center that there is an integration of the thirst mechanism, osmolality detection, and ADH release.

The osmosodium receptors respond to changes in osmolality (sodium concentration) in the ECF. An increase in osmolality excites the osmoreceptors. They signal the neurohypophyseal tract that ADH is needed. The posterior pituitary (neurohypophysis) releases the ADH that it has stored. In the presence of ADH, the distal convoluted tubules and the collecting ducts reabsorb water. The reabsorption of the water leaves a hypertonic urine. This cycle will continue until the concentration of the ECF compartment and fluid homeostasis are returned to normal.

If osmolality of the ECF decreases, ADH release is inhibited because the osmoreceptors are not stimulated. Without ADH, the distal tubules and collecting

ducts are impermeable to water. Urine will be very dilute because the water cannot be reabsorbed. Dilute urine will continue until the loss of water has raised the concentration of the ECF solutes to normal.

Countercurrent Mechanism. The countercurrent mechanism is used to concentrate urine and excrete excessive solutes. Excreting dilute urine is no problem for the kidney unless there is a neurological dysfunction, an endocrine dysfunction, or traumatic injuries. These conditions may result in an inappropriate release and affect normal kidney function of ADH, aldosterone, and/or cortisol. Concentrating urine to excrete waste solutes is a complex interaction between the long loops of Henle, the peritubular capillaries, and the vasa recta.

The countercurrent multiplier mechanism functions constantly in a loop cycle, with fresh filtrate continuously entering the loop of Henle. At the entry to the loop, the filtrate has a concentration of 300 mosm/liter. The medulla increases this concentration so that at the tips of the papillae in the pelvic tip of the medulla, the concentration of the filtrate is 1200 to 1400 mosm/liter.

It is essential for the medullary interstitium to be hyperosmolar. There are four steps in concentrating the solutes to produce this hyperosmolality (Fig. 29-5).

In step 1, chloride ions are actively transported

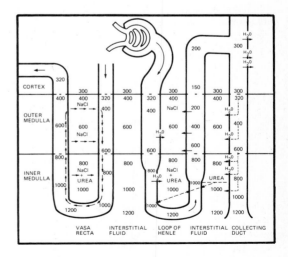

Figure 29-5. Countercurrent multiplier mechanism for maintaining medullary interstitial hyperosmolality and concentrating urine.

from the thick portion of the ascending limb of the loop of Henle into the upper medullary interstitial fluid. The active transport of chloride pulls sodium and some potassium, magnesium, and calcium also.

In step 2, the collecting ducts actively transport sodium into the medullary interstitial fluid. Chloride follows along passively. Steps 1 and 2 increase medullary interstitial fluid hyperosmolality by about 500 mosm.

In step 3, the collecting duct yields urea to the lower medullary interstitial fluid if ADH is present. The hormone makes the collecting duct mildly permeable to urea and very permeable to water. Water leaves the collecting duct to enter the medullary interstitium, resulting in a high concentration of urea in the collecting duct. Urea, following concentration gradients, then diffuses out into the medullary interstitial fluid. This increases the medullary osmolarity by about another 200 to 400 mosm.

In step 4, water osmosis occurs from the thin (descending) segment of the loop of Henle because of the high urea concentration in the lower medullary interstitial fluid. As the water moves from the loop of Henle, sodium ion concentration in the thin limb increases. Because of the high concentration, sodium and chloride passively diffuse out of the collecting duct into the lower medullary interstitium. This increases the osmolarity of the medullary interstitial fluid to between 1000 and 1200 mosm.

Excess solutes concentrated in the medullary interstitium must not be allowed to reenter the bloodstream via the peritubular capillary network. This is prevented by sluggish blood flow in these capillaries and a very small amount of blood being present (less than 2% of the total renal blood supply), keeping ion movement to a minimum. Throughout the countercurrent multiplier activity, ion movement from the loop of Henle into the medullary interstitium has been by ionic secretion (ions moving from the tubule lumen) either actively or passively and by diffusion or osmosis.

The ion solutes present in the medullary interstitial fluid must move into the ascending limb of the loop of Henle so that they can be excreted with the urine. This is accomplished by the countercurrent exchange mechanism. The vasa recta are essentially straight tubes forming a long, slender U-shaped blood vessel. Because both sides of the U are highly permeable, fluids and solutes readily exchange places in the high-concentration gradients of the lower medullary interstitium.

As the blood in the vasa recta flows back up the ascending loop of Henle, excess sodium and urea diffuse out of the blood in exchange for water diffusing into the blood. The blood leaves the medulla with almost the same osmolarity as when it entered the descending loop.

The fluid in the loop of Henle becomes more concentrated in the presence of ADH, since water has diffused out. In the ascending thick limb of the loop of Henle and the diluting segment of the distal convoluted tubule, the osmolarity of the filtrate drops. In the distal convoluted tubules and the collecting ducts, the osmolarity depends upon the presence of ADH and aldosterone. If these hormones are present, sodium and water will be absorbed and the tubule fluid will remain concentrated as it passes through the collecting ducts to the renal pelvis to enter the ureter. If the hormones are not present, water will be secreted and a more dilute urine will enter the ureter. Only juxtamedullary nephrons have long loops of Henle; they are responsible for concentrating and diluting the filtrate as urine is formed.

EXCRETION OF METABOLIC WASTE PRODUCTS

The metabolic waste products handled by the kidneys are estimated to be in excess of 200 different substances. These waste products are classified as threshold substances, nonthreshold substances, electrolytes, water, and other substances that may be reabsorbed or excreted by the kidneys according to individual fluctuating needs.

Threshold substances are those that are entirely reabsorbed by the kidneys unless the substances are present in excessive concentration in the blood. Glucose is the most common threshold substance. Amino acids are also threshold substances.

Nonthreshold substances are not reabsorbed by the kidney tubules. Creatinine is the most abundant nonthreshold substance. Urea is included in this category even though urea passively diffuses back into the kidney bloodstream. Proteins and acids of disease processes (lactic acid, ketones) are nonthreshold substances. Water and most electrolytes will be absorbed or secreted according to individual needs.

There are two commonly used tests to determine efficiency of kidney function in handling waste products, blood urea nitrogen (BUN) and creatinine.

The BUN measures the level of urea, a nitrogen

waste product of protein metabolism. The BUN is an unreliable test of renal function because the BUN level is affected by many factors. In the presence of liver disease, the BUN will remain low because the liver cannot synthesize urea at a normal rate. Conversely, with normal kidney function, dehydration, GI bleeding, sepsis, trauma, drugs, diet, and changes in catabolism may elevate the BUN markedly, to as much as 50 mg/100 mL. Food in the digestive tract may also falsely elevate the BUN.

Serum creatinine is a more reliable index of kidney function. Creatinine is a waste product of muscle metabolism and is freely filtered. The nephron tubules neither reabsorb nor secrete creatinine. The normally functioning kidney filters creatinine from the blood at a rate equal to the GFR. Since the amount of creatinine produced each day is constant and is proportional to the body's muscle mass, serial serum creatinines are valuable indices of kidney function except in septic patients and patients with muscle-wasting diseases.

Normally, a BUN-to-creatinine ratio of 10:1 is present in serum. A ratio of 20:1 or more is indicative of prerenal insufficiency (water and salt depletion), a high protein catabolism, or low renal perfusion pressures.

An elevation of both BUN and creatinine above the normal ratio indicates renal disease. In these patients, a creatinine clearance is usually performed. Creatinine clearance is probably the most reliable index of kidney function available. Normal creatinine clearance is 125 mL/minute. Urine is collected for 12 or 24 hours or for a specified period of time, and a blood serum sample is drawn halfway through the urine collection. If the BUN, creatinine, and creatinine clearance tests are normal, the kidneys are functioning adequately in excreting metabolic waste products from the body.

REGULATION OF ACID-BASE BALANCE

The body acid-base balance is maintained by the lungs, blood buffers, and the kidneys. The kidneys regulate acid-base balance by controlling the bicarbonate ion (HCO_3^-) and, in much lesser quantity, the hydrogen ion (H^+).

A normal diet contains some acids (phosphates and sulfates) that must be excreted. In addition, protein catabolism is markedly increased in the critically ill. Protein catabolism adds to the acid load of the body.

Products of protein catabolism are eliminated by the kidneys.

Four mechanisms provide for the excretion of acid and regulation of acid-base balance by the kidneys.

The first mechanism is direct excretion of hydrogen ions. Hydrogen ion is excreted in a very minute amount (less than 1 mEq of hydrogen ion per day) and has only a minor role in acid-base control. A passive secretion of hydrogen ion occurs in the proximal tubules. An active secretion of hydrogen ion occurs in the distal tubules.

The second mechanism is excretion of hydrogen with urine buffers. Nonvolatile acids are excreted in this process. The glomerulus filters these acids and bicarbonate. The phosphate acids filtered are an example of the process for excreting hydrogen ion with a urine buffer.

$$H_2CO_3 + Na_2HPO_4 \rightarrow NaHCO_3 + NaH_2PO_4$$

carbonic acid	bisodium phosphate	sodium bicarbonate	sodium biphosphate

The carbonic acid combines with disodium phosphate and yields sodium bicarbonate and sodium biphosphate. The sodium bicarbonate breaks down into sodium and bicarbonate and is reabsorbed as needed. The sodium biphosphate adds a hydrogen ion to become a molecule and is excreted in urine. The net result of the phosphate and sulfate wastes filtered by the glomerulus is the addition of a hydrogen ion per molecule excreted. Up to 20 mEq per day may be excreted with these buffers.

The third mechanism of acid-base control by the kidneys is excretion of acids by using ammonia (NH_3). Chemically, ammonia is produced in renal tubular cells and diffuses into tubular fluid, where carbonic acid combines with ammonia and actually produces two factors that benefit acid-base control.

$$NH_3 + H_2CO_3 \rightarrow NH_4 + HCO_3$$

ammonia	carbonic acid	ammonium ion	bicarbonate ion

Ammonium (ammonia with one additional hydrogen ion) combines with anions.

$$2NH_4HCO_3 + NA_2SO_4 \leftrightarrow 2NaHCO_3 + (NH_4)_2SO_4$$

ammonium bicarbonate	sodium sulfate	sodium bicarbonate	ammonium sulfate

The ammonium sulfate, which now has two hydrogen ions, is excreted in the urine. The sodium bicarbonate is available to buffer in the body as needed. Up to 50 mEq of acid per day may be excreted by using ammonia.

In the fourth mechanism, production and reabsorption of bicarbonate, new bicarbonate ion is manufactured in the distal convoluted tubule as needed. The formula is:

$$H_2O + CO_2 \overset{CA}{\leftrightarrow} H_2CO_3 \overset{CA}{\leftrightarrow} H^+ + HCO_3^-$$

water carbon carbonic hydrogen bicarbonate
      dioxide acid ion ion

The process of forming a new bicarbonate can start in the distal tubule. Carbon dioxide results from dissolved carbon dioxide in the renal venous blood. The carbon dioxide combines with water present in the distal tubule to form carbonic acid. This is termed the hydration of carbon dioxide with the catalyst carbonic anhydrase (CA).

Carbonic anhydrase speeds up the chemical reaction without actually entering into the chemical reaction. The brush border of the proximal convoluted tubule contains a great deal of carbonic anhydrase; the distal convoluted tubule does not. The formation of carbonic acid is very rapid in the proximal tubule. The carbonic acid produced ionizes more slowly in the distal tubule.

The carbonic acid ionizes into hydrogen ion and bicarbonate ion to buffer as needed. If the body is acidotic, the hydrogen ion is excreted in the urine. The bicarbonate is absorbed into the ECF along with sodium. If the body is in acid-base balance, the carbonic acid dissociates into water and carbon dioxide. The water joins the urine, and the carbon dioxide rapidly diffuses into the ECF.

In acidotic states, there is an increase in hydrogen ion secretion in the distal tubule that accompanies an increased excretion of acid buffers, phosphates, and sulfates. Ammonium formation is the predominant control mechanism. Because more acid is being excreted in the urine, urine pH may be as low as 4.4.

In alkalotic states, there is a decrease in hydrogen ion secretion in the distal tubules. This is accompanied by an excess bicarbonate excretion in the urine, resulting in urine that is alkaline (pH greater than 7.0).

REGULATION OF BLOOD PRESSURE

The kidneys participate in regulation of blood pressure through four different mechanisms: by maintaining ECF volume and composition, by regulating aldosterone, through the renin-angiotensin mechanism, and by regulating prostaglandin synthesis.

Maintaining Extracellular Fluid Volume and Composition

The autoregulatory system of the afferent and efferent arterioles responds to change in blood pressure to maintain consistent perfusion of the glomerulus. When this system fails, plasma flow may increase by the remaining three mechanisms. Vasoconstriction will maintain or elevate the blood pressure for a short period of time. If no more defense mechanisms exist, then only intravenous fluids, plasmanate, albumin, and such will alter the volume flow or composition of the plasma and the ECF. As the flow of plasma decreases, the patient becomes hypotensive, hypoxic, and hypoperfused. As the plasma flow deficit and the extracellular deficits are corrected, the patient becomes more closely normotensive.

Aldosterone Effect on Blood Pressure

The main effect of aldosterone is to maintain normal sodium concentration in the ECF. As sodium is the most abundant cation in the ECF, all other cations and anions will be present in varying ratios to the sodium. Aldosterone promotes reabsorption of sodium in both the distal convoluted tubule and the collecting ducts of the kidneys. Sodium will "drag along" water, bicarbonate, chloride, and other ions as it is reabsorbed. This mechanism helps to restore extracellular and intracellular fluid volumes, alter the composition of the compartments as needed, and subsequently, in a normal healthy kidney, maintain the blood pressure.

Renin-Angiotensin Mechanism

Any factor that decreases the glomerular filtration rate will activate the renin-angiotensin system. The most potent effect is upon systemic blood pressure.

Once activated, the juxtaglomerular apparatus (JGA), located adjacent to the glomeruli, releases inactive renin. Factors triggering the release of inactive renin (e.g., decreased blood pressure and decreased sodium content in the distal tubule) reflect a diminished GFR. Once released, the inactive renin acts on angiotensinogen to split away the vasoactive peptide, angiotensin I. Angiotensin I is split to angiotensin II in the presence of a converting enzyme found primarily in the lung and liver but also located in the kidney and all blood vessels.

Angiotensin II is a potent vasoconstricting agent. Angiotensin II in the circulatory system causes a severe constriction of peripheral arterioles and a milder constriction in the venous system. It also causes a constriction of renal arterioles. This results in the kidneys reabsorbing sodium and water and expanding the ECF volume.

Angiotensin II also stimulates the release of aldosterone to enhance sodium and water reabsorption, thus supporting an increase in circulating volume. This increase in sodium stimulates the thirst mechanism in an effort to reestablish circulating blood volume.

On rare occasions, some factors initiate the release of renin and the release is never turned off. The continuous presence of renin may maintain an active system known as malignant hypertension. The key to treating malignant hypertension is to cut off the release of renin.

Prostaglandins

It was once thought that prostaglandins were originally located in the seminal vesicles and produced by the prostate gland (thus their name). Prostaglandins are unsaturated fatty acids found in most cells but highly concentrated in the kidneys, brain, and gonads. Prostaglandins or their precursors are synthesized in the medullary interstitial cells and the collecting tubules of the kidneys. Prostaglandins promote a vasodilation of the renal medulla to maintain renal perfusion during severe or prolonged systemic hypoperfusion.

RED BLOOD CELL SYNTHESIS AND MATURATION

Renal erythropoietic factor is an enzyme that is released by a hypoxic kidney as a result of decreased oxygen supply. After being released into the bloodstream, the erythropoietic factor reacts with a glycoprotein to break away as erythropoietin. Erythropoietin circulates in the blood for about 24 hours. During this time, it stimulates red blood cell production by the bone marrow. After five or more days, a maximum rate of red blood cell production is achieved. The life of the red blood cell is approximately 120 days.

Either the kidney itself or some other factor that is the precursor of erythropoietin synthesizes the erythropoietic factor by releasing an enzyme called renal erythropoietin factor. Bone marrow by itself does not respond to hypoxia by producing new red blood cells.

Patients with chronic renal failure have hemoglobins of 5 and 6 grams. The diseased kidneys are unable to respond to hypoxia and cannot produce erythropoietin factor. It is believed that possibly 10% of erythropoietin is formed in some place other than the kidney.

CHAPTER 30

Renal Regulation of Electrolytes and Electrolyte Imbalances

Editor's Note

This chapter contains information from the CCRN section on life-threatening electrolyte imbalances. You will find more detail in this chapter than the test requires. However, understanding this detail is helpful in answering the questions presented on the exam. Expect two to four questions from this chapter on the exam.

One of the major functions of the kidney is to maintain electrolyte homeostasis. Within one hour of cessation of kidney function, physiological deterioration of the body begins due to a lack of electrolyte regulation. Electrolytes are in a precarious balance in the critically ill patient. Continuous monitoring is essential to recognize imbalances early, to prevent generalized deterioration, and to assist the kidneys in reestablishing homeostasis.

The electrolytes of major concern are sodium, potassium, calcium, phosphate, and magnesium. Electrolyte imbalances are a result of (1) excessive ingestion or reabsorption of an electrolyte or (2) the lack of ingestion or excessive excretion of an electrolyte. Most body fluid imbalances are caused by a dysfunction in the regulation of electrolytes and water by the kidney.

SODIUM

Sodium Regulation

Sodium (Na^+) is the most prevalent cation in the body's extracellular fluid compartment. Na^+ directly influences the fluid (water) load of the body and exists in the body in combination with an anion, usually chloride. Sodium is important in maintaining extracellular fluid osmotic pressure, serum osmolarity, and acid-base balance. Intracellularly, it plays a major role in chemical pathways. Sodium also stimulates reactions within nerve and muscle cells. The normal serum sodium level ranges between 135 and 145 mEq/L. To maintain this level, sodium is reabsorbed from four parts of the kidney. The majority of filtered sodium is reabsorbed in the proximal convoluted tubules; lesser amounts are reabsorbed in the loop of Henle, in the distal convoluted tubule, and in the collecting ducts. Reabsorption of sodium increases with a decreased glomerular filtration rate (GFR) as seen with hypoperfusion states (shock, myocardial infarction).

Aldosterone has the greatest influence on sodium excretion. Aldosterone is a mineralocorticoid secreted by the adrenal cortex. It is the most potent natural inhibitor of sodium excretion. Aldosterone production and release is stimulated by high potassium levels, steroids (ACTH), and angiotensin II. Aldosterone acts on the distal convoluted tubule and the collecting duct to promote reabsorption of sodium and excretion of potassium. Without aldosterone present, the distal tubule and the collecting ducts cannot closely regulate the amount of sodium reabsorbed. The increased reabsorption of sodium in the presence of aldosterone also results in reabsorption of water.

Diuretic therapy is usually thought of in relation to potassium. However, the loop diuretics (Lasix, Edecrin, and Bumex) block the chloride pump in the thick portion of the ascending limb of the loop of Henle. When chloride reabsorption is blocked, sodium cannot diffuse out of the ascending limb. Other factors that can increase the excretion of sodium include an increased GFR, decreased aldosterone secretion, and increased antidiuretic hormone (ADH) levels.

Hypernatremia

A serum sodium level above 145 mEq/L is termed hypernatremia. Most cases of hypernatremia are due not to Na^+ disturbances but to fluid disturbances. Hypernatremia maybe seen with dehydration. Treatment is centered on giving fluid, not removing sodium. If there is a pure water loss or decreased intake causing the hypernatremia, the hematocrit will be elevated, serum chloride will be above 106 mEq/L, urine specific gravity will be greater than 1.025, and urine sodium levels will be low. Hypernatremia may also be associated with fluid volume excess with a gain of both sodium and water, but a relatively greater gain of sodium. Hypernatremia is a significant electrolyte disturbance due to the neurologic and endocrine disturbances that result. Hypernatremia may cause some depression of cardiac function.

Etiology. With the exception of disturbances in vascular fluid levels, any condition leading to polyuria with conservation of sodium results in hypernatremic dehydration. The most common cause is the lack of or insufficient ADH secretion (e.g., diabetes insipidus). Increased insensible water loss (e.g., from severe burn injuries) and hypertonic enteral feedings may lead to hypernatremia. Potassium depletion (from vomiting, diarrhea, or nasogastric suction) and uncontrolled diabetes mellitus may also create a hypernatremia.

The comatose patient is a high-risk patient for hypernatremia, since the thirst mechanism cannot be recognized or expressed. Excessive administration of osmotic diuretics and sodium bicarbonate (in treating lactic acidosis) may also cause an iatrogenic hypernatremia. Overuse of high sodium-containing laxatives and antacids may also precipitate a hypernatremia. Hypernatremia may also be seen with renal dysfunction. If the kidneys are too damaged to filter and excrete sodium, sodium and fluid retention may result.

Clinical Presentation. Hypernatremia generally occurs with dehydration. Signs include dry, sticky mucous membranes, thirst, oliguria, fever, tachycardia, and agitation. The patient may demonstrate behavior changes, hypotension, decreased cardiac output, convulsion, or coma; death may result. As long as renal function is intact, hypernatremia rarely produces increased mortality. Patients with hypernatremia associated with sodium and fluid volume excess present with edema, increased blood pressure, and weight gain.

Treatment. Fluid administration with free water (nonelectrolyte solutions like D_5W) in a dehydrated patient is the key to diluting the sodium and halting the progression toward hypovolemic shock. Identifying and treating the underlying cause is the key to success-ful treatment of hypernatremia with fluid retention. The challenge is to stabilize the patient's hypertension, prevent pulmonary edema, and maintain neurologic stability. Diuretics and limitation of fluid intake are indicated.

Hyponatremia

Hyponatremia is present when the serum sodium level is less than 130 mEq/L. Usually, the plasma chloride will be less than 98 mEq/L. Hematocrit may be decreased due to water excess.

Etiology. Hyponatremia is due to either (1) an excessive amount of water or (2) sodium depletion. Excessive amounts of water can occur in many situations. The postgastric or postintestinal surgery patient who has nasogastric suction in use and who is receiving intravenous (IV) D_5W may become hyponatremic in only two or three days. Repeated tap water enemas may result in hyponatremia. Occasionally, patients drink too much plain water.

The syndrome of inappropriate ADH (SIADH) release may precipitate a hyponatremia. In this instance, the stimulus that activated ADH release is never turned off. The presence of ADH results in the kidneys reabsorbing water continuously and diluting the body's sodium levels. Water retention diluting serum sodium levels may also occur with congestive heart failure, cirrhosis of the liver, or nephrotic syndrome. A low cardiac output precipitates water retention by the kidneys.

Hypovolemic hyponatremia due to sodium depletion or loss is commonly caused by the overuse of the thiazide diuretics and furosemide (Lasix). Diarrhea, Addison's disease, gastric suction, hyperglycemia (with a glucose-induced diuresis), vomiting, and extreme diaphoresis without IV replacement of sodium may also cause hypovolemic hyponatremia.

Clinical Presentation. The clinical presentation of hyponatremia depends on the magnitude, rapidity of onset, and cause. In general, the faster the serum sodium drops and the lower the serum sodium level, the more likely that symptoms will be severe.

Hyponatremia with Water Retention. In hyponatremia with water excess, signs of water intoxication are usually present. They include apathy, coma, confusion, headache, generalized weakness, hyporeflexia, convulsions, and death. Increased blood pressure and edema are usually present.

Hyponatremia with Dehydration. If the hyponatremia is associated with decreased extracellular fluid, the symptoms are essentially the same as for heat prostration. Apprehension and anxiety are followed by a feeling of impending doom. The patient is weak, is confused or stuporous, and may have abdominal cramps and muscle twitching. In some cases, convulsions follow the muscle twitching rather quickly. Mucous membranes are dry. Azotemia develops and progresses to oliguria. In severe cases, vasomotor collapse occurs with hypotension, tachycardia, and shock.

An interesting clinical presentation exists in cases of hyponatremia associated with dehydration. As dehydration progresses, fluid moves from the extracellular to the intracellular compartment. A finger pressed over the sternum will result in a fingerprint. This "fingerprinting of the sternum" indicates that much extracellular fluid has been excreted and plasma fluid has moved into the intracellular spaces from the vascular system. Without appropriate intervention, the patient may die very quickly. In less severe cases, symptoms may include lassitude, apathy, headache, anorexia, nausea, vomiting, diarrhea, muscle spasms, and cramps.

Treatment. The goal of treatment is to reestablish normal serum sodium levels as rapidly as possible while avoiding a fluid overload. Fluid restriction or diuretic therapy is the treatment of choice if the hyponatremia is due to excess vascular fluid. Diuretics, if used, are given cautiously to avoid cerebral injury. Cerebral injury could occur from too rapid expansion of brain cells from the water removal. In instances except SIADH, replacement of sodium with normal or hypertonic saline may also be indicated. Close monitoring of all system, along with monitoring of serial serum sodium levels, is essential during this period.

In SIADH, the treatment is to restrict water intake while attempting to aid the kidneys in excreting water normally. In susceptible SIADH patients, hypertonic saline administration may induce congestive heart failure.

POTASSIUM

Potassium Regulation

Potassium (K^+) is the most prevalent intracellular cation in the body. The normal serum potassium level is 3.5 to 5.0 mEq/L. Potassium maintains osmolarity and electrical neutrality inside the cell and helps maintain acid-base balance. Intracellular homeostasis is needed for converting carbohydrates into energy and for reassembling amino acids into proteins. Transmission of nerve impulses is dependent upon potassium. The muscles of the heart, lungs, intestines, and skeletal muscles cannot function normally without potassium.

All of the potassium filtered by the glomeruli is reabsorbed in the proximal convoluted tubule. Potassium that is excreted is secreted from the interstitial medullary space into the distal convoluted tubules. It amounts to about 10 to 12% of the original potassium volume of the ultrafiltrate in the proximal convoluted tubules. The amount of potassium excreted depends largely upon the volume of urine. About 85% of the potassium is excreted in the urine, and about 15% is excreted in the intestines. Even in hypokalemia (decreased potassium), a large urine volume will contain potassium, further compounding problems. Sodium and potassium will compete with each other for reabsorption. The normal ratio of potassium to sodium ion reabsorption is 1:35.

Sodium and potassium are intimately related, and factors that affect sodium reabsorption and excretion also affect the potassium level. Potassium levels are commonly raised by intravenous fluids containing potassium chloride. Although the kidneys act readily to conserve sodium, potassium is poorly conserved, especially in patients who are critically ill.

Factors that enhance excretion of potassium include an elevated intracellular potassium level, which may be caused by an acute metabolic or respiratory alkalosis that forces potassium into the cells and hydrogen out of the cells. Diuretics and other factors resulting in high-volume flow rates in the distal convoluted tubule result in increased excretion of potassium. Aldosterone functions as a feedback mechanism on the distal convoluted tubule and collecting ducts to reabsorb sodium and excrete potassium when the extracellular fluid potassium level is increased. The enhancement of sodium reabsorption may force potassium excretion.

Potassium maintains an extracellular-to-intracellular fluid gradient. This gradient is affected by the adrenal steroids, hyponatremia, glycogen formation, testosterone, and pH changes. The most significant of these influences is the pH. Serum potassium moves inversely to the pH. If the pH falls, potassium concentration increases. If the pH rises, potassium concentration decreases due in part to the ionic charge of potassium and hydrogen. Serum potassium must be evaluated with the arterial blood gases to avoid compounding problems of potassium therapy.

Hyperkalemia

Hyperkalemia is a potassium level greater than 5.5 mEq/L. It is due to an inability of the kidney tubules to excrete potassium ions. Tubular damage or increased potassium load that exceeds the kidney's ability to handle the quantity of potassium results in hyperkalemia.

Etiology. Hyperkalemia may be due to acute and chronic renal disease, low cardiac output states, acidosis, sodium depletion, or large muscle mass injury. Any factor that destroys cells (e.g., burns, trauma, or crush injuries) will release the intracellular potassium, causing hyperkalemia. Excessive ingestion of potassium chloride (found in antacids and salt substitutes), adrenal cortical insufficiency, and the hemolysis of banked blood may also cause hyperkalemia.

Clinical Presentation. Hyperkalemia causes a dilated and flaccid heart accompanied by a bradycardia. Generalized muscle irritability or flaccidity, which may be severe enough to be a flaccid paralysis, and numbness of extremities are present. There may be abdominal cramping, nausea, and diarrhea. Generally, the patient is apathetic and may be confused.

ECG tracings show a tall, peaked or tent-shaped T wave with potassium levels of 5.5 to 7.5 mEq/L. In marked hyperkalemia (potassium of 7.5 to 9 mEq/L), there is a flattening and widening of the P wave, a prolonged PR interval, and usually depression of the ST segment. In severely advanced hyperkalemia (potassium of 8 to 9 mEq/L and often more than 10 mEq/L), the P waves disappear and intraventricular conduction disturbances occur, producing intraventricular and supraventricular dysrhythmias progressing to ventricular tachycardia, ventricular standstill, or fibrillation and death.

Treatment. A serum potassium level above 5.5 mEq/L requires immediate intervention. Treatment is initiated to prevent increasing bradycardia and cardiac arrest. The objective of treatment is to reduce the serum potassium to a safe level as rapidly as possible. Cardiac monitoring is essential.

Intravenous 10% glucose with regular insulin will induce a cellular deposition of potassium with glycogen. Intravenous sodium bicarbonate will buffer cellular hydrogen and allow potassium to move intracellularly. Calcium chloride will oppose the cardiotoxic effects of hyperkalemia. However, calcium therapy is contraindicated in patients on digoxin. Kayexalate is given orally or via the rectum to rid the body of potassium. Kayexalate forces a one-for-one exchange of sodium for potassium in the intestinal cell wall; however, the patient must be monitored for sodium retention. Sorbitol is used to induce an osmotic diarrhea through semiliquid stools.

These measures are all emergency procedures to provide time to ascertain the cause of the hyperkalemia. If the cause is physiological or if the hyperkalemia is refractory, dialysis is indicated. If the cause is overingestion, the emergency measures may be sufficient and the patient may need only additional conservative treatment, close monitoring, and instruction on how to prevent recurrences.

Hypokalemia

Hypokalemia is a serum potassium level of less than 3.5 mEq/L. Hypokalemia occurs when potassium loss is greater than potassium intake.

Etiology. Hypokalemia may be due to alkalosis, which stimulates hydrogen ion retention and potassium ion secretion in the distal convoluted tubules of the kidney. Diuretic therapy, without potassium replacement, endocrine dysfunction (increased ACTH, thyroid storm) and renal dysfunction (tubular acidosis) may all cause hypokalemia.

High potassium losses, gastric and intestinal surgery, nasogastric suctioning, and intestinal diseases predispose the patient to hypokalemia unless replacement therapy is maintained.

Clinical Presentation. Hypokalemia has many of the same signs as hyperkalemia. There is a general malaise and muscle weakness which may progress to a flaccid paralysis. Anorexia, nausea, and vomiting may accompany a paralytic ileus. Mental status may range from drowsiness to coma. Hypotension may be present and may lead to cardiac arrest. If the patient is on digitalis, signs of digitalis toxicity may be present because hypokalemia potentiates the effect of digitalis.

Cardiac dysrhythmias are most commonly atrial unless the hypokalemia is profound, in which case premature ventricular beats are found. Other ventricular dysrhythmias are rare unless digitalis toxicity is present. ECG tracings most commonly show a prominent U wave. Depression or flattening of the ST segment or inversion of the T wave may be apparent. An inverted T wave may fuse with the U wave, giving the appearance of a prolonged QT interval. There is a generalized irritability of the heart in hypokalemic states.

Weakness of the muscles results in shallow respiration that may progress to apnea. In hypokalemia, death may be due to respiratory arrest.

Treatment. Emergency treatment of severe hypokalemia is the slow intravenous administration of potassium chloride (approximately 10 to 20 mEq/hour) while monitoring the patient's ECG patterns for dysrhythmias due to hyperkalemia. Monitoring of symptoms, serum potassium levels, and arterial blood gases is imperative to prevent an iatrogenic hyperkalemia.

Nonemergency treatment is to replace potassium with intravenous fluids containing potassium chloride or with oral potassium supplements. Oral supplements should be diluted to prevent gastrointestinal irritation and to facilitate absorption. The patient is monitored for adequate intake and output, cardiac status, potassium levels, and signs of alkalosis or impending digitalis toxicity.

CALCIUM

Calcium Regulation

The normal serum calcium (Ca^{2+}) concentration is 8.5 to 10.5 mg/dL. Calcium, with phosphorus, makes bones and teeth rigid and strong. Calcium is integral to determining the strength and thickness of cell membranes. Calcium exerts a quieting action on nerve cells, thus maintaining normal transmission of nerve impulses. Calcium also activates specific enzymes of the blood-clotting process and those involved in the contraction of the myocardium.

Ninety-eight percent of calcium filtered by the kidneys is reabsorbed along the same pathways as sodium. There are four major factors influencing calcium reabsorption: parathyroid hormone (PTH), vitamin D, corticosteroids, and diuretics.

Parathyroid Hormone. If the serum PTH level is increased, there is increased reabsorption of ionized calcium from renal tubules. Reciprocally, the PTH increases phosphate excretion and increases calcium absorption from the gastrointestinal tract. PTH will mobilize calcium from the bones when the kidneys cannot or do not reabsorb sufficient calcium.

Vitamin D. Vitamin D must be present in an activated form to promote absorption of calcium from the small intestines. Vitamin D is ingested in food, especially milk. The vitamin must then be activated by ultraviolet (sun) light changing a chemical in the skin. This vitamin is additionally changed in the liver. Finally, the kidneys convert the vitamin to 1,25-dihydroxycholecalciferol, also known as activated vitamin D. The activated vitamin D promotes absorption of calcium from the small intestines. PTH stimulates this activation process, since a low serum level of calcium precludes an increase of calcium absorption in the kidney without PTH.

Corticosteroids. Corticosteroids are suspected of interfering with the activation of vitamin D, possibly in the liver, and decreasing the amount of calcium absorbed from the small intestines.

Diuretics. Diuretics can cause increased excretion of calcium and the other electrolytes. If a fluid volume loss results in a decreased total body fluid volume, there will be a decreased GFR, resulting in reduced calcium excretion.

Hypercalcemia

Etiology. Hypercalcemia exists when the serum calcium level is above 10.5 mg/dL. Increased renal reabsorption of calcium may cause hypercalcemia. It may also be the result of increased intestinal absorption of calcium due to excessive dietary calcium intake or excessive vitamin D ingestion.

Hyperparathyroidism caused by parathyroid adenoma will cause hypercalcemia by increasing bone release of calcium and by continuously stimulating the kidneys to reabsorb calcium. This also occurs in carcinoma of the parathyroid glands. Milk-alkali syndrome can occur in peptic ulcer patients treated for a prolonged period with milk and alkaline antacids, particularly calcium carbonate.

Multiple myelomas and metastatic carcinoma of the bone cause hypercalcemia secondary to the release of calcium from the bone into the serum. Prolonged bedrest or immobilization potentiates the movement of calcium from the bones, teeth, and intestines. This process is more conspicuous in patients with Paget's disease. Frequently, the calcium is deposited in joints, in muscle tissue close to joints, and in the kidneys as calcium stones.

Drugs, especially thiazide diuretics, inhibit calcium excretion leading to hypercalcemia in susceptible patients. Renal tubular acidosis, thyrotoxicosis, and hypophosphatemia may all cause hypercalcemia in susceptible patients.

Clinical Presentation. Neurological changes include subtle personality changes in early and mild hypercalcemia progressing to lethargy, confusion, and coma as the severity of the hypercalcemia increases. Neuromuscular changes progress from weakness and hypotonicity to flaccidness.

The renal system may be affected by the formation of calcium calculi with varying amounts of urine output, dependent upon the location of the calculi, which may cause thigh or flank pain. Polyuria and polydipsia are often present because the increased calcium inhibits the action of ADH on the distal tubules and the collecting ducts.

Gastrointestinal symptoms include anorexia, nausea, vomiting, and constipation. Hypercalcemia stimulates gastric acid secretion and may lead to peptic ulcers. The hypotonicity caused by hypercalcemia results in decreased intestinal motility and constipation.

Cardiac changes are less common in hypercalcemia than in hyperkalemia. The earliest ECG change is a shortening of the QT interval due to shortening of the ST segment. Digitalis and calcium are synergistic. Sudden death in hypercalcemia is often attributed to ventricular fibrillation due to this synergism.

An ocular abnormality known as band keratopathy may occur due to deposition of calcium crystals in the cornea. Calcium is deposited at the lateral borders of the cornea in the shape of parentheses. If the calcification is extensive, calcium will be deposited in semilunar bands across the cornea connecting the parentheses. This band keratopathy may be seen by the naked eye.

Treatment. The objective of treatment is to reduce the serum calcium level. Normal saline IVs and diuretics will increase the GFR and thus excretion of calcium, provided there are no obstructive calculi. These treatments require accurate intake and output monitoring.

Drug therapy includes corticosteroids (which antagonize vitamin D and decrease gastrointestinal absorption of calcium), mithramycin (which actually depresses mobilization of calcium from the bones), and phosphates (which will bind to calcium in the intestines and precipitate calcium when administered intravenously).

Neurological and cardiac monitoring are essential in assessing the efficacy of treatment. Some underlying causes (such as multiple myeloma) will tend to make hypercalcemia refractory to treatment. In such cases, the goal of therapy becomes keeping the calcium level as low as possible.

Hypocalcemia

Etiology. Hypocalcemia is a clinical condition in which the serum calcium level is less than 8.5 mg/dL. Hypocalcemia usually develops from an excessive loss of calcium as a result of, for example, diarrhea, use of diuretics, malabsorption syndromes, or hypoparathyroidism. Chronic renal failure is probably the most common cause of hypocalcemia. If calcium is lost in peritoneal dialysis or hemodialysis, a hyperphosphatemia may occur. This enhances a peripheral deposition of calcium. Calcium deposits keep calcium from being available to raise serum levels. There is also an inability of the patient with chronic renal failure to absorb calcium from the intestines secondary to a lack of activated vitamin D. Alkalosis can cause a hypocalcemia because the calcium becomes bound to albumin and thus remains inactive in the serum.

Chronic malabsorption syndromes may cause a hypocalcemia. These syndromes are found following gastrectomies, in small bowel diseases, in patients with a high fat diet (fat impairs calcium absorption), and in patients with a magnesium deficiency (magnesium inhibits PTH).

Malignancies may also cause hypocalcemia. These include osteoblastic metastases (whereby calcium is used for abnormal bone synthesis) and medullary carcinoma of the thyroid (causing an increased secretion of thyrocalcitonin, which in turn stimulates osteoblasts and prevents calcium from entering the serum).

Hypoparathyroidism of any etiology causes hypocalcemia, since there is a decreased secretion of PTH. The most common causes are surgical removal of the parathyroid glands, adenoma of the parathyroid glands, depleted magnesium levels (inhibits PTH), and idiopathic hypoparathyroidism.

A vitamin D-deficient state (or nonactivated vitamin D) is often seen in chronic renal failure, liver failure, and rickets. Without activated vitamin D, calcium is not absorbed from the intestines. Acute pancreatitis causes a precipitation of calcium in the inflamed pancreas and in intra-abdominal lipids.

In hyperphosphatemia, phosphates and calcium bind together and precipitate in tissues. This is commonly found in chronic renal failure due to decreased excretion of phosphates. Increased oral intake of phosphates rarely causes hyperphosphatemia if renal function is normal.

Clinical Presentation. Neuromuscular irritability is the overwhelming symptom present and the most dangerous. Muscle tremors and cramps are present in mild hypocalcemia. As the calcium level drops, tetany and generalized tonic-clonic seizures occur. Neuromuscular irritability causes labored, shallow respirations. Wheezing will be present if bronchospasms have occurred. Bronchospasms may lead to laryngospasm and tetany of the respiratory muscles, resulting in respiratory arrest. Monitoring of the neurological status by testing Chvostek's and Trousseau's signs is important.

To test Chvostek's sign, tap your finger over the supramandibular portion of the parotid gland, which is located in the subcutaneous tissue of the cheek. If the upper lip twitches on the side of stimulation, the test is positive. To test Trousseau's sign, apply a blood pressure cuff to the arm and inflate it until a carpopedal spasm occurs. If no spasm appears in three minutes, the test is negative. To test this result, remove the blood pressure cuff and have the patient hyperventilate (>30 breaths/minute). The respiratory alkalosis that develops may produce the carpopedal spasm. This indicates a positive test.

The neuromuscular irritability frequently causes a decreased cardiac contractility leading to a cardiac arrest. The earliest ECG change is a lengthening of the QT interval due to a lengthening of the ST segment. Significant dysrhythmias due to hypocalcemia are extremely rare. The neuromuscular irritability may also cause biliary colic and paralytic ileus.

An alteration in blood clotting may be seen in hypocalcemia. Since calcium is necessary for normal blood clotting, hypocalcemia is often accompanied by bleeding dyscrasias.

Treatment. The aim of treatment is to raise the calcium level to normal as rapidly as possible to halt or prevent tetany.

In cases of tetany or impending tetany, intravenous 10% calcium gluconate or calcium chloride is administered. The patient must be on a cardiac monitor because a rapid infusion may enhance digitalis toxicity and because hypocalcemic patients are often also hyperkalemic. Vitamin D supplements are administered if a deficiency is present.

Monitoring serum calcium, phosphate, and potassium levels along with ECG monitoring and neuro-

logic monitoring (using Chvostek's and Trousseau's signs) will evaluate the efficacy of patient treatment.

PHOSPHATE

The normal serum level of phosphate (PO_4) is 3.0 to 4.5 mg/dL. The phosphate ion is found in bones and is a major factor in intracellular production of ATP (energy). Phosphate combines with proteins and lipids to form important intracellular molecules. Intracellular phosphate ions may react with DNA and RNA molecules. Phosphate acts as a buffering agent for urine, is responsible for bone growth, promotes white blood cell phagocytic action, and is important in platelet structure and function.

Phosphate Regulation

Phosphate levels are influenced by two major factors, PTH secretion (increases renal excretion of phosphate ions) and calcium concentration. Calcium and phosphate have a reciprocal relationship. If calcium levels increase, phosphate levels decrease; conversely, if calcium levels decrease, phosphate levels increase.

Reabsorption of phosphates occurs actively in the proximal convoluted tubule in the presence of sodium. Without sodium, phosphates will not be reabsorbed.

Excretion of phosphates is regulated by PTH and the GFR. PTH inhibits reabsorption of phosphates in the proximal tubule, so phosphates will be excreted. With a decrease in the GFR, phosphate excretion will increase; with an increase in the GFR, phosphates excretion will decrease.

Hyperphosphatemia

Etiology. A serum phosphate level above 4.5 mg/dL constitutes hyperphosphatemia. Inability to excrete phosphates or excessive ingestion of phosphates are the two pathologic processes of hyperphosphatemia. The inability to excrete phosphates may be due to a decreased GFR or to renal failure.

Excessive ingestion of phosphates may be due to routine use (or abuse) of phosphate-containing laxatives and enemas or use of cytotoxic agents for the treatment of leukemias and lymphomas. Hypoparathyroidism causes hyperphosphatemia secondary to the effects of PTH on the kidney. Occasionally, overadministration of intravenous or oral phosphates will induce a hyperphosphatemia.

Clinical Presentation. Clinical presentation of hyperphosphatemia is the same as for hypocalcemia. Elevated phosphate levels enhance the movement of calcium into bone. If seizures occur, they are due to hypocalcemia caused by hyperphosphatemia. Remember that calcium and phosphate have a reciprocal relationship.

Metastatic calcification occurs when calcium and phosphates chemically combine to form calcium phosphate, which then precipitates in arteries, soft tissue, and joints.

Treatment. The objective of therapy is to decrease the serum phosphate level. This is accomplished by giving aluminum hydroxide gels or calcium antacids that combine with phosphate, limiting the amount of phosphate available for absorption in the intestines.

Hypophosphatemia

Etiology. Hypophosphatemia is a serum phosphate level of less than 3.0 mg/dL. Any factor that increases the cellular uptake to form sugar phosphates will decrease serum levels of phosphate. For example, prolonged intense hyperventilation can depress serum phosphate by inducing respiratory alkalosis. A decreased phosphate absorption from the intestines (malabsorption syndromes), loss of proximal convoluted tubular function with renal phosphate wasting as seen in Fanconi's syndrome, and rickets that are vitamin D resistant may also cause hypophosphatemia.

Chronic alcoholism results in a dietary deficiency of phosphates and may interfere with the absorption of any phosphates present. Abuse (including overuse) of phosphate-binding gels such as Amphojel and hyperparathyroidism (causing renal phosphaturia) cause hypophosphatemia.

Long-term hyperalimentation may contribute to hypophosphatemia if phosphates are not included in the solution in adequate amounts. Use of the high glucose content in hyperalimentation solutions requires phosphates. This is no longer a common etiology.

Clinical Presentation. Complaints of general malaise, anorexia, and vague muscle weakness may be of chronic or acute onset. With chronic onset, muscle wasting is apparent. With acute onset, rhabdomyolysis (a diffuse muscle-wasting necrosis) is due to a depletion of intracellular ATP and a concurrent decrease in all ATP-mediated processes. Hypercalcemia and hypercalciuria, with associated symptoms, are indicators

of acute phosphate depletion due to hyperparathyroidism (PTH increases serum calcium by removing it from bone and decreases serum phosphate by excretion in the urine).

Hypoxia occurs because of a deficit in red blood cell phosphate content necessary for the formation of 2,3-DPG. With a decrease in 2,3-DPG, a decrease in the dissociation of oxygen from hemoglobin is seen and tissue hypoxia results.

Complicating hypophosphatemia may be osteomalacia, severe metabolic acidosis, and insulin resistance resulting in hyperglycemia. This syndrome is rare and usually seen in chronic alcoholism. It is a severe intravascular hemolysis caused by a phosphate depletion that results in a decrease of 2,3-DPG in red blood cells.

Treatment. The objective of therapy is to replace the phosphates, first by intravenous administration and then orally. Use of phosphate-binding gels is discontinued, and then treatment of the underlying cause of hypophosphatemia is started.

MAGNESIUM

The normal serum level of magnesium (Mg^{2+}) is 1.5 to 2.5 mEq/L. The magnesium ion is the second major intracellular cation. Magnesium acts as a coenzyme in the metabolism of carbohydrates and proteins. It regulates neuromuscular excitability and phosphate levels. It is stored in bone, muscle, and soft tissue.

Magnesium Regulation

Renal reabsorption of magnesium is essentially the same as for calcium. The presence of sodium directly affects the reabsorption in the proximal tubules. Without sodium, there is no reabsorption of magnesium. PTH appears to have a minimal effect on reabsorption. Reabsorption processes of calcium and magnesium are mutually suppressive.

Hypermagnesemia

Etiology. Hypermagnesemia is a serum magnesium level above 2.5 mEq/L. This is extremely rare. Reabsorption is similar to the calcium process. Absorption of excessive sodium (due to any cause) in the renal tubules may "drag" an excessive amount of magnesium back into the blood.

Chronic renal disease and untreated diabetic acidosis are the usual causes. Addison's disease, hyperparathyroidism, excessive magnesium administration, and overuse of magnesium-containing antacids are other causes of hypermagnesemia.

Clinical Presentation. Lethargy, coma, impaired respirations, hyporeflexia, and hypotension are the usual symptoms. All of the symptoms of hyperkalemia may be present. ECG changes consist first of prolonged PR intervals, followed by widening of the QRS complex as the magnesium concentration rises. Death usually occurs with a concentration of 6 mEq/L or more.

Treatment. Attempts to lower magnesium levels by hemodialysis with a hypomagnesium dialysate have been successful.

Hypomagnesemia

Etiology. A magnesium level of less than 1.5 mEq/L is a state of hypomagnesemia. Any inhibition of absorption of magnesium from the gastrointestinal tract or of reabsorption from the renal system may account for hypomagnesium. Severe malabsorption syndromes, acute pancreatitis, chronic alcoholism, primary aldosteronism, diabetic ketoacidosis, diuretic therapy, and renal disease are the usual causes.

Clinical Presentation. Neuromuscular and central nervous system hyperirritability characterize hypomagnesemia. Muscle tremors, delirium, convulsion, and coma are seen. Positive Chvostek's and Trousseau's signs, tachycardia, increased blood pressure, depressed ST segments, and prolonged QT intervals are also seen. Hypomagnesemia may result in digitalis-induced dysrhythmias.

Treatment. The objective of treatment is simply to provide sufficient magnesium to raise the serum level. This can be achieved by intravenous administration of fluids with magnesium or orally by a diet high in magnesium.

CHLORIDE (Cl)

Chloride Regulation
Normal serum chloride level is 98 to 106 mg/dL. Chloride is reabsorbed by the kidney at all of the sites for sodium reabsorption. Chloride moves freely with the gastric and intestinal fluids and is reabsorbed accordingly.

Anion Gap
Excretion of chloride is influenced by the acid-base balance. In acidosis, chloride is excreted while bicar-bonate is reabsorbed. In alkalosis, chloride is reabsorbed while bicarbonate is excreted. Chloride can be used in combination with bicarbonate and sodium to obtain an estimated "anion gap." While an anion gap never really exists, since cations and anions must balance to maintain electrochemical neutrality, an anion gap appears to be present if only sodium, bicarbonate, and chloride are measured. A normal anion gap is less than 15 mEq and is obtained by subtracting bicarbonate and chloride from sodium. For example, a patient with a sodium of 140, bicarbonate of 25, and chloride of 100 would have an anion gap of 15 ($140 - [(100 + 25)/\backslash] = 15$.

The value in computing an anion gap is simple. If an anion gap exceeds 15, a specific type of metabolic acidosis exists. If the anion gap exceeds 15, either a lactic, keto, or chronic renal failure acidosis exists. The reason the anion gap appears to increase is due to the loss of bicarbonate to buffer the acidosis without the simultaneous increase in chloride. In lactic, keto, and chronic renal failure, acidosis anions other than chloride increase to offset the loss of bicarbonate.

Hyperchloremia

Etiology. Hyperchloremia is a serum chloride level above 106 mg/dL. An excessive ingestion of chloride or an excessive kidney reabsorption of chloride ions are the pathophysiological changes in hyperchloremia.

Clinical Presentation. The symptoms are the same (or very similar) to hypernatremia.

Treatment. The objectives of treatment are to reduce the chloride level, which is most often achieved by the treatment for metabolic acidosis.

Hypochloremia

Etiology. Hypochloremia is a serum chloride level of less than 98 mg/dL. Chloride ions are lost through excessive vomiting or gastric suction without replacement of electrolytes. This results in a physiological metabolic alkalosis. The bicarbonate ion and chloride ion normally balance each other in kidney function.

Clinical Presentation. Syptoms of hypochloremia include changes in sensorium, possible neuromuscular irritability, and usually slow, shallow respirations.

Treatment. The objective of treatment is to replace the lost chloride ions either orally or intravenously and to treat the metabolic alkalosis to re-establish acid-base balance.

CHAPTER 31

Acute Renal Failure

DEFINITION

Acute renal failure (ARF) refers to a sudden loss of renal function that may or may not produce oliguria or anuria with a concurrent increase in plasma creatinine and blood urea nitrogen (BUN). Oliguria is present if less than 400 cc of urine is produced per day. This is an obligatory water loss, i.e., the minimum amount of urine needed to rid the body of its daily wastes. The mortality rate for ARF ranges from 40 to 70%.

PATHOPHYSIOLOGY

ARF can be classified as prerenal, intrarenal, or postrenal.

Prerenal ARF is defined as a decreased renal perfusion secondary to decreased cardiac output. Decreased renal perfusion causes a decrease in renal artery pressure leading to a reduced afferent arteriole pressure. Afferent arteriole pressures of less than 100 mm Hg may decrease the glomerular filtration rate (GFR), resulting in oliguria and/or anuria. Hypovolemia is the most common cause of acute renal failure in the critically ill patient.

Intrarenal ARF is caused by disease or injuries of the nephron from the glomerulus to the collecting duct.

The most common cause of intrarenal failure is acute tubular necrosis (ATN). Subsequently, these intrarenal conditions can be cortical or medullary in nature.

Cortical conditions involve swelling of the renal capillaries and cellular proliferation. Infectious, vascular, and/or immunologic processes cause edema and some resultant cellular debris that obstructs the glomeruli, resulting in a fall in urine output.

Medullary involvement specifically affects the tubular portions of the nephron, causing necrosis. The extent of medullary damage differs depending upon nephrotoxic injury or ischemic injury. Tubular necrosis, which occurs in a local, patchy pattern, is the result of nephrotoxic injury. Nephrotoxic injury affects the epithelial cells, which can regenerate after the nephrotoxic injury is resolved. Ischemic injury extends to involve the tubular basement membrane and may involve peritubular capillaries and other parts of the nephron. Ischemic injury is more serious, since the tubular basement membrane cannot regenerate. Ischemic injury occurs when the mean arterial pressure falls below 60 mm Hg for over 40 minutes secondary to massive hemorrhage or shock.

Postrenal ARF usually indicates an obstruction at or below the level of the collecting ducts. The obstruction may be partial or complete. If the obstruction is complete, the blockage and subsequent backup of urine flow involve both kidneys. Eventually, urine output is decreased due to decreased glomerular filtration.

ETIOLOGY

Prerenal failure has many causes. One major cause is hemorrhage resulting in hypovolemia with fluid and electrolyte imbalance. Other causes include excessive use of diuretics and decreased glomerular perfusion after an acute myocardial infarction or congestive heart

TABLE 31-1. CAUSES OF INTRARENAL FAILURE

Cortical Nephron Failure	Medullary Nephron Failure
Infections	Nephrotoxic causes
Post streptococcal	Heavy metals
glomerulonephritis	Pesticides
Acute pyelonephritis	Fungicides
Goodpasture's syndrome	X-ray contrast media
Severe hypercalcemia	Antibiotics
Systemic lupus erythematosus	Aminoglycosides
Malignant hypertension	Cephalosporins
	Tetracyclines
	Penicillins
	Ischemic causes
	Crush injuries
	Burns
	Sepsis
	Cardiogenic shock
	Postsurgical hypotension
	Hemorrhage with multiple trauma
	Hemolysis of blood transfusion reaction

failure. Occasionally, following anesthesia and surgery, increased renal vascular resistance and/or the hepatorenal syndrome occurs. Septicemia progressing to gram-negative septic shock results in vasodilation and a resultant hypovolemia. Embolism or thrombosis may cause a bilateral renal vascular obstruction, resulting in decreased or no perfusion.

Intrarenal failure etiologies can be fairly well categorized as either cortical or medullary. Table 31-1 summarizes the multiple causes of cortical and medullary intrarenal failure.

Causes of postrenal ARF are obstructive in nature and include prostatic hypertrophy; bladder, pelvic, or retroperitoneal tumors; renal calculi; ureteral blockage (after surgery or instrumentation); urethral obstruction; bladder infections; or a neurogenic bladder.

PHASES

There are three phases in the cycle of ARF: oliguric, diuretic, and recovery. The first phase is preceded by a precipitating event. Renal blood flow and urine volume decrease.

Oliguric Phase

The oliguric phase reflects the obstruction of tubules from edema, tubular casts, and cellular debris. Damage to the tubules makes absorption and secretion of

solutes variable. If the obstruction and damage are severe enough, a backleak of filtrate through the epithelium may occur, returning the filtrate into the circulation.

During the oliguric phase, laboratory reports will indicate rising levels of urea, creatinine, and potassium. Serum and urine osmolality are increased. The fluid and electrolyte imbalances caused by retention of the metabolic waste products are the greatest dangers to the patient. This phase lasts 8 to 14 days.

Diuretic Phase

The diuretic phase indicates the beginning of the return of tubular function. The diuretic phase lasts about ten days. The greatest danger to the patient in this phase is excessive loss of water and electrolytes. Extreme diuresis is due to the osmotic diuretic effect produced by the elevated BUN and the inability of the tubules to conserve sodium and water, resulting in an output of 3000 cc or more of urine per 24 hours. Hypokalemia is usually present.

Recovery Phase

The recovery phase begins when the diuresis is no longer excessive. There is a gradual improvement in kidney function. This improvement may continue for 3 to 12 months. The end result may be a permanent reduction in the GFR, which may or may not be sufficient to maintain adequate renal function without dialysis. AFR may progress to chronic renal failure, but this is uncommon unless the patient has an underlying kidney disease or is of advanced age.

CLINICAL PRESENTATION

Clinical signs and symptoms may be overlooked during the first few days due to the primary illness. Oliguria may or may not be present. Fifty percent of ARF patients and many ATN patients are anuric. Therefore, urine volume alone is not an adequate guide to renal function. Progressive azotemia (an excess of urea or other nitrogenous bodies in the blood) occurs as a result of decreased GFR in spite of apparently adequate urine output. ARF should be diagnosed before uremic signs are present. Table 31-2 summarizes the uremic signs of ARF.

DIAGNOSIS

Diagnosing ARF or ATN may be difficult, especially in the nonoliguric patient. Factors that must be considered in a diagnosis include urinary volume, urinary sediment, BUN levels, serial serum creatinines, cre-

atinine clearance, arterial blood gases, trauma, and postsurgical status.

Urinary Volume

Normal urinary output is about 0.5 cc/kg/hour. Complete anuria suggests obstruction or cortical necrosis. It may occur in acute glomerulonephritis and complete postrenal obstruction but is very rare otherwise. Daily urine output may be constant or may gradually increase in acute renal parenchymal disease. Different degrees of obstruction are suggested by large and irregular daily urine volumes. Partial obstruction can cause progressive azotemia, even though there may be normal or increased urine volume.

Laboratory Data

In prerenal failure, urine volume is decreased. Urinary Na^+ is less than 10 mEq/L as the kidneys attempt to conserve Na^+ and water. Urinary osmolality, which reflects the concentrating ability of the kidney, is elevated. Urinary osmolality is usually greater than 500 mosm (normal level is 300 to 900 mosm). Specific gravity, a less sensitive indicator of concentrating power than osmolality, is also elevated. Specific gravity is greater than 1.020. There is minimal or no proteinuria. The BUN increase is greater than the cre-

TABLE 31-2. UREMIC SIGNS OF ARF

Respiratory	Metabolic
Deep or rapid respiratory rate (metabolic acidosis)	Electrolyte imbalance
Bilateral rales	
Pulmonary edema	
Cardiovascular	Integument
Tachycardia	Dry skin
Dysrhythmias	Uremic frost (excretion
Pericarditis	of urea)
Friction rub	Pruritus
	Increased susceptibility to infection
Neurological	Hematological
Decreased LOC	Anemias
Confusion	Uremic coagulopathies
Lethargy	Bruising
Stupor	
Gastrointestinal	
Nausea	
Vomiting	
Anorexia	
Constipation or diarrhea	
Abdominal distension	

atinine increase (normal rate is 10:1). Normal serum creatinine is about .8–1.8 mg/dL and normal BUN is about 10–20 mg/dL. The fractional excretion of sodium (FeNa) is less than 1 in prerenal failure.

$$FeNa = \frac{\dfrac{Urine}{Na} \Big/ \dfrac{Plasma}{Na}}{\dfrac{Urine}{Creatinine} \Big/ \dfrac{Plasma}{Creatinine}}$$

In cortical intrarenal failure, urinary sodium is less than 10 mEq/L. Specific gravity will vary with moderate to heavy proteinuria. Serum BUN and creatinine will be elevated. Hematuria is present with erythrocyte casts and leukocytes. In medullary intrarenal failure or ATN, urinary sodium is greater than 20 mEq/L, an abnormal sign when urine output is low. Normally the kidneys conserve sodium in an attempt to maintain extravascular water. In ATN when urine output is low, the expected conservation of sodium fails to occur, resulting in a normal urinary sodium level (40 to 220 mEq/L). Urinary osmolality decreases (below 500 mosm), reflecting the inability of the kidneys to concentrate the urine. Simultaneously, the specific gravity also decreases, usually below 1.010 to 1.015. Minimal to moderate proteinuria is present with an elevated serum BUN and creatinine. The FeNa is >1 in ATN.

In postrenal failure there are scanty sediment, rare white cells, red cells, hyaline casts, and fine granular casts. Urinary sodium is elevated, specific gravity varies, and BUN and creatinine are elevated.

MANAGEMENT OF PATIENT CARE PROBLEMS

There are four major problems of patient care in renal failure: an increase in the products of catabolism, severe electrolyte imbalance with associated acidosis, fluid overload, and infection.

Increase in the Products of Catabolism

Protein catabolism increases in the critically ill and stressed patient. A decrease in proteins available for catabolism will retard the rate of azotemia, decrease the incidence and severity of acidosis, and decrease the occurrence and levels of hyperkalemia in the serum.

Caloric requirements of the patient must be met mainly through an adequate carbohydrate diet intake.

Serum Electrolyte Imbalance and Acidosis

Sodium intake is restricted unless there is a serum sodium deficit. No salt substitutes are used because of their potassium content. Careful management of fluids and sodium intake will prevent overhydration, congestive heart failure, hyponatremia, and water intoxication.

Hyperkalemia is a significant imbalance seen in ARF. Hyperkalemia is further compounded as a result of catabolism associated with fever. It also occurs as a result of decreased potassium excretion caused by volume depletion or drugs. Metabolic acidosis can also cause hyperkalemia. The fall of the pH forces hydrogen ions into the cells and potassium into the extracellular fluid.

Fluid Overload

It is essential to determine the patient's state of hydration and to continually monitor this state. Indicators of overhydration include weight gain, edema, anasarca, ascites, increased blood pressure, JVD (jugular vein distension), and dyspnea. Indicators for dehydration include weight loss, decreased blood pressure, poor skin turgor, no evidence of JVD, and decreased central venous pressure.

Fluids are restricted to amounts equal to urine output plus 400 cc for insensible fluid loss. It is vitally important that accurate daily weights be taken using the same scales. It is also important to remember that 1000 cc of fluid weighs about 2.2 lb or 1.0 kg.

Infection

Since proper kidney function affects all body systems, the chance of infection is greatly increased in renal failure patients. The body defense systems do not function properly, and the patient is predisposed to urinary tract infections, septicemia, pneumonia, and wound or skin infections (due to the severe pruritis that some patients experience). A good nutritional intake for the patient and proper hygiene will help prevent infections. If fever develops, culture and sensitivities of blood, urine, sputum, or any wound should be performed to identify the invading organism. Once the organism is identified, appropriate antibiotic therapy is started with antibiotic doses adjusted to renal function.

CHAPTER 32

Dialysis

Editor's Note

This chapter is designed to help answer questions regarding treatment modalities for acute renal failure and electrolyte disturbances. More content is given than is required for the exam. However, if you understand the major concepts in this chapter (do not focus on details), you should be prepared to address any questions regarding dialysis in the treatment of acute renal failure or life-threatening electrolyte disturbances.

As the patient develops systemic symptoms of renal failure, the need for dialysis is assessed. The purposes of dialysis are to (1) remove the by-products of protein metabolism, including urea, creatinine, and uric acid, (2) remove excess water, (3) maintain or restore the body's buffer system, and (4) maintain or restore the body's concentration of electrolytes. Dialysis is defined as the diffusion of dissolved particles from one fluid compartment to another across a semipermeable membrane. Three principles are utilized in dialysis: osmosis, diffusion, and filtration.

Osmosis is the movement of fluid across a semipermeable membrane from a less concentrated solution to a more concentrated solution. Diffusion is the movement of particles (or solutes) across a semipermeable membrane from a more concentrated solution to a less concentrated solution. Filtration is the movement of particles or solutes across a semipermeable membrane through the utilization of hydrostatic pressure.

PERITONEAL DIALYSIS

In peritoneal dialysis, the peritoneum is the semipermeable membrane. The peritoneum is a strong, smooth, colorless, serous membrane that lines the abdominal cavity with a parietal layer and wraps the abdominal organs with a visceral layer (Fig. 32-1).

The dialysate is instilled into the abdominal cavity between these two layers of peritoneum. The visceral peritoneum is contiguous with the intestinal wall and the capillary beds of the intestines. The dialysate is instilled into the peritoneal space, bathing the intestines. Osmosis, diffusion, and filtration occur readily after "dwelling" in the abdomen.

Indications
There are many instances in which peritoneal dialysis may be used. In acute renal failure, peritoneal dialysis may be used to treat the renal failure or to prevent uremia while ascertaining an underlying cause or while stabilizing a patient for surgery.

Chronic renal failure patients who have had a recent infection may undergo peritoneal dialysis to prevent localization of the infection at the fistula site.

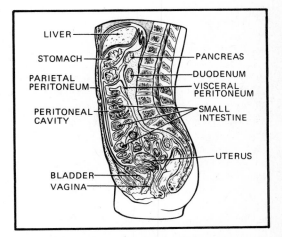

Figure 32-1. The peritoneal space (female).

Patients in whom there is no vascular access route for hemodialysis may undergo peritoneal dialysis until an access route is available.

Circulatory overload from renal impairment with congestive heart failure is amenable to peritoneal dialysis. Refractory hyperkalemia and metabolic acidosis and intoxication from diazable drugs and poisons are also indicators for peritoneal dialysis.

In chronic renal failure, peritoneal dialysis may postpone the need for chronic hemodialysis. In patients with diabetes, chronic hemodialysis may cause blindness associated with diabetic retinopathy. Patients awaiting renal transplantation may utilize peritoneal dialysis because it is less expensive than hemodialysis. Some patients undergo peritoneal dialysis instead of hemodialysis because of religious beliefs and the desire to avoid blood transfusions associated with hemodialysis emergencies.

The use of peritoneal dialysis in peritonitis is a controversial topic. Some nephrologists believe in adding antibiotics to the dialysate in addition to using oral or intravenous antibiotics. The rationale is to bathe the infected area itself with antibiotics. Other nephrologists believe that peritonitis is justification for stopping peritoneal dialysis. The rationale here is to treat the patient with intravenous antibiotics to prevent septic shock from developing or to prevent weakening (to the actual point of rupture) of an inflamed, infected visceral peritoneum and the contiguous intestinal wall.

Contraindications

Any patient with blood-clotting dyscrasias should not undergo peritoneal dialysis until the blood-clotting problems have been resolved. Patients with fresh postoperative vascular prostheses, such as a fresh femoral-popliteal bypass, are not candidates for peritoneal dialysis. The procedure may result in graft failure at the site of anastomosis, resulting in exsanguination.

Patients who have had recent peritoneal surgery or those with postoperative abdominal drains are not able to undergo peritoneal dialysis. The peritoneum may not be strong enough to hold the dialysate without rupture or tearing of the peritoneum, and abdominal drains preclude any dwell time since the dialysate would flow out of the drains.

Abdominal adhesions or any other condition where a danger of puncturing viscera exists is a contraindication to peritoneal dialysis. Pregnant women should not undergo peritoneal dialysis due to the increased risk for fetal distress.

Advantages

Peritoneal dialysis can be performed at the bedside. The expensive, elaborate equipment and highly skilled personnel utilized for hemodialysis are not needed in peritoneal dialysis. Because it requires more time to effectively remove metabolic wastes and restore electrolyte and fluid balance, it is less stressful for pediatric and elderly patients and can be initiated quickly. There is no need for systemic anticoagulation.

Disadvantages

Peritoneal dialysis is slower to rid the body of waste products than hemodialysis. It takes 48 to 72 hours to complete peritoneal dialysis, as opposed to 3 to 4 hours for hemodialysis. Prolonged peritoneal dialysis results in a protein depletion and may result in ascites, poor wound healing, and decreased resistance to infection. Peritonitis, usually due to staphylococcus or gram-negative organisms, may develop with repeated treatments. With peritonitis, some physicians will stop the peritoneal dialysis and others will continue with the addition of an antibiotic to the dialysate.

Dialysate

The dialysate solution concentration is selected by the physician. The more concentrated the solute concentration, the greater the osmotic forces exerted to remove fluid and waste products. Osmotic forces are determined by the concentration of glucose in the dialysate, usually ranging from 1.5 to 4.25%. During the administration of 4.25% dialysate, the serum glucose must be monitored because glucose can diffuse into the serum.

The temperature of the dialysate influences the effectiveness of peritoneal dialysis; urea clearance is 35% greater at body temperature (98.6°F) than at room temperature (75°F). Body temperature dialysate will also enhance patient comfort.

The volume of the dialysate influences effectiveness. An exchange volume of 3 liters of dialysate in one hour almost doubles the urea clearance achieved with 1 liter per hour. Most adults are comfortable with 2 liters per exchange, and a few can tolerate 3 liters.

The physician will order the amount of heparin to be added to the dialysate to prevent fibrin or blood from clotting the catheter. The amount of potassium chloride added depends on the patient's serum potassium level, state of digitalization, and arterial blood gases.

Some physicians add lidocaine, usually 50 mg/2

liters of dialysate, for generalized abdominal discomfort. Some physicians also add antibiotics if peritonitis is present or suspected.

Procedure and Nursing Care

To help obtain the patient's cooperation, the nurse should explain the procedure, making the patient aware of the discomforts of, limited mobility during, and duration of the procedure. The patient should be weighed before the procedure and either daily or after the last exchange.

The patient should void or be catheterized immediately before the physician inserts the catheter. Using strict sterile technique at the bedside, the physician inserts the catheter midline of the abdomen between the umbilicus and the symphysis pubis. Once the catheter is in place, 2 liters of warmed dialysate is unfused and drained as soon as it is instilled to ensure patency of the catheter. Outflow should drain in a steady stream.

When catheter patency is confirmed, the warmed dialysate is infused, allowed to dwell in the abdomen, usually for 20 to 45 minutes, and then allowed to drain via gravity as completely as possible. One exchange usually takes about an hour. Turning the patient side to side may enhance the drainage of dialysate.

At the end of the dwell time, the dialysate is assessed for color. Normally, it is clear, pale yellow. If the drainage is cloudy, suspect infection or peritonitis. If it is brownish, suspect bowel perforation. Blood-tinged dialysate during the first four exchanges is normal. However, if after four exchanges the dialysate is still bloody, discontinue and notify the physician. The patient may have abdominal bleeding or a uremic coagulopathy.

Periodic cultures of the dialysate drainage are obtained to assess for infection, and the tip of the catheter is cultured when it is removed.

Monitoring of vital signs every 15 minutes during the first hour and then every one to two hours is the usual procedure if the vital signs are stable. The outflow period is the most likely time for abnormal or changing vital signs. Signs of impending shock, fluid overload, and pulmonary edema will be most apparent in this outflow period.

One of the most important aspects of peritoneal dialysis is the intake-output record maintained by the nurse. Hospital policies vary in the format for recording peritoneal dialysis intake and output. Information needed is the time the exchange was started, the number of the exchange, the amount of fluid infused, the dwell time, the amount of fluid drained, and the fluid balance.

Fluid balance is crucial. If 2000 cc is instilled and only 1750 cc drains out, the patient fluid balance is +250 cc. If the next exchange instills 2000 cc and drains 1900 cc, the patient fluid balance for the exchange is +100 cc. The present balance is now +350 cc. Assume that the third exchange is with a 4.5% dialysate (hypertonic solution). The amount instilled was 2000 cc, and the output drainage was 2275 cc. The patient balance for this exchange is −275 cc. The patient gave back more fluid than was instilled in this exchange. However, in the continuous fluid balance columns, the patient is still at a fluid balance of +75 cc. Intake-output records are maintained for each exchange and overall for total exchanges.

Complications

Infection is one of the most common complications of peritoneal dialysis. Insertion of the catheter under sterile technique and closed sterile instillation and drainage of dialysate will help reduce infection. Nursing intervention of daily sterile changes of the dressing over the tube insertion site helps decrease the chance of infection. Perhaps the most effective way to prevent infection is to keep the procedure time to 36 hours or less.

Volume depletion occurs if the dialysis is too effective and removes several hundred milliliters of fluid per exchange. This will result in hypotension. Water removal may cause hypernatremia if the 4.25% glucose dialysate is used. Nursing intervention includes monitoring for signs of increasing sodium retention.

Volume overload may occur during peritoneal dialysis. When the patient is severely hyponatremic, sodium and water move into the third space. As third spacing resolves by sodium and water returning to the intravascular bed, cardiovascular overload may occur. Shortening the dwell time and repositioning the patient may help. If not, the patient may need hemodialysis.

Hyperglycemia may be severe if hypertonic fluid is used in the diabetic patient. Hyperosmolar coma and death have occurred. If hyperglycemia develops, the dialysis is discontinued until the blood sugar is controlled. Suspect hyperglycemia if the patient complains of thirst or if there is a deterioration in the patient's level of consciousness.

Metabolic alkalosis may occur if dialysis is continued for a long time. Dialysate fluid contains sodium lactate or acetate (45 mEq/L), which is converted to sodium bicarbonate in the body.

Digitalis intoxication is a serious complication. It is a result of lowering the serum potassium and at the same time correcting hypocalcemia, hyponatremia, and acidosis. The dose of the digitalis is usually reduced in uremic patients. Serum levels of cardiac glycosides are not affected by routine dialysis. Disequilibrium syndrome occurs more often in hemodialysis and will be covered in the discussion of hemodialysis.

Respiratory insufficiency may occur as the 2 liters of dialysate are infused into the abdomen and push the abdominal viscera against the diaphragm, resulting in decreased depth of respirations. There is also an increased risk for atelectosis and pneumonia.

Severe pain at the end of inflow or outflow must be assessed. The pain may be caused by the temperature of the dialysate, incomplete draining of the previous exchange, early-stage development of peritonitis, or instillation of too much dialysate.

HEMODIALYSIS

Hemodialysis is a process of removing metabolic waste products of the body by use of extracorporeal circulation. The patient's blood is transferred by tubing from the patient to a machine that functions like a kidney to filter out waste products and then return the filtered blood to the patient by another tube. Hemodialysis uses the same principles of osmosis, diffusion, and filtration that are used in peritoneal dialysis.

Indications

Hemodialysis has the same indications as peritoneal dialysis. Other reasons for performing hemodialysis include acute renal failure due to trauma or infection, chronic renal failure no longer controlled by medication and diet, when rapid removal of toxins, poisons, and drugs is essential, and when peritoneal dialysis is contraindicated.

Contraindications

Labile cardiovascular states that would deteriorate with rapid changes in extravascular fluid volume are the major contraindications to hemodialysis.

In the past, patients who could not tolerate systemic heparinization could not be hemodialyzed. Today, however, the heparin is infused into the dialysis machine to keep blood anticoagulated within the machine. Before the blood is returned to the patient, protamine is infused to neutralize the heparin as the blood is returned to the patient. This process is called regional heparinization (Fig. 32-2).

For the patient without a condition that would be worsened by heparin, intermittent heparinization is used. In these cases, 2000 to 5000 units of heparin are infused at the start of hemodialysis, and 1000 to 2000 units of heparin are added for each hour that the patient is on the machine. These patients must be monitored closely for signs of bleeding.

There are three ways to access a patient's blood for hemodialysis: an arteriovenous (AV) shunt, single- or double-lumen catheters, and an AV fistula. The AV shunt (Fig. 32-3) consists of two Silastic catheters; one is inserted in an artery, and the other is inserted into a nearby vein. Blood is channeled from the artery to the dialysis machine and back to the vein. Part of the shunt lies subcutaneously, and part lies outside the skin.

When the patient is not undergoing hemodialysis, blood flows directly from the artery through the shunt and into the vein. Shunts are inserted under local anesthesia. The favored sites are the arm, wrist, legs, and ankles. In the upper extremity, the preferred vessels are from the radial artery to the cephalic vein. In the lower extremity, the preferred vessels are from the posterior tibial artery to the great saphenous vein.

Shaldon catheters (Fig. 32-4) are short-term shunts. They can be placed in the femoral vein or subclavian vein. With femoral access, one or two cannulas may be placed in the femoral vein. During dialysis, one catheter is used to channel blood to the dialysis machine and the other catheter is used to channel blood from the dialysis machine back to the patient. One bifurcated catheter can also be used. Peripheral pulses must be frequently assessed in the cannulized extremity. The patient must be maintained on bedrest. Assessment for signs of bleeding or hematoma formation is done frequently. If the catheter(s) is to remain after dialysis, low-dose heparin is utilized to maintain catheter potency.

Subclavian access also provides immediate short-term or long-term access. One bifurcated catheter is utilized with heparin irrigations to maintain catheter potency between dialysis treatments. Patient activity is not restricted with subclavian access. However, the patient must be monitored for signs of a pneumothorax.

Fistulas have a longer life span than do AV shunts

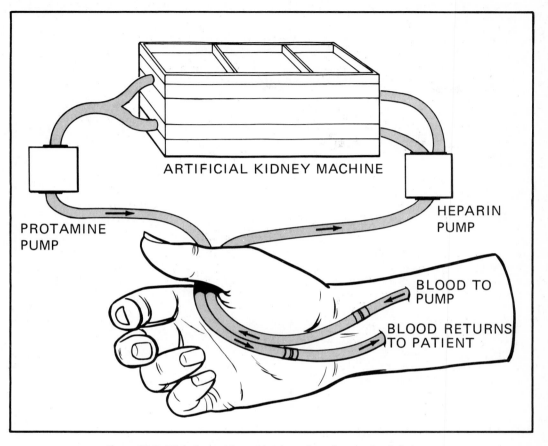

Figure 32-2. Dialysis machine with a heparin and protamine infusion.

and tend to preserve the blood vessels in which they are placed. Fistulas are less restrictive than other forms of vascular access and therefore offer greater freedom to the patient. The fistula can be formed by the patient's vessels or by a graft (Fig. 32-5). Examples of graft materials are bovine carotid, woven Dacron, and umbilical vein. If grafts are used, they are tunneled under the skin in a U shape (Fig. 32-6). The surgical procedure involves anastomosis of the artery directly to the vein, utilizing most frequently a side-to-side technique. Fistulas need to mature over a 10- to 14-day period. During this time, the vein adapts to the high pressure of the arterial blood by dilatation and thickening of the venous wall. When the fistula matures, the

vein will be able to withstand the insertion of large-bore needles (14 to 16 gauge). The insertion of needles in the arterial and venous arms of the fistula permits attachments to the dialysis machine.

Complications associated with the AV fistula are infection, clotting, venous hypertension, and steal syndrome. Infection at the fistula site has direct access to systemic circulation and can precipitate septicemia. Localized infections present as reddened, tender, warm areas over the fistula, particularly at the anastomosis or needle puncture sites. Clotting sometimes causes severe pain and numbness in the affected arm; it can be confirmed by the absence of the bruit and thrill at the fistula site.

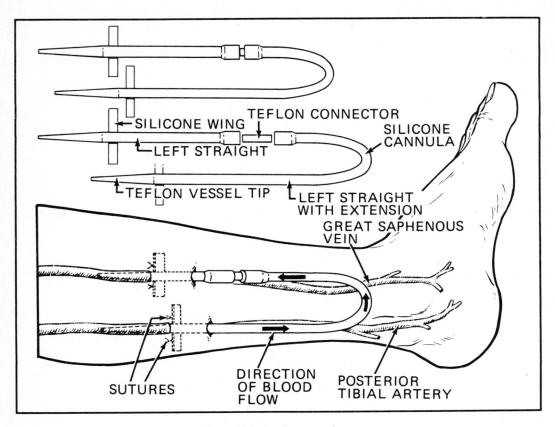

Figure 32-3. Arteriovenous shunt.

In venous hypertension, there is too much blood in the extremity distal to the fistula. This may cause ulcerations and may necessitate a fistula revision. In the steal syndrome, there is insufficient blood to the extremity due to excessive diversion of arterial blood to the vein at the anastomosis. Symptoms include coldness and poor function of the extremity. In severe cases, gangrene with necrosis of the extremity tips may develop. The steal syndrome is corrected by revising the fistula.

Once an access site is available, an evaluation of the patient's most recent electrolytes is made to determine what adjustments in the dialysate bath are to be made. An accurate predialysis weight of the patient is determined daily. By weighing the patient postdialysis, it is possible to calculate exactly how much fluid was removed or added.

Nursing Care

Infection is prevented by cleaning the shunt site daily using sterile technique and also by cleaning the fistula site until the incision is healed. If the shunt or fistula becomes infected, culture and sensitivity tests are done to identify the infecting organism. Once the organism is identified, intravenous antibiotics are started. If the shunt or fistula remains infected, it is removed and a new shunt or fistula is created.

The prevention of thrombosis is always a challenge. Anything that decreases blood flow increases the chance of thrombosis. Some examples are hypotension, hypovolemia, tourniquets, blood pressure cuffs, tight clothing and jewelry, heavy handbags and packages, and dehydration.

If the shunt is patent, one can see bright red blood flowing freely through it and it feels warm to touch.

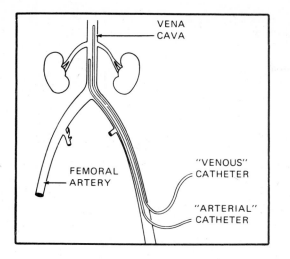

Figure 32-4. Shaldon catheters.

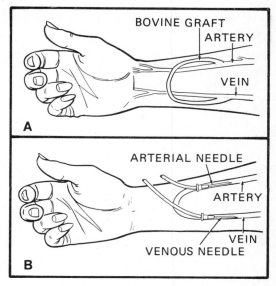

Figure 32-6. A graft in place (**A**) and placement of needles in a graft for hemodialysis (**B**).

There should not be any layering of the blood components (cells at the bottom, clear serum at the top). Proximal to the insertion site, one should feel a thrill (the turbulence of the arterial blood). With a stetho-

scope, one should hear a bruit (arterial blood turbulence). If either the thrill or bruit is absent, notify the physician immediately.

If the shunt becomes clotted, the physician may insert a catheter to remove the clot. After patency has been established, routine use of heparin will maintain patency.

To prevent hemorrhage due to shunt disconnection, clamps are attached to the dressing to ensure immediate availability. If the catheter becomes unconnected, the arterial cannula is clamped first to control excessive blood loss from the arterial system and then the venous cannula is clamped.

The precautions taken for shunts are also taken for fistulas. A thrill and bruit should be present. The arm with a fistula is not used for intravenous fluids, blood pressure monitoring, venipuncture, or injections. The fistula is cleansed daily using sterile technique. Bleeding, skin discoloration, or drainage is reported to the physician.

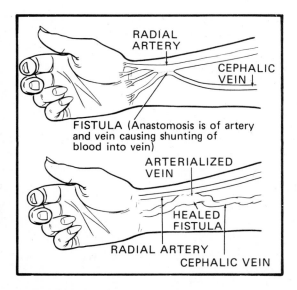

Figure 32-5. Anastomosis to form an arteriovenous fistula.

Complications

Problems associated with hemodialysis occur most often during the initial stages or during a procedure lasting more than four hours. Hypotension is caused by dehydration, sepsis, or blood loss. The patient may already be hypotensive or may rapidly become hypotensive when dialysis is initiated. This is treated by reducing the blood flow, discontinuing ultrafiltration (fluid removal), and giving fluids. If the patient does not respond to this method of treatment, dialysis is discontinued.

Cardiac dysrhythmias may be caused by potassium intoxication, but usually no specific electrolyte derangement can be identified. In some instances, dysrhythmias may be related to the development of transient myocardial ischemia as evidenced by premature ventricular contractions. Treatment consists of decreasing the blood flow and using appropriate medication as indicated. The dialysis procedure must be stopped if the dysrhythmia is severe or does not respond to treatment. Congestive heart failure in most instances is secondary to fluid overload, which can be reversed by ultrafiltration.

Air embolism may occur through an arterial or venous site. With arterial air embolism, air travels the arterial system to a point distal to the entry site. In the head, the emboli enters the small vessels of the brain. Death will occur if critical areas of the brain are destroyed.

Venous emboli migrate back to the lungs and may cause a pulmonary emboli. In the sitting patient with dialysis access in the lower extremities, air enters the venous system of the leg and travels to the inferior vena cava, then up through the right atrium to the superior vena cava, and then finally to the head. In this case, the symptoms are the same as for arterial emboli in the brain.

If the patient is lying flat when air is introduced, the air enters the right atrium and moves into the right ventricle. Essentially, the air is trapped in the right ventricle and cannot be propelled from the heart. Blood cannot enter the pulmonary system. The lack of pulmonary blood return to the left atrium quickly stops the pumping of blood into the systemic circulation.

The symptoms are deep respiration, coughing, cyanosis, unconsciousness, and then cessation of breathing. Auscultation over the heart reveals a "mill wheel" sound during both phases of contraction. This is the sound of air turbulence in the heart.

Once air embolism has occurred, rapid corrective action is imperative. There are several important differences in the resuscitation of a patient with an air embolism as compared with the usual cardiopulmonary resuscitation. The patient must be placed in Trendelenburg's position and turned on the left side. Once resuscitated, the patient must be kept in the Trendelenburg's left side position until the air is absorbed. This will prevent movement of the air into the cerebral tissues and heart and promote movement toward the feet (air will be higher than fluid). The absorption time will vary, but it usually takes from days to weeks; the mortality rate is extremely high.

Editor's Note

The topic of continuous arteriovenous hemofiltration, including concepts such as slow continuous ultrafiltration (SCUF) and continuous arteriovenous hemodialysis is not covered in this text. While the topic is of interest and of importance to a segment of the critically ill population, it does not seem like this information is to be covered on the CCRN exam. If this topic is of interest to you, please refer to several excellent nursing articles on this topic in the past few years. As a matter of interest, we did include a question on this topic in the practice test questions, but we doubt the actual CCRN exam will address this content area.

BIBLIOGRAPHY

Baer, C.L., & Lancaster, L.E. (1992). Acute renal failure. *Crit Care Nurse Q, 14,* 4, 1–21.

Calhoun, K.A. (1990). Serum potassium concentration abnormalities. *Crit Care Nurse Q, 13,* 3, 34–38.

Graves, L. (1990). Disorders of calcium, phosphorus, and magnesium. *Crit Care Nurse Q, 13,* 3, 3–13.

Guyton, A. (1986). *Textbook of Medical Physiology,* 7th ed. Philadelphia: W.B. Saunders Co.

Hudak, C., Gallo, B., & Benz, J. (1990). *Critical Care Nursing,* 5th ed. Philadelphia: J.B. Lippincott Co.

Innerarity, S.A. (1990). Electrolyte emergencies in the critically ill renal patient. *Crit Care Clin North Am, 2,* 1, 89–99.

Isley, W.L. (1990). Serum sodium concentration abnormalities. *Crit Care Nurse Q, 13,* 3, 82–88.

Kinney, M.R., Packa, D.R., & Dunbar, S.B. (1988). *AACN's*

Clinical Reference for Critical Care Nursing. St. Louis: McGraw-Hill Book Co.

Mars, D.R., & Treloar, O. (1984). Acute tubular necrosis-pathophysiology and treatment. *Heart Lung, 13,* 2, 194–201.

Metheny, N.M. (1992). *Fluid and Electrolyte Balance: Nursing Considerations,* 2nd ed. Philadelphia: J.B. Lippincott Co.

Norris, M.K. (1989). Acute tubular necrosis: Preventing complications. *DCCN, 8,* 1, 16–26.

PART 6

Endocrine

Teresa Halloran, RN, MSN, CCRN

CHAPTER 33
Introduction to the Endocrine System

Editor's Note

About 4% of the CCRN test (eight questions) addresses the endocrine system. According to the CCRN guideline from the AACN Certification Corporation, the key areas covered in the exam regarding endocrine dysfunctions include the following five areas: diabetes insipidus, inappropriate secretion of antidiuretic hormone, hyperglycemic hyperosmolar nonketotic coma, diabetic ketoacidosis, and acute hypoglycemia. Considering that the CCRN exam will probably contain only eight questions on these five areas, it is unlikely that any of the areas will be covered in great detail.

While the CCRN exam has not specifically addressed items that have been on the exam in the past, such as thyrotoxic crisis, myxedema coma, and acute adrenal insufficiency/ pheochromocytoma, we have left these chapters in for two reasons. First, a review of these chapters may give you insight into endocrine disturbances in general. Second, even though the exam may not specifically address these disorders, an understanding of the content may help answer questions that are indirectly related to these concepts.

As you review the following chapters, focus on key concepts rather than minor details. The endocrine system is a difficult area for many nurses taking the CCRN exam. Do your best to acquaint yourself with the information in these chapters while also noting patients in your units with endocrine disturbances. Using both this text and observations of patients will strengthen your ability to recall key concepts in endocrinology and increase the likelihood of correctly answering most of the exam questions on endocrinology.

HORMONAL PURPOSE

The primary function of the endocrine system is to regulate metabolic functioning of the body. Metabolic functioning includes chemical reactions and the rates of these reactions, growth, transportation of chemicals, secretions, and cellular metabolism.

A close interrelationship exists between the nervous system (responsible for integration of body processes) and the endocrine system (responsible for appropriate metabolic activity). Neuronal stimulation is required for some specific hormones to be secreted and/or to be secreted in adequate amounts.

The endocrine system is composed of specific glands (Fig. 33-1) that secrete their chemical substances directly into the bloodstream. The major single endocrine glands are the pituitary (also called the hypophysis) and the thyroid (Fig. 33-2). The parathyroids are usually four glands, not two sets of paired glands. The adrenals are one pair of endocrine glands. Other glands exist that contain endocrine components and function in both the endocrine system and another system. These glands are the ovaries and testes (collectively termed the gonads) and the pancreas. The thymus gland has a major role in immunology but is sometimes included in the endocrine system.

All endocrine glands are very vascular. The endocrine glands function by extracting substances from the blood to synthesize into complex hormones. Hormones are released from the specific endocrine glands into the veins that drain the glands themselves. The circulatory system is used to transport endocrine substances to target glands and tissues throughout the body.

Classification of Hormones
The substances secreted by endocrine glands are chemicals called hormones. Hormones exert a physiological control on body cells. Local hormones are those released in specific areas (or tissues), and they exert a

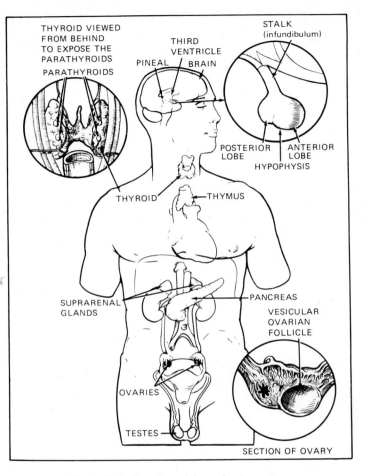

Figure 33-1. Overview of the endocrine system.

limited, local effect. Acetylcholine is an example of a local hormone having physiological control at some synapses in the nervous system. General hormones are secreted by a specific endocrine gland and transported by the vascular system to a specific, predetermined site.

Types of Hormones
Hormones may be amines, peptides, proteins (or protein derivatives), or steroids. Prostaglandins are often considered tissue hormones. The first three types of hormones are water soluble and do not require a carrier molecule for transportation throughout the body. Steroids and thyroxine are not water soluble and must have a carrier substance to transport them to their site

of action. The site of action for a hormone is known as the target cell.

Prostaglandins are unsaturated fatty acids of which three types have been identified according to their chemical structure. They are synthesized in the seminal vesicles, brain, liver, iris, kidneys, lungs, and thymus. Prostaglandins have a potent effect but are considered local, not general, hormones. Their major effects occur by diffusing to cells adjacent to those from which they are secreted. Only tiny amounts actually enter the bloodstream.

Important General Hormones
All of the general hormones are important for regulating functions in the body. However, dysfunctions of

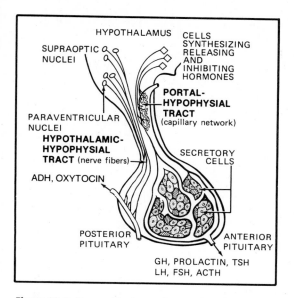

Figure 33-2. Paraventricular nucleus and supraoptic nucleus of the hypothalamus.

certain hormones would rarely, if ever, be a reason for admission to a critical-care area. These hormones include oxytocin, follicle-stimulating hormone, luteinizing hormone, prolactin, melanocyte-stimulating hormone, corticosterone, deoxycorticosterone, and androgens (including estrogens, progesterone, and testosterone). These hormones will not be discussed in this text. The general hormones that may precipitate an admission to a critical-care area because of dysfunction are listed in Table 33-1 and will be covered in the following three chapters.

Editor's Note

Although the actions of the hormones are important, remember that you should concentrate on general concepts rather than specific information. Terms such as amine hormones are for purposes of explanation. Do not expect to see this type of information on the CCRN exam.

Action of Hormones

Amine, Protein, and Peptide Hormones. These hormones include growth hormone, adrenocorticotropin, thyroid-stimulating hormone, parathyroid hormone, calcitonin, insulin, the catecholamines, glucagon, antidiuretic hormone, follicle-stimulating hormone, luteinizing hormone, and prolactin. Since these hormones do not require a carrier substance because they are water soluble, their concentrations may fluctuate rapidly and widely. These hormones are thought to react with specific surface receptors on the target cell membrane. This alters the membrane enzymes and leads to a change in the intracellular concentration of an enzyme. The hormone is called the first messenger, and the intracellular enzyme is called the second messenger. This second messenger is cAMP (cyclic 3′,5′-adenosine monophosphate). cAMP (within the cell) activates enzymes, causes protein synthesis, alters cell permeability, causes muscle relaxation and contraction, and causes secretion. It is by the action of cAMP that many hormones exert control over the cells.

TABLE 33-1 ENDOCRINE GLANDS AND HORMONES OF SIGNIFICANT IMPORTANCE

Glands	Hormones
Adenohypophysis (anterior pituitary)	Adrenocorticotropin, somatotropin or growth hormone, thyroid-stimulating hormone
Neurohypophysis (posterior pituitary)	Antidiuretic hormone, oxytocin
Thyroid	Thyroxine, triiodothyronine, calcitonin
Parathyroid	Parathyroid hormone (parathormone)
Adrenal medulla	Epinephrine, norepinephrine
Adrenal cortex	Glucocorticoids (cortisol), mineralocorticoids (aldosterone)
Pancreas	Insulin, glucagon

Steroids and Thyroxine. Steroids include the sex hormones, mineralocorticoids (aldosterone) and glucocorticoids (cortisol and corticosterone). Steroids and thyroxine are lipid soluable and are able to cross the cell membrane easily and then bind with an intracellular receptor. The hormone-receptor complex reacts with chromatin in the cell nucleus to synthesize specific proteins. Because these hormones are lipid chemicals, the reactions take longer to occur, but are no less potent than the amine, protein, and peptide hormone reactions.

Negative Feedback System

Some hormones are needed in very minute amounts in the body for variable amounts of time; some have prolonged action periods; and some affect and interact with other hormones, producing a very complex, intricate system to control. A control system must exist to maintain this complex system.

Most control systems, including the endocrine system, act by a negative feedback mechanism. When there is an increased hormone concentration, physiological control is increased and a stimulus is received in the hypothalamus. This results in an inhibition of hormone-releasing factors. In the same manner, when there are deficient or absent hormone concentrations, a stimulus is received in the hypothalamus that results in an increased release of hormone-stimulating factors. This again is a negative (or opposite) response to the stimulus sent to the hypothalamus. The greater the need for the hormone, the greater the intensity of the stimulus; similarly, the greater the concentration of the hormone, the less the intensity of the stimulus.

When a hormone concentration is deficient, as more hormone is produced and/or secreted, the physiological control of the body cells increases. With an increase in physiological control, the feedback stimulus relayed to the endocrine gland decreases in intensity and release of the hormone decreases as homeostasis is achieved. The reverse process applies when the hormone concentration is excessive.

It is known that the hypothalamus produces releasing and inhibiting hormones (or factors) whose single target is the anterior pituitary gland, the so-called master gland. It is believed that all hormones have releasing and inhibiting factors produced by the hypothalamus, but only eight are known at this time (Table 33-2).

The principles of achieving regulatory control are similar for all of the hormones listed in Table 33-1, with the exception of the hormones of the adrenal medulla. The hormones of the adrenal medulla (epinephrine and norepinephrine) are under control of the autonomic nervous system. The hormones of the neurohypophysis (the posterior pituitary) are controlled by the concentration of the substance released from the target cell "feeding back" to the hypothalamus. The release of the hormone leads to a change in a plasma constituent that regulates hypothalamic activity rather than the gland itself. Tropic hormones, secreted only by the adenohypophysis (anterior pituitary), cause an increase in size and secretion rates of other endocrine

TABLE 33-2 RELEASING AND INHIBITING FACTORS PRODUCED BY THE HYPOTHALAMUS

Releasing Hormones	Inhibiting Hormones	Peripheral Hormones
Growth hormone-releasing hormone	Growth hormone-inhibiting hormone	Growth hormone
Prolactin-releasing hormone	Prolactin-inhibiting hormone	Prolactin
Corticotropin-releasing hormone	—	Adrenal steroids
Follicle-stimulating hormone-releasing hormone	—	Gonadal steroids
Luteinizing hormone-releasing hormone	—	Gonadal hormones
Thyrotropin-releasing hormone	—	Thyroid hormones

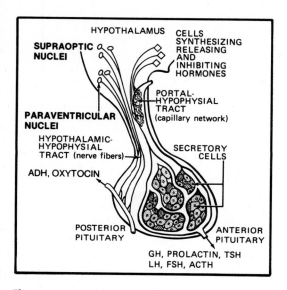

Figure 33-3. Portal-hypophysial tract and hypothalamic-hypophysial tract of the hypothalamus.

glands and are controlled by the negative feedback system as well as other factors.

All adenohypophysial hormone-releasing and -inhibiting factors (except the adrenal medulla) are car-ried by the hypothalamic-hypophysial tract from the hypothalamus into the median eminence (Fig. 33-3) and then into the pituitary stalk.

Editor's Note

Remember, aspects of anatomy such as the pituitary stalk are usually not addressed on the CCRN exam. It may be helpful to understand basic concepts of anatomy for general understanding, but do not spend too much time attempting to memorize this type of detail.

In the stalk, the portal-hypophysial system carries the releasing and inhibiting factors into the adenohypophysis for storage until needed.

The two neurohypophysial hormone-releasing and -inhibiting factors are formed in the paraventricular nucleus and supraoptic nucleus in the hypothalamus (Fig. 33-3). They are then carried by nerve fibers into the neurohypophysis for storage.

CHAPTER 34

Anatomy, Physiology, and Dysfunction of the Pituitary Gland

Editor's Note

As you review the functions of the pituitary gland, do not attempt to memorize basic anatomical features. Rarely would anatomy questions, such as the type of tissue from which the pituitary arises, be on the CCRN exam. Skim these areas with the goal of acquainting yourself with terms and concepts. Focus your attention on the key functions of the gland and how they may cause clinical disturbances.

The pituitary gland is often referred to as the master gland of the body since its hormones control and regulate many other endocrine glands. The pituitary gland is now often called the hypophysis. It has two lobes: the anterior pituitary, known as the adenohypophysis, and the posterior pituitary, known as the neurohypophysis. A mnemonic may help keep these names straight. The anterior pituitary starts with an "a," as does the adenohypophysis (anterior = adeno).

ANATOMY OF THE PITUITARY GLAND (HYPOPHYSIS)

The hypophysis develops from two types of tissues. The adenohypophysis is an outgrowth of the pharyngeal tissue, which grows upward toward the brain in the embryo. The neurohypophysis is an outgrowth of the hypothalamus, which grows downward in the embryo.

Location and Size

The hypophysis is located in the sella turcica, which is a hollow depression in the sphenoid bone (Fig. 34-1)

of the brain. It is a small gland weighing 0.5 to 1 gram and is about 1 cm in diameter. The hypophysis gland is attached to the hypothalamus by the hypophysial stalk.

Lobes of the Hypophysis

The two lobes of the hypophysis are separated by the pars intermedia (Fig. 34-2). The pars intermedia is almost avascular and is a small band of fibers between the hypophysial lobes. The function of the pars intermedia, other than to separate the anterior lobe of the hypophysis from the posterior lobe, is unknown.

Structure of the Adenohypophysis

The adenohypophysis is composed of epithelial-type cells (embryologic extension of pharnygeal tissue). Many different types of these epithelial cells have been identified for each hormone formed.

In the adenohypophysis are microscopic blood

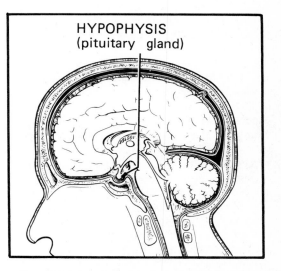

Figure 34-1. Location of the hypophysis (pituitary gland).

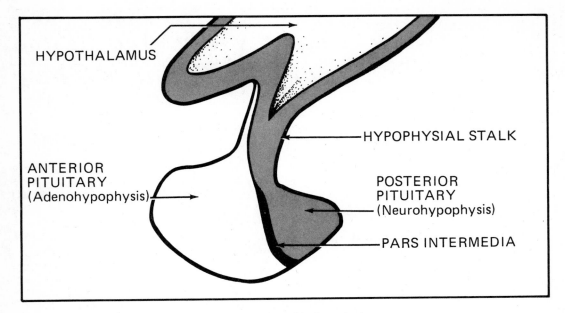

Figure 34-2. Lobes of the hypophysis.

vessels composing the hypothalamic-hypophysial portal vessels (Fig. 34-3). These vessels connect the hypothalamus and the adenohypophysis (by passage through the pituitary stalk) and terminate in the anterior pituitary sinuses.

Substances carried in the hypothalamic-hypophysial vessels are actually hormone factors and not hormones per se. These factors are releasing and inhibiting factors (see Table 33-2). For each adenohypophysial hormone, there is an associated releasing factor. For some adenohypophysial hormones, there are inhibitory factors.

Structure of the Neurohypophysis

Many cells of the neurohypophysis (posterior pituitary) are called pituicytes. Pituicytes are like the glial cells of the nervous system. The pituicytes provide supporting tissue for nerve tracts that arise from the supraoptic nuclei and paraventricular nuclei of the hypothalamus. The supraoptic nuclei and the paraventricular nuclei form the neurohypophysis hormones. These hormones are carried by the nerve tracts through the hypophysial stalk and terminate in bulbous knobs in the neurohypophysis. The knobs lie on the surface of capillaries. As hormone that were formed in the hypothalamus and stored in the bulbous knobs are needed, exocytosis

occurs. Exocytosis is the discharge of substances from a cell that are too large to diffuse through the cell membrane. The hormone is thus secreted from the bulbous knobs onto the capillaries and is absorbed into the vascular system. The adenohypophysis has a vascular relationship to the hypothalamus, whereas the neurohypophysis has a neural relationship.

PHYSIOLOGY OF THE PITUITARY GLAND (HYPOPHYSIS)

The action of the various hormones is to control the activity of the target glands and target tissues. Hormones exert an effect on target tissues by altering the rates at which cellular processes occur. There are two basic mechanisms of hormone action: cyclic AMP (cAMP) and genetic activation. cAMP initiates actions characteristic of the target cell. For example, parathyroid hormone cells activated by cAMP form and secrete parathyroid hormone (parathormone); specific cells in the pancreas activated by cAMP form and secrete glucagon. Known hormones affected by cAMP include secretin, glucagon, parathormone, vasopressin, catecholamines, adrenocorticotropin, follicle-

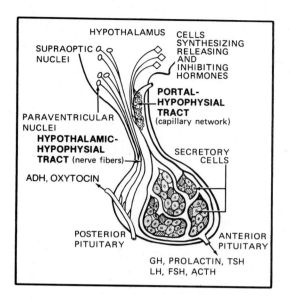

Figure 34-3. The hypothalamic-hypophysial portal vessels.

stimulating hormone, thyroid-stimulating hormone, and hypothalamic releasing factors.

Hormones of the Adenohypophysis

Eight hormone factors, all formed in the hypothalamus, are secreted by the adenohypophysis:

1. Thyrotropin-releasing hormone, which causes the release of thyroid-stimulating hormone.
2. Growth hormone-releasing hormone, which causes release of growth hormone or somatotropin. Growth hormone-inhibiting hormone or somatostatin inhibits the release of growth hormone.
3. Corticotropin-releasing hormone, which causes the release of adrenocorticotropin.
4. Follicle-stimulating hormone-releasing hormone, which causes release of follicle-stimulating hormone.
5. Luteinizing hormone-releasing hormone, which causes release of luteinizing hormone.
6. Prolactin-inhibiting hormone, which causes inhibition of prolactin secretion.
7. Human chorionic gonadotropin.
8. Human placental lactogen.

Action of Adenohypophysial Hormones

All of the major adenohypophysial hormones except growth hormone have an effect upon a target gland. Thyroid and parathyroid hormonal action is discussed in Chapter 35. Hormonal action of the adrenal gland is discussed in Chapter 36. Hormonal action of the pancreas is discussed in Chapter 37.

Growth Hormone and Metabolism

Growth hormone, also called somatotropin, has a general effect upon bones, organs, and soft tissues and is therefore considered a peripheral hormone. It influences the growth of body tissues.

Growth hormone has an important role in all aspects of metabolism. Growth hormone increases the rate of intracellular protein synthesis throughout the body. It is a factor in the mobilization of fatty acids from adipose tissue and in the conversion of these fats into energy. Growth hormone conserves carbohydrates by decreasing glucose utilization in the body.

Growth Hormone Factors

There are specific factors that stimulate or inhibit the release of growth hormone. The most common factors inhibiting the release of growth hormone include hyperglycemia, sustained corticosteroid therapy at high levels, and the release of growth hormone-inhibiting factor from the hypothalamus. Common factors promoting the release of growth hormone include pituitary tumors, hypoglycemia, exercise, decreased amino acid levels, and the release of growth hormone-releasing hormone from the hypothalamus.

Growth hormone secretion follows a diurnal pattern, with most release occurring in the first two hours of deep sleep. This follows the non-REM stage of sleep pattern.

Growth Hormone and Bones

Once the epiphyses of the long bones have united with the bone shafts, there can be no increase in the length of the bones. The thickness of the bones can still increase, however.

If there is oversecretion of growth hormone (commonly tumor related) prior to adolescence, all body tissues grow rapidly, including bones. The result is gigantism in which a height of 8 to 9 feet is not uncommon. Most giants are hyperglycemic, and 10% will develop diabetes mellitus. Giants who do not receive treatment usually die in early adulthood due to deterioration of the hypophysis. Since most gigantism is due to a tumor in the adenohypophysis, treatment is surgical removal of the tumor if possible. Radiation therapy may be tried if surgery is not feasible.

If there is oversecretion of growth hormone after adolescence, the result is acromegaly (Fig. 34-4). In acromegaly, soft tissues (especially the tongue, lips, liver, and kidneys) become greatly enlarged. Bones grow in thickness. The most affected bones are the membranous bones—the cranium, nose, lower jaw-

bone, forehead, and small bones of the hands and feet. Overgrowth of vertebrae may cause a kyphosis (hunchback). Treatment of acromegaly is directed toward arrest of the disease process by excising a pituitary tumor if possible. Reversal of the process is not usual.

Inadequate secretion of growth hormone results in dwarfism (growth retardation). In most cases, body growth is proportional but markedly decreased (Fig. 34-5). Mental retardation is not usual. If growth hormone is the only pituitary deficiency (true in 10%

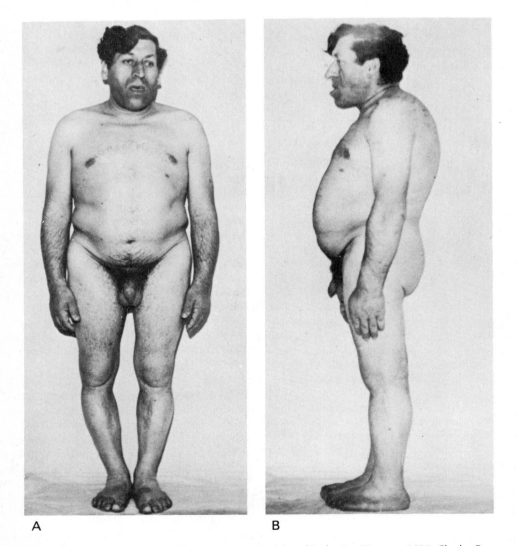

A   **B**

Figure 34-4. (**A** and **B**) Acromegaly. From Kosowicz, Atlas of Endocrine Diseases. 1978, Charles Press.

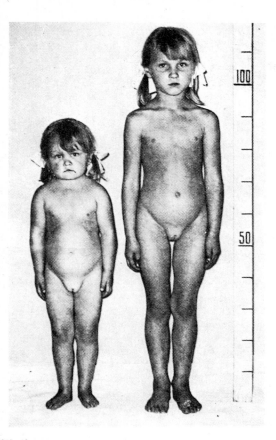

Figure 34-5. Dwarfism in two sisters, 8 years old (left) and 6 years old.

of the cases), the dwarf will experience puberty and may reproduce.

Hormones of the Neurohypophysis
Two hormones are released by the neurohypophysis: antidiuretic hormone (ADH), also called vasopressin, and oxytocin. Oxytocin will not be discussed in this text.

ADH is formed mainly in the supraoptic nuclei of the hypothalamus. (The paraventricular nuclei mainly form oxytocin. The ration of ADH to oxytocin formed in the supraoptic nuclei is 6:1, whereas the ratio is 1:6 in the paraventricular nuclei.) ADH is transported from the supraoptic nuclei by neurophysins. Neurophysins are protein carriers that bind very loosely with ADH and oxytocin to transport these hormones to the neurohypophysis for storage until needed.

Editor's Note:

One or two questions may be expected on ADH influence on clinical conditions.

Action of Antidiuretic Hormone
ADH alters the permeability of the distal convoluted tubules and the collecting ducts of the kidney. Without ADH, the tubules and ducts are impermeable to water. In the presence of ADH, these tubules and ducts become permeable to water, thus allowing large quantities of water to leave the tubules and collecting ducts and reenter the hypertonic medullary interstitial fluid. This helps to conserve and balance the fluid content of the body.

Control of Antidiuretic Hormone
Serum sodium levels and extracellular fluid osmolality exert a major influence on ADH. Osmoreceptors shrink when hypertonicity of the extracellular fluid exists. The osmoreceptors emit impulses to the hypothalamus, and ADH is released from the neurohypophysis to reabsorb water from the kidneys and reestablish homeostasis. When body fluids become diluted, stimulated osmoreceptors result in the inhibition of ADH, and water is not reabsorbed from the kidneys. ADH is controlled by many factors in addition to serum sodium and extracellular osmolality. Inadequate blood volume stimulates volume receptors in the periphery, the carotid sinus, the left atrium of the heart, and the aortic arch, stimulating release of ADH. ADH response is much greater in hemorrhagic states than in altered osmolality states. Trauma, anxiety, pain, and specific drugs enhance ADH release. ADH release is inhibited by a decreased serum osmolality and pituitary surgery.

NEUROHYPOPHYSIAL DYSFUNCTION

There are two main neurohypophysial disorders: diabetes insipidus and the syndrome of inappropriate ADH (SIADH).

Diabetes Insipidus
When there are decreased levels of ADH, diuresis and dehydration occur. Decreased levels of ADH occur

when there is damage or destruction of the ADH neurons in the supraoptic and paraventricular neurons of the hypothalamus. Diabetes insipidus results.

Etiology. The two leading etiologies of diabetes insipidus are hypothalamic or pituitary tumor and closed head injuries with damage to the supraoptic nuclei and/or hypothalamus. Postoperative diabetes insipidus is usually transient. Other causes include inflammatory and degenerative systemic conditions, but these are not common.

Clinical Presentation. Symptoms of diabetes insipidus include dilute urine (until severe dehydration occurs) with a specific gravity between 1.001 and 1.005. Urinary output varies from 4 to 15 liters per day. Polyuria is often of sudden onset. Polyuria may not occur until one to three days after injury due to the utilization of stored ADH in the neurohypophysis. Polydipsia will occur unless the thirst center has been damaged. There is an increased serum osmolality and a decreased urine osmolality. A relative diabetes insipidus may occur in cases of high-dose, lengthy steroid therapy with a specific gravity of the urine ranging from 1.000 to 1.009, urine osmolality less than 500 mosm, and urinary volume about 6 to 9 liters per day.

Treatment. The objective of therapy is first to prevent dehydration and electrolyte imbalances while determining and treating the underlying cause. A variety of replacement therapy modalities are available. Aqueous pitressin may be given as an intravenous bolus, as a continuous infusion, and subcutaneously. It is a short-acting ADH therapy. Desmopressin acetate (DDAVP) is a synthetic ADH and can be used as an intravenous or nasal spray therapy. The advantage of DDAVP is a longer duration of action. Vasopressin tannate in oil can be given by subcutaneous or intramuscular injection. The substance must be warmed and vigorously shaken prior to administration. Following head trauma or neurosurgery, an aqueous vasopressin of 5 to 10 units subcutaneously may be used to decrease the risk of water intoxication. Diabetes insipidus may resolve in only a few days in these conditions.

Nursing Intervention. Of prime importance is maintaining an accurate intake and output record of the patient. Monitoring of body weight, electrolytes, urine specific gravities, blood urea nitrogen, and signs of

dehydration and shock will allow for early intervention in cases prone to deterioration.

SYNDROME OF INAPPROPRIATE SECRETION OF ADH

SIADH is the second dysfunction of ADH. In SIADH, there is either increased secretion or increased production of ADH. This increase is unrelated to osmolality and causes a slight increase in total body water. There is severely decreased sodium (hyponatremia) and osmolar (hypo-osmolality) concentration in extracellular fluid and serum.

Etiology
SIADH is occasionally caused by pituitary tumor, but much more commonly by a bronchogenic (oat cell) or pancreatic carcinoma. Head injuries, other endocrine disorders (Addison's disease and hypopituitarism), pulmonary disease (such as pneumonia or lung abcesses), central nervous system infections (and tumors), and drugs such as tricyclics, oral hypoglycemic agents, diuretics, and cytotoxic agents are all possible etiologies.

Clinical Presentation and Complications. Symptoms produced by SIADH reflect the interaction between the underlying condition and excessive water retention. Symptoms are mainly neurologic and nonspecific. The most common symptoms of SIADH are personality changes, headache, decreased mentation, lethargy, nausea, vomiting, diarrhea, anorexia, decreased tendon reflexes, seizures, and coma. Complications of SIADH include seizures, coma, and death.

Laboratory Recognition of SIADH. The cardinal laboratory abnormality in SIADH consists of plasma hyponatremia and hypo-osmolality occurring simultaneously with inappropriate hyperosmolarity of the urine. Another feature that separates SIADH from other conditions that produce hyponatremia is the appropriately high urinary sodium excretion. Other laboratory findings are nonspecific.

Treatment. The first step in treating SIADH is to restrict fluid intake to prevent water intoxication. Then, the objective of therapy is to correct electrolyte imbalances. In severe cases, 3% hypertonic saline and intravenous furosemide (Lasix) are used. Supplemental potassium is usually necessary. Demeclocycline (less than 2400 mg/day) and lithium carbonate (up to 900 mg/day) have proven useful by interfering with the normal ADH effect of increasing cAMP in the distal tubules and collecting ducts.

Nursing Intervention.

With SIADH, it is necessary to maintain strict fluid restrictions and to monitor the patient for electrolyte imbalances as indicated by confusion, weakness, lethargy, vomiting, and/or seizures. If the patient is comatose, turning, suctioning as needed, and standard nursing care procedures are required. Cardiac monitoring will allow for early identification of impending hyperkalemia and its associated cardiac problems. Nutritional needs of the patient must be met without increasing fluid intake. Emotional support of the alert patient by stating that this condition can be treated successfully will help to obtain cooperation from the patient unless there is an untreated psychological problem.

CHAPTER 35

Anatomy, Physiology, and Dysfunction of the Thyroid and Parathyroid Glands

Editor's Note

The most recent CCRN guidelines do not discuss the care of patients with thyroid and parathyroid disturbances as part of the CCRN exam. However, understanding their function is useful for understanding other clinical conditions, particularly electrolyte and cardiovascular responses. You may be able to concentrate less heavily on this chapter, however, than in the past.

ANATOMY OF THE THYROID GLAND

Location and Shape

The thyroid gland is in the anterior portion of the neck at the lower part of the larynx and the upper part of the trachea (Fig. 35-1). The thyroid has two lobes which, with a little imagination, resemble a butterfly's wings. The lobes lie on either side of the trachea and are connected by a narrow band of tissue called the isthmus, which lies across the second and third tracheal rings.

Internal Structures

Each lobe of the thyroid is divided into lobules by dense connective tissue. Each lobule (Fig. 35-2) is composed of saclike structures called follicles. The follicles are lined with cuboidal epithelium.

The follicular sacs are filled with a thick, viscous material called colloid. Colloid is actually thyroglobulin, which is converted to thyroxine as needed. Storage, synthesis, and release of thyroxine are controlled by the hypothalamic releasing hormone (factor)

and the thyroid-stimulating hormone of the adenohypophysis.

PHYSIOLOGY OF THE THYROID GLAND

The thyroid gland secretes three important hormones: thyroxine, triiodothyronine, and calcitonin. Approximately 90% of the hormone is thyroxine (T4) and 10% is triiodothyronine (T3). In peripheral tissues, thyroxine is converted to triiodothyronine. The functions of these two hormones are essentially the same. The in-

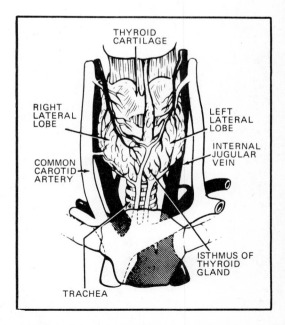

Figure 35-1. Location and shape of the thyroid gland.

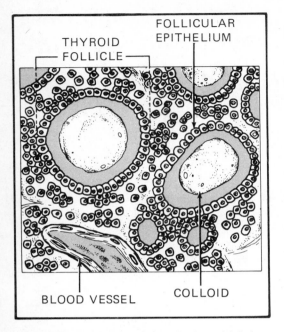

Figure 35-2. Internal structure of the thyroid follicles.

tensity, speed of action, and formation of these hormones are different.

Iodide Trapping (the Iodide Pump)

To form thyroid hormones, iodides must be removed from blood and extracellular fluids and transported into the thyroid gland follicles. The basal membrane of the thyroid gland has the ability to transfer iodide into the thyroid cells. The iodide then diffuses throughout the thyroid cells and follicular sacs. This process is known as iodide trapping. The iodide is stored until thyroglobulin in needed. It then becomes ionized by the enzyme peroxidase and hydrogen peroxide, converting the iodide into iodine at the point where thyroglobulin is released intracellularly. If the peroxidase system is blocked, thyroid hormone production ceases.

Organification of Thyroglobulin

Thyroglobulin is the major component reacting with iodide to form thyroxine. Thyroid cells synthesize the glycoprotein thyroglobulin, which is the colloid filling the follicular sacs. The binding of iodide with the glycoprotein is termed the organification of thyroglobulin, and the iodide is then an oxidized iodine. The oxidized iodine will slowly bond with tyrosine (an amino acid). In the presence of enzymes, this bonding is very rapid.

Chemical reactions progress to yield thyroxine and triiodothyronine. The thyroid hormones are stored in an amount that is equal to the normal body requirements for one to three months.

Release of Thyroxine and Triiodothyronine

These two thyroid hormones separate from the thyroglobulin molecules. Separation is a multistep process involving several intermediate chemicals. The end result is that thyroxine and triiodothyronine are lysed from the glucoprotein. Once freed, these thyroid hormones enter the venous circulatory system of the thyroid gland itself and are carried into the systemic circulation. The strongest stimulation for release of these hormones is cold temperature. Thyrotropin-releasing hormone factors will stimulate release of thyroid-stimulating hormone, and thyroxine and triiodothyronine will be released from the thyroid gland (but not in as rapid a response as to cold).

The release of these hormones is inhibited by heat, insufficient hypothalamic releasing factors (which result in insufficient thyroid-stimulating hormones), and/or increases in plasma glucocorticoids.

Action of Thyroxine and Triiodothyronine

An interesting "rule of four" exists. Once these two hormones are in the peripheral tissues, triiodothyronine is four times as strong in initiating metabolic activities as thyroxine. Thyroxine's effect upon the tissues will last four times as long as triiodothyronine's effect. Thus, these two hormones balance each other very well.

Thyroxine Function

Approximately 1 mg of iodine per week is needed for normal thyroxine formation. Iodides are absorbed from the gastrointestinal tract. Two-thirds of ingested iodides are excreted in the urine, and the remaining one-third is used by the thyroid gland to form the glycoprotein thyroglobulin.

The major effect of the thyroid hormones is to increase all of the metabolic activities of the body, excluding the brain, spleen, lungs, retina, and testes. In children, the thyroid hormones also promote growth.

Production, Release, and Action of Calcitonin

Calcitonin is manufactured in special thyroid cells called parafollicular cells or C cells. These cells are found in the interstitial tissue between the follicles of the thyroid gland.

An increase in plasma concentration of calcium stimulates the release of calcitonin, as will the ingestion or administration of magnesium and/or glucagon.

Calcitonin functions in a relationship with parathyroid hormone more so than with the thyroid hormones. Calcitonin's major effect is on bones. Calcitonin reduces plasma calcium levels by an immediate decrease in osteoclast activity, a transient increase in osteoblastic activity, and a prolonged prevention of new osteoclast formation. Calcitonin also interacts with parathormone in the urinary excretion of calcium, magnesium, phosphates, and other electrolytes.

ANATOMY OF THE PARATHRYOID GLANDS

Size and Location
Four small, flat, roundish glands are located on the posterior surface of the lateral lobes of the thyroid (Fig. 35-3). Usually one parathyroid gland is located at the superior end of each thyroid lobe, and another gland is located at the inferior end of each lateral lobe of the thyroid. This location may vary considerably. It

is normal to have four glands; however, there may be fewer or more than four glands.

Internal Structure
Two types of cells have been identified in the adult parathyroid glands. Chief cells (Fig. 35-4) are the main cells in the adult. Oxyphil cells (Fig. 35-4) are present in adults but are frequently absent in children. The function of oxyphil cells is unknown. There is the possibility that oxyphil cells are modified chief cells.

PHYSIOLOGY OF THE PARATHYROID GLANDS

Hormone Secretion
The parathyroid glands secrete a hormone termed parathormone. If two of the glands are inadvertently removed during a subtotal thyroidectomy, the remaining glands will produce sufficient parathormone for the body's needs. Some parathyroid tissue should be preserved. This tissue will hypertrophy and continue to secrete parathormone. Chief cells in the parathyroid

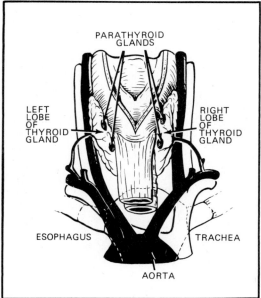

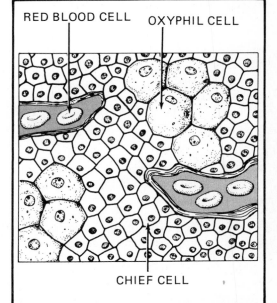

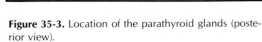

Figure 35-3. Location of the parathyroid glands (posterior view).

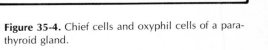

Figure 35-4. Chief cells and oxyphil cells of a parathyroid gland.

gland are responsible for the secretion of parathormone. Oxyphil cells may also secrete some hormones.

When hypothalamic releasing factors are stimulated by a decreased serum calcium level or an increased serum magnesium/phosphate concentration, a series of reactions occurs, resulting in the secretion of parathormone.

Parathormone release is also inhibited by hypothalamic factors when serum calcium is increased or when there is an excessive concentration of vitamin D.

Action of Parathyroid Hormone

The main action of parathormone and calcitonin is conservation of normal blood calcium levels. Parathormone decreases renal tubular reabsorption of phosphates, sodium, potassium, and amino acids. It increases reabsorption of calcium, magnesium, and hydrogen ions.

Activated vitamin D is essential for parathormone to function appropriately. The release of parathyroid hormone is controlled by a negative feedback mechanism between the blood calcium levels, the hypothalamus, and the parathyroid glands.

Target cells of the parathyroid glands include all bones (in a reciprocal relationship with calcium), kidney cells, and the gastrointestinal tract, if there is sufficient ingestion of vitamin D.

THYROID DYSFUNCTION

Common thyroid disorders result from too little (hypothyroidism) or too much (hyperthyroidism) of the thyroid hormone secretions. Hypothyroidism, also called myxedema, results from a lack of thyroid hormones. Myxedema coma is the result of severe deficiency or total absence of thyroid hormones. Hyperthyroidism is also called Graves's disease. The fulminant form of hyperthyroidism is called thyroid storm or thyrotoxic crisis. Storm or crisis may occur at any time.

Hypothyroidism (Myxedema)

Hypothyroidism is present when there is insufficient secretion of thyroid hormone. In hypothyroidism, the thyroid gland is usually small and consists of large amounts of fibrous tissue. Some 60% of all cases have autoantibodies present, caused by an autoimmune process.

Hypothyroidism is a chronic disease that is ten times more common in females than in males and occurs in all age groups, but most commonly after the age of 50. Physiological signs and symptoms of hypothyroidism are the same regardless of the etiologic basis.

Etiology. Hypothyroidism can result from a thyroidectomy. More common etiologies include inadequate dosage of thyroid medications in the known hypothyroid patient and postthyroidectomy patient. Lack of compliance with the prescribed medical regimen, cessation of medication, pituitary tumors, autoimmune processes, and idiopathic factors are other causes of hypothyroidism. Myxedema coma can develop from a decompensation of a preexisting hypothyroid state due to infection, trauma, exposure to cold, administration of sedatives, physical stress, or anesthesia.

Clinical Presentation. A common symptom is edema of the face and a puffiness of the eyelids (Fig. 35-5). Bloating of the face produces a broad, round shape. Lips become thickened and develop a cyanotic hue. Weakness, fatigability, exertional dyspnea, sensitivity of cold, paresthesia of the fingers, and loss of hearing are frequent symptoms. Lethargy, lack of concentration, failing memory, and alteration in mentation occur. Skin and hair changes are often early signs of hypothyroidism. The skin becomes dry and scaly; the hair becomes friable and dry and falls out. Total body hair may be involved. These signs increase as the condition progresses to myxedema coma.

Complications. The most serious complication of hypothyroidism is its progression to myxedema coma and death if untreated. Hypothyroidism is associated with an increased incidence of early, severe arteriosclerosis. Anemia and increased sensitivity to hypnotic and sedative drugs may become serious problems. Resistance to infection is suppressed, and response to treatment of infection is poor. Angina and myocardial infarction are especially common after replacement thyroid therapy is started. The therapy improves and increases myocardial action, but the arteriosclerosis prevents increased delivery of oxygen to the myocardium. Commonly, this results in ischemia and infarction.

Treatment. The optimum treatment for hypothyroidism is early intervention. The only possibility for pre-

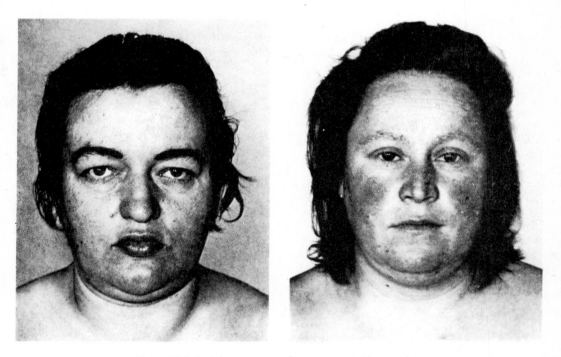

Figure 35-5. Facial appearance of two patients with myxedema.

vention of complications is the early recognition of hypothyroidism and close monitoring of medication therapy for the remainder of the patient's life. This, of course, necessitates the patient's compliance with the medical regimen.

Usual thyroid hormone replacement may be accomplished with the following:

1. Desiccated thyroid extract (thyroid USP) in daily doses of 60 mg per os (PO), with an increase every 15 to 30 days to a daily maximum of 180 mg PO.
2. Levothroxine sodium of L-thyroxine sodium (Synthroid) in doses of 0.025 to 0.1 mg PO daily, with an increase to 0.05 to 0.1 mg every one to four weeks until the patient is stable. The maintenance dose is 0.1 to 0.4 mg daily PO.
3. Liothyronine sodium (T3) (Cytomel), 25 mcg daily PO, increased to 12.5 to 25 mcg daily every one to two weeks until the patient is stable. The usual maintenance dose is 25 to 75 mcg daily PO.

Editor's Note

Do not attempt to remember all of these dosages. For the CCRN test, keep in mind basic concepts such as that hypothyroidism (if addressed at all) simply requires thyroid hormone replacement.

Myxedema Coma
Myxedema coma is a life-threatening emergency that is fatal without treatment.

Clinical Presentation. Myxedema coma is characterized by hypothermia, hypoventilation, hyponatremia, hyporeflexia, hypotension, and a bradycardia. The crisis occurs more commonly in winter than in summer due to exposure to cold. Myxedema crisis also occurs frequently following trauma, infection, and central nervous system depression.

The most frequent complication not already mentioned is seizures, which may be almost continuous as death becomes imminent.

Treatment. A multiple-systems approach must be used in treating this emergency. Mechanical ventilation is used to control hypoventilation, carbon dioxide narcosis, and respiratory arrest. Intravenous hypertonic normal saline and glucose will correct the dilutional hyponatremia and hypoglycemia. Hydrocortisone (100 mg daily) may be used to treat a possible adrenocortical insufficiency (a commonly associated problem). Thyroid therapy is started immediately without waiting for laboratory confirmation of the diagnosis. Levothyroxine sodium (L-thyroxine sodium) is the most commonly used drug in this emergency. Intravenous doses of 0.2 to 0.5 mg during the first 24 hours may be followed by an additional 0.1 to 0.3 mg intravenously if required after 24 hours. Oral doses may then be tolerated. Vasoactive drugs may be used to support blood pressure. Bradycardia may require treatment with drugs or with a temporary pacemaker.

Hyperthyroidism

Toxic goiter and thyrotoxicosis are synonyms for hyperthyroidism. Hyperthyroidism due to Graves's disease is thought to be an autoimmune process, although the terms are used interchangeably.

Etiology. In hyperthyroidism, the thyroid gland enlarges, usually to two or more times the normal size. This releases excess thyroid hormones into the body, increasing the systemic adrenergic activity. Hyperthyroidism is thought to be caused by a failure of the negative feedback system. Some cases are due to thyroid adenomas, goiters, or familial traits.

Clinical Presentation. Exophthalmos (protruding eyeballs) is a clinical sign of hyperthyroidism or Graves's disease (Fig. 32-6). The common signs and symptoms are marked fatigue accompanied by insomnia, tachycardia, heat intolerance, emotional lability, irritability, nervousness, and weight loss (often extreme).

Diagnosis. The diagnosis is confirmed by T3 and T4 test results and an increased ^{131}I uptake by the thyroid. Some physicians feel that the ^{131}I test is the only reliable index, along with the patient's symptoms, to establish a diagnosis of hypo- or hyperthyroidism.

Complications. Heart failure, malnutrition, and ventilatory failure (due to exhaustion) are common. A more life-threatening complication is thyroid storm.

Treatment. Treatment may be medical or surgical. Propylthiouracil or methimazole is given orally for six weeks to decrease synthesis and secretions of hormones from the thyroid. After the patient is euthyroid, ^{131}I or a subtotal thyroidectomy may be used as definitive therapy. The patient usually requires daily thyroid medication (for life) after surgery.

Thyrotoxic Crisis (Thyroid Storm)

Thyrotoxic crisis is a metabolic emergency and has a greater than 20% mortality rate.

Pathophysiology. Pathophysiology is the same as for hyperthyroidism.

Etiology. Any factor that increases synthesis and secretion of thyroid hormones may cause a storm. Etiologic factors include subtotal thyroidectomy (due to release of thyroid hormones during the surgery), ketoacidotic states, abrupt cessation of antithyroid drugs, or overdose of thyroid medications (intentional or otherwise). Trauma, stress, or infection may precipitate a crisis.

Clinical Presentation. The thyroid storm syndrome characteristically includes hyperthermia (up to 105°F), tachydysrhythmias, diarrhea, dehydration, diaphoresis, and altered neurologic status, including agitation, tremors, hyperkinesia, delirium, and stupor or coma. Nausea and vomiting with weight loss are common.

Complications. If untreated, thyroid storm results in heart failure, exhaustion, coma, and death. With treatment, the sequence is frequently the same. Thyroid storm is most often seen in the summer in undiagnosed or inadequately treated hyperthyroid persons. The presence of stress, infection, nonthyroid surgery, diabetic ketoacidosis, and trauma may result in thyroid storm so intense that it is not amenable to reversal.

Treatment. Treatment of thyroid storm is of an emergency nature. Treatment is started without waiting for laboratory confirmation of the diagnosis. The first objective is to support vital functions, which necessitates respiratory, cardiac, and renal monitoring.

Second, a reversal of the peripheral effects of ex-

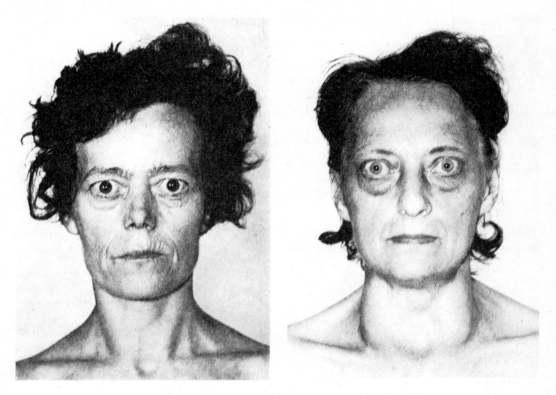

Figure 35-6. Facial appearance of two patients with hyperthyroidism.

cessive thyroid hormone is achieved by intravenous propranolol hydrochloride (Inderal) to decrease the hypermetabolic activity. Propranolol is a beta-adrenergic blocker used to control tachycardias, which are often resistant to digitalis therapy. Propranolol is changed to oral doses as soon as possible, since effects may last four to eight hours. Reserpine in doses of 0.5 to 1 mg intramuscularly and then 1 to 2.5 mg intramuscularly every four to six hours helps reverse peripheral effects, provides sedation, decreases anxiety, and may help reduce the tachycardia. The maximum dose is 4 mg. When tolerated, 0.1 to 0.5 mg PO daily is given for maintenance.

Third, reduction of the available and circulating thyroid hormones must be achieved. Iodine solutions may slow the release of thyroid hormones. The two most commonly used are Lugol's solution and sodium iodide. Lugol's solution is 30 drops of iodine mixed in milk or juice and given orally through a straw to prevent staining of the teeth. If Lugol's solution cannot be used, slow intravenous administration of 1 to 2 grams of sodium iodide may achieve the desired results. Pro-

pylthiouracil in doses of 900 to 1200 mg orally will reduce synthesis of thyroid hormones.

Fourth, high doses of hydrocortisone will help support body functions in this extreme stress situation. Doses as high as 300 mg per day may be needed.

Fifth, large amounts of vitamin B complex are required, along with glucose, protein, and carbohydrates, to provide the body with the nutrients necessary for the extreme catabolic state it is in.

Sixth, antipyretic agents are found to be effective only during the mild febrile stage of thyroid storm. Aspirin should be avoided, as salicylates are thought to interfere with the binding of T3 and T4, which may exacerbate the already existing hypermetabolism.

Nursing Intervention. General symptomatic supportive care is appropriate. A quiet environment with limited visitors helps decrease external stress. Physiologic stress is often treated with hydrocortisone daily.

Cooling blankets are useful in hyperpyrexia. Cooling to the extent of shivering and piloerection (hair on arms standing up, such as with goose bumps) may have a rebound effect of raising the temperature even higher and increasing metabolic activity.

Fluids, electrolytes, and glucose are given to prevent dehydration and imbalances and to provide energy for meeting metabolic needs. Iodine may be given by nasogastric tube or intravenously to prevent release of thyroid hormones.

PARATHYROID DYSFUNCTION

A major parathyroid dysfunction is hypoparathyroidism. This state is a metabolic crisis. Hypoparathyroidism is often seen with hypocalcemia.

Pathophysiology
A deficiency of parathormone causes a hypocalcemic state resulting in abnormal neuromuscular activity (calcium level less than 8.5 mg/dL). It is thought that this deficiency occurs secondary to a dysfunction in the calcium and the phosphate concentration feedback loop control systems.

Etiology
Acute hypocalcemia is usually secondary to ischemia or damage of the parathyroid gland during a thyroidectomy. Very rarely, radiation therapy (^{131}I) of the thyroid may cause a hypoparathyroidism, as can acute pancreatitis. It may also be idiopathic.

Clinical Presentation
Nausea, vomiting, and abdominal cramps are common. Dyspnea may be accompanied by a laryngeal stridor and cyanosis. Neurological signs and symptoms are prominent. There may be confusion, emotional lability, paresthesias of fingers and toes, and muscular twitching progressing to tetany and convulsions.

Diagnosis
Laboratory blood work will show a hypocalcemia. Urine tests will reveal a hypophosphaturia and perhaps a hypocalcuria. Two signs are a positive Trousseau's sign and a positive Chvostek's sign, although these signs are not always present.

Complications. Complications include seizures, tetany, shock, and death. A quiet environment with supportive equipment (ventilator, pacemaker) on standby may be useful in preventing potential complications.

Treatment
The objective of treatment is to raise serum calcium levels to normal. If seizures and tetany have not developed, oral calcium supplements are indicated, with additional vitamin D to promote calcium absorption. (Calcium may be given with food but not with milk, since milk products will decrease calcium absorption.)

Some types of calcium chloride should be given only through a central line, as infiltration in a peripheral line will result in tissue necrosis and sloughing. Calcium cannot be infused in saline due to precipitation formation with sodium bicarbonate, forcing calcium ion excretion in the kidneys.

Cardiac status must be monitored, especially if the patient is on digitalis. Digitalis and calcium have a synergistic action.

Nursing Interventions. Preventive nursing care in hypoparathyroidism may avoid the complications of seizures and tetany. The environment should be modified to be as quiet as possible, including the limiting of visitors, until the patient is well stabilized.

A respirator on standby will provide for immediate intervention in the event of hypoventilation or deteriorating respiratory status as shown by serial arterial blood gases. Emotional and physical stress often cause hyperventilation. In turn, hyperventilation causes alkalosis, which may precipitate tetany.

Cardiac monitoring is essential, since calcium therapy may alter cardiac conduction times with resultant dysrhythmias. Standard monitoring of intake and output, response to medication therapy, neurological status, and such are applicable to these patients, as the medication therapy will cause a change in the patient's electrolytes and fluid balance.

Administration of calcium as ordered, with special attention to possible infiltration and precipitation if the calcium is given intravenously and avoidance of milk products if it is given orally, will help ensure maximum benefit with minimal side effects of the drugs. Trousseau's sign is elicited by occluding circulation to the arm. This is done by maintaining a BP cuff pressure just above the systolic level. If the response is positive, the patient's hand will develop a carpopedal spasm within three minute. A carpopedal spasm results in a hollow palm position and fingers rigid and flexed at the metacarpophalangeal joints. Chvostek's sign is elicited by lightly tapping the facial nerve in front of the ear. If the response is positive, there is a unilateral contraction of the facial muscles.

CHAPTER 36

Anatomy, Physiology, and Dysfunction of the Adrenal Glands

Editor's Note

As with thyroid disturbances, adrenal dysfunction is unlikely to be addressed on the CCRN exam. If it is addressed, it is usually in conjunction with another system. Consequently, read this chapter for the purpose of introducing yourself to key concepts and becoming familiar yourself with major functions of the adrenal glands.

ANATOMY OF THE ADRENAL GLANDS

The adrenal glands are a pair of glands located on the top of each kidney (Fig. 36-1). Each pair of adrenal glands is identical to the other.

The adrenal gland is composed of two separate parts (Fig. 36-2). The adrenal cortex is the outer two-thirds of the gland. The adrenal medulla is the inner one-third of the gland. A mnemonic for remembering where each part lies in the letter "m," which stands for the medulla and the middle.

Adrenal Cortex

The adrenal cortex is composed of three distinct regions or zones (Fig. 36-3). The outermost zone is the zona glomerulosa. The middle zone is the zona fasciculata. The innermost zone is the zona reticularis. The zona glomerulosa functions by itself. The zona fasciculata and zona reticularis function together as a unit.

The zona glomerulosa is a thin zone located on the outer part of the cortex, directly under the capsular covering. The cells in this zone are arranged in clumps. Regulation of the hormone (aldosterone) secreted in the zona glomerulosa is completely independent of the regulatory controls over the zona fas-

ciculata and the zona reticularis. The regulatory control of the zona glomerulosa is the release of adrenocorticotropic hormone (ACTH)-releasing factors from the hypothalamus and ACTH-stimulating factors from the adenohypophysis.

The zona fasciculata is the largest of the three zones. Its cells are arranged in straight rows. The zona reticularis is composed of an anastomosing network of cells. These two zones function together to regulate cortisol and androgen hormones and are controlled by the same regulatory mechanisms of the adenohypophysis.

Adrenal Medulla

Cells of the adrenal medulla (Fig. 36-2) develop from the same embryological source as the sympathetic neurons. The cells are also called chromaffin cells because of their histologic staining characteristics. Because of their origin, the adrenal medulla cells are related functionally to the sympathetic nervous system.

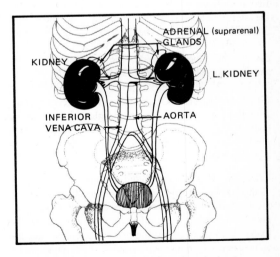

Figure 36-1. Location of the adrenal glands.

or flight" body response to stress. These actions would include positive effects on the cardiac muscle, shifting blood to certain muscles, decreasing gastrointestinal function, bronchiole dilatation accompanied by hyperpnea and tachypnea, and an increase in the serum glucose level.

Epinephrine is released by sympathetic nervous system stimulation and other hormones such as insulin and histamine.

Norepinephrine. Norepinephrine accounts for 20% of catecholamines secreted by the adrenal medulla. Norepinephrine excites mainly alpha receptors and to a slight degree beta receptors. Norepinephrine action is similar to adrenaline action with two notable exceptions. The effect of norepinephrine is not as intense as the effect of adrenaline on cardiac and metabolic functions. Also, norepinephrine has a more intense action than does adrenaline on skeletal muscle vasculature. This increases peripheral vascular resistance due to the increased vasoconstriction.

The sites of action for norepinephrine are body cells and vascular beds, and releasing factors for norepinephrine are the same as for epinephrine.

ADRENAL GLAND DYSFUNCTION

Adrenal insufficiency is a major life-threatening dysfunction of the adrenal cortex. It is also known as hypoadrenalism or hypocorticism.

Addison's Disease

Addison's disease is a chronic dysfunction of the adrenal glands resulting in an inadequate adrenal secretion of cortisol and aldosterone (adrenal insufficiency).

Pathophysiology. The adrenal cortex dysfunction results in a deficiency of mineralocorticoids and glucocorticoids.

Mineralocorticoids decrease results in an aldosterone deficiency. Without aldosterone, there is an increased excretion of sodium chloride and water in the urine. The depletion of sodium leads to dehydration and hypotension. At the same time, there is a retention of potassium. If the potassium concentration increases sufficiently, there is first a flaccidity of the cardiac myocardium following by cardiac cell paralysis as the potassium level rises. Hemoconcentration, acidosis,

decreased cardiac output, shock, and death due to the cardiac paralysis occur.

A decrease in glucocorticoids results in a cortisol deficiency with normal blood glucose concentrations between meals. Anorexia, nausea, vomiting, and abdominal pain result in weight loss. The neurological effects of cortisol deficiency include fatigue, lethargy, apathy, confusion, and psychoses. Cardiovascular effects include an impaired response to the vasoactive catecholamines. Energy-producing mechanisms are altered; examples are decreased glucogenesis (causes hypoglycemia) and fat mobilization. The decreased cortisol level stimulates the pituitary to secrete ACTH unrestrained. There is a decreased resistance to both physical and psychogenic stress.

Melanin pigmentation (Fig. 36-4) is increased in most cases of Addison's disease. The increased pigmentation is unevenly distributed and is probably due to increased secretion of melanocyte-stimulating hormone and ACTH from the adenohypophysis.

Etiology. The most frequent cause is a primary atrophy of the adrenal cortex. This may be an autoimmune process. Often tubercular destruction of the cortex or a cancerous tumor causes Addison's disease. Stress may be a factor.

Complications. Addisonian crisis may be fatal. A crisis may occur any time there is an increase in stress, since the adrenal cortex cannot increase it production of cortisol. Steroids should be increased in patients with Addison's disease who are under stress. Even a slight cold necessitates increased steroid hormone levels. The only successful treatment of Addisonian crisis is massive doses of glucocorticoids. Often as much as ten or more times the normal dose must be used to prevent death.

Treatment. If untreated, the patient dies within a period of a few days to a few weeks. Replacement therapy of small amounts of mineralocorticoids and glucocorticoids may prolong life for years.

Strict adherence to a diet low in potassium and high in sodium will help prevent complications. If a tumor is the etiological factor, surgery is performed.

Acute Adrenal Insufficiency

Adrenal crisis and Addisonian crisis are synonyms for acute adrenal insufficiency and may be used interchangeably.

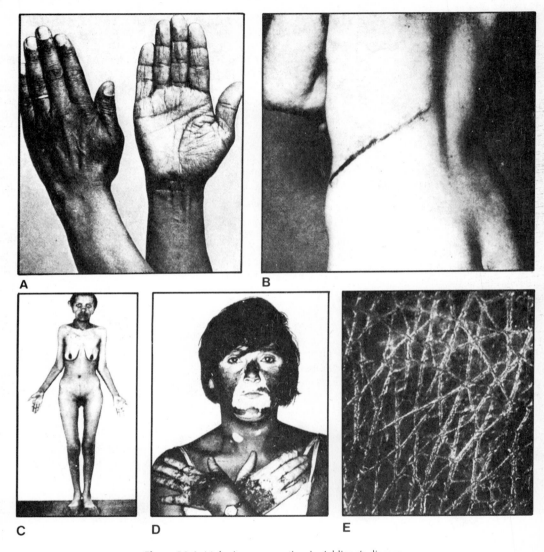

Figure 36-4. Melanin oversecretion in Addison's disease.

Etiology. Usually an underlying chronic condition (Addison's disease) is present before a crisis. In addition to this chronic disease, an infection, trauma, a surgical procedure, or some extra stress occurs, and the patient develops acute adrenal insufficiency. Less common causes of acute adrenal insufficiency are adrenalectomy, Waterhouse-Friderichsen syndrome, abrupt cessation of steroid therapy, chemotherapy, and hypothalamic diseases. An autoimmune response may be a factor.

Clinical Presentation. Anorexia, nausea, vomiting, diarrhea, and abdominal pain lead to increased fluid and electrolyte disturbances. Fever may lead to alterations in consciousness. Hypotension precedes shock and coma.

Diagnosis. Patient history, physical examination, and presenting symptoms are usually sufficient to provide a tentative diagnosis and to indicate the need for immediate treatment. Definitive laboratory studies are those evaluating endocrine function and identifying resultant system dysfunction or imbalances in the electrolytes.

Complications. Death is the common complication, although it is usually preceded by dysrhythmias, hypovolemia, shock, and coma.

Treatment. Adequate circulatory volume is vital. Continuous monitoring of vital signs to identify developing dysfunction provides for early intervention. Glucocorticoids must be replaced. An intravenous glucocorticoid such as hydrocortisone should be given. Physical and psychological stress should be avoided.

Nursing Intervention. Continuous monitoring of the respiratory system with a ventilator on standby is indicated. If serial arterial blood gases show deteriorating respiratory status, the patient may be intubated and placed on the respirator. Standard nursing procedures for all artificially ventilated patients should be instituted.

Cardiac and hemodynamic monitoring will reveal early signs of impending dysrhythmias and shock, providing an opportunity for early intervention. Intake and output records will indicate renal function. Emotional support of the patient and family is of utmost importance in an attempt to decrease exogenous stress as much as possible.

Hypercorticism (Cushing's Syndrome)

Hypercorticism is a marked increase in the production of mineralocorticoids, glucocorticoids, and androgen steroids resulting in the condition known as Cushing's syndrome (not to be confused with Cushing's triad).

Etiology. Cushing's syndrome is usually due to adrenal tumors or a pituitary tumor. A pituitary tumor causes increased release of ACTH that results in hyperplasia of the adrenal cortex.

Clinical Presentation. Increased glucocorticoids (cortisol) cause increased glucogenesis, resulting in hyperglycemia. This condition causes increased protein tissue wasting. It also causes increased fat, resulting in the typical "moon face" and increased trunk fat (Fig. 36-5). The increased cortisol causes mood swings ranging from euphoria to depression.

Increased mineralocorticoids (aldosterone) result in increased potassium excretion, causing dysrhyth-

mias, renal disorders, and muscle weakness. The increased aldosterone causes a decrease in sodium secretion. The increased sodium causes an increase in fluid retention, resulting in edema and usually an increase in blood pressure. (Eighty percent of patients with Cushing's syndrome have hypertension.) Increased sex hormones (androgens) cause increased facial hair and acne.

Diagnosis. Patient history, physical examination, and presenting symptoms are usually sufficient to provide a tentative diagnosis. Definitive laboratory studies are those evaluating endocrine function and identifying resultant system dysfunction or imbalance.

Treatment. Treatment consists of removing the tumor, if possible, which will necessitate steroid replacement. A diet low in sodium and high in potassium is required.

Nursing Intervention. Routine postsurgical nursing care is required. In addition, the patient must be assessed for endocrine imbalance indicating a need for replacement therapy. The patient's immune system will have been depressed because of the increased steroid levels prior to surgery, so signs of infection must be closely monitored. Education relating to diet therapy and medication regimens is essential to prevent endocrine crises in the future.

Note: The increase in mineralocorticoids may also cause Conn's syndrome (increased blood pressure and decreased potassium levels due to a benign aldosterone-secreting tumor).

Hypofunction of the Adrenal Medulla

Hypofunction of the adrenal medulla does not cause systemic problems because the sympathetic nervous system will compensate for decreases in epinephrine and norepinephrine.

Hyperfunction of the Adrenal Medulla

Hyperfunction of the adrenal medulla can be life threatening primarily due to the possibility of cerebral vascular accidents and congestive heart failure. In hyperfunction, epinephrine increases blood pressure, cardiac output, pulse, and metabolism. Norepinephrine increases the blood pressure more than epinephrine does. Hyperfunction may be precipitated by stress or exertion.

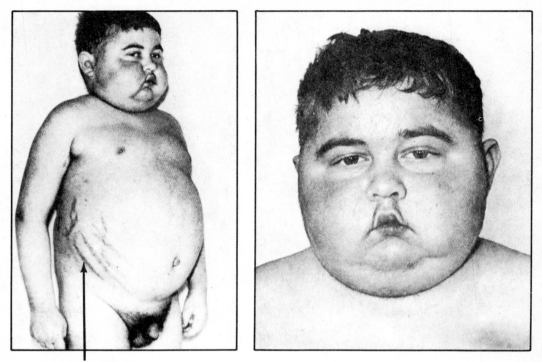

PURPLE STRIAE

Figure 36-5. Cushing's syndrome showing "moon face," trunk fat, and purple striae.

Pheochromocytoma

Hyperfunction of the adrenal medulla is the most common cause of pheochromocytoma. Pheochromocytoma is an encapsulated, vascular tumor of chromaffin tissue of the adrenal medulla.

Diagnosis. Signs and symptoms are the major diagnostic clues. However, hyperfunction of the adrenal medulla often resembles other disorders, which must be ruled out. These include diabetes mellitus, essential hypertension, and psychoneurosis.

Clinical Presentation. The outstanding symptom is the extremely high blood pressure secondary to the excessive medulla hormones. Other signs and symptoms include increased sympathetic nervous activity, sweating, headache, palpitations, apprehension, nausea and vomiting, tremor, pallor or flushing of the face, abdominal and/or chest pain, and hyperglycemia.

Treatment. Treatment is surgical removal of the pheochromocytoma. A preoperative diet low in sodium and carbohydrates is usual.

Nursing Intervention. Preoperatively, the nurse should promote rest and decrease patient apprehension. Postoperative routine procedures are instituted; in addition, the patient must be closely monitored for shock, hypotension (due to decreased levels of epinephrine and norepinephrine), hypoglycemia, and hemorrhage (the adrenal glands are very vascular).

CHAPTER 37

Anatomy, Physiology, and Dysfunction of the Pancreas

Editor's Note

According to the CCRN exam blueprint, specific questions regarding pancreatic function are less likely to be addressed than are questions regarding acute hyper- and hypoglycemia. Focus your attention on disturbances in blood glucose and the clinical conditions associated with abnormal blood glucose levels. Bear in mind, however, that only two to four questions are likely in the content area covered by this chapter.

The pancreas has a dual classification. It is considered an accessory digestive gland since it produces many enzymes essential to digestion. These enzymes are released through exocrine glands (glands that release substances through ducts). The pancreas (Fig. 37-1) is also classified as an endocrine gland because it releases two hormones, insulin and glucagon, directly into the bloodstream.

ANATOMY OF THE PANCREAS

There are two major types of tissues found in the pancreas: the acini and the islets of Langerhans. The acini secrete digestive enzymes into the duodenum by exocrine glands. The islets of Langerhans cells are scattered throughout the pancreas and may be called pancreatic islets by some texts.

Islets of Langerhans

Three structurally and functionally different cells comprise the islets of Langerhans: alpha, beta, and delta cells (Fig. 37-2).

Alpha cells are located within the clusters of islet cells. Alpha cells secrete the hormone glucagon, which is often called the hyperglycemic factor. Alpha cells secrete directly into the venous system of the pancreas.

Beta cells are located within the clusters of islet cells and are slightly smaller than alpha cells. Beta cells secrete insulin. The insulin molecules are very complex amino acid structures.

Delta cells are located within the clusters of the islet cells. Delta cells secrete a recently identified hormone called somatostatin. Somatostatin is the same as the growth hormone-inhibiting hormone secreted by the hypothalamus. Somatostatin has an effect upon glucagon and insulin secretion.

PHYSIOLOGY OF THE PANCREAS

Glucagon

The alpha cells of the islets of Langerhans secrete the hormone glucagon, which affects many body cells, especially the liver cells. Glucagon is secreted when

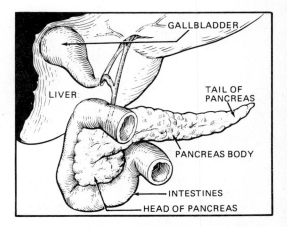

Figure 37.1. The pancreas.

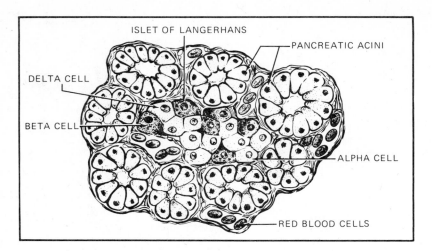

Figure 37.2. Cells of the pancreas.

blood amino acid levels rise and in the presence of a decreased blood glucose level.

Glucagon acts primarily as an antagonist to insulin, and its primary site of action is the liver. The most important aspect of this action is to increase blood glucose levels. Glucose metabolism is altered by two important actions of glucagon: glycogenolysis (the breakdown of liver glycogen stores), which release glucose for use in the body; and gluconeogenesis (the formation of glucose from other substances), which provides new glucose for the body. There is also an increase in fatty acid oxidation and in urea formation as a natural response to glucagon.

Insulin
This is a small protein of two amino acid chains. If the chains become separated, insulin loses its effectiveness. Once secreted into the circulatory system, insulin is removed by the liver and degraded. Most insulin circulates for only about ten minutes before the degradation process occurs. This allows control and rapid initiation or cessation of insulin action when it is being administered intravenously.

The target cells for insulin action are skeletal muscle, adipose tissue, the heart, and certain smooth muscle organs such as the uterus and especially liver cells. Factors that facilitate secretion of insulin are an increase in blood glucose levels and the growth hormone levels. A decreased insulin level results in hypoglycemia, ketosis, and acidosis.

Insulin action includes transporting glucose across cell membranes, increasing fatty acid storage, enhancing protein synthesis, and decreasing the breakdown of triglycerides in cells.

GLUCOSE METABOLISM DYSFUNCTION

Dysfunctions of glucose metabolism treated in critical-care areas include diabetic ketoacidosis (DKA), hyperosmolar coma, and insulin shock.

Diabetic Ketoacidosis
The digestion of carbohydrates raises the blood glucose level, which stimulates the pancreas to secrete insulin. If insulin cannot be secreted or is secreted in insufficient amounts, hyperglycemia develops.

Pathophysiology. A lack of insulin prevents peripheral cell utilization of available blood glucose. The liver inhibits the production of glycogen, and glycogen that is available is rapidly degraded. This releases free glucose into the blood, further raising the blood sugar level.

Since the cells cannot utilize the free glucose, protein stores release amino acids, and adipose tissue releases fatty acids. The amino acids and free fatty acids are synthesized by the liver, which is producing excessive amounts of acetyl coenzyme A. The acetyl coenzyme A is rapidly degraded into keto, acetoacetic, and beta-hydroxybutyric acids. These acids are produced faster than the kidneys and lungs are able to dispose of them, causing a metabolic acidosis. Ketones (keto acids or ketoanions) are excreted by the kidneys, producing a positive urine acetone test. Acetoacetic acid and beta-hydroxybutyric acid are oxidized into acetone. The acetone is exhaled and is responsible for the sweet, fruity smell of the breath. (It is the acetone of the acetoacetic acid that has the odor; beta-hydroxybutyric acid is odorless.)

Etiology. The most common causes of DKA are failure to take insulin, increased stress due to illness, trauma, surgery, cardiac conditions, and occasionally psychogenic trauma. Pregnancy and pancreatitis may also precipitate a diabetic ketoacidotic state.

Clinical Presentation. The most common symptoms are polydipsia', polyuria, polyphagia (usually with weight loss), dyspnea, and a generalized malaise. Nausea, vomiting, anorexia, and abdominal pain may be present. Signs of dehydration, tachycardia, orthostatic hypotension, and weakness are usually present. Respirations are Kussmaul in character and may have an acetone smell. Mentation ranges from lethargy to coma.

Diagnosis. Serum glucose levels are above 300 mg/dL. Urine tests reveal glycosuria and acetone. DKA should be ruled out in any patient who is comatose and dehydrated and is having deep, labored respirations.

Complications. Acidosis, electrolyte imbalances, acute renal failure, pulmonary edema, cerebral edema, seizures, cerebrospinal fluid acidosis, shock, and coma are the major complications of DKA.

Treatment. The objectives of treatment are to correct acidemia, hyperglycemia, hypovolemia, hyperosmolality, potassium deficit (if present), and ketonemia. Underlying conditions responsible for the diabetic ketoacidosis such as infections must be treated concurrently.

Resolving the DKA is the most effective method of restoring normal acid-base balance.

Hypovolemia is corrected by rapid infusions of 0.9% normal saline or 0.45% normal saline. Isotonic or hypotonic fluids are administered to counter the hyperosmolality that accompanies DKA. When the serum glucose level is decreased to 250 mg/dL, the fluids should be changed from saline to 5% glucose in 0.5% normal saline. This change will help avoid hypoglycemia, hypokalemia, and cerebral edema caused by the glucose diuresis. Correcting the hypovolemia usually corrects the hyperosmolality and, over a period of hours, the ketonemia. Patients may move from DKA coma to insulin shock without regaining consciousness. The addition of glucose by intravenous fluids helps prevent this.

Hyperglycemia is corrected by insulin administration. Normally, an intravenous bolus of insulin is administered, followed by slow continuous intravenous infusion. Insulin may be administered by subcutaneous injections of 10 to 100 units per hour. Intramuscular injection is not advocated in the crisis stage of DKA due to poor peripheral absorption.

Potassium deficits and other electrolyte imbalances may precipitate cardiac and/or neurological disturbances. Potassium is usually added to intravenous fluids, as the insulin forces potassium from the plasma back into the cells, producing a hypokalemia. However, the patient's potassium levels may be normal or high. Continuous monitoring and gradual changes to effect a correction over a 24-hour period are safer than massive, rapid changes. The exception to this is the patient whose life is threatened by extremes of hypo- or hyperkalemia.

Nursing Intervention. Maintaining a patent airway and suctioning as required to prevent aspiration are essential. Monitoring respiratory status by observation and arterial blood gases will identify impending hypoxia.

Cardiac monitoring due to electrolyte imbalances will reveal early dysrhythmias. With hypokalemia, U waves are normally present. In hyperkalemia, peaked or tented T waves are present. There may be a tachycardia that converts to a bradycardia if the hyperkalemia increases.

Monitor urinary output and listen to lung sounds frequently to identify pulmonary edema, especially in the presence of underlying cardiac diseases. Check urine hourly for acetone and sugar. The objective is to achieve a 1+ glycosuria (ensuring that the patient is not going into insulin shock). Once adequate urinary output is present, electrolytes are often added to the intravenous fluids to correct imbalances.

Blood sugar may be monitored hourly by bedside blood glucose monitoring to guide in the administration of regular insulin. Long-acting insulin is not used in DKA crisis.

Potassium is checked frequently, since initially it moves from the cells into the blood and much is excreted in the urine. When insulin is given, potassium shifts back into the cells. In addition to the laboratory results, the cardiac monitor will show whether the patient's serum potassium is low, normal, or high.

Neurologic status is assessed hourly. Hyperglycemia does not have a deleterious effect upon brain cells, but other electrolyte imbalances and cerebral edema will affect the cells.

Controversy exists over the use of bicarbonate to correct the acidosis present in DKA. Bicarbonate given intravenously does not cross the blood-brain barrier. It causes a shift in the bicarbonate/carbonic acid ratio, which releases carbon dioxide. Carbon dioxide crosses the blood-brain barrier, dissolving in the spinal fluid. This raises the carbonic acid level and increases cerebral acidosis, which may prolong diabetic coma.

Hyperosmolar Coma—HHNK

In hyperosmolar, hyperglycemic, nonketotic coma (HHNK), there is enough insulin being released in the body to prevent ketosis, but there is not enough insulin to prevent hyperglycemia.

Pathophysiology. Hyperglycemia increases the solutes in the extracellular fluid, causing a hyperosmolality. Cellular dehydration occurs because of the hyperosmolality, which is also the cause of diuresis. Without treatment, an osmotic gradient develops between the brain and the plasma, resulting in dehydration and central nervous system dysfunction. The end result of dehydration is a decreased glomerular filtration rate and the development of azotemia.

Typically, the HHNK patient is over 50 years old, becomes ill, and has a general malaise. Due to this, the patient is anorexic and eats and drinks poorly, which leads to dehydration. Since the patient is not eating, the body uses protein and fat for energy to maintain body processes. Almost the same pathophysiologic pattern of DKA appears in HHNK. The difference is that in HHNK, a sufficient amount of insulin is released to prevent the development of ketosis. The patient may be stuporous or comatose before being seen by a physician.

Etiology. One of the common causes of HHNK is undiagnosed or untreated diabetes. Frequently, a mild diabetic state exists without any problems until the diabetic patient is under stress. Iatrogenic causes account for some cases of HHNK due to hyperalimentation, the administration of hypertonic intravenous fluids, and the administration of steroids.

Clinical Presentation. Usually the patient is over 50 years old. The patient is lethargic or comatose. Symptoms include polyuria, polydipsia, nausea, vomiting, and weight loss. Eventually, the urinary output begins to fall as fluid depletion becomes more severe. Dehydration is evidenced by dry skin and mucous membranes. A tachypnea is present. Tachycardia, hypotension, and glycosuria are present.

Diagnosis. The three outstanding symptoms may well be the blood sugar level (commonly over 1000 mg), the plasma hyperosmolarity (as high as 450 mosm/kg), and an extremely elevated hematocrit. Urine and plasma are both negative for acetone. The blood urea nitrogen is usually elevated, and there is a marked leukocytosis.

Complications. Shock, coma, acute tubular necrosis, and vascular thrombosis are common complications. High mortality rates can be associated with HHNK if treatment is not quickly initiated.

Treatment. Correcting the fluid balance is one of the first objectives of treatment. It is essential that fluids be administered in order to correct the hyperosmolality and hypovolemia. The hypoinsulinemia may be corrected by the use of insulin. Hyperglycemia is not known to have deleterious effects upon the brain, but hyperosmolar dehydration may cause seizures. Return of the anion gap to normal levels may be used as an indication of success in the use of insulin therapy.

If metabolic acidosis is present, it is usually corrected by the administration of sodium bicarbonate. This is controversial for the same reasons as in DKA. Any electrolyte imbalances, such as a hypokalemia, should be corrected. As much as 200–400 mEq of potassium during the first 24 to 48 hours to correct the potassium imbalance may be required. Close and continuous monitoring is necessary to identify further changes or deterioration in the patient's electrolyte status. Cardiac monitoring and hourly neurological checks will provide clues to changing status.

Nursing Intervention. The primary nursing responsibility is the administration of intravenous fluids to correct both the dehydration and hyperosmolality without putting the patient into pulmonary edema. As much as 20 liters of isotonic or hypotonic (controversial) fluids is given over the first 48 hours. The nurse must monitor breath sounds hourly to determine whether pulmonary edema is developing.

Cardiac monitoring is continuous to identify dysrhythmias due to electrolyte imbalances, especially hypo- or hyperkalemia. Also, one must monitor the patient to detect early signs of congestive heart failure.

Administration of insulin to correct hyperglycemia is usually accomplished by a loading intravenous dose of insulin followed by repeated doses as indicated by the blood glucose level. Continuous insulin infusion is used with caution. The nurse may monitor the patient's glucose level by blood glucose monitoring hourly.

Neurologic status should be evaluated hourly to provide information on the efficacy of treatment. Skin care and mouth care are important aspects of preventing infection and keeping the patient comfortable.

Hypoglycemic Reaction (Insulin Shock)

Pathophysiology. A decreased blood level of glucose is the criterion for a diagnosis of hypoglycemic reaction or insulin shock. The decrease may be due to a defect in the process of forming glucose, either gluconeogenesis or glycogenolysis, or by the removal of glucose by the use of adipose, muscle, or liver tissues.

Etiology. Causes of hypoglycemia include an intolerance of fructose, galactose, or amino acids. Postgastrectomy patients may have hypoglycemia. A broad range of drugs, such as alcohol, insulin, and sulfonylurea drugs, may be the origin. Endocrine dysfunctions, liver disease, severe congestive heart failure, and pregnancy may cause hypoglycemia. In diabetic patients, overdoses of insulin and exercising without adjustment of the insulin dosage are the common causes of insulin shock.

Clinical Presentation. The early signs and symptoms are restlessness, diaphoresis, tachycardia, and hunger. (Propranolol hydrochloride [Inderal] may mark these signs and symptoms.) If the hypoglycemia progresses to less than 50 mg/dL, the central nervous system is affected and the patient may exhibit behavior that ranges from bizarre to a coma. Headache, weakness, tremors, nausea, and personality changes are common signs and symptoms.

Complications. The brain obtains almost all of its energy from glucose metabolism. If the glucose level is maintained below 45 to 50 mg/dL, cerebral ischemia, edema, and neuronal hyperexcitability occur. If the blood glucose level drops to 20 to 40 mg/dL, clonic convulsions may occur. If the blood glucose level drops below 20 mg/dL, coma develops. If not promptly reversed, the low blood glucose levels may cause irreversible brain damage, myocardial ischemia, infarction, and death.

Diagnosis and Treatment. A glucose level of less than 45 mg/dL with blood glucose monitoring is sufficient to warrant infusion of 50 mg of 50% dextrose intravenously. The patient will usually respond within one to two minutes. A sample of blood should be drawn before the glucose is given to confirm the diagnosis by laboratory tests. If hypoglycemia is present in a *non*diabetic patient, additional tests must be performed to rule out endocrine disorders or tumors. If hypoglycemia is present in a known diabetic patient, the underlying cause of the insulin shock must be identified and corrected.

Somogyi Effect

When too much insulin is administered, hypoglycemia occurs. The hypoglycemia alerts the body's defense systems, which overreact. With hypoglycemia, certain anti-insulin hormones are secreted. These include epinephrine, glucagon, glucocorticoids, and growth hormones. Because of these hormones, hyperglycemia occurs. Most often a cycle occurs. Hypoglycemia one day may be followed by one or more days of hyperglycemia. In some patients, the cycle is so short that periods alternate within the same day. Symptoms of hypoglycemia in a hyperglycemic patient may indicate a Somogyi effect. Blood sugar levels may reach dangerously high levels because of this rebound effect.

BIBLIOGRAPHY

Besser, G.M., & Cudworth, A.G. (1987). *Clinical Endocrinology: An Illustrated Text*. Philadelphia: J.B. Lippincott.

Chernow, B., Wiley, S.C., & Zaloga, G.P. (1989). Critical care endocrinology. In *Textbook of Critical Care*. Ed.

Shoemaker, W.C., et al. Philadelphia: W.B. Saunders.

Chipps, E. (1992). Transphenoidal surgery for pituitary tumors. *Crit Care Nurse 12,* 1, 30–39.

DeGroot, L.J. (1989). *Endocrinology.* Philadelphia: W.B. Saunders.

Lindamann, C. (1992). S.I.A.D.H.: Is your patient at risk. *Nursing 22,* 6, 104–109.

O'Riordan, J.L.H., Malan, P.G., & Gould, R.P. (1988). *Essentials of Endocrinology.* Oxford: Blackwell Scientific Publications.

Reichlin, S. (1987). Neural control of the pituitary gland: Normal physiology and pathophysiologic implications. *Current Concepts.* Kalamazoo: Upjohn Co.

Sabo, C.E., & Michael, S.R. (1989). Diabetic ketoacidosis: Pathophysiology, nursing diagnosis and nursing interventions. *Focus Crit Care 16,* 1, 21–28.

Sheppard, M.C., & Franklin, J.A. (1988). *Clinical Endocrinology and Diabetes.* Edinburgh: Churchill Livingstone.

Watts, N.B., & Keffer, J.H. (1989). *Practical Endocrinology.* Philadelphia: Lea & Febiger.

PART 7

Immunology and Hematology

Paula Goldberg, RN, MSN
Nelda K. Martin, RN, MSN, CCRN

CHAPTER 38

Introduction to Immunology and Hematology

Editor's Note

Immunologic and hematologic concepts account for 4% of the CCRN exam (eight questions). The major content areas covered under immunology and hematology include organ transplantation, disseminated intravascular coagulation (DIC), and immunosuppression. To correctly answer the questions on anaphylactic shock and immunosuppression, one must have a working knowledge of immune response principles. To answer questions on DIC, normal coagulation concepts must be known. The following chapters present key information normally encountered on the CCRN exam regarding both the four major concepts and the principles necessary to achieve the understanding required on the CCRN exam.

As with most other chapters, concentrate on key principles rather than on details or pure anatomy and physiology points. Nurses often find immunology and hematology is a difficult area of the CCRN exam due to lack of clinical familiarity with the concepts. Study this chapter and then try to apply the information during your work. The more you can integrate the information after reading it, the more likely the information will be retained for the test.

IMMUNE SYSTEM

The immune system is a dynamic system, consisting of many cell types and structures. In fact, approximately 1 in every 100 of the body's cells is an immune cell. It is dynamic, not only in the sense that it does not necessarily remain in one place as does, say, the heart, but also in the sense that its many components are in a constant state of dynamic interaction.

The mature immune system is capable of performing three general types of functions: defense, homeostasis, and surveillance. In providing defense, resistance to infection is facilitated by both nonspecific innate mechanisms and more specific acquired immune responses that bring about the destruction of foreign antigens (anything recognized by the body as non-self, e.g., microorganisms, proteins, and cells of transplanted organs). Maintaining immunologic homeostasis involves keeping a balance between immune protective and destructive responses and the removal of senescent immune cells from the body. Although the function of the immune system is inherently protective, there are conditions in which natural immune responses become destructive to the host. Examples of such conditions are the numerous autoimmune diseases as well as allergic and anaphylactic reactions. Surveillance involves the recognition of microorganisms or cells bearing foreign antigens on their membranes. Some of the immune cells, lymphocytes in particular, are highly mobile and travel throughout the vascular and lymphatic systems in search of potentially harmful antigens. Some types of cancer cells, in particular, are sought out and destroyed by immune cells in this way.

Immune responses can be classified into two major types: natural or innate responses and acquired responses. Both types of responses play critical roles in host defense.

INNATE IMMUNE SYSTEM

The innate immune system consists of natural or nonspecific mechanisms for the protection of an individual against foreign antigens. These natural defenses are present from birth and do not necessarily require exposure to specific antigens to develop. Natural defenses, the body's first line of defense, consist of anatomic, chemical, and cellular defenses against microbial invasion. Anatomic defenses include the skin, mucous membranes, and ciliated epithelia. Chemical defenses include gastric acid, lysozymes, natural immunoglobulins, and the interferons. Cellular defenses include leukocytes.

ANATOMICAL AND CHEMICAL DEFENSES

The skin provides the initial physical barrier to external environmental antigens. The outermost skin layer, the stratum corneum, is the main barrier to microbial invasion. Certain conditions (pH, humidity, and temperature) influence the growth of potentially pathogenic organisms on the skin. Alterations in normal conditions related to these factors favor the development of infection. The normally acid pH of the skin inhibits the growth of microorganisms. When the acid-base balance of the skin is altered in favor of a higher pH, this protective mechanism is lost. When water loss from epidermal cells exceeds intake, the stratum corneum can dry and crack, predisposing the host to microbial invasion. On the other hand, excessive moisture decreases barrier efficiency.

Skin cells are constantly exfoliating, and in this process organisms are sloughed along with dead skin cells. In addition, the skin is colonized with normal flora (mainly aerobic cocci and diphtheroids), which, through various mechanisms, prevents the colonization of potentially pathogenic organisms. The resident flora maintains the skin's pH in the acidic range and competes effectively for nutrients and binding sites on epidermal cells, making it difficult for nonresident flora to survive. It is when the normal flora is altered, such as occurs with long-term or broad-spectrum antibiotic therapy and with the use of disinfectants or occlusive dressings, that potentially pathogenic organisms become opportunistic. Opportunistic organisms take advantage of the lack of competition for nutrients and epidermal binding sites, and multiply to cause infection.

The sebaceous glands, mammary glands, respiratory epithelium, gastrointestinal mucosa, genitourinary mucosa, and conjunctivae all secrete a protective immunoglobulin (another word for antibody) called secretory IgA. Ciliated respiratory epithelial cells also facilitate the removal of bacteria and other foreign antigens from the respiratory tract; the low pH of the gastric mucosa prevents bacterial growth in the stomach.

Leukocytes

All leukocytes (white blood cells [WBCs]) develop as stem cells in the bone marrow. Leukocytes develop along two major lineages: the myeloid lineage and the lymphoid lineage. The myeloid lineage includes all leukocytes except the lymphocytes. The lymphoid lineage consists of T and B lymphocytes. Myeloid cells make up the backbone of the natural or innate defense system. Myeloid leukocytes can be further classified into two major groups: granulocytes and monocytes. The major function of both is phagocytosis.

Granulocytes

Granulocytes, commonly referred to as polymorphonuclear granulocytes (PMNs) or polymorphs, are produced in the bone marrow at the rate of approximately 80 million per day, and their average life span is about two to three days. Sixty to seventy percent of all leukocytes are PMNs. These cells are sometimes called polymorphs because their nuclei are multilobed; they are called granulocytes because they contain intracellular granules. These intracellular granules contain hydrolytic enzymes that are cytotoxic to foreign organisms. Furthermore, granulocytes are classified, according to the histologic staining reactions of the granules, into three more distinct types: neutrophils, eosinophils, and basophils. Granulocytes may leave the circulation to become tissue phagocytes (Fig. 38–1).

Neutrophils. Neutrophils are the most abundant cells in the bone marrow and blood, comprising about 90% of all granulocytes. Three forms of neutrophils can be identified in the peripheral blood: segmented neutrophils, bands, and metamyelocytes. Segmented neutrophils are fully mature, bands are slightly immature, and metamyelocytes are completely immature neutrophils. Neutrophils are strongly phagocytic; that is, they ingest microorganisms or other cells and foreign particles, and they digest the ingested material within their phagocytic vacuoles.

In conditions such as infection, there is an increased demand for neutrophils. The bone marrow responds by releasing more neutrophils into the circulation, and in this process immature cells are released along with the mature cells. As a result, the percentage of bands in the peripheral blood is increased. This condition is referred to as a "shift to the left" and indicates acute inflammation or infection. In more serious conditions, metamyelocytes will also appear in increased numbers in the peripheral blood. The normal neutrophil count in the adult is between 1000 and 6000 cells/mm³ blood, or approximately 60% of the differential WBC count. Bands normally number about 600 cells/mm³ blood, or approximately 0 to 5% of the differential WBC count. Metamyelocytes should not be present in the peripheral blood.

Eosinophils

Eosinophils are weakly phagocytic cells that are seen in increased numbers in the circulation specifically during parasitic infections and allergic reactions. Eosinophils degranulate (release their cytotoxic granules) upon antigenic stimulation and kill organisms extracellularly. The normal eosinophil count is about 200 cells/mm³ blood, or between 2 and 5% of the differential WBC count.

Basophils. Basophils are responsible for anaphylactoid reactions to allergens. Like eosinophils, basophils are capable of releasing their cytotoxic granules when stimulated by certain antigens to effect extracellular killing. Basophils are morphologically identical to mast cells but can be differentiated from mast cells in that basophils are bloodborne and mast cells reside in tissues outside of the circulation. In other words, when a basophil migrates out of the circulation to reside in tissue, it becomes a mast cell. The normal basophil count is about 100 cells/mm³ blood, or about 0.2% of the differential WBC count.

Monocytes. PMNs can be differentiated from monocytes by their multilobed nuclei and many intracellular granules. Monocytes are mononuclear cells and do not contain cytotoxic intracellular granules. They do, however, release the prostaglandin PGE₂, which is a mediator of the inflammatory response. The normal monocyte count is about 200 to 1000 cells/mm³ blood, or about 5% of the differential WBC count.

A specific type of monocyte is the antigen-presenting cell (APC). APCs are formed in the epidermis, where they are called Langerhan's cells, and in the lymphoid system. APCs play an important role in linking the innate immune system with the acquired immune system. APCs carry foreign antigens that enter the host via the respiratory or gastrointestinal tract, or the skin, through the lymphatic system and present them to lymphocytes in the lymph nodes and spleen,

thereby triggering cellular and humoral immune responses.

Phagocytosis

Monocytes, like granulocytes, may leave the circulation to become tissue macrophages. Together, blood and tissue macrophages comprise a highly mobile network of cells for first-line defense called the reticuloendothelial system. These cells are strategically and conveniently located in the liver, spleen, lymph nodes, kidney, lung, peritoneum, brain, and synovia.

Phagocytosis, which means "cell eating," is the first step in host defense. Phagocytes (or macrophages) have surface receptors that allow them to seek out and attack nonspecific foreign organisms, engulf them, and ultimately destroy them (Fig. 38-2). Phagocytosis is the process by which excess antigen and dead cells are removed from the body. Phagocytosis is also essential in the initiation of cellular and humoral immune responses by T and B lymphocytes.

Inflammation

Inflammation is an attempt to restore homeostasis. It is the body's initial reaction to injury and the first step in the healing process. Wound healing cannot occur if the inflammatory response is fully inhibited. During the

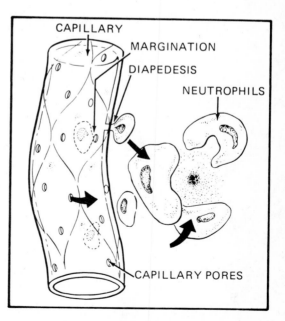

Figure 38-1. Diapedesis of WBCs.

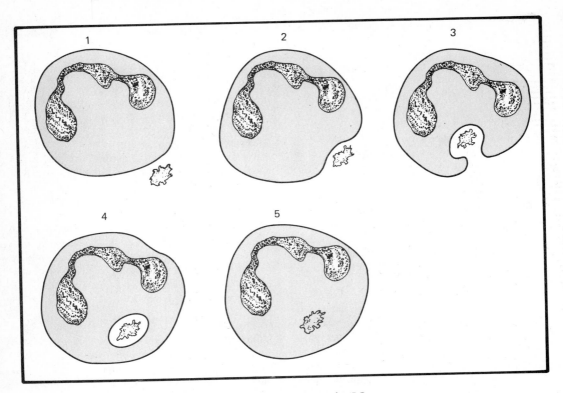

Figure 38-2. Phagocytosis of WBCs.

inflammatory response, a series of cellular and systemic reactions is triggered; these responses serve to localize and destroy the offending antigen, maintain vascular integrity, and limit tissue damage.

Tissue injury provides the initial stimulus for activation of inflammatory mechanisms and results in the cellular release of vasoactive substances such as histamine, bradykinin, and serotonin. The circulatory effects are vasodilatation and increased blood flow to the affected site, increased vascular permeability that facilitates diapedesis of immune cells from the circulation to the tissues, and pain. The clotting system is activated in an attempt to "plug up" the injury. Increased blood flow and capillary permeability lead to local interstitial edema and swelling. Leukocyte migration occurs as phagocytes are attached to the affected site (chemotaxis), and dying leukocytes release pyrogens, which stimulate the hypothalamus to produce a state of fever. Pyrogens also stimulate the bone marrow to release more leukocytes, thus perpetuating the process.

Finally, the complement system is activated. The complement system consists of a complex set of approximately 20 interacting proteolytic enzymes and regulatory proteins found in the plasma and body fluids that attack antigens. The complement system is conceptually similar to the coagulation system in that complement proteins react sequentially in a series of enzymatic reactions in a cascading manner. Several factors are responsible for activation of the complement system: the formation of insoluble antigen-antibody complexes, aggregated immunoglobulin, platelet aggregation, release of endotoxins by gram-negative bacteria, the presence of viruses or bacteria in the circulation, and the release of plasmin and proteases from injured tissues. Complement proteins can mediate the lytic destruction of cells, including red blood cells (RBCs) and WBCs, platelets, bacteria, and viruses.

The inflammatory response can be altered or suppressed in many situations: the administration of corticosteroids or other immunosuppressive drugs, malnutrition, advanced age, chronic illness, and prolonged stress. Conversely, the inflammatory response can become exaggerated in conditions such as anaphylaxis and septic shock.

The innate immune mechanisms just discussed will be called upon as the first line of defense in ridding the host of foreign antigens. However, if these mechanisms are not entirely successful, a second set of defenses, the acquired immune system, is activated to work in concert with the innate immune system. The acquired immune system is composed of lymphocytes and other lymphoid structures necessary for specific immune responses.

ACQUIRED IMMUNE SYSTEM

The lymphoid system matures during the fetal and neonatal periods, when lymphoid stem cells differentiate into T and B lymphocytes. At this time, the mechanisms for conferring genetic specificity to lymphocytes develop. This property of specificity is what differentiates the lymphoid cell from the myeloid cell, which can react with any antigen. The process of lymphopoiesis (lymphocyte origination and differentiation into functional effector cells) begins in the yolk sac and then continues later in life in the thymus gland, the liver, the spleen, and finally the bone marrow, which is the primary site of lymphopoiesis in the full-term neonate.

Primary Lymphoid Tissue
Primary lymphoid tissue consists of central organs that serve as major sites of lymphopoiesis. Lymphoid stem cells originate in the bone marrow. These cells give rise to the various components of the acquired immune system.

Secondary Lymphoid Tissue
Secondary lymphoid tissue is peripheral tissue that provides an environment for lymphocytes to encounter antigens and proliferate if necessary. Secondary lymphoid tissue consists of the bone marrow, spleen, lymph nodes, thymus, liver, and mucosal associated lymphoid tissue in the tonsils, respiratory tract, gut, and urogenital tract. Localization of secondary lymphoid tissue is not coincidental, as all of these structures provide major portals for the entry of foreign microorganisms into the body. Once in secondary lymphoid tissue, lymphocytes may migrate from one lymphoid structure to another by vascular and lymphatic channels.

Lymphatics. The lymphatic system consists of (1) a capillary network, which collects lymph (a clear, watery fluid in the interstitial spaces); (2) collecting vessels, which carry lymph from the lymphatic vessels back to the vascular system; (3) lymph nodes; and (4) lymphatic organs, such as the tonsils. Lymphatic channels provide a major transit system for lymphocytes while they carry out specific functions related to immunologic surveillance. Both superficial and deep lymphatics empty into the large thoracic duct, which drains into the left subclavian vein (Fig. 38-3).

Lymph Nodes. Lymph nodes are small, oval-shaped bodies of lymphatic tissue encapsulated by fibrous tissue that are situated in the course of lymphatic vessels. The interior of the lymph nodes resembles a matrix of connective tissue that forms compartments that are densely populated with lymphocytes. Afferent

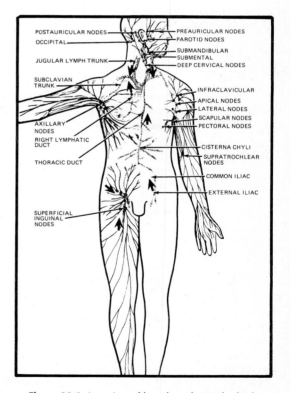

Figure 38-3. Location of lymph nodes in the body.

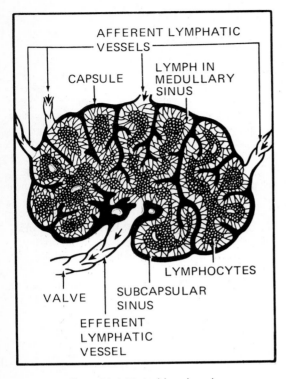

Figure 38-4. Typical lymph node.

lymphatics carry lymph to the lymph nodes, and efferent lymphatics serve as exit routes for lymphocytes from lymph nodes (Fig. 38-4). Lymph nodes are located at the junctions of lymphatic vessels and form a complete network for the draining and filtering of extravasated lymph from interstitial fluid spaces.

Spleen. The spleen is a soft, purplish, highly vascular, coffee bean-shaped organ in the left upper quadrant. It lies between the fundus of the stomach and the diaphragm. It is covered by a fibroelastic membrane that invests the organ at the hilum to form fibrous bands (trabeculae) that constitute the internal framework of the spleen and contain the splenic pulp.

During fetal and neonatal life, the spleen gives rise to RBCs. The physiologic function of the spleen in adult life is not completely understood. However, a major function of the spleen seems to be in the removal of particulate matter from the circulation. It is known that it has reticuloendothelial, immunologic, and storage functions. The spleen produces monocytes, lym-

phocytes, opsonins, and IgM antibody-producing plasma cells.

Blood flow within the spleen is sluggish, which allows phagocytosis to occur. The spleen clears the blood of encapsulated organisms (*Neisseria meningitidis, Haemophilus influenzae, Streptococcus pneumoniae*), and antigens in the rest of the body are phagocytosed and carried to the spleen to be eradicated by antibodies.

Postsplenectomy sepsis syndrome is seen predominantly in young immunosuppressed individuals who have been splenectomized, but this syndrome can occur in the healthy adult after splenectomy. The etiology of this often fatal syndrome is the loss of particulate filtering, coupled with IgM and opsonin production by the spleen.

Normally about 30% of the total platelet population is sequestered in the spleen, but this can increase to 80% with splenomegaly. Increased numbers of red and white blood cells will also be sequestered and destroyed in splenomegaly. Therefore, pancytopenia (anemia, leukopenia, and thrombocytopenia) occurs during splenomegaly.

Thymus. The thymus is a prominent organ in the infant, occupying the ventral superior mediastinum. In the older adult, it may be scarcely visible due to atrophy. The thymus is composed mostly of lymphocytes. Its only known function is the production of lymphocytes.

LYMPHOCYTES

Lymphocytes are the primary defenders of the acquired immune system. Lymphocytes have surface receptors that are specific for surface molecules (antigens) located on the surfaces of foreign proteins and are therefore the only cells that have the intrinsic ability to recognize specific antigens.

There are two major types of lymphocytes: T lymphocytes (T cells) and B lymphocytes (B cells). T cells are involved in immunologic regulation and mediate what is called the cellular immune response. B cells produce antibodies and mediate what is called the humoral immune response.

T Lymphocytes (T Cells)

Under the influence of thymic hormones, immature T cells develop. As mediators of the cellular immune response, T cells defend against viruses, fungi, and some neoplastic conditions, and they destroy transplanted organs by mediating accelerated and acute rejection responses. T-cell function is inhibited by viral and parasitic infections, malnutrition, prolonged general anesthesia, radiation therapy, uremia, Hodgkin's disease, and advanced age.

T cells are divided into four functionally distinct but interactive cell populations or subtests: cytotoxic, helper (T4), suppressor (T8), and memory T cells.

Effector Cells. Cytotoxic and memory T cells are referred to as effector cells because they have a specific cytotoxic effect on antigen-bearing cells. Cytotoxic T cells bind to target cells and facilitate their destruction via substances known as lymphokines, which stimulate inflammatory cells, and via the production of cytolytic proteins.

Lymphokines. Lymphokines are one of the two soluble products of lymphocytes, the other being antibodies. Lymphokines are inflammatory and regulatory hormones of the immune system that serve a variety of functions, such as the recruitment of macrophages to antigen sites (chemotaxis), augmentation of T-cell function in general, and inhibition of viral replication.

Lymphokines carry molecular signals between immunocompetent cells for the purpose of amplification of the immune response. Their role in amplification of the T-cell response is crucial to cellular immunity. Two of the most important lymphokines are interleukin-1 (IL-1) and interleukin-2 (IL-2). IL-1 stimulates T-cell proliferation, induces fever, stimulates the liver to produce acute-phase proteins, and stimulates the release of prostaglandin. IL-2 (T-cell growth factor) also stimulates T-cell proliferation. The reaction of T cells with IL-1 is necessary for the production of IL-2.

Memory T cells are T cells that have been sensitized to a specific antigen and then cloned to remember the antigen. Memory cells remain present in the body for many years and are therefore available for defense upon repeated exposure to an antigen. Repeated exposure to an antigen that the host has been previously sensitized to will result in a more rapid and accelerated immune response than on the first exposure.

Regulatory Cells. Helper and suppressor T cells are regulatory in nature. Helper T cells are active in lymphokine-mediated events. They produce multiple lymphokines that promote the proliferation and activation of other lymphocytes and macrophages. Although the B cell can produce antibody by direct interaction with surface antigen on a macrophage, the assistance of helper T cells is required for the majority of antibody production. They recruit cytotoxic T cells to antigen sites and interact with macrophages in the spleen and lymph nodes to facilitate antibody production by B cells. Helper and suppressor T-cell activity is normally balanced to maintain immunologic homeostasis. Too much suppressor T-cell function, for instance, will inhibit helper T-cell function.

B Lymphocytes (B Cells)

B cells are effector cells that mediate the humoral immune response through the production of antibodies, which is their major function. B cells are important in defense against pyrogenic bacterial infections and can destroy transplanted organs by mediating hyperacute graft rejection. When a B cell is stimulated by a particular antigen, it differentiates into a lymphoblast. The lymphoblast differentiates into a plasmablast, which further differentiates into a plasma cell. Plasma cells, which are capable of producing and releasing antibody, do so until the antigen is destroyed. Memory of the offending antigen is retained for at least several months.

Antibodies are also referred to as immunoglobulins. Immunoglobulins are specifically modified proteins present in serum and tissue fluids that are capable of selectively reacting with inciting antigens. The body produces several million antibodies that are capable of reacting with just as many antigens. However, each is specific and can usually recognize only one antigen. When viruses or bacteria, for instance, enter the body, their structural surface features are recognized by the body as not belonging to it. Antibodies are then formed and attracted to these foreign structures, for which they have identical matching receptors. In this way, antibodies are able to bind with antigens in a process called antigen-antibody complex formation. Mechanisms of antigen interaction by antibody include agglutination, precipitation, neutralization, and lysis.

Antibodies can be divided into five major classifications: IgM, IgG, IgA, IgD, and IgE. IgM is the principal mediator of the primary immune response. IgM is a natural antibody; i.e., there is no known contact with the antigen that stimulated its production. About 10% of all antibodies are of the IgM type. IgG is the principal mediator of the secondary immune response, which requires repeated exposure to the same antigen. IgG is the major antibody against bacteria and viruses. About 75% of all antibodies are of the IgG type. IgA is the secretory immunoglobulin present in bodily secretions and offers natural protection against nonspecific foreign antigens. About 15% of all antibodies are of the IgA type. The function of IgD is not known, but about 1% of antibodies are of this type. Although only about 0.002% of antibodies are of the IgE type, IgE antibodies present on basophils and mast cells play a significant role in inflammatory and immune reactions.

Lymphocyte Responses

All cells express foreign antigens. Foreign cells, of course, express antigens that are genetically different from those of the host. It is through specific receptors on the surfaces of lymphocytes that B and T cells can be differentiated, and it is also through these receptors that B and T cells are able to recognize foreign antigens. During lymphocyte maturation, each B and T cell acquires specific cell membrane surface receptors that allow the cell to "match up" with certain foreign antigens. This matching between host lymphocytes and foreign antigens is the recognition phase of the acquired immune response. When this occurs, lymphocytes are activated to differentiate, proliferate, and then quickly mount an effective immune response against the offending antigen.

CELLULAR IMMUNE RESPONSE

The cellular immune response is the immune response mediated by T cells. T cells recognize foreign antigens only after they are displayed on the surfaces of macrophages or APCs. The cellular immune response can be summarized as follows:

1. Naturally, the presence of a foreign antigen is necessary to initiate the response.
2. Initially, macrophages encounter the antigen and begin to phagocytize it. Antigenic fragments are released and then carried to T cells in the lymph nodes by APCs.
3. Resting virgin or memory T cells are activated when the antigen-APC complex binds with the T-cell surface receptor.
4. APCs are stimulated to produce IL-1, which summons helper T cells.

5. Helper T cells are then responsible for a number of actions, including the release of IL-2, which causes the differentiation and proliferation of T cells. The helper T cells also stimulate antibody production by B cells.
6. Clonal expansion greatly increases the sensitized T-cell population.
7. Ultimately, the antigen-bearing cells are destroyed by the direct cytotoxic effect of effector T cells. Some sensitized T cells are returned to the lymphoid system with the memory of the antigen for future challenge.

Examples of cellular immune responses include tumor cell surveillance, defense against viral and fungal infections, acute organ rejection, graft-versus-host disease, and autoimmune diseases.

HUMORAL IMMUNE RESPONSE

The humoral immune response is mediated by B cells. Antigens trigger B cells by stimulating immunoglobulins on their surfaces. The humoral immune response can be summarized as follows:

1. Naturally, as with the cellular immune response, the presence of a foreign antigen is necessary to initiate the process. Unlike T cells, B cells can recognize an antigen in its native configuration.
2. Initially, macrophages encounter the antigen and begin to phagocytize it. Antigenic fragments are released and then carried to B cells in the lymph nodes and spleen by APCs. Resting virgin or memory B cells are activated when antigen binds to surface immunoglobulin.
3. IL-1 is released by APCs, and helper T cells stimulate the sensitization and clonal proliferation of effector B cells. B cells are activated to differentiate and produce antibody when antigen binds to their receptors.
4. Antigen-antibody complexes form, and ultimately the antigen-bearing cells are destroyed.
5. As in the cellular immune response, some of the plasma cells with specific memory of the antigen are cloned and returned to the lymphoid system.

In addition, B cells can process and present antigen to T cells. Examples of humoral immune responses include resistance to encapsulated pyrogenic bacteria such as pneumococci, streptococci, meningococci, and *H. influenzae,* hemolytic transfusion reactions, and hyperacute organ rejection.

The first exposure of an antigen to an activated lymphocyte evokes a primary immune response. Repeated exposure of the identical antigen to activated lymphocytes evokes an accelerated secondary response. In the secondary immune response, the latent period is shorter and the amount of antigen required to initiate the response is less.

IMMUNOSUPPRESSION

Immunosuppression is an alteration in normal immune protective responses, a state of decreased responsiveness of the immune system. The individual who cannot mount an effective immune response is said to be anergic. Anergy can occur as a natural phenomenon in the life cycle, as in the cases of the very young and the elderly, or it can occur as a result of intentional and unintentional immunosuppression.

Opportunistic Infection

Immunosuppressed individuals are vulnerable to opportunistic infections. Opportunistic infections are caused by organisms that are ubiquitous in the environment (internal and external) but rarely cause disease in the immunocompetent host. Organisms responsible for opportunistic infections include bacteria (*Pseudomonas, Serratia, Proteus,* and *Enterobacter* spp.), fungi (*Candida* spp.), viruses (the herpesvirus family), and parasites (*Pneumocystis carinii, Toxoplasma gondii*). Natural protection from opportunistic infection depends on the presence of normal and intact innate and acquired immune mechanisms.

Etiologies of Immunocompromise and Infection in the Critically Ill

The three major determinants of nosocomial infection are the hospital environment, microorganisms, and host defense. Hospitalization and the critical-care environment alone predisposes an individual to an increased risk of infection. Hospitalization initiates the conversion of normal cutaneous flora to colonization of a new microbial population, that which is prevalent in the hospital. Colonization by itself is not harmful to the individual. However, when the first lines of defense are broken or bypassed, colonization leads the way for infection.

Fifty percent of patients admitted to intensive-care units become colonized with gram-negative bacteria within 72 hours. The major vector of these bacteria is the human hand. Nosocomial infections occur in 25 to 50% of patients admitted to intensive-care units. Infection is more prevalent in teaching hospitals and on surgical services. The most frequent types of nosocomial infections are urinary tract infections, wound infections, respiratory infections, and septicemia, in that order.

Other factors that predispose critically ill patients to infection include surgery, trauma, endotracheal intubation, shock, malnutrition, renal failure, liver failure, splenectomy, broad-spectrum antibiotic or corticosteroid therapy, and obesity.

HYPERSENSITIVITY REACTIONS

When an adaptive immune response occurs in an exaggerated or inappropriate form, causing tissue damage, a hypersensitivity reaction is said to occur. Hypersensitivity reactions occur on second exposure to the causative antigen. Four types of hypersensitivity reactions are described.

Type I

Type I hypersensitivity reactions (allergic or anaphylactic) are immediate in nature. This antibody (IgE)-mediated response results in the release of histamine by mast cells, which produces an acute inflammatory reaction. The distinguishing clinical feature of a type I hypersensitivity reaction is an immediate wheal and flare reaction.

Type II

Type II hypersensitivity reactions are caused by the presence of preformed circulating cytotoxic antibodies. These antibodies destroy the target cells on contact.

Examples of type II hypersensitivity reactions are transfusion reactions, autoimmune hemolytic anemia, and hemolytic disease of the newborn (HDNB). In a transfusion reaction, antibodies (IgM) to ABO antigens cause agglutination, complement fixation, and intravascular hemolysis. A direct Coombs test will confirm the presence of antibody on the RBCs. An indirect Coombs test measures the degree of hemolytic activity. In autoimmune hemolytic anemia, antibodies against the body's own RBCs are produced. This reaction is provoked by allergic reactions to drugs, when a drug and antibody to the drug form a complex that attacks the RBCs. HDNB occurs during the pregnancy of a mother who has been sensitized to blood group antigens on a previous infant's RBCs and makes IgE antibodies to them. The antibodies cross the placenta and react with the fetal RBCs, causing destruction. Rhesus D (Rh factor) is the most commonly involved antigen.

Type III

Type III hypersensitivity reactions are immune complex-mediated reactions. In this condition, large quantities of antigen-antibody complexes are deposited in the tissues and cannot be cleared from the body by the reticuloendothelial system. This leads to a condition known as serum sickness. Causes are persistent infection, autoimmune disease, and environmental antigens.

Type IV

In type IV (delayed-type) hypersensitivity reactions, when the host comes into contact with a foreign antigen, antigen-sensitized T cells release lymphokines that destroy the antigen. Allergic contact dermatitis, acute allograft rejection, and delayed hypersensitivity skin testing are examples of type IV hypersensitivity reactions.

ANAPHYLACTIC

Anaphylactic Shock

Anaphylaxis is an acute, generalized, and violent antigen-antibody reaction that may be rapidly fatal even with prompt emergency treatment.

Pathophysiology. Upon first exposure to an antigen, antibodies (of the immunoglobulin IgE) are formed and attach to mast cells in tissues and basophils in the vascular system. Once antibodies have been formed, a second exposure to the antigen results in an immune reaction (releasing histamine) that may vary from mild to fatal. In its severe form, the reaction is called anaphylactic shock.

The reaction of anaphylactic shock is primarily a histamine reaction, setting off a chain of multiple chemical reactions that causes further reactions. The more reactions that occur, the more severe the anaphylaxis and the greater the mortality.

The release of histamine results in vasodilatation of the capillaries (causing hypotension) and a markedly increased cellular permeability. The increase in intracellular fluid alters the cell shape, leaving spaces between the previously compact cells. This promotes movement from the vascular system, thus increasing the colloid osmotic pressure. As more colloids move into interstitial spaces, edema and a decreased circulating volume of blood occur. This has the effect of decreasing cardiac output.

Histamine occurs in two forms, H1 and H2. H1 causes vasoconstriction of the bronchi and intestines. H2 increases gastric acid secretion and minor cardiac stimulation. Both H1 and H2 are responsible for vasodilatation.

The release and action of histamines result in the release of other amines into the bloodstream. Bradykinin, serotonin, slow-reacting substances, a chemotactic factor attracting eosinophils, prostaglandins, and acetylcholine all play a role in the physiologic development of anaphylaxis. These chemicals may also activate the complement system. These amines increase arteriolar and venous dilatation, capillary permeability, and abnormal shift of fluid from the vascular tree into the interstitial compartment. This shift decreases circulating blood volume but does not decrease total blood in the body. With blood remaining in the microcirculation, decreased systolic and diastolic pressure occurs. These substances and H1 and H2 cause an intense bronchiolar constriction that leads to a general hypoxemia.

Etiology. Drugs, especially antibiotics, are the major allergens in anaphylaxis. Other drugs, iodine-based contrast dye, and blood transfusions are also involved in anaphylaxis.

Aside from medications injected or ingested, bites and stings from insects are the major causes of anaphylaxis. Of these, the stings of bees and yellow jackets are the most common, but wasps and hornets may also cause anaphylaxis.

Clinical Presentation. The major symptoms resulting from release of histamine and other chemicals are anxiety, severe dyspnea (the patient may have cyanosis), and angioedema. Angioedema is edema in membranous tissues and is most easily seen in the eyes and mouth. It also occurs in the tongue, hands, feet, and genitalia. There is a diffuse erythema occurring more in the upper body parts than in the lower. Occasionally, abdominal cramps, vomiting, and/or diarrhea may occur. Unconsciousness occurs early in severe anaphylaxis.

As fluid shifts from the capillaries into the interstitial tissue, edema of the uvula and larynx occurs. This edema may produce an acute respiratory obstruction. Laryngeal edema is accompanied by impaired phonation and a barking or high-pitched cough. If the patient is alert, he or she will show signs of increased anxiety and complain of air hunger.

Cardiovascular effects of anaphylaxis are the same as those associated with other types of shock—mainly hypotension, tachycardia, and changes in the ECG similar to those that occur in myocardial injury. Temporary changes in the ST segment and the T wave suggest coronary ischemia. However, the serum enzymes are normal.

The changes in ventilation (causing hypoxia) and decreased circulating blood may result in convulsions and unconsciousness. Circulatory failure and laryngeal edema are the usual causes of death in anaphylaxis.

Complications. Myocardial infarction secondary to venous dilation and a decreased blood pressure may occur. With decreased blood pressure, increased tissue hypoxia occurs. Increased tissue hypoxia results in increased tissue anoxia and destruction. Hypoventilation occurs due to the decreased venous return of blood to the heart and increased tissue hypoxia.

Pulmonary status, already compromised by bronchiolar constriction, may be further damaged due to overadministration of the intravenous fluids that are used to compensate for the decreased vascular volume. Chemical reactions causing further imbalances may lead to central nervous system convulsions and coma. If the pulmonary, cardiac, or vascular system is refractory to treatment, anaphylaxis is fatal.

Treatment. The primary objective of treatment is to dilate the bronchioles, which is accomplished by the administration of epinephrine either subcutaneously or intramuscularly. Antihistamines may help control local edema and itching, but they cannot alter the circulatory failure and bronchoconstriction to a significant degree. After administration of epinephrine, the respiratory system should be supported by mask, intubation, or tracheostomy with the use of a ventilator.

The second goal of therapy is to improve the patient's circulatory status. Promoting the movement of fluid from the interstitial compartment back into the vascular compartment is usually achieved through the use of intravenous fluids. Vasopressors may be used to cause constriction of the blood vessels. However, this can make tissue anoxia more severe, and use of vasopressors is controversial. The third-space loss of fluid is believed to be caused by leakage through the injured capillary walls. Glucocorticoids help to decrease cellular damage, reduce the severity of anaphylaxis, and prevent inflammation of the damaged tissues. Hydrocortisone given intravenously is the drug usually used. Steroids stabilize the membrane of the basophils, reducing the chemical reactions in anaphylaxis.

In addition to maintaining respiratory status, using epinephrine, and administering glucocorticoids (both those formed by the body in response to stress and synthetic forms), intravenous fluid will increase the circulating blood volume. Intravenous fluids may have electrolytes added to control acid-base imbalances.

Nursing Intervention. Assessment of the symptoms in all body systems is extremely important. Research has shown that laryngeal edema and hypotension are major factors causing death.

Anaphylaxis may occur in susceptible patients immediately or as much as an hour after injection of an antigen (drug, blood). Respiratory assessment includes identifying signs of stridor, the use of auxiliary muscles for breathing, and or cynosis; auscultating lung fields for rales, rhonchi, or wheezes; and measuring arterial blood gases. Mechanical ventilation should be on standby if not already in use. Normal nursing interventions for patients on respirators are applicable for these patients.

Monitoring the patient's cardiac and circulatory status is best achieved by using a pulmonary artery catheter. Death can occur within minutes if there is circulatory failure or pulmonary edema. These parameters must be observed continuously until the patient is stable and then at very frequent intervals (at least every 15 minutes for four times, then every 30 minutes for four times, and then every one to two hours).

Antihistamines are not usually helpful in altering circulatory failure and bronchoconstriction. The use of antihistamines does not affect the release of histamine but they do occupy receptor sites, thus preventing the attachment of histamine. Administration of these drugs requires close observation due to their depressive effects on the central nervous system. If epinephrine is used intravenously, monitoring for hypertension and cardiac dysrhythmias is essential.

Renal status is monitored by Foley catheter to prevent fluid overload as the extracellular fluid moves back into the vascular system with appropriate drugs. In severe anaphylaxis, the patient is frequently comatose, and establishing the monitoring and support systems may leave little, if any, time for psychosocial support. As the patient's condition stabilizes and his or her level of consciousness returns to normal, emotional support is essential. Explaining to the patient what has happened, what all the monitoring equipment is being used for, and that these monitors will be removed as his or her condition improves will help to alleviate the patient's fear.

RED BLOOD CELL FORMATION AND ANEMIAS

Hematopoiesis

The bone marrow is a spongy substance within the bone where maturation of blood cells occurs. In the adult, bone marrow is primarily located in the long, flat bones (skull, ribs, sternum, pelvis, shoulder girdles, vertebrae, innominates). The mature erythrocyte, leukocyte, and thrombocyte all begin as a primitive cell called a stem cell. In response to specific stimuli, called colony stimulating factors, a stem cell becomes "committed" to a particular cell line and matures to perform the functions of either an RBC, WBC, or platelet. Once the stem cell is committed, it is no longer capable of mitosis. It matures within the bone marrow and is released into the peripheral blood. The following diagram illustrates the relationship of the stem cell to the mature blood cells seen in the peripheral blood (Fig. 38-5). Stem cells increase in number during times of increased demand (hypoxia, infection) in order to increase production of the needed blood cell type.

RBC production is stimulated by the hormone erythropoietin. Erythropoietin is released by the kidney in response to tissue hypoxia. This hormone results in increased erythrocyte production by (1) increasing the number of stem cells placed into the maturational process, (2) decreasing maturational time, (3) increasing hemoglobin synthesis, and (4) causing a premature release of reticulocytes from the bone marrow. Reticulocytes may appear in the peripheral blood within two days of increased demand, but an increase in mature erythrocytes is not apparent until six to eight days. An increase in the peripheral reticulocyte count is an indication of increased RBC production.

The primary function of the RBC is the transportation of oxygen and carbon dioxide. Hemoglobin is the molecule responsible for this function. It is produced throughout most of the maturation of the RBC. Normal hemoglobin production is dependent upon sufficient iron supply, protoporphyrin, and globin.

The life span of the mature RBC in the circulation is approximately 120 days. As the cell becomes older, it is no longer able to traverse the microvasculature, and then it is phagocytized by the reticuloendothelial tissue.

Anemia

Definition and Etiology. Anemia is the most common problem of the erythrocyte. It is a clinical sign defined as (1) a reduction in the number of RBCs, (2) a reduction in the quantity of hemoglobin, and/or (3) a reduction in the volume of RBCs. There are numerous causes of anemia. Table 38-1 outlines the classification of anemias.

Clinical Presentation. The signs and symptoms of anemia are the result of tissue hypoxia or the compensatory mechanisms activated to prevent damage resulting from hypoxia. Persons are symptomatic at varying levels. Someone with mild anemia may be asymptomatic. Anemia may be the first indication of a serious underlying disease such as cancer or renal failure. If it occurs gradually, adaptation allows for minimal signs and symptoms. A person with rapid onset of anemia may be very symptomatic. The signs and symptoms associated with anemia are as follows: increased pulse, respiration, and pulse pressure; decreased blood pressure; palpitations; chest pain; dyspnea on exertion; fatigue; weakness; vertigo; bone tenderness; and delayed wound healing.

Diagnosis. Laboratory findings that are indicative of anemia are (1) decreased hemoglobin and hematocrit, (2) decreased RBC indices, (3) increased reticulocyte count, and (4) decreased erythrocyte count.

Nursing Intervention. Nursing interventions for the patient with anemia are based upon the principles of minimizing complications, conserving energy, and

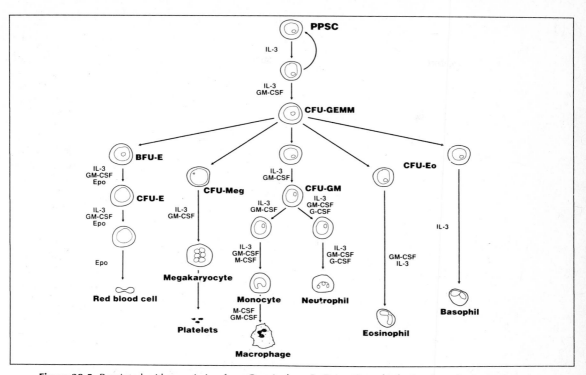

Figure 38-5. Reprinted with permission from Cunningham R. Prevention of infection in patients receiving myelosuppressive chemotherapy. New York: Triclinica Communications, 1992.

instituting medical therapies. The key interventions include the following:

1. History
   a. Signs of blood loss
   b. Bleeding tendencies
   c. Exposure to marrow toxins (drugs, radiation, chemicals)
   d. Previous history of anemia
   e. Surgical history (e.g., gastric resection)
   f. Changes in nutritional status
2. Physical assessment
   a. Oxygenation: Vital signs, lung sounds, tolerance of activity
   b. Skin, mucous membranes: Pallor, jaundice, purpura, petechiae, IV sites, wounds, indwelling catheters, stomatitis
   c. Gastrointestinal: Ascites, splenomegaly
   d. Mobility: Parathesias, impaired sensation, bone pain (sternum, ribs, vertebrae)
3. Minimize energy expenditure by:

   a. Organizing activities according to patient tolerance
   b. Planning rest periods
   c. Limiting external stimulation
   d. Preventing chills
4. Maintain skin integrity
5. Promote a diet adequate in protein, iron, vitamins, and minerals
6. Maintain physical safety (e.g., assist with ambulation if the patient is dizzy)
7. Institute an appropriate oral hygiene program

Platelet Production

Platelet production is thought to be regulated by the hormone thrombopoietin. Platelets mature in the bone marrow and migrate to the spleen. They travel between the spleen and circulatory system in order to maintain a steady state of circulating platelets. Platelets contribute to hemostasis by the formation of a plug over an area of damaged endothelium. Plug formation requires an

TABLE 38-1. CLASSIFICATION OF ANEMIA

I. Blood loss
   A. Acute
   B. Chronic
II. Deficient RBC production
   A. Iron deficiency
   B. Vitamin B_{12} deficiency
   C. Folic acid deficiency
   D. Bone marrow failure or suppression
      1. Myelofibrosis
      2. Aplastic anemia
      3. Marrow toxin (drugs, radiation)
      4. Infectious agents
III. Excessive RBC destruction
   A. Hemolytic anemia
   B. Defective glycosis (G6PD deficiency)
   C. Membrane abnormalities
   D. Physical causes (prosthetic heart valves)
IV. Defective hemoglobin synthesis
   A. Thalassemias
   B. Sickle cell anemia
V. Anemias of chronic disease
   A. Renal disease
   B. Liver disease
   C. Endocrine disorders
   D. Cancers

adequate number of functioning platelets as well as vascular integrity. Platelets are a source of phospholipids, which are necessary in the coagulation process.

Thrombocytopenia

Thrombocytopenia is a quantitative decrease in the number of circulating platelets. The risk of bleeding increases as the platelet count decreases. Normal platelet count is 100,000 to 300,000/mm³. Usually persons are placed on bleeding precautions when the platelet count falls below 50,000/mm³. The risk of spontaneous bleeding increases at a platelet count of less than 20,000/mm³. Table 38-2 outlines causes of thrombocytopenia.

Clinical Presentation. Signs and symptoms associated with thrombocytopenia include petechiae, bruising, ecchymosis, hematemesis, hemoptysis, hematuria, vaginal bleeding, rectal bleeding, blood in stools, anemia, and active bleeding from mucous membranes, wounds, indwelling catheters, and sites of invasive procedures.

Treatment. Platelet transfusions are administered to thrombocytopenic patients who are actively bleeding, undergoing invasive procedures, or at increased risk of spontaneous bleeding. Platelet transfusions can be a random donor pooling or a single donor HLA-matched product. Upon exposure to an increasing number of platelet transfusions, the patient may become refractory to the benefits of the transfusion as a result of antibody formation to platelets. A person with fever usually has increased destruction of platelets. A one- to two-hour post-transfusion platelet count is performed to document the effectiveness of the platelet transfusion. Reactions or complications of platelet transfusions are similar to those of whole blood transfusions.

Nursing Intervention. Nursing interventions are based upon (1) protection of the patient from bleeding and associated complications and (2) early detection of bleeding. Most institutions have policies (bleeding precautions, platelet precautions) that are instituted when the platelet count is less than 50,000/mm³. A sign is placed near the patient to alert all health team members that the patient is at risk of bleeding. Key interventions include:

1. Bleeding precautions for a platelet count of less than 50,000/mm³
2. Assessment of sites of potential bleeding
   a. Skin
   b. Mucous membranes
   c. Indwelling catheter sites
3. Assessment of bodily excrement for occult and frank bleeding
   a. Urine
   b. Stool
   c. Sputum
   d. Pad count in menstruating females
4. Routine neurological assessment
5. Prevention of trauma
   a. Use soft toothbrushes or toothettes for oral hygiene
   b. Use electric razors
   c. Coordinate blood sampling to avoid multiple venipunctures
   d. Institute bowel routine to prevent constipation
   e. Avoid intramuscular injections
   f. Avoid prolonged use of tourniquets

TABLE 38-2. CAUSES OF THROMBOCYTOPENIA

Symptom	Cause
Decreased production	Leukemia
	Lymphoma
	Multiple myeloma
	Metastatic cancer
	Chemotherapy
	Radiation therapy
	Drugs (thiazides, estrogen)
	Alcohol
Increased destruction	Autoimmune disorders
	Idiopathic thrombocytopenia purpura
	Malignant disorders
	Disseminated intravascular coagulation
	Infectious agents
Abnormal platelet function	Aspirin
Decreased availability	Sequestration of spleen

g. Avoid use of urinary catheters
h. Use soft restraints only when absolutely necessary
i. Use padded siderails when the patient is in bed
j. Assist the patient with ambulation, if indicated
k. Institute measures to minimize vomiting

6. Avoid use of aspirin or aspirin-containing compounds
7. Control of temperature elevations
8. Monitoring of pertinent laboratory data
   a. Hemoglobin
   b. Hematocrit
   c. Platelet count
   d. Pre- and post-platelet transfusion counts

CHAPTER 39

Blood and Component Therapy

Editor's Note

This chapter is supplemental to other chapters in this book, providing more information for CCRN content areas of hypovolemia and coagulopathies. No specific questions generally come from this chapter, although questions may be derived indirectly from the content of this chapter. Read this chapter to improve your general understanding of the reasons for use of blood component therapy.

The primary reason for transfusing blood is to increase the oxygen available for preventing tissue hypoxia. Blood is administered primarily when the hemoglobin/hematocrit levels are low (generally when hemoglobin levels are below 7 g/dL), when intravascular volume is low, and to replace deficient or utilized substances such as protein, platelets, and clotting factors.

TRANSFUSION WITH WHOLE BLOOD

One unit of whole blood is approximately 500 cc of blood cells, serum, platelets,, proteins, and other intravascular nutrients and substances. Whole blood is the best substance to transfuse in hemorrhage bleeds, since it replaces both volume and elements.

Normally, during the administration of a blood transfusion, the cold (due to storage) donor blood is rapidly warmed as it mixes with circulating blood at normal infusion rates. Rapid replacement with cold blood predisposes the patient to a cardiac arrest. When massive, rapid transfusions are necessary, the blood can be passed through a warmer to reach body temperature, thus reducing the danger of cardiac arrest.

Red Blood Cells (Packed RBCs)

Packed RBCs provide the advantage of less blood volume (200 to 250 cc) to infuse, thereby decreasing the chance of fluid overload. Packed RBCs are used in severe anemias without blood loss, in patients with congestive heart failure (CHF), and cautiously in patients with underlying cardiac disease or with renal failure.

Fresh Frozen Plasma

Fresh frozen plasma (FFP) is the fluid portion of blood after centrifugation to remove the RBCs. Due to freezing the plasma, all clotting factors (especially V and VII) are preserved except for platelets.

Administration of plasma is indicated when there is a coagulopathy or hypovolemia with little or no actual blood loss, for example, in burns and crush injuries. In an emergency, FFP may be used as a volume expander in hypovolemic bleeds until fresh whole blood is available.

Cryoprecipitates

Cryoimmunoglobulins are serum proteins that precipitate at temperatures below 20°C. Cryoimmunoglobulins must be obtained and processed at temperatures above 20°C and ideally before refrigeration, which may cause cryoproteins to be caught in the blood clots. Many authorities feel that cryoprecipitates are antigen-antibody protein compounds.

Cryoprecipitates usually consist of 20 to 30 cc/unit of blood and must be infused immediately after thawing. Cryoprecipitates contain factors VIII, factor XIII, and fibrinogen. It is not uncommon to infuse as many as 30 bags of cryoprecipitates at one time, using a special transfusion administration set.

The administration of cryoprecipitates is indicated in disseminated intravascular coagulation (DIC), hemophilia A, and von Willebrand's disease.

Platelets

Less than 40,000 to 50,000 platelets/mm³ is considered inadequate for hemostasis. Prolonged bleeding time is a better index of the need for platelet transfusion than an actual platelet count. There is an approximate increase of 10,000/unit (platelet)/mm³. A postplatelet transfusion bleeding time is the most accurate index of response to therapy.

In thrombocytopenia, splenomegaly, and DIC, platelet transfusions are useful until more definitive therapy can be instituted. Alloimmunity may require cross-matching to have any value for platelet transfusion. Platelets can be safely kept at room temperatures for up to three days and are inactivated if refrigerated.

Volume Expanders

Albumin, hetastarch (Hespan), and, in some institutions, dextran 40 and dextran 70 are used as volume expanders.

Salt-Poor Albumin. This is a concentrate of human serum albumin packaged in 50-cc ampules with a total protein of 12.5 g in 50- to 100-cc amounts. It is not low in sodium content, nor does it supply any clotting factors. Its sole value is its blood volume expansion, increasing colloid osmotic pressure for up to 24 hours (time may be a low as 4 hours).

Hetastarch (Hespan). Hetastarch is a large, glucose-based colloidal volume expander. It has approximately the same molecular weight as albumin and similar volume expansion properties. Only about 20% of the volume of crystalloid solutions (lactated Ringer's or normal saline) is necessary with hetastarch to achieve similar hemodynamic responses. Normally, hetastarch is administered in a 6% solution. Hetastarch is cleared via renal excretion in about 24 to 36 hours. While similar to albumin in volume expansion, it has the advantage of only costing about one-third as much as albumin.

Dextran. This is commercially available in two forms: dextran 70 (Macrodex) or dextran 40 (low-molecular-weight dextran [LMWD]).

Dextran 70 is a 6% solution in 0.9 normal saline or D5W composed of both small and large molecules. It has colloid effects similar to those of plasma.

Dextran's greatest value lies in its expansion properties in addition to its lowering of blood viscosity. The lower blood viscosity is due to a lower hematocrit

and reduction of platelet and RBC aggregations, which improve tissue perfusion. LMWD may help prevent a vascular thrombus occlusion of a vessel or graft.

Major complications of dextran use are allergic reactions, impaired coagulation (due to interference with platelet aggregation), and difficulty in future type-matching and cross-matching attempts for whole blood infusions. The allergic reactions may range from urticaria to anaphylaxis, which may occur immediately or after more than 30 minutes. Nausea, vomiting, and hypotension may occur.

Dextran therapy is not indicated in oliguric patients, CHF patients, and patients with blood-clotting dyscrasias. Its use has markedly decreased over the past years.

Granulocytes

Centers performing leukopheresis have the ability to filter out granulocytes. Each unit is about 200 to 300 cc, and the recipient must be compatible with the donor. An infusion of granulocytes improves phagocytosis from the marginal cells, not increasing the already circulating white blood cell pool. The marginal cells are those being released from the bone marrow.

It is common for the patient to have fever and chills during granulocyte infusion. Steroids and antihistamines given before the infusion will help control the fever, whereas meperidine hydrochloride (Demerol) will control the chills.

REACTIONS TO BLOOD AND COMPONENT THERAPY

In spite of meticulous procedures for blood and component therapy, reactions do occur. There are four major reactions.

1. Circulatory overload occurs when too much fluid or too rapid an infusion is administered to patients with underlying cardiac, renal, liver, pulmonary, or hematologic disease. With proper monitoring and assessment, circulatory overload should not occur. If it does occur, prompt and appropriate intervention will remove sufficient fluid to restore the normal fluid status.

2. A bacterial reaction to transfusion therapy is the most common reaction and is characterized by the development of a fever in a previously

afebrile patient. If the patient is febrile, a rising temperature may indicate a reaction.

3. Allergic reactions may occur with almost any product transfused. A slight reaction may be manifested by a mild urticaria. A severe allergic reaction is indicated by anaphylaxis that may or may not be reversible.

4. A hemolytic reaction usually occurs within the first 30 minutes of the transfusion. It results in actual hemolysis of the RBCs, and the transfusion must be stopped.

Clinical Presentation

The signs and symptoms will differ with the type of reaction, length of transfusion, substance being infused, and intensity of the reaction. Common signs and symptoms may include chills, fever, hives, hypotension, cardiac palpitations, tachycardia, flushing of the skin, headache, loss of consciousness, nausea and vomiting, shortness of breath, back pain, and hemoglobinuria. In some instances, warmth along the vein carrying the infusion may be detected.

Nursing Intervention

The nurse must immediately stop the infusion (saving the substance being transfused) and keep the vein open with 0.9 normal saline. Accurate assessment of patient status must be completed quickly and efficiently for a comparison with pretransfusion baseline data. The physician and the blood bank are notified of the reaction, and physician's orders are carried out. If the reaction is anaphylactic, emergency resuscitative measures are instituted while personnel contact the doctor and laboratory and save the substance being transfused.

Nursing support of the patient and family is best achieved by rapid but efficient and professional conduct in instituting all necessary interventions. Education as to the cause of the reaction may prevent a recurrence.

CHAPTER 40
Normal Coagulation and Pathologic Hematologic Conditions

Editor's Note

This chapter contains supplemental information helpful in answering CCRN questions addressing the concepts of disseminated intravascular coagulation and thrombolytic therapy. Understanding concepts in this chapter will be useful in answering several questions on the exam. Use this chapter to supplement your understanding of clinical conditions requiring thrombolytic treatment and coagulopathies.

Three sequential events occur to aid in preventing bleeding. Vasoconstriction and platelet aggregation are the first two events in hemostasis. The third hemostatic mechanism is coagulation.

NORMAL COAGULATION

Normal coagulation is dependent upon the presence of all clotting factors and the appropriate functioning of other separate, but interrelated components. These components are the extrinsic cascade, the intrinsic cascade, and the common final pathway.

Clotting Factors

Confusion often occurs with the nomenclature assigned to the specific clotting factors. Consequently, an international committee agreed that all clotting factors would be designated by roman numerals for the inactive clotting factors. It was further agreed that once activated, the clotting factors would be identified by the roman numeral and a subscript "a." Table 40-1 lists the clotting factors and their synonyms. There is no designated factor VI.

Most of the clotting factors are found in circulating blood, the blood elements and tissues surrounding and within the microcirculatory system. Clotting factors I (fibrinogen), II (prothrombin), and V, VII, IX, and X are synthesized in the liver. Factors XI and XIII may also be synthesized in the liver. Factor VIII is most likely synthesized by macrophages in the spleen. Lymphocytes and the bone marrow may work in conjunction with the macrophages to form factor VIII.

Four clotting factors, factors II, VII, IX, and X, are dependent upon vitamin K for synthesis by the liver. Research indicates that factor XI may also be vitamin K dependent. It is known that at least 30 sub-

TABLE 40-1. CLOTTING FACTORS AND THEIR SYNONYMS

Factor	Synonym
I	Fibrinogen
Ia	Fibrin
II	Prothrombin
IIa	Thrombin
III	Thromboplastin
IV	Calcium
V	Acglobulin (labile factor, proaccelerin)
VII	Proconvertin (autoprothrombin I)
VIIa	Convertin
VIII	Antihemophiliac globulin
IX	Christmas factor (autoprothrombin II), plasma thromboplastin component
IXa	Activated plasma thromboplastin component
X	Stuart-Prower factor (autoprothrombin III)
XI	Plasma thromboplastin antecedent
XII	Hageman factor
XIIa	Activated Hageman factor
XIII	Fibrin-stabilizing factor

stances may be connected with the clotting process; however, the 17 listed in Table 40-1 are the most significant.

Cascades

A cascade is similar to a row of dominoes standing on their ends. When the first domino falls, it strikes the next domino, starting a chain reaction that continues until all of the dominoes have been toppled. This necessitates positioning the dominoes so that each will connect with the next. Within the circulating blood, there is a plethora of clotting factors to continue a cascade once initiated. It is interesting to note that there is at least one specific spot in each of the three cascades (extrinsic, intrinsic, and final common pathway) that requires calcium ions (Ca^{2+}, factor IV) to continue activation of these cascades. These sites are identified in Fig. 40-1, which shows the normal coagulation process.

Extrinsic Cascade. This cascade (Fig. 40-2) is activated by injury to vessels and tissue. The end result of this cascade is the release of thromboplastin into the circulatory system.

A second mechanism for activating clotting factors is the release of phospholipids from platelets and damaged tissue. This is thought to increase the rate of blood coagulation through both extrinsic and intrinsic cascades.

Intrinsic Cascade. This cascade (Fig. 40-3) is initiated when factor XII (the Hageman factor, the surface substance) comes into contact with collagen or the basement membrane of the blood vessel's damaged endothelium.

Common Final Pathway Cascade. Both the extrinsic and intrinsic cascades react to completion and, in the presence of calcium ions, join to form the common final pathway (cascade) shown in Fig. 40-4.

Syneresis is the final step in coagulation and the first step in clot stability. Syneresis is the process of particle suspension in a gel that begins to aggregate and form a compact mass—the clot. Clot retraction occurs soon after syneresis is complete. Platelets contain an enzyme called thromboplastin. This enzyme causes the fibrin strands and cells in the clot to be drawn together, expressing a clear, serous fluid. Clot retraction is responsible for drawing the edges of damaged vessels together, which fosters healing.

ANTICOAGULATION

When the vascular damage has been repaired, dissolution of the clot begins. This is termed fibrinolysis. Up to this point, the various cascades have clotted the injured vessels but have not caused massive intravascular clotting. Massive clotting is avoided because of excess thrombin is carried away from the clot site by the circulating blood and antithrombin III is released from mast cells.

There are actually two mechanisms to prevent excessive clotting: the fibrinolytic system and the antithrombin system.

Fibrinolytic System

In this system, plasminogen is converted to plasmin. Plasmin lyses the clot. Clot lysis (fibrinolysis) is accomplished by two mechanisms: clearance of activated clotting factors by the reticuloendothelial system and the actual lysis of the fibrin structure in the clot. Lysis of the clot is initiated by either the internal or external pathway. In the internal pathway, factor XII is activated to XIIa upon contact with an abnormal or irregular vascular lining. At the same time, XIIa catalyzes prekallikrein to kallikrein (a blood plasminogen activator). The extrinsic system provides tissue plasminogen activators from damaged vascular areas. Both types of plasminogen activators convert plasminogen to plasmin. Plasmin breaks the fibrin structure, causing the mesh holding blood components, such as platelets, to weaken and dissociate as a stable unit. The breakdown of the fibrin structure causes an increase in fibrin degradation products (or fibrin split products). An increase in fibrin degradation products may signal the onset of a coagulopathy such as disseminated intravascular coagulation (DIC).

Fibrinolytic Therapy

Fibrinolytic therapy in the treatment of acute myocardial infarction and pulmonary emboli employs the principles of normal clot lysis. Normally, the fibrinolytic system converts plasminogen to plasmin, which degrades fibrin into soluble fragments. In the presence of large thrombi, this system cannot dissolve the large fibrin mass. However the introduction of exogenous plasminogen activators produces more plasmin, which depletes circulating fibrinogen and promotes lysis. Exogenous plasminogen activator also destroy coagulation factors V and VIII, causing a systemic lytic state that increases the potential risk of bleeding.

The fibrinolytic agents used most frequently in-

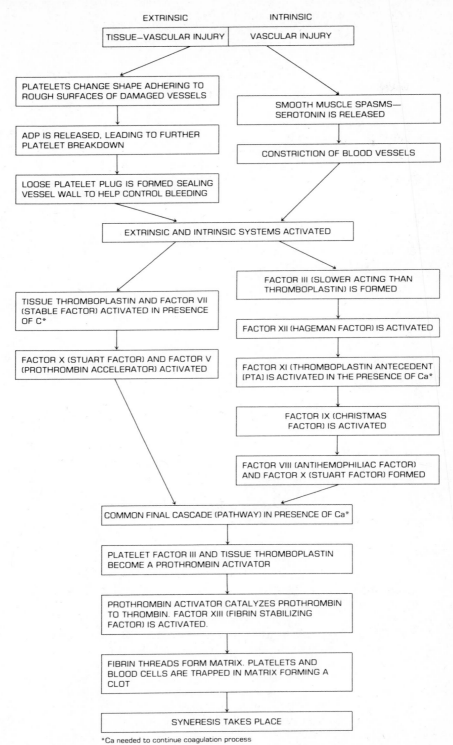

EXTRINSIC   INTRINSIC

TISSUE—VASCULAR INJURY | VASCULAR INJURY

PLATELETS CHANGE SHAPE ADHERING TO ROUGH SURFACES OF DAMAGED VESSELS

SMOOTH MUSCLE SPASMS— SEROTONIN IS RELEASED

ADP IS RELEASED, LEADING TO FURTHER PLATELET BREAKDOWN

CONSTRICTION OF BLOOD VESSELS

LOOSE PLATELET PLUG IS FORMED SEALING VESSEL WALL TO HELP CONTROL BLEEDING

EXTRINSIC AND INTRINSIC SYSTEMS ACTIVATED

FACTOR III (SLOWER ACTING THAN THROMBOPLASTIN) IS FORMED

TISSUE THROMBOPLASTIN AND FACTOR VII (STABLE FACTOR) ACTIVATED IN PRESENCE OF C*

FACTOR XII (HAGEMAN FACTOR) IS ACTIVATED

FACTOR X (STUART FACTOR) AND FACTOR V (PROTHROMBIN ACCELERATOR) ACTIVATED

FACTOR XI (THROMBOPLASTIN ANTECEDENT [PTA] IS ACTIVATED IN THE PRESENCE OF Ca*

FACTOR IX (CHRISTMAS FACTOR) IS ACTIVATED

FACTOR VIII (ANTIHEMOPHILIAC FACTOR) AND FACTOR X (STUART FACTOR) FORMED

COMMON FINAL CASCADE (PATHWAY) IN PRESENCE OF Ca*

PLATELET FACTOR III AND TISSUE THROMBOPLASTIN BECOME A PROTHROMBIN ACTIVATOR

PROTHROMBIN ACTIVATOR CATALYZES PROTHROMBIN TO THROMBIN. FACTOR XIII (FIBRIN STABILIZING FACTOR) IS ACTIVATED.

FIBRIN THREADS FORM MATRIX. PLATELETS AND BLOOD CELLS ARE TRAPPED IN MATRIX FORMING A CLOT

SYNERESIS TAKES PLACE

*Ca needed to continue coagulation process

Figure 40-1. Normal coagulation process.

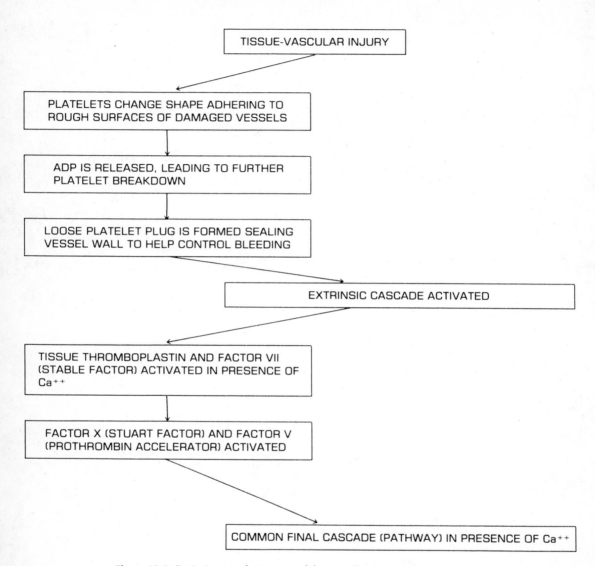

Figure 40-2. Extrinsic cascade segment of the overall normal coagulation process.

clude streptokinase (SK), urokinase (UK), and tissue plasminogen activator (TPA). SK is derived from beta-hemolytic streptococci and activates the fibrinolytic process by forming an activator complex with plasminogen. SK depletes fibrinogen and other coagulants factors predisposing the patient to systemic bleeding. Allergic, anaphylactic reactions can be induced upon a second exposure to the drug due to its nature as a bacterial protein.

UK is a naturally occurring human enzyme that acts directly on the circulating plasminogen to produce plasmin. TPA is also a naturally occurring human enzyme that activates plasminogen only after plasminogen has bound to fibrin contained in the thrombus. Relatively little circulating plasmin is produced, and clotting factors are not depleted. The risk of systemic bleeding is lessened.

Neither UK nor TPA produces allergic reactions because they are naturally occurring within the human body. TPA is shorter acting (ten minutes) than streptokinase (several hours) or urokinase (approximately one hour).

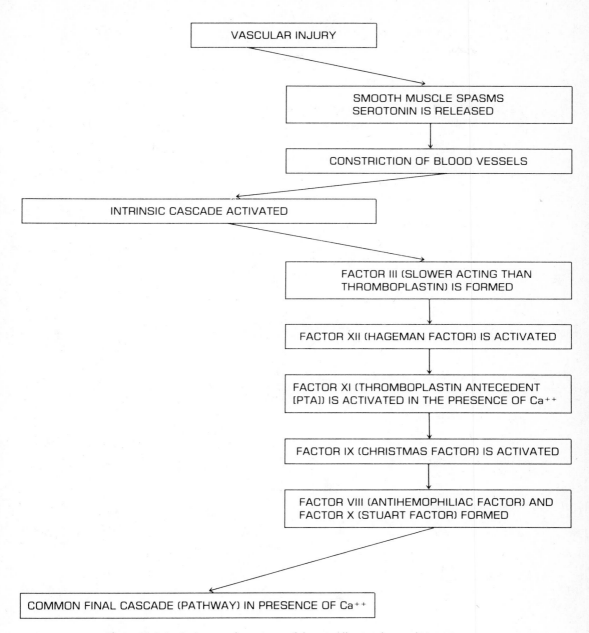

Figure 40-3. Intrinsic cascade segment of the overall normal coagulation process.

Antithrombin System

This system protects our bodies from excessive intravascular clotting by neutralizing the clotting capability of thrombin. Antithrombin III is the neutralizing agent. Heparin functions as an antithrombin III and inhibits all serine proteases in all cascades. These include Xa,

Ha, Vt12, and thrombin. It interrupts the action of thrombin on fibrinogen.

When clot retraction is complete, profibrinolysis is activated by factor XII. This activation results in fibrinolysin (plasmin), which phagocytizes the clot and other clotting factors present in excess of the normal

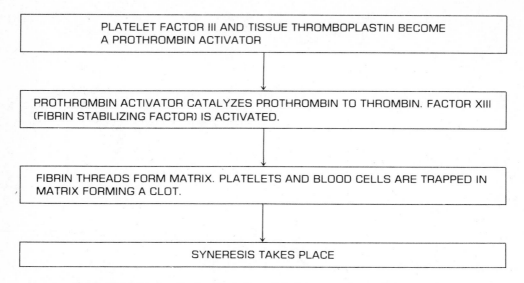

Figure 40-4. Common final pathway (cascade) of the normal coagulation process.

amount. In this way, both intravascular clotting and bleeding are controlled.

HEMOSTATIC SCREENING TESTS

Specific tests can be performed to evaluate blood-clotting activity, to identify abnormalities, and to ascertain patient response to therapy.

Prothrombin Time
The prothrombin time (PT) measures the activity level and patency of the extrinsic cascade and the common final pathway. The PT measures factors I, II, V, VII, and X. Normal values are the same as control values (should be 11 to 16 seconds). Coumadin effectiveness is assessed with the PT.

Activated Partial Thromboplastin Time
The activated partial thromboplastin time (aPTT) measures the activity level and patency of the intrinsic cascade and common final pathway. Normal values of 20 to 35 seconds are used to assess all clotting factors except VII and XIII. Heparin effectiveness is assessed with the aPTT.

Bleeding Time
Platelet plug formation time is measured with the bleeding time. Normal values are less than four min-

utes (Ivy), one to four minutes (Duke), and one to nine minutes (Mielke).

Platelet Count
This is a specific count of platelets seen in a blood smear. Normal values are 150,000 to 450,000 platelets/mm^2. Values below 100,000 platelets/mm^2 are pathognomonic for thrombocytopenia, the cause of which must be determined. A lower platelet count results in excessive bleeding since there is an insufficient number of platelets to clot. Counts less than 20,000 are associated with spontaneous bleeding.

In summary, normal clotting has three stages: (1) vascular injury activates thromboplastin activity in both the extrinsic and intrinsic pathways, (2) thromboplastin converts prothrombin to thrombin, and (3) thrombin converts fibrinogen in the plasma at the site of injury to form a fibrin plug.

DISSEMINATED INTRAVASCULAR COAGULATION

Disseminated intravascular coagulation (DIC) is a state of hypercoagulability utilizing all of the clotting factors. The exhaustion of these clotting factors results in hemorrhage.

Pathophysiology

Regardless of the etiology, specific pathophysiological signs occur in DIC. The common denominator is the release of procoagulants into the circulatory system. Free hemoglobin, cancer tissue fragments, amniotic fluid, and bacterial toxins are some procoagulants that may activate the clotting cascade. Activation of the cascade results in diffuse intravascular fibrin formation. Fibrin is then deposited in the microcirculation.

With the clotting of the capillaries, blood is shunted to the arteriovenous anastomoses. This shunting causes the capillary tissue to use anaerobic metabolism. With the production of lactic and pyruvic waste products and blood stagnation in the microcirculation, acidemia develops.

Three procoagulant factors develop in capillary blood as a result of the DIC disease process. Acidosis acts as a strong procoagulant along with the "normal" procoagulants in the blood. The third factor is the concentration of procoagulants, which increases secondary to the stagnation of blood. All of these processes result in massive sequestration of clotted blood in the capillaries (Fig. 40-5).

DIC develops rapidly, so coagulating factors are

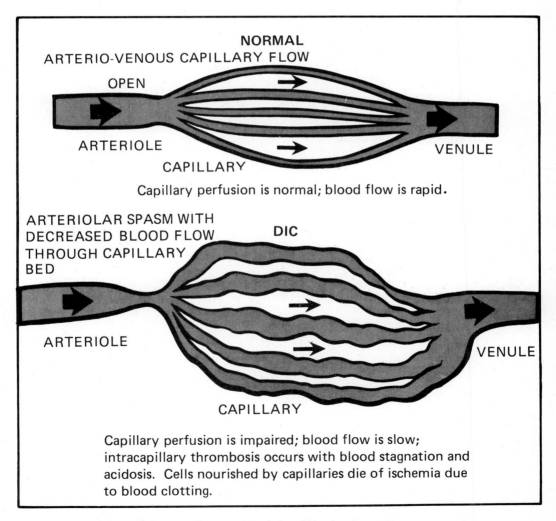

Figure 40-5. Sequestration of clotted blood in the capillaries.

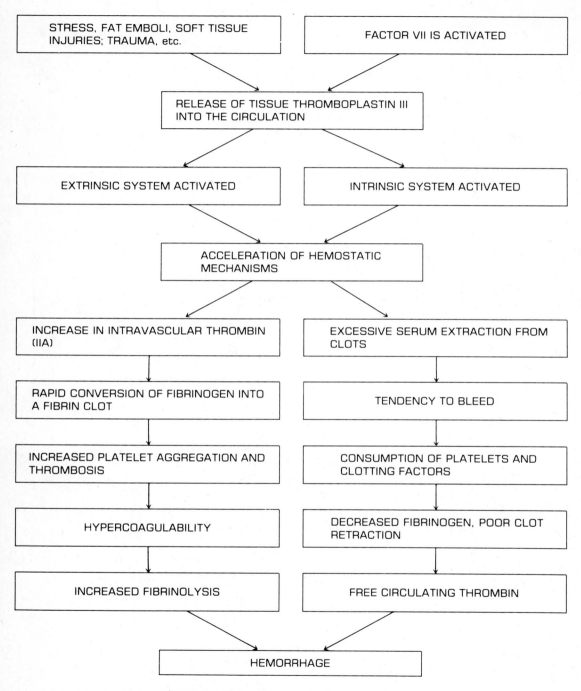

Figure 40-6. Alteration the coagulation process in DIC.

depleted in the microcirculation faster than the clotting factors can be replenished. Without circulating co-agulant factors, hemostasis cannot be maintained (Fig. 40-6) and the patient begins to bleed.

Etiology

Many factors may precipitate DIC, including multiple trauma, crush injuries, hemorrhagic shock, malignant hypertension, incompatible blood transfusion, any and all cancers, burns, and coronary bypass surgery. DIC does not occur in isolation; it is always a sequelae of some initiating event.

Clinical Presentation

In most cases of DIC, arterial hypotension occurs secondary to the arteriovenous anastomoses. The anastomoses are caused by arterial vasoconstriction of the precapillary sphincter and vasodilatation of the capillaries.

Bleeding occurs after injections or venipunctures, from incisions, in the mucosa of the mouth, in the respiratory system, in the gastrointestinal system, and in the genitourinary system. It is common for several of these systems to be bleeding simultaneously; rarely is only one system involved.

Despite the complete depletion of circulating fibrinogen, some circulating thrombin still exists, since fibrinogen is not present to convert it to fibrin. Activation of the clotting process produces thrombin and thereby fibrin. Fibrin and thrombin convert plasminogen to plasmin. Antithrombins (especially anti-thrombin III) destroy thrombin function. In DIC, thrombin production exceeds antithrombin III production and thereby promotes uncontrolled coagulation.

The initiation of fibrinolysis results in dissolution of clots and degrades fibrin into its fractions, which further adds to the bleeding.

In an attempt to restore hemostasis, the liver produces more fibrinogen or the patient is transfused with blood, plasma, or fibrinogen. This perpetuates the process, making the DIC more severe and intractable.

Pulmonary compromise may require intubation. Following the trend of ABGs and observing for signs and symptoms of hypoxemia will show when suctioning and/or mechanical ventilation is indicated.

Monitor fluid balance especially if the patient receives multiple blood transfusions and other fluids or if the patient has another pre-existing disease.

Skin care to preserve skin integrity is very important. Care must be taken to treat the patient very gently and to maintain good body alignment with adequate support. Sufficient but not excessive pressure is applied to sites of intramuscular injections or venipunctures by laboratory personnel to prevent hematoma formation.

Petechiae are pinpoint flat lesions that appear as reddish purple spots on the skin, buccal mucosa, and conjunctivae. Purpura is characterized by reddish brown spots usually evidencing presence of fluid. Ecchymoses are black and blue bruises.

Psychosocial support is extremely important to decrease the anxiety of the patient who is aware and frightened by all the lost blood and the flurry of activity around him or her. Very brief explanations should be given; for example, "I'm giving you some medicine through the vein to help stop your bleeding."

Being honest with the patient's family as well as with the patient will help to decrease anxiety and foster a positive relationship between all parties involved.

Treatment of DIC

The primary treatment of DIC is to treat the underlying disease which is easier said than done in the face of a patient hemorrhaging.

The second treatment is to halt the DIC. This is accomplished by several concurrent actions. It is necessary to replace the clotting factors so the serum is converted back to plasma. At the same time, the effects of thrombin must be stopped. Also at the same time, correction of acidosis, hypotension, hypovolemia, and hypoxia must be attempted since these four conditions act as procoagulants to continue utilization/depletion of clotting factors. Vitamin K (formation of prothrombin) and folic acid (thrombocytopenia) are administered to correct these deficiencies.

The use of heparin remains controversial since it is difficulty to assess its effectiveness. Heparin neutralizes free circulating thrombin by combining with anti-thrombin III which inactivates the thrombin. Heparin functions as an anticoagulant to prevent further thrombus formation in the microcirculatory system. (It does not alter the thrombi already formed.) Heparin prevents the activation of factor X. Heparin also inhibits platelet aggregation.

Caution: If used, heparin should be given intravenously, not subcutaneously. Factors affecting subcutaneous heparin include the absorption rate which is dependent on the amount injected, the depth of injection, body temperature, and cardiovascular status. If a hematoma develops at the injection site, absorption is markedly altered. The amount of heparin needed may be too much for subcutaneous administration. The delay in reaching a therapeutic blood level may be too long with subcutaneous administration.

After heparin therapy is started, whole blood, fresh frozen plasma, and/or platelet transfusion are administered.

Complications

DIC may become an exsanguinating hemorrhage. Death is not uncommon.

Nursing Interventions

Assessment of patients at high risk of DIC include looking for development of petechiae, purpura, and ecchymosis. Oozing of blood from injection sites, I.V. lines, and invasive monitoring lines all may indicate the onset of DIC.

Cardiac status must be monitored for dysrhythmias secondary to acidosis, hypovolemia, hypervolemia, and electrolyte imbalances. Early recognition and treatment of dysrhythmias may prevent progression to more serious dysrhythmias. Renal problems develop due to fluid overload, fluid depletion, and hypotension. The oliguric or anuric patient cannot eliminate heparin adequately, so the dose must be titrated to match the patient's utilization and excretion of the drug.

Monitor the amount of bleeding and identify the system involved. All drainage should be tested for blood. Observe for frank bleeding.

Watch for signs of thrombus formation. If thrombi develop, the symptoms will vary according to the system involved. The kidneys are most often involved (oliguria or anuria).

Intracranial bleeding may be identified by altered level of consciousness; orientation to person, place, and time; pupil reactions; and extremity movement. These must be checked frequently. Any change will indicate a possible bleed.

Avoid infection. The DIC patient is at high risk for infection primarily due to all the entry ports for bacteria. Development of a fever is an indication to culture blood, urine, sputum, and any other drainage. If the bacteria is identified, appropriate antibiotics are started.

Editor's Note

It is unlikely that the following two conditions will be on the CCRN exam. This section is included simply to provide a more complete description of abnormal coagulation concepts.

HEMOPHILIA AND VON WILLEBRAND'S DISEASE

Hemophilia is the name given to three inherited disorders that have bleeding in common. The bleeding is due to a lack of or deficiency in a plasma clotting factor. Von Willebrand's disease is included in this section since it also involves a deficient clotting factor.

Etiology

Hemophilia A and B are sex-linked recessive disorders. They affect men mainly, but do occur rarely in women. It is more common that the female is a "carrier" and genetically transmits these diseases to the male. Hemophilia C is an autosomal trait. Von Willebrand's disease is an autosomal dominant mode of inheritance, so it should occur equally among men and women. Von Willebrand's disease is an actual lack of factor VIII. A complete absence of this factor may occur or there may be a reduced amount of structurally normal factor.   Hemorrhaging may occur in a muscle mass, forming an extremely painful hematoma. These hematomas (masses) press against nerves, resulting in transient motor and/or sensory loss. Gastrointestinal bleeding is the next most common symptom, in which there is often no evidence of ulceration to account for the bleed. Epistaxis is also common.

Joint deformity with eventual crippling may occur. Hematuria is often present in hemophiliacs and may continue for weeks without a known cause.

Hemorrhage into the central nervous system (CNS) is rare in hemophiliacs but is extremely severe when it does occur. It is not uncommon for these patients to die secondary to hemorrhage into the CNS. This bleeding is often caused by trauma.

Hemophiliacs seem to fluctuate in the frequency and severity of the bleed during the year. Hemophiliacs tend to bleed less with age. The reasons for these two variables are unknown at this time. All of these symptoms except hemarthrosis also occur in von Willebrand's disease also.

Diagnosis

A familial tendency to excessive bleeding is known, and the family frequently reports the diagnosis as "the bleeding disease." The clinical condition can be verified by laboratory tests. The PTT is prolonged. Factor assays reveal decreased factor VIII in hemophilia A and normal to decreased factor VII in von Willebrand's disease. Factor IX is decreased in hemophilia B. Platelet aggregation is normal in hemophilia but decreased in von Willebrand's disease.

Treatment

The goal of therapy is to prevent crippling deformities and prolong life expectancy. A cure is not available at this time. Stopping the bleed and increasing the plasma levels of the deficient factors will help prevent the degenerative stages of joint destruction.

In hemophilia A, cryoprecipitated antihemolytic factor (AHF) is administered to raise the factor to 25% of normal to allow coagulation. Surgery requires increasing the AHF to 50% of normal. If the AHF is not available, fresh frozen plasma or plasma fraction, rich in AHF, may be administered.

In hemophilia B, administration of fresh frozen plasma or of factor IX itself will increase the blood level of factor IX.

In von Willebrand's disease, the infusion of cryoprecipitates or blood fractions rich in factor VIII and VWF will shorten the bleeding time. Prior to surgery or in bleeding states, an intravenous infusion of cryoprecipitate or fresh frozen plasma is needed to raise the factor VIII level to 50% of normal.

A patient with hemophilia or von Willebrand's disease needs the care of a hematologist for surgical procedures and dental extraction.

Nursing Intervention

During hemophiliac bleeds, administration of the deficient clotting factor or plasma is ordered. AHF is effective for 48 to 72 hours. This means that repeat transfusions may be required to stop the bleed.

Apply cold compresses to the injured area, raise the injured area if possible, and cleanse any wounds. Thrombin-soaked fibrin or sponge may be utilized for wound care in some institutions. Restrict activity for 48 hours after the bleeding is controlled to prevent recurrence. Control pain with analgesics such as acetaminophen (Tylenol), propoxyphene hydrochloride (Darvon), codeine, or meperidine hydrochloride (Demerol). Avoid intramuscular injections to prevent a he-

matoma at the injection site. Aspirin is contraindicated because it affects platelet aggregation. If the patient bleeds into a joint, immediately elevate the joint and immobilize it in a slightly flexed position. Watch for signs of further bleeding such as increased pain and swelling, fever, or possible shocklike symptoms. Monitor the patient's PTT.

In von Willebrand's disease, monitor the patient's bleeding time for 24 to 48 hours after surgery and observe for signs of new bleeding. During a new bleed, elevate the injured part and apply cold compresses and gentle pressure to the bleeding site.

Education as to the causative factors and treatment of minor injuries is indicated, as well as discussion of conditions for which the patient should seek medical attention.

Educate the patient and parents (if the patient is a child) in how to control minor trauma and warn against using aspirin or aspirin-containing drugs. Refer the parents to a genetic counseling service.

The National Hemophilia Society, local hemophiliac groups, genetic evaluation, or psychotherapy may be useful for fostering better acceptance of the disease and forming an association with other patients who are managing successfully.

Editor's Note

Sickle cell disease is not likely to be on the CCRN exam. It is included primarily to give a better picture of abnormal coagulation conditions.

SICKLE CELL DISEASE

Sickle cell disease is also referred to as sickle cell anemia because of the pathophysiology.

Pathophysiology

With an abnormal hemoglobin S, the RBCs become insoluble when hypoxic. Because of this, RBCs become rigid, rough, and elongated. The hemoglobin becomes shaped like a crescent or sickle.

Sickling hemolyzes and altered cells collect in the capillaries and small vessels. This impairs normal circulation and results in pain, swelling, tissue infarctions, and anoxia. This increases blood viscosity, causing further impairment of circulating blood. Blockages extend on the capillaries and small vessels, leading to further sickling obstruction. A vicious cycle has started.

Etiology

This congenital hemolytic anemia occurs most often in blacks. The causative factor is a defective hemoglobin molecule referred to as hemoglobin S.

There is a homozygous and a heterozygous inheritance. Homozygous inheritance involves an amino acid valine submitting for glutamic acid in the beta hemoglobin chain, resulting in the disease itself. In heterozygous inheritance, the patient carries the sickle cell trait but may be asymptomatic.

Clinical Presentation

Several types of crises occur, but common to all are the symptoms and physical findings of tachycardia, cardiomegaly, murmurs, pulmonary infarctions, chronic fatigue, dyspnea (with or without exertion), hematomegaly, jaundice or pallor, aching bones, chest pain, ischemic leg ulcers, and increased susceptibility to infection. Infection, stress, dehydration, and hypoxic states (e.g., strenuous exercise) may induce a crisis.

The most common crisis is the painful crisis. This is a vaso-occlusive or infarctive crisis. It does not usually develop for the first five years but then appears sporadically. It is a result of RBCs obstructing blood vessels by rigid, tangled sickle cells. Tissue anoxia and possible necrosis occur, causing severe thoracic, abdominal, muscular, and bone pain. Jaundice may occur along with dark urine and a low-grade fever. After the crisis resolves, infection may occur within from four days to several weeks secondary to occlusion and necrosis of the blood vessel.

Autosplenectomy occurs with long-standing disease. Autosplenectomy is the process of splenic damage and scarring, inducing shrinkage of the spleen such that it is no longer palpable. After autosplenectomy, the patient is very susceptible to diplococcal pneumonia, which is rapidly fatal without immediate aggressive treatment. Lethargy, sleepiness, fever, and/or apathy occur as signs and symptoms of infection.

Aplastic (megaloblastic) crisis is a result of bone marrow suppression and is often associated with a viral infection. Signs and symptoms include fever, markedly decreased bone marrow activity, pallor, lethargy, dyspnea, possible coma, and RBC hemolysis.

Acute sequestration develops in some children from eight months to two years old. There is a sudden, massive entrapment of RBCs in the liver and spleen. Symptoms of this rare crisis are lethargy and pallor. If not treated, it progresses to hypovolemic shock and death. This is the leading cause of death in sickle cell children under one year old.

A hemolytic crisis is rare and is usually confined to those who have a glucose-6-phosphate dehydrogenase deficiency. This crisis usually occurs as an infectious response to complications of sickle cell disease rather than to the disease itself.

Diagnosis

A family history and the clinical picture point toward sickle cell disease. A blood smear shows sickle-celled RBCs rather than normal RBCs. Hemoglobin electrophoresis showing hemoglobin S is pathognomonic.

Treatment

Treatment is palliative, since no cure and no reversible treatment have been established for this disease. Usually home care will suffice, but in a crisis state, hospitalization is needed.

Treatment of aplastic crisis includes transfusion of packed RBCs, oxygen, and supportive therapies. In sequestration crisis, treatment includes whole-blood transfusion, oxygen, and large amounts of oral or intravenous fluids.

Nursing Intervention

Supportive care during exacerbations will help avoid such crises and provide a more normal life. During the crisis, apply warm compresses to painful areas and cover the child with a blanket. Avoid cold compresses, since their use may result in vasoconstriction and prolong the crisis. Encourage bedrest and administer analgesics, antipyretics, and antibiotics as ordered.

Patient and family education will help avoid some crises. Such education would include avoidance of drinking large amounts of cold fluids, swimming in cold water, clothing that restricts circulation, and any activity that would produce hypoxia, such as flying in small (unpressurized) aircraft. A large fluid intake will prevent dehydration and decrease blood viscosity, reducing the chance of another crisis. Stress the importance of childhood immunizations and prompt treatment for infections.

CHAPTER 41

Disorders of the Immune System

Editor's Note

The CCRN exam may contain two to eight questions on disorders of the immune system. Although specifics of different types of diseases, such as cancers, are not likely to be addressed on the exam, it is important to understand the general concepts presented in this chapter. Immunologic concepts are sometimes difficult to apply clinically, but the major concepts are important to the assessment and therapeutic interventions associated with critical-care immunology.

CELLS OF THE IMMUNE SYSTEM

Inflammatory Response

The body's inflammatory response constitutes a nonspecific response to diverse stimuli, including tissue injury and microorganisms. Predominant in this response are neutrophils, also referred to as segmented neutrophils (segs) and polymorphonuclear leukocytes. The first cells to respond to tissue damage, neutrophils, are phagocytic and effective primarily against many bacteria and some fungi, including *Candida* species. Banded neutrophils (bands), an immature form of neutrophil, are released from the bone marrow during times of increased demand after the depletion of neutrophils from the storage pool.

Monocytes, which normally appear in the peripheral blood, are immature cells that increase in number late in acute infection or during chronic infection. Monocytes leave the blood, travel to tissue, and mature into macrophages. Macrophages are phagocytic and also secrete chemical mediators that serve to stimulate lymphocytes and activate the immune response. It is significant to note two limitations of phagocytosis: (1)

certain bacteria, almost all viruses, and many fungi are able to resist digestion after being engulfed by phagocytes, and (2) organisms can multiply within phagocytes and the infection can spread.

Immune Response

The immune response is a specific response to an antigen or foreign substance. These precise reactions are dependent upon the ability to distinguish self, the body's own tissues, from non-self, the antigen. The cells with this capability are the lymphocytes, which increase in number late in the infectious process.

Humoral Immunity

There are two major types of lymphocytes, B and T cells. B cells constitute approximately 20% of all lymphocytes. It is believed that they mature in the bone marrow, from which they are released to migrate to lymph tissue. B cells, when activated, transform into plasma cells that produce immunoglobulins or antibodies. Five major types of immunoglobulin are produced, although millions of antibody variations are possible to combat the spectrum of antigens that may be encountered (Table 41-1). Upon encountering an antigen, the antibody combines with it, much like a lock and key fit together. This antigen-antibody complex, sometimes with the aid of the complement system, can cause the death of the antigen directly or make it a better target for other cells of the immune system. This B-cell immune response is referred to as humoral immunity, since the antibodies are carried by the blood and lymph. It is most effective against pyogenic bacteria and some viruses.

Cell-Mediated Immunity

T-cell lymphocytes are so called because they mature in the thymus before migrating to peripheral lymph tissues. The T-cell response to antigen comprises cell-mediated immunity because of the ability of cytotoxic

TABLE 41-1. TYPES AND FUNCTIONS OF IMMUNOGLOBULINS

Type	Function
IgM	First antibody in fetal life First antibody after exposure to a new antigen
IgG	Major antibody of adult life Produced after repeated exposure to the same antigen
IgA	Found in secretions: tears, saliva, mucous secretions in GI and respiratory tracts Meets antigen at port of entry
IgE	Mediates allergic reactions
IgD	Function unclear, but may be regulatory in nature

T cells, a specific subset of T cells, to directly induce lysis of antigens. Cell-mediated immunity is protective against intracellular bacteria, most viruses, fungi, and protozoa.

Cytotoxic T cells act under the direction of T4 (CD4) and T8 (CD8) cells, two major subdivisions of T cells that serve important regulatory functions within the entire immune system. The T4 cell, also known as a helper cell, is vital in activating the immune response, whereas the T8, or suppressor, cell functions to suppress the immune response. The complex coordination of the immune response is based on an elaborate system of communication and interaction that occurs among T cells, B cells, and macrophages largely due to chemical mediators called lymphokines, which are secreted by the T4 cells. Table 41-2 summarizes the functions of B and T cells.

IMMUNOSUPPRESSION

Etiology

Immunodeficiencies can occur with congenital conditions or may be acquired secondary to disease, injury, treatments, medications, and other factors such as age, stress, and nutritional status. The effect of these disorders is an impairment in one or more of the major components of immunity, through either an insufficient number of immune cells or ineffective functioning of the immune mechanisms. Immunosuppression, ranging from mild to severe, is present in almost every person who is critically ill. Refer to Table 41-3 for a listing of some of the major causes of immunosuppression.

Infection

The ultimate effect of immunodeficiency is an impaired ability of the body to defend against foreign antigens. This leads to an increased susceptibility to infection and certain other diseases believed to sometimes be linked to an impaired immune status, such as cancer and autoimmune disorders. The incidence of infection, the most common complication of immunosuppression, increases with both the duration and the severity of the immunodeficiency. In fact, the highest risk of infection occurs when the WBC count is less than 1000 cells/mm^3 and the neutrophils number less than 500 cells/mm^3. The infections that develop are related to the underlying immune defect and the organisms to which the individual is now most susceptible. Most infections associated with immunosuppression are opportunistic or secondary to endogenous organisms that do not cause infection in the presence of a normal functioning immune system. However, many of the organisms colonizing a hospitalized patient are actually acquired during the hospitalization. Also, the infections that develop in immunosuppressed patients tend to be more severe, to be of longer duration, and to have a greater potential for dissemination than those seen in the general population. The lung is the most common site of serious infectious complications. Refer to Table 41-4 for a review of common infections in the immunocompromised host.

Treatment

Antimicrobials. At the first indication of infection, the patient is pan-cultured and then started on a combination of antimicrobials. On an empirical basis, antimicrobial coverage is generally aimed at bacterial infection, although other drugs, including antifungals, are usually added or substituted as indicated by the clinical status of the patient. Of course, once culture results are obtained, the antimicrobial regimen can be individualized. Refer to Table 41-5 for a listing of commonly used antimicrobials. Some of the undesirable side effects possible with these agents include bone marrow suppression, a change in the normal body flora allowing colonization by more pathogenic hospital-acquired organisms, and development of resistance by the organism.

TABLE 41-2. COMPARISON OF B- AND T-CELL IMMUNITY

Characteristic	B Lymphocyte	T Lymphocyte
Type of immunity	Humoral	Cell-mediated
Immune functions	Antibody formation Immediate hypersensitivity	Direct cytotoxicity Delayed hypersensitivity Immune surveillance (destruction of cancer cells) Graft rejection Immune regulation

Organisms protective against	Pyogenic bacteria
	  Staphylococcus
	  Haemophilus
	  Neisseria
	
	Viruses
	  Hepatitis B virus
	  Adenovirus
	  Enterovirus
	  Echovirus
		Intracellular bacteria
		  Pseudomonas
		  Listeria
		  Mycobacteria
		
		Viruses
		  Herpes simplex virus
		  Herpes varicella-zoster virus
		  Cytomegalovirus
		  Epstein-Barr virus
		  Retrovirus (excluding HIV)
		
		Fungi
		  Candida
		  Cryptococcus
		  Aspergillus
		
		Protozoa
		  Pneumocytis carinii
		  Toxoplasma gondii

Immunotherapy. A major area of investigation is that of immunotherapy, which consists of substances called biological response modifiers. These are naturally occurring substances that act to augment the immune response. Most of the biological response modifiers are lymphokines, the chemical mediators secreted by the T4 cell. Examples include interferon, interleukin, and granulocyte-macrophage colony-stimulating factor. When given for therapeutic purposes, these substances are man-made through genetic technology and administered in much higher doses than occur naturally. The desired effect is to enhance the immune response and enable it to combat the existing disorder associated with the immunodeficiency. Thus far, the majority of clinical trials have been undertaken with cancer patients.

Nursing Care

Nursing care of the patient who is immunosuppressed is based on the nursing diagnosis of potential for infection related to specific, and many times multiple, immunodeficiencies or a disruption in the natural protective barriers to microorganisms. The patient requires frequent and thorough physical assessments because the signs and symptoms of infection are often subtle in the immunocompromised host. Important points regarding assessment and interventions are the following.

Assessment

History

- Age
- Past infections
- Medications, noting those which are immunosuppressive
- Treatment which can be immunosuppressive (for example, radiation therapy)
- Presenting signs and symptoms
- Coexisting systemic symptoms (weight loss, malaise, etc.)

TABLE 41-3. ETIOLOGY OF ACQUIRED IMMUNODEFICIENCY

Etiologic Condition	Immune Defect
Injury/Disease	
Burns	Disruption of natural barrier Impaired phagocytosis Deficient delayed hypersensitivity
Uremia	Abnormal neutrophil function Impaired cell-mediated immunity
Diabetes mellitus	Impaired neutrophil function
Cancer	
Solid tumors	Deficiency in cell-mediated immunity Impaired neutrophil function
Leukemias	Deficiency in humoral and cell-mediated immunity
Hodgkin's disease	Impaired cellular immunity
Non-Hodgkin's lymphoma	Impaired humoral or cellular immunity (depends on type of lymphocyte involved)
Multiple myeloma	Impaired humoral immunity
AIDS	Impaired cell-mediated immunity with subsequent deficiency in humoral immunity
Certain infections (influenza, cytomegalovirus, Epstein-Barr virus, mononucleosis, tuberculosis, candidiasis)	Depression of lymphocyte and monocyte function
Treatment/Medication	
Surgery	Disruption of natural barriers Lymphopenia
Splenectomy	Impaired humoral immunity
Radiation therapy	Neutropenia Lymphopenia
Anesthetic agents	Inhibition of phagocytosis Impaired humoral and cell-mediated immunity
Cytotoxic drugs (cancer chemotherapy)	Disruption of natural barriers (mucositis) Neutropenia Deficiencies in humoral and cell-mediated immunity
Steroids	Anti-inflammatory Suppressed functioning of neutrophils Deficiencies in humoral and cell-mediated immunity
Immunosuppressive agents (azathioprine, cyclosporin, antilymphocyte globulin)	Impaired cell-mediated immunity
Certain antibiotics (pentamidine, gentamicin, Septra)	Leukopenia Neutropenia

(continued)

TABLE 41-3. (*Continued*)

Etiologic Condition	Immune Defect
Miscellaneous	
Extremes of age	Deficiencies in humoral and cell-mediated immunity
Protein-calorie malnutrition	Impaired phagocytosis Deficiencies in humoral and cell-mediated immunity
Stress	Exact mechanism of immunodeficiency unknown

Physical Examination

1. Inspect skin carefully, particularly noting conditions of skin folds, pressure points, and perirectal area (frequent site of infection in the immunocompromised host). Observe for:
   a. Localized redness or swelling (may not be present with neutropenia or lymphopenia)
   b. Excoriation
   c. Lesions, infections, or Kaposi's sarcoma
   d. Lymphadenopathy
2. Closely inspect the mouth and throat, a frequent

TABLE 41-4. COMMON INFECTIONS IN THE IMMUNOCOMPROMISED HOST

Site of Infection	Bacteria	Viruses	Fungi	Protozoa
Skin	Staphylococcus aureus Staphylococcus epidermidis	Herpes simplex virus Herpes varicella-zoster virus	Candida	
Oropharynx		Herpes simplex virus	Candida	
GI tract	Gram-negative rods Mycobacterium avium-intracellulare	Herpes simplex virus (esophagitis) Cytomegalovirus	Candida	Giardia lamblia Cryptosporidium Entamoeba histolytica
Urinary tract	Gram-negative rods		Candida	
Lungs	Gram-negative rods Mycobacterium tuberculosis Mycobacterium avium-intracellulare	Cytomegalovirus	Candida Aspergillus Histoplasma capsulatum	Pneumocystis carinii Toxoplasma gondii
CNS	Listeria monocytogenes Streptococcus pneumoniae Pseudomonas aeruginosa Haemophilus influenzae	Herpes varicella-zoster virus Herpes simplex virus	Cryptococcus neoformans Aspergillus	Toxoplasma gondii
Blood	Gram-negative rods		Candida	

site of infection in the immunocompromised host. Note:

  a. Condition of teeth and gums (if infected, can cause sepsis)

  b. Lesions (candidiasis, herpes simplex, Kaposi's sarcoma)

3. Monitor temperature and note pattern of elevation.

  a. An elevated temperature is the best indication of infection in the immunosuppressed.

  b. A temperature over 38°C for 12 or more hours is probably indicative of infection.

  c. Fever is also part of the disease process of some disorders associated with immunosuppression (leukemia, lymphona, human immunodeficiency virus [HIV] infection).

4. Assess breath sounds

  a. Adventitious sounds are frequently absent or minimal at the onset of infection in the immunosuppressed patient.

  b. Note respiratory rate, presence of cough, and character of sputum.

  c. Be prepared with ventilator support, since rapid deterioration in respiratory status can occur.

5. Note complaints of tenderness and localized pain, as they may be indicators of infection.

  a. Back pain

  b. Burning on urination

  c. Rectal discomfort with bowel movements

TYPE 41-5. ANTIMICROBIALS COMMONLY USED AGAINST INFECTIONS IN THE IMMUNOCOMPROMISED HOST

Type of Infection	Antimicrobial
Bacterial	Penicillin
	Cephalosporin
	Aminoglycoside
	Vancomycin
Fungal	Nystatin (oral candidiasis)
	Ketoconazole
	5-Flucytosine
	Amphotericin B
Viral	Acyclovir
	Ganciclovir (cytomegalovirus infections)
Protozoal	Trimethoprim/sulfamethoxazole (Septra)
	Pentamidine

Laboratory Data

1. WBC (leukopenia or leukocytosis)

  a. WBC differential

  b. Absolute granulocyte count, especially if less than 500 cells/mm^3.

  c. Lymphocyte count

2. T4 count; T4:T8 ratio (indicators of immune status in patients with AIDS)

Interventions

1. Meticulous personal hygiene

  a. Prevent skin breakdown by turning the patient and using pressure-relieving devices.

  b. Avoid injury (will provide a port of entry for microorganisms), keep nails trim, use electric razor.

  c. Provide meticulous perirectal care.

    (i) Avoid taking rectal temperatures and using rectal suppositories and enemas because of fragile rectal mucosa and the possibility of causing a break in the mucosa.

    (ii) Initiate a bowel regimen to avoid constipation or control diarrhea.

2. Good oral hygiene

  a. Brush oral cavity, using a soft toothbrush or toothettes.

  b. Moisturize lips and mucosa with water-soluble lubricant.

  c. If stomatitis is present, rinse mouth with normal saline every two to four hours.

  d. Avoid commercial mouthwashes.

  e. Advise patient to avoid smoking and use of alcohol.

  f. Encourage a soft bland diet and cool foods or provide nutritional support.

  g. Control pain.

    (1) Viscous xylocaine

    (2) Mixture of sodium bicarbonate (5 ml), Maalox (5 ml), 2% viscous xylocaine (5 ml), and Benadryl (5 mg). Swish in mouth for three minutes and swallow every four hours.

  h. Obtain order for appropriate antimicrobials if secondary infection is present.

3. Utilize aseptic technique with all invasive procedures.

  a. Minimize invasive procedures.

b. Use smallest-gauge lumens possible on all invasive devices.

c. Provide meticulous care of vascular access.

d. Coordinate blood studies.

e. Keep all systems closed as much as possible.

f. Avoid transparent, occlusive dressings over drainage wounds (require the presence of WBCs collecting under the dressing to clean out the wound).

4. Manipulate the environment to minimize exposure to organisms.

a. Eliminate sources of stagnant water (sources of gram-negative bacteria).

  (i) Change disposable tubing on ventilators daily.

  (ii) Avoid cold mist humidifiers.

b. Remove live plants and flowers from the room (sources of *aspergillus*).

c. Institute protective isolation when the WBC count is less than 1000 cells/mm³ or the absolute granulocyte count is less than 500 cells/mm³.

d. Restrict exposure to persons with infection.

e. Evaluate the appropriateness of a low bacterial diet.

  (i) Eliminate raw, unpeeled fruits and vegetables and uncooked eggs and meat from the diet.

  (ii) Effectiveness in decreasing the incidence of infection is controversial.

5. Ensure adequate nutrition.

a. Nutritional intake may be compromised by anorexia, fatigue, stomatitis, dysphagia, nausea and vomiting, and taste changes due to some medications, including chemotherapy.

b. Encourage a high-calorie, high-protein diet.

c. Enteral feedings are preferable to parenteral nutrition because of decreased risk of infection.

6. Alleviate the patient's stress as much as possible.

a. Allow rest periods.

b. Maintain day/night schedule as much as possible.

c. Minimize environmental noise.

d. Maximize comfort.

e. Attend psychosocial needs.

With this overview of immunosuppression to serve as a background, a few diseases that are associated with severe and multiple immunodeficiencies will be reviewed in more detail.

ACQUIRED IMMUNODEFICIENCY SYNDROME

AIDS, or acquired immunodeficiency syndrome, is the end point of infection by HIV, a retrovirus found in the body fluids of infected individuals. HIV is transmitted by sexual contact (either heterosexual or homosexual), blood-to-blood contact, and perinatally. The profile of the high-risk groups affected by the disease to date include male homosexuals and bisexuals, IV drug users, hemophiliacs, blood transfusion recipients prior to 1985, and sexual partners of any of these individuals.

Since recognition of the disease in 1981, much has been learned about the spectrum of HIV infection. Individuals who are infected may range from being asymptomatic to having systemic symptoms such as generalized persistent lymphadenopathy, fever, night sweats, diarrhea, and weight loss. AIDS itself is diagnosed when specific "indicator" diseases (i.e., diseases that indicate an underlying immunodeficiency) are present. The diagnosis, under most circumstances, also requires the person to be HIV seropositive. This is determined by enzyme-linked immunosorbent assay and Western blot laboratory tests, which screen for the antibody to HIV. The antibody develops an average of 6 to 12 weeks after exposure to the virus. Thus far, the pattern of disease seems to be that the virus remains latent for an average of seven years before symptoms appear. It is not known whether everyone infected will eventually develop AIDS.

Clinical Presentation

The immunodeficiency of AIDS is multifaceted. HIV primarily infects the T4 cell, and because of the rule of the T cell as the main coordinator of the immune response, devastating deficiencies occur in both the cell-mediated and humoral immune responses. The viral effects on the immune system include a profound lymphopenia and a reverse T4:T8 ratio (less than 1). As a result, the person with AIDS develops opportunistic infections. Typical of infections seen in the immunocompromised host, the opportunistic infections associated with AIDS tend to be severe and become disseminated, but they also tend to recur upon discontinuation of antimicrobial therapy. Most patients with AIDS die as a result of infection due to an organism normally protected against by T cells.

Some of the infections frequently seen with AIDS include cytomegalovirus retinitis, cryptococcal meningitis, and, most commonly, *Pneumocystis carinii* pneumonia (PCP). The onset of PCP is usually insidious, characterized by a gradually increasing shortness of breath, dry cough, fever, and on chest x ray, pulmonary infiltrates. The respiratory status of a patient with PCP can deteriorate rapidly and necessitate admission to a critical-care unit. Hypoxemia and dyspnea may require ventilatory support. Drug therapy usually includes administration of a 21-day course of intravenous pentamidine or trimethoprin/sulfamethoxazole (Septra). If these drugs are ineffective, one alternative is an investigational drug that is a much stronger folate antagonist than trimethoprin. Occasionally, high-dose steroids are given. In many patients, it may take seven to ten days for a clinical response to be seen. It is not unusual for a relapse of PCP to occur; when it does, it is often fulminant in nature and associated with a mortality ratio of approximately 40%. For this reason, patients are commonly started on prophylactic therapy, which may consist of maintenance doses of oral Septra or aerosolized pentamidine.

Secondary cancers, namely, Kaposi's sarcoma and non-Hodgkin's lymphoma (NHL), can also occur in association with AIDS. Kaposi's sarcoma, which arises from the endothelium of either the lymphate vessel or blood vessel, is characterized by skin and mucosal lesions ranging in color from dark red or purple to nearly black. The lesions also tend to develop in the oropharynx, lymph nodes, gastrointestinal (GI) tract, and lungs. NHL is typically high grade, of B-cell origin, and present in extranodal sites. In approximately 20% of those with NHL, the cancer presents as a primary lymphoma of the brain, a very rare occurrence in the general population. Generally, the AIDS-related malignancies are much more aggressive and respond more poorly to therapy than when the same cancers develop in the general population.

Neuropsychiatric manifestations accompany AIDS in over 60% of patients and in some cases are diagnostic for the disease. The most common disorder of this type is AIDS dementia complex, a subcortical dementia manifested by changes in cognition, behavior, and motor functioning. Symptoms initially include memory loss, difficulty in concentrating, and lethargy and may progress to withdrawal, aphasia, ataxia, paresis, and seizures. The condition is thought to occur secondary to HIV infiltration of the brain. The virus is known to inflict macrophages, which themselves are not destroyed by the virus but serve to transport HIV across the blood-brain barrier.

Also identified as part of the clinical picture asso-

ciated with AIDS is the HIV wasting syndrome. This is defined as loss of over 10% of the usual body weight, accompanied by diarrhea, weakness, or fever of a chronic nature. Multiple factors may contribute to development of the syndrome, including difficulty in maintaining adequate nutrition. However, like the cachexia seen with cancer, muscle wasting seems to exceed what is expected.

Treatment

Treatment is aimed at the secondary diseases that develop with AIDS. Appropriate antimicrobial coverage is initiated for the specific opportunistic infection (see Table 41-5). Systemic NHL, usually widely disseminated at the time of diagnosis, necessitates treatment with an intensive chemotherapy regimen that is fairly toxic and usually poorly tolerated by the patient with AIDS. Primary lymphoma of the brain usually has a good initial response to cranial radiation, but relapse soon occurs, generally within the central nervous system (CNS). Therapy for Kaposi's sarcoma, commonly initiated when the patient develops pain or lymphatic obstruction or when the lesions are cosmetically disturbing, is palliative and consists of chemotherapy and/or radiation. These cancer therapies, particularly chemotherapy, induce myelosuppression and compound the already existing immunodeficiencies of AIDS, making the patient even more susceptible to the development of infection.

Zidovidine, also known as AZT or Retrovir, is an antiretroviral agent that helps control the replication of HIV. It appears to increase the median survival of patients with advanced AIDS by approximately one year. Because it is able to cross the blood-brain barrier, it frequently results in improvement of symptoms associated with AIDS dementia complex. Side effects of zidovidine include headache and weakness, hepatotoxicity, and unfortunately bone marrow suppression. Transfusion-dependent anemia as well as granulocytopenia and thrombocytopenia can result. When patients are receiving other therapy that is myelosuppressive, such as antibiotics for a life-threatening infection or chemotherapy, treatment with zidovidine may need to be suspended. The efficacy of zidovidine in early-stage HIV infection is currently being studied in clinical trials.

Nursing Intervention

In addition to requiring nursing care relevant to immunosuppression, patients with AIDS, especially those with PCP, require aggressive pulmonary care and close monitoring of ABGs. Decisions regarding intubation and ventilation should be made prior to severe respiratory dysfunction. As impaired cognitive functioning can occur secondary to hypoxemia, AIDS dementia, opportunistic infection, or CNS malignancy, a close assessment of mental status is required in order to detect any changes from baseline. If impaired concentration and memory are noted, it is necessary to provide simple explanations and directions as well as a safe environment for the patient. Nutritional support measures must also be addressed. If diarrhea is present, a common problem due to either HIV enteropathy or opportunistic infection, enteral feedings may not be possible. As is evident, the patient with AIDS presents an array of problems with complex etiologies, requiring advanced nursing skills in assessment and symptom management.

LEUKEMIAS

Leukemias are a group of malignancies that occur when immature WBCs proliferate uncontrollably and accumulate in the bone marrow and peripheral blood. Leukemias are classified according to the type of cell that is predominant and whether they are acute or chronic in nature. The four general categories of leukemia are acute lymphocytic or lymphoblastic (ALL), acute nonlymphocytic or myelogenous (ANLL or AML), chronic lymphocytic (CLL), and chronic myelogenous (CML).

The accumulation of leukemic cells, which do not function normally, impedes the adequate production of normal RBCs, WBCs, and platelets. This, along with infiltration of other organs by the leukemic cells, is the rationale for the clinical presentation of leukemia. Refer to Table 41-6 for a summary of the signs and symptoms.

Complications

The patient with leukemia requires a critical-care setting when complications, either due to the disease or to its treatment, arise. Both the disease itself and the intensive chemotherapy used to treat it are associated with severe and often prolonged myelosuppression. The total WBC count may be less than $100/mm^3$ for a period of one or more weeks after high-dose chemotherapy. As a result, infection is the major cause of morbidity and mortality in the patient with leukemia. Sepsis is common and must be treated immediately and aggressively.

TABLE 41-6. MANIFESTATIONS OF LEUKEMIA

Rationale	Signs and Symptoms
Bone marrow failure	Anemia Thrombocytopenia Leukocytosis (primarily blast cells) Granulocytopenia (if ALL, CLL) Lymphopenia (if ALL, CML)
Organ infiltration	Bone pain Lymphadenopathy Splenomegaly Hepatomegaly Testicular mass or swelling Headache, nausea, vomiting (CNS involvement)
Hyperleukocytosis	Stroke Adult respiratory distress syndrome Splenic infarction
Hypercatabolism and rapid cell turnover (tumor lysis syndrome)	Disseminated intravascular coagulation Hyperuricemia Hyperkalemia Hypocalcemia Weight loss

Also contributing to the likelihood of infection is the disruption that can occur in the natural barriers of the skin and mucous membranes, allowing easy entry by microorganisms. The chemotherapy, depending on the drug and the doses, can cause severe stomatitis and mucositis. In patients who have received bone marrow from a donor, graft-versus-host disease (GVHD) can occur as the transplanted marrow recognizes the host tissue as foreign. One of the tissues that the engrafted T cells attempt to reject is the skin. In acute GVHD, this usually starts as a rash and may progress to desquamation. The treatment for GVHD includes immunosuppressive drugs, thus compounding the already existing immunodeficiencies.

Another reason for admission of a leukemia patient to the critical-care unit is severe bleeding and hemorrhage. This can occur secondary to thrombocytopenia, induced by the disease process and/or the chemotherapy. It is not unusual for the platelet count to be under $20,000/mm^3$, which puts the patient at risk for spontaneous bleeding. Of particular concern is the possibility of an intracranial hemorrhage. Because of the multiple platelet transfusions required, single-donor, leukocyte-poor products are administered.

Bleeding may also be seen in association with

disseminated intravascular coagulation (DIC), a complication of leukemia, especially progranulocytic leukemia, a subtype of AML. It is caused by the release of tissue thromboplastin from tumor cells. The clotting cascade is triggered, leading to accelerated coagulation and the formation of excessive thrombin. With the ongoing coagulation, the fibrinolytic system is activated. Thus, clotting and bleeding continue until the cycle is interrupted by treating the cause. Besides hemorrhage, organ dysfunction can occur due to thromboemboli. Chemotherapy should be initiated immediately. Heparin, although its use is controversial with other etiologies of DIC, has been found to be an effective supportive therapy in acute progranulocytic leukemia.

Leukostasis can also be life threatening. Leukostasis can occur with a WBC count of over 100,000/mm^3, consisting of mostly blasts. Leukemia blasts plug capillaries, causing rupture, bleeding, and organ dysfunction. Intracerebral hemorrhage is the most common and most lethal complication. Management includes the administration of fluids and allopurinol, to counteract the hyperuricemia associated with cell lysis. Appropriate chemotherapy must be initiated. As an emergency measure, leukopheresis may be necessary.

Treatment

The acute leukemias require immediate treatment with chemotherapy. Treatment is approached in three phases. The initial phase, called induction therapy, consists of a combination of chemotherapy drugs given in high doses in order to achieve remission. Complete remission occurs when the number of leukemic cells is below detection, hematopoiesis is restored, and signs and symptoms of the disease are no longer present. However, since leukemic cells remain, even though they are microscopically undetectable, a consolidation phase of therapy is necessary to further decrease or eliminate these cells. This cycle of chemotherapy, also very intensive, is usually administered six to eight weeks after induction. The third phase, maintenance therapy, involves the administration of moderate doses of chemotherapy over a prolonged time. Given with the intent of maintaining remission, its effectiveness is controversial.

By comparison, chronic leukemia is treated with oral chemotherapy agents with much less associated toxicity. More aggressive therapy may be initiated as the disease progresses, particularly in patients with CML who undergo an end-stage blast crisis, which resembles an acute leukemia.

The rate of relapse, i.e., the recurrence of detect-able leukemic cells, either in the bone marrow, peripheral blood, or extramedullary sites, varies with the type of leukemia. However, once it occurs, it is more difficult to induce a second remission. One treatment alternative that is available to patients with ALL, ANLL, and CML who meet specific criteria is bone marrow transplantation. Bone marrow transplantation involves administration of dosages of chemotherapy and radiation therapy that, though ablative to the bone marrow, are also more cytotoxic to cancer cells. Prior to the cytotoxic therapy, bone marrow cells are harvested from the patient or a matched donor. If the patient is to receive his or her own marrow, special techniques are used in an attempt to completely eliminate all leukemic cells before infusion. The bone marrow is reinfused at the time the blood counts reach their lowest point. Engraftment of the bone marrow and functional immune recovery takes approximately four weeks.

Nursing Intervention

In the patient with leukemia, nursing care centers around the diagnosis of potential for infection and potential for injury (bleeding), discussed elsewhere in this chapter. In addition to the assessments previously reviewed, assessment of neurological status is important because of the possibility of CNS complications, including intracranial bleeding or stroke. Fluids and electrolyte balance must also be carefully monitored because of the large volume of fluids given and the possibility of tumor lysis syndrome or septic shock. Multisystem failure can occur due to leukemic infiltration, leukostasis, DIC, sepsis, or the toxicity of cancer chemotherapy. In addition to the continual assessments, the nurse will administer the extensive supportive therapy required, including multiple antibiotics, blood and blood product transfusions, and usually total parenteral nutrition. Nursing care of the patient with leukemia is a challenge, particularly in terms of protecting the patient from infection amid all of the critical-care interventions.

OTHER MALIGNANCIES ASSOCIATED WITH IMMUNODEFICIENCY

Lymphomas

Lymphomas, in which the malignant cell is a lymphocyte, are broadly classified as either Hodgkin's disease (HD) or non-Hodgkin's lymphoma (NHL). Though similar in many respects, the distinguishing feature of HD is the presence of Reed-Sternberg cells, whose origin and nature are uncertain. The incidence of HD peaks during the second and third decades and again after the age of 60. MHL occurs primarily in older individuals and is four times more common than HD.

The pathology of lymphomas is the transformation of the lymphocyte into a malignant cell at some stage of its development, which accounts for the different histologic subtypes of both HD and NHL. What triggers this transformation is unknown, although there is evidence linking HD to a viral etiology, particularly when it occurs in the young. In the case of NHL, there is a strong association with a preexisting immunodeficiency. Regardless of the histology, the lymphocytes proliferate uncontrollably and invade body organs, although the degree of aggressiveness varies.

The disease usually presents as one or more enlarged lymph nodes, usually in the cervical region. Occasionally, the initial site of disease is the GI tract. Approximately one-third of patients also exhibit systemic symptoms consisting of fever, night sweats, and loss over 10% of the usual body weight. Staging procedures are done to determine the extent of disease, as this has implications for treatment. HD tends to spread from one lymph node group to an adjacent group, whereas NHL tends to skip to noncontiguous groups. The workup must determine the involvement, if any, of lymph node groups, the bone marrow, liver, and spleen. Sometimes an explanatory laparotomy may be necessary, especially with HD.

If the lymphoma is localized, radiation therapy is initiated. In HD, this consists of total nodal irradiation and radiation to the spleen (if not removed at laparotomy). For early-stage disease, radiation is given with curative intent, although it is generally more effective in HD than in NHL. Chemotherapy is given for more widespread systemic disease, and sometimes in the case of NHL is recommended as the treatment of choice for localized disease. Both chemotherapy and radiation therapy, if given to areas of major bone marrow activity, are myelosuppressive. Another side effect that is sometimes associated with the chemotherapeutic treatment of NHL is tumor lysis syndrome.

Cure is expected in over 50% of patients with lymphoma. However, if the disease recurs, therapy is more poorly tolerated because of the depressed bone marrow reserve as a result of the initial therapy. Potential complications representing oncologic emergencies that can occur with progressive disease are superior vena cava syndrome and spinal cord compression. In superior vena cava syndrome, the vena cava is obstructed by tumor or enlarged nodes. The impaired

TABLE 41-7. CLINICAL MANIFESTATIONS OF MULTIPLE MYELOMA

Rationale	Signs and Symptom
Bone marrow involvement by plasmacytomas (plasma cell tumors)	Anemia (common) Leukopenia Thrombocytopenia
Skeletal involvement by plasmacytomas and tumor activation of osteoclasts	Bone pain Osteolytic lesions Pathologic fractures Hypercalcemia
Production of light chains called Bence Jones protein (part of immunoglobulin)	Proteinuria Renal insufficiency due to tubular damage
Hyperviscosity	Occlusion of small vessels Headache Mental status changes Visual disturbances Retinal hemorrhage Intermittent claudication
Hypervolemia	Congestive heart failure

venous drainage causes cough, dyspnea, neck vein distension, and facial, trunk, and arm edema. Immediate treatment with radiation is required to relieve pressure on the superior vena cava. The other complication treated on an emergency basis is spinal cord compression, usually due to lymph node extension into the epidural space. Paraplegia can result if treatment is not initiated with radiation therapy or, if the neurological deterioration is rapid, a decompression laminectomy.

Multiple Myeloma

Multiple myeloma is a relatively uncommon malignancy of the plasma cell, the antibody-producing form of the B cell. In this disease, excessive amounts of a single type of immunoglobulin are produced. Refer to Table 41-7 for the clinical manifestations of myeloma. The disease, commonly advanced at the time of diagnosis, is treated palliatively with chemotherapy. Infection, usually bacterial in origin, is the most common cause of death due to the impaired production of normal, functional antibodies.

BIBLIOGRAPHY

Abernathy, E. (1984). How the immune system works. *Nursing 87,* 4, 456–469.

Barrick, B. (1988). Caring for AIDS patients: A challenge you can meet. *Nursing 88 18,* 11, 50–60.

Bellanti, J.A. (ed.). (1985). *Immunology III*. Philadelphia: W.B. Saunders.

Brandt, B. (1988). A nursing protocol for the client with neutropenia. *Oncol Nurs For 11,* 2, 24–28.

Breathnach, S.M. (1988). The skin as an immunologic barrier. In *The Physical Nature of the Skin*. Ed. Marks, R.M., Barton, S.P., & Edwards, C. Lancaster, England: MTP Press Limited, pp. 53–60.

Dinarello, C.A., & Mier, J.W. (1987). Current concepts. Lymphokines. *N Eng J Med 317,* 940–945.

Ellerhorst-Ryan, J.M. (1985). Complications of the myeloproliferative system: Infection and sepsis. *Semin Oncol Nurs 1* 4, 244–250.

Foon, K.A. (1988). Biotherapy of cancer with interleukin-2, colony-stimulating factors, and monoclonal antibodies. *Oncol Nurs For 15*(Suppl. 6), 13–22.

Gallin, J.I., Goldstein R.M., Snyerman, R. (1992). *Inflammation: Basic Principles and Clinical Correlates,* 2nd ed. New York: Raven Press.

Grady, C. (1988). Host defense mechanisms: An overview. *Semin Oncol Nurs 4,* 2, 86–94.

Graziano, F.M., & Bell, C.L. (1986). The normal immune response and what can go wrong. *Med Clin North Am 69,* 440–451.

Griffin, J.P. (1986). *Hematology and Immunology Concepts for Nursing*. New York: Appleton-Century-Crofts.

Griffin, J.P. (1986). Nursing care of the immunosuppressed patient in an intensive care unit. *Heart Lung 15,* 2, 179–186.

Groenwald, S.L. (1987). *Cancer Nursing: Principles and Practice*. Boston: Jones and Bartlett Publishers.

Gurevich, I., & Tafuro, P. (1986). The compromised host: Deficit-specific infection and the spectrum of prevention. *Cancer Nurs 9,* 5, 263–275.

Harnett, S. (1989). Septic shock in the oncology patient. *Cancer Nurs 12,* 4, 191–201.

Hillman, R., & Finch, C. (1985). *Red Cell Manual*. Philadelphia: F.A. Davis Co.

Kemp, D.K. (1986). Development of the immune system. *Crit Care Q 9,* 1–6.

Larson, E. (1985). Infection control issues in critical care. *Heart Lung 14,* 149–156.

McNally, J., Staci, J.C., & Somerville, E. (eds.). (1985). *Guidelines for Cancer Nursing Practice*. New York: Grune & Stratton, Inc.

Nily, G. (1988). AIDS: Opportunistic diseases and their physical assessment. *J Adv Med Surg Nurs 1,* 1, 27–36.

Nossal, G.J.V. (1987). The basic components of the immune system. *New Engl J Med 316,* 21, 1320–1325.

Philpot, C.M. (1988). The skin as a microbial barrier. In *The Physical Nature of the Skin*. Ed. Marks, R.M., Barton, S.P., & Edwards, C. Lancaster, England: MTP Press Limited, pp. 61–68.

Piel, J. (ed.). (1988). What science knows about AIDS. *Sci Am 259,* 4, 41–152.

Roitt, B.J., & Male, D. (eds.). (1985). *Immunology*. St. Louis: C.V. Mosby Company.

Siegrist, C.W., & Jones, J.A. (1985). Disseminated intravascular coagulopathy and nursing implications. *Semin Oncol Nurs 1,* 4, 273–243.

Smith, S.L. (1986). Physiology of the immune system. *Crit Care Q 9,* 7–13.

Virella G. (1993). *Introduction to Medical Immunology*. New York: Marcel Dekker, Inc.

Wiernik, P. (1989). Neutrophil function in infection. *Mediguide Infect Dis 9,* 1, 1–8.

Wormser, G.P. (1992). *AIDS and Other Manifestations of HIV Infection,* 2nd ed. New York: Raven Press.

Yarnelli, B., & Gurevich, I. (1988). Infection control in critical care. *Heart Lung 17,* 596–600.

PART 8

Multisystem Patient Care Problems

Patricia A. Ahrens, RN
Thomas Ahrens, RN, DNS, CCRN
Donna Prentice, RN, MSN (R), CCRN, TNS

CHAPTER 42

Burns and Toxicology

This chapter contains a large amount of information that is likely to be addressed only superficially on the CCRN exam. Do not be concerned if you do not understand or remember everything in this chapter. Try to remember major assessment categories and therapeutic maneuvers. This approach should prepare you for the few questions relating to burns and toxicology on the CCRN exam.

Burn care is one of the new areas on the CCRN exam. Questions on the CCRN exam are likely to center on immediate postburn care, which is the focus of this chapter. It is possible to encounter anywhere from two to four questions on burns on the exam.

BURNS

Burns are among the most devastating injuries that a nurse can encounter. Burns can affect multiple organ systems, beyond what appears to be the area involved. Unfortunately, burns are relatively common and are the third leading cause of accidental deaths in adults.

Burns can be the result of thermal, chemical, electrical, or inhalation injury. According to the American Burn Association, more than 2.5 million people in the United States experience thermal injury each year. Approximately 100,000 of those are hospitalized, and 12,000 will die. Burn mortality has improved: a 70% body surface area (BSA) burn today has the same 50% mortality that a 30% BSA burn had in 1970. The best survival exist for persons between the ages of 5 and 34. The very young and very old have the worst prognosis. The median age for a burn victim is 22. Due to the loss of body image and self-esteem, burns can leave both physical and emotional scars that prevent a person from returning to or becoming a productive member of society. Burns typically require a prolonged rehabilitation phase. The medical and societal costs of burns are truly great.

The common variable in all burn injuries is skin damage. The skin is one of our largest organ systems. It is composed of two layers, the epidermis and dermis. The epidermis is the outer, thinner layer. The dermis is a deeper, thicker layer that contains the hair follicles, sweat glands, sebaceous glands, and sensory fibers. (Fig 42–1)

The skin is our first defense against infection and injury. It protects us from the environment, prevents loss of body fluids, regulates body temperature, and provides sensory contact with the environment through pain, touch, pressure, and temperature.

Burns are classified by the extent of BSA affected and the depth of skin damage. The extent of a burn is a product of the temperature generated by the heat source and the exposure time. The center of the burn wound has the most contact with the heat source. The cells have been coagulated and are necrotic. This area is referred to as the zone of coagulation. Lying next to the zone of coagulation is the zone of stasis. This area has cells that have been injured but are not necrotic. If proper resuscitation occurs, these cells will survive; however, they will usually become necrotic within 24 to 48 hours and extend the severity of the burn. The outermost area of the burn wound is the zone of hyperemia. These cells have suffered the least injury and usually recover in seven to ten days. The rule of nines formula is used to estimate the BAS involved (Figure 42-2), but this method gives only a gross estimate. More exact BSA involvement can be calculated with the use of more detailed charts (e.g., Lund and Browder); however, the charts must be available for use and are not easily committed to memory. BSA can also be estimated with the use of the victim's palm, which is equal to 1% of the BSA. This is a useful method with scattered or irregular patterns of burns. The extent of BSA involved is used to calculate the patient's fluid replacement needs.

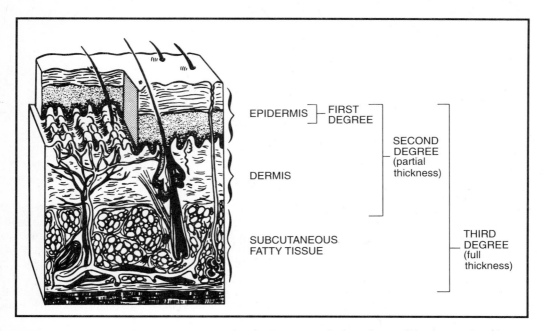

Figure 42-1. Anatomy of the skin. The depth of injury determines whether a burn will heal or require skin grafting. (Adapted from Rue III, L. and Cioffi, W. (1991). Resuscitation of Thermally Injured Patients. *Critical Care Clinics of North America,* 3(2), 183.)

Classification

Depth of the burn will determine to what degree or whether any skin grafting is needed. Variable destruction of skin can occur. Formerly burns were classified as first, second, or third degree. More recently, burns have been subdivided into partial- and full-thickness wounds (Table 42-1 and Fig. 42-1). The partial-thickness wounds are further divided into superficial and deep wounds. First-degree burns damage the epidermis or superficial layer of the skin. The wounds appear pink, dry (no blistering), and slightly edematous and are painful. Clinically, first-degree burns are of little importance and are not typically considered in fluid replacement.

Second-degree or partial-thickness burns destroy the epidermis and varying degrees of the dermis. The wounds appear blistered and are painful, and blanching will be detected.

Third-degree or full-thickness burns destroy both the epidermis and dermal layers of the skin. These burns may extend into the subcutaneous tissue to muscle and may even reach bone. The wounds appear dry, hard, and leathery, and no blanching is detected due to destruction of the capillary bed. A common misconception is that the wound is painless since the nerve endings are destroyed. However, the patients may experience deep somatic pain from ischemia or inflammation. Wound edges may also be hypersensitive in making the transition from third-degree to less severely burned areas.

Initial Management

The initial management of a burn victim is to stop the burning process. This is usually accomplished before the patient receives hospital care, but, depending on the type of burn, irrigation may still be necessary once the patient reaches the hospital. All clothing must be removed, including jewelry, which can retain heat and have a "tourniquet-like" effect on limbs and cause neurovascular compromise. As with all trauma patients, attention must then be given to airway management, assistance with breathing, and support of circulation as needed. The possibility of other injuries must also be assessed, with management as appropriate. Since major burn victims are often intubated at the scene or in the emergency room, a history must be obtained from either witnesses, scene responders, or family members.

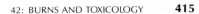

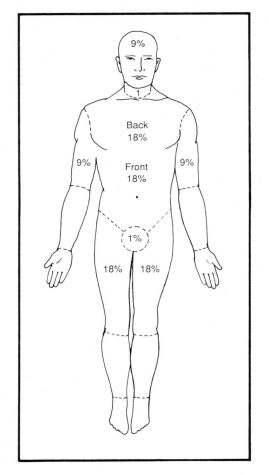

Figure 42-2. The rule of nines. (From Kravitz, M. (1988). Thermal injuries. In: *Trauma Nursing,* p. 709. Cardona, V.; Hurn, P.; Mason, P.; et al., eds. Philadelphia: W.B. Saunders Co.)

Burn Shock

Burn shock has both a cellular and a hypovolemic component. Burns of less than 20% BSA have primarily a local response, whereas major burns of greater than 20 to 25% BSA have a systemic response. The greater the percentage of burn, the greater the systemic response.

Initially, burn patients experience a rise in capillary hydrostatic pressure and an increase in capillary permeability. Rapid fluid shifts occur, with fluid moving from the intravascular space to the interstitium, causing edema formation within the wound and a decrease in circulating blood volume. The cardiac output can decrease as much as 50% in the first hour if ade-

quate resuscitation is not initiated. Catecholamine release may further compromise cardiac output by causing the heart to pump against increased systemic vascular resistance. The greatest fluid shifts occur during the first six to eight hours postburn. Adequate and rapid fluid replacement is required to prevent hypovolemic shock. As a result of decreased cardiac output, the systemic vascular resistance increases in an attempt to preserve some organ perfusion and protect the blood pressure. This increase in systemic vascular resistance, however, further depresses cardiac output. Myocardial depressant factors may also play a role in lowering cardiac output, but attempts to isolate them have been inconclusive.

Fluid requirements are based on the percentage of BSA burned. The clinician must keep in mind that this is only an estimate, and the patient's response to therapy must be closely monitored to assist with fluid replacement and adjust fluid rates accordingly. Many formulas exist to calculate fluid replacement (Table 42-2). The most frequently used calculation is the Parkland formula, which is 4 cc/kg per % BSA of lactated Ringer's solution. Most agree that colloids are not to be used during the first 24 hours since the degree of capillary leakage is so severe that the large colloid molecules will also pass through the capillaries. Fifty percent of the calculated fluid requirement is given in the first 8 hours postburn; the remaining 50% is given over the last 16 hours. It may be necessary for the critical-care nurse to catch up on fluid requirements that have not been adequately met early in the patient's care. Remember that fluid replacement is based on the first 24 hours after injury, not after hospital admission. The nurse must inquire about prior fluid administration and time of injury as well as obtain an accurate weight. Clinical indicators of adequate fluid resuscitation are maintenance of a stable blood pressure with a urine output of 0.5 to 1.0 cc/kg per hour. Invasive hemodynamic monitoring is usually required only in high-risk patients who have underlying cardiopulmonary disorders or those who are not responding as predicted. Patients who may require higher than expected fluid requirements are those with inhalation injury, underlying dehydration preburn, or electrical burns. The most common reason for low urine output and low blood pressure is inadequate fluid resuscitation. However, if invasive hemodynamic monitoring indicates that fluid volume is adequate, inotropic agents may be necessary. Due to the large catecholamine released postburn, larger than normal doses of inotropic agents may be necessary since some down regulation of the receptors may occur.

TABLE 42-1. CLASSIFICATION OF BURN DEPTH

Degree of Burn	Depth of Tissue Penetration	Characteristics
First degree	Partial thickness	Injury to the superficial epidermis, usually caused by over-exposure to sunlight or brief heat flashes. Classically, can be described as a sunburn. Wounds are red, dry, blanch, and are painful to touch, although superficial blisters may be present. Wounds will heal within 7 days, shedding the dead skin layers, and will leave no residual scar.
Second degree	Superficial partial thickness	Injury is to the epidermis and upper layers of the dermis. Wounds characteristically appear red, wet, or blistered, blanchable, and extremely painful. Will heal within 3 weeks from epidermal regeneration from remaining remnants found in the tracts of hair follicles and sweat and sebaceous glands. Will not scar unless unduly manipulated or infected.
	Deep partial thickness	Injury is through the epidermis and may affect isolated areas of the deep dermal strata from which cells arise. This wound may appear red and wet or white and dry, depending upon the extent of deep dermal damage. It heals without grafting but requires > 3 weeks and closes with suboptimal cosmesis. Excision and split-thickness skin grafting are recommended for optimal and timely wound closure.
Third degree	Full thickness	Injury has destroyed both the epidermis and the dermis. The wound appears white, will not blanch, and is anesthetic. Tough, nonelastic and tenacious coagulated protein (eschar) tissue may be present on the surface. This wound will not heal without surgical intervention, unless it is extremely small and healing can occur through contracture. Excision of the nonviable tissue with split-thickness skin grafting is necessary to close the wound optimally and to minimize contracture.

(With permission from Desai, M. & Herdon, D. (1991). Burns. In: *Current Therapy of Trauma*, pp. 317. Trunkey, D. & Lewis F., eds. St. Louis: B.C. Decker.)

Capillary integrity returns to normal by 24 to 36 hours postburn, resulting in decreased loss of fluid and protein into the wounds. If fluid resuscitation has been adequate, cardiac output will return to normal and then proceed to a hyperdynamic level at which CO is above normal. The goal of fluid therapy changes as compared with the first 24 hours and is now meant to maintain organ perfusion. Inadequate fluid resuscitation can lead to acute tubular necrosis, stress ulcers, and conversion of partial-thickness wounds to full-thickness wounds. Colloids may now be given to help replace the plasma volume deficit. Due to the large sodium load given in the first 24 hours, patients usually have a whole-body excess of sodium. Fluid management is aimed at helping the patient excrete the large sodium and water load obtained during initial resuscitation. Rapid sodium shifts should be avoided, since cerebral edema may result. The patient's weight and serum sodium level are used to guide fluid replacement.

Overresuscitation should be avoided, since it can have serious consequences such as pulmonary edema or excessive wound edema inhibiting perfusion either locally or distally to the wound. Decreased local wound perfusion can cause conversion of wounds from partial to full thickness. Decreased perfusion distally can lead to neurovascular compromise of extremities.

Current research is looking into alternatives in fluid resuscitation. One possibility is the use of high-osmolar solutions such as hypertonic lactate saline, 7.5% sodium chloride, or 6% dextran 70. In theory, high-osmolar solutions will cause a rapid shift of fluid from the intracellular compartment to the intravascular space, expanding plasma volume. This improvement in cardiovascular performance, however, may be only transient. The potential risks of high-osmolar solutions are cellular dehydration and hypernatremia. Research has not yet proven any benefit in decreased wound edema. Further research is needed in this area.

TABLE 42-2. FORMULAS FOR FLUID REPLACEMENT/RESUSCITATION

	FIRST 24 HOURS			SECOND 24 HOURS		
	Electrolyte	*Colloid*	*Glucose in Water*	*Electrolyte*	*Colloid*	*Glucose in Water*
Burn budget of F.D. Moore	1000–4000 mL lactated Ringer's solution and 1200 mL 0.5N saline	7.5% of body weight	1500–5000 mL	1000–4000 mL lactated Ringer's solution and 1200 mL 0.5N saline	2.5% of body weight	1500–5000 mL
Evans	Normal saline, 1mL/kg/% burn	1.0 mL/kg/% burn	2000 mL	One half of first 24-hr requirement	One half of first 24-hr requirement	2000 mL
Brooke	Lactated Ringer's solution, 1.5 mL/kg/% burn	0.5 mL/kg/% burn	2000 mL	One half to three quarters of first 24-hr requirement	One half to three quarters of first 24-hr requirement	2000 mL
Parkland	Lactated Ringer's solution, 4 mL/kg/% burn				20–60% of calculated plasma volume	
Hypertonic sodium solution	Volume to maintain urine output at 30 mL/hr (fluid contains 250 mEq Na/L)			One third of salt solution orally, up to 3500 mL limit		
Modified Brooke	Lactated Ringer's solution, 2 mL/kg/% burn				0.3–0.5 mL/kg/% burn	Goal: maintain adequate urinary output
Burnett Burn Center	Isotonic or hypertonic alkaline sodium solution/% burn/kg			D_5 1/4 NS maintenance	Colloid 0.5 mL/% burn/kg	D_5W (% burn) (TBSAm^2)

(Hudak C, Gallo B, Berg J. Critical Care Nursing, 5th ed, p. 766. Philadelphia, JB Lippincott, 1990; with permission.)

Fluid Remobilization Phase

Fluid remobilization or diuresis usually begins 48 to 72 hours postburn and lasts one to three days. Fluid shifts from the interstitial space into the intravascular compartment, causing great increase in blood volume. As a result, urine volume will increase. Caution should be used with fluid volume replacement, since giving large amounts during this phase may lead to fluid overload. The nurse must assess the patient for signs of volume overload such as venous distension, crackles, and frothy sputum. Patients with impaired renal or cardiovascular function are at high risk during this time, since they may be less likely to handle the large fluid shifts. Most patients return to preburn weight by postinjury day 10. Remember that loss of skin integrity will increase water loss by evaporation.

Other Initial Management

Patients with a greater than 15% BSA burn should have a nasogastric tube inserted and hooked to low intermittent suction. These patients are prone to paralytic ileus. Gastric prophylaxis should be initiated, since burn patients are prone to stress ulcers.

Pain relief is an essential treatment for burn victims. Typically, narcotics are given intravenously in small doses until pain relief is achieved. Due to the unpredictability of circulation and absorption, intramuscular and subcutaneous routes should not be utilized.

Edema formation related to initial fluid shifts occurs both locally at the wound sites and systemically in burns of greater than 20% BSA. Edema formation may cause neurovascular compromise to the extremities; therefore, frequent assessments are necessary to evaluate pulses, skin color, capillary refill, and sensation. Arterial circulation is at greatest risk on circumferential burns. The Doppler flow probe may be one of the best ways to evaluate compromise. Elevating extremities may help decrease some of the edema formation. An escharotomy may be required to restore arterial circulation, prevent ischemia and necrosis, and allow for further swelling. Eschar, which forms from third-degree burns, is tight, leathery, and nondistensible and does not have pain fibers. The escharotomy can be performed at the bedside, utilizing a sterile field and scapel. (Figure 42-3) Care should be taken to avoid major nerves, vessels, and tendons. The incision should extend through the length of the eschar, over joints, and down to the subcutaneous fat. The incision is placed laterally or medially on the extremity. If a single incision does not restore circulation, bilateral incisions will be required.

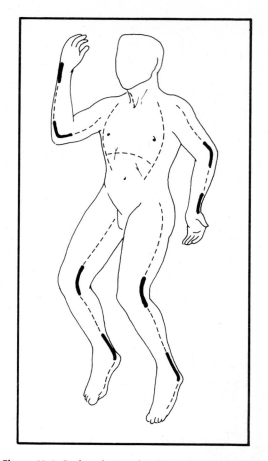

Figure 42-3. Preferred sites of escharotomy incisions. (Redrawn from Rye, L.W., Cioffi, W.S. Resuscitation of Thermally Injured Patients. *Critical Care Nursing Clinics of North America*, 1991:3; 181–189.)

Circumferential burns can also cause problems when they occur on the chest. Adequacy of respiration must be assessed continually. Ventilatory excursion may be restricted, requiring a chest escharotomy. Bilateral incisions should be made down the anterior axillary line. If burns are extensive, the incision may be extended onto the abdomen. The incisions are then connected by a transverse incision along the costal margin.

Wound Management

Treatment of other life-threatening conditions take priority over burn wound management. Initially, the burn wound should be covered with clean sheets. Ice is never used to treat burns due to the susceptibility to hypothermia or frostbite. If transfer to a burn center is

TABLE 42-3. BURN CLASSIFICATIONS BY THE AMERICAN BURN ASSOCIATION

Injury Severity	Identifying Criteria	Recommended Treatment Facility
Minor burns	Partial thickness of $\leq$ 15% TBSA No full thickness No involvement of eyes or ears	Emergency rooms—outpatients
Moderate burns	Partial thickness of 15–25% TBSA Full thickness of $<$ 10% TBSA not involving the hands, face, eyes, ears, feet, or genitalia	General hospital or may be outpatients
Major burns	Partial thickness of $>$ 25% TBSA Full thickness of $>$ 10% TBSA True electrical injuries Injury to hands, face, eyes, ears, feet, or genitalia Concomitant injuries, e.g., inhalation injury, fractures, or other trauma High-risk patients, e.g., $<$ 2 years old, $>$ 50 years old, or with pre-existing conditions	Burn unit or center

(From Desai, M. and Herdon, D. (1991). Burns. In: *Current Therapy of Trauma*, p. 317. Trunkey, D. and Lewis, F. St. Louis: B.C. Decker.)

anticipated, (Table 42-3) it is not necessary to debride or apply topical antimicrobial agents within the first 24 hours.

Besides hypovolemia, the major threat to the patient is sepsis of the burn wound. The incidence of infection varies with burn size, patient's age and current health, and type of bacteria. None of the topical antimicrobials sterilizes the wound, but they do control bacterial proliferation and provide the best control over bacterial growth. The most common topical antimicrobial agents include silvadene, silver maleate, and sulfidine. The nonviable eschar is an ideal environment for bacterial growth. Systemic antibiotics have little control over this bacterial growth, since they are unable to reach the injured tissue.

Once a patient is hemodynamically stable, wound care begins. All burned area are cleansed once or twice daily with normal saline or an antimicrobial liquid detergent. Loose and necrotic tissue is gently removed, with care taken not to damage viable tissue or cause excessive bleeding. Large blisters are debrided. Once the wounds are cleansed, a topical antimicrobial agent is applied. One of two methods is utilized, depending on the philosophy of the burn center. The open method applies the antimicrobial agent sterilely and leaves the wound open to the air. Advantages of this method are that it allows for constant wound assessment, eliminates painful dressing changes, and may limit bacterial proliferation. The closed method also applies an antimicrobial agent, but then covers the wound with a gauze dressing. Advantages include less heat loss and faster eschar separation.

Inhalation Injury

With any burn situation the clinician must consider the possibility of an inhalation injury since 80% of all fire victims die of smoke inhalation. Death at the scene of a fire is almost always a result of smoke inhalation. The degree of thermal injury however is not an indication of presence or absence of inhalation injury. Inhalation injury can occur from direct thermal injury or inhalation of carbon monoxide or other toxic gases that result from incomplete combustion.

Patients at risk for smoke inhalation are anyone with the history of being in a closed space where fire was present and/or flame burns of the face, neck and chest. Early recognition and intervention is critical to the patient's early survival. Suspect smoke inhalation if you observe singed nasal hairs, mucosal burns of the nose, lips, mouth or throat, carbonaceous or sooty material in sputum or hoarseness. If inhalation injury is suspected the patient should be intubated immediately. Airway edema can occur rapidly making it impossible to insert an endotracheal tube.

Direct thermal damage occurs usually just to the upper respiratory tract. Heat is dissipated by the upper respiratory tract in the nasal pharynx and upper airways. Cellular damage occurs leading to tissue swelling and edema. Airway obstruction can result. Direct thermal injury below the glottis is rare but may occur with steam exposure. Pulmonary edema develops in 5 to 30% of inhalation injury patients. The lower respiratory tract injury is most often the result of inhalation of noxious gases. Destruction of surfactant can occur resulting in a high incidence of adult respiratory distress syndrome.

Carbon monoxide (CO) is a product of incomplete hydrocarbon combustion. CO has a 200 times greater affinity for hemoglobin than oxygen. As a result, CO attaches to hemoglobin displacing oxygen making less oxygen available to the cells. The oxyhemoglobin dissociation curve shifts to the left so the oxygen on the hemoglobin is not readily given up to the cells. CO also attacks the cytochrome oxidase system which affects mitochondrial activity further decreasing cellular oxygenation. The result can be massive tissue hypoxia. A pulse oximeter will provide an inaccurate assessment of hemoglobin oxygen saturation. The pulse oximeter sees oxyhemoglobin and carboxyhemoglobin as the same so the SpO_2 reading will be falsely elevated. Carboxyhemoglobin levels should be drawn on admission to the emergency department and repeated every four hours until the level returns to normal.

Treatment of inhalation injuries includes first the maintenance of a patent airway. Prophylactic intubation carries little risk when compared to the danger of complete airway obstruction. The greatest risk of laryngeal and upper airway edema is 12 to 36 hours post injury. Oxygen therapy should be instituted early. Carbon monoxide elimination can be decreased from four hours to 45 minutes with an inspired oxygen concentration of 100%. Hyperbaric oxygen therapy can shorten the time even greater. Ventilatory support with PEEP and CPAP will be required since the patient often experience decreased lung compliance and atelectasis. Following airway edema and pulmonary edema the third stage of an inhalation injury is bronchopneumonia. Bronchopneumonia occurs 3 to 10 days post exposure in 15 to 60% of the patients and carries a mortality rate of 50 to 80%. A high incidence of sepsis is associated with the development of bronchopneumonia. Antibiotics should be given for documented infections.

Editor's Note

Toxicology is another new area for the CCRN exam and will probably engender only one to four questions. Questions are likely to center on the immediate critical-care setting, although a knowledge of emergency room care may be useful. This section provides a brief but intense review in the area of toxicology. The information provided may be more than you will need for the CCRN exam; however, since this area is new to the CCRN exam, it may be best to overprepare. The other option is not to study this area in any depth and

take the risk of missing these few questions; the choice is yours. Once again, do not focus on minor details but try to understand the major concepts in assessing and managing the acute-overdose patient.

TOXICOLOGY

Toxic emergencies are grouped in four categories: poisonings, overdoses, drug abuse, and alcoholism. Of the more than one million poisonings that are reported in the United States each year, 75% involve children under the age of 5. Most are caused by household products and constitute 10% of all emergency room visits.

A poison is defined as any substance which, when introduced into an organism, acts chemically upon the tissue to produce serious injury or death. There are four routes of entry: ingestion, inhalation, injection, and surface absorption. This chapter will focus primarily on ingestion.

Poisonings most commonly involve household products such as petroleum-based agents, cleaning agents, and cosmetics. Medications are the next most frequent source, followed by toxic plants and contaminated food. Table 42-4 lists agents that are the leading causes of death by poisoning.

Toxic effects of ingested substances can be delayed or immediate. Delayed effects are dependent on the rate of absorption from the gastrointestinal (GI) tract. Since most absorption occurs in the small intestine, toxins may remain in the stomach for up to several hours if a large amount of food is present. Medications or other substances that slow GI motility may interfere. Some medications or toxins are more rapidly absorbed than others. Immediate effects of a toxin can be seen with the ingestion of corrosive substances such as strong acids or alkalis or with highly toxic and rapidly absorbed toxins such as organophosphates (pesticides) or cyanide.

Assessment

Patient assessment begins with the taking of a history. This should include the five Ws: (1) who (patient age and previous medical history, including allergies and current therapies); (2) what (inquire about the suspected agent[s] or toxin[s] to which the patient has access, then obtain management information from local poison control centers); (3) when (determine the approximate time of ingestion, corroborating with

TABLE 42-4. AGENTS RESPONSIBLE FOR THE HIGHEST POISONING MORTALITY

Category	No. of Deaths/year	Percent of All Exposures in Category
Antidepressants	140	0.559
Analgesics	126	0.078
Stimulants and street drugs	64	0.320
Sedatives/hypnotics	78	0.153
Cardiovascular drugs	70	0.345
Alcohols	53	0.122
Gases and fumes	46	0.225
Asthma therapies	34	0.265
Hydrocarbons	31	0.053
Chemicals	27	0.051
Cleaning substances	25	0.016
Pesticides (including rodenticides)	14	0.023

Adapted from Litovitz, TL, Schmitz BF, Bailey KM. 1989 Annual Report of the American Association of Poison Control Centers, National Collection System. *Am J Emer Med,* 1990: 8; 394–42.

others in contact with the patient); (4) where (it is important to know the surroundings or circumstances in order to prepare for complications, as in the case of an overdose that takes place in a running car in a garage or in a tub full of water); and (5) why (assess the patient's psychiatric stability to account for inaccuracies in history or the intent of the depressed patient to deliberately mislead).

These questions are important tools in assessment because many initial intake histories are incorrect concerning agent, time, or amount.

Emergency Versus Hospital Admissions. Criteria for an intensive care unit admission may vary, but as a general rule, an emergency admission referral is made based on certain criteria: (1) overdose is substantial or highly toxic chemical is involved; (2) patient exhibits signs of acute poisoning; (3) patient is asymptomatic, but the suspected agent is rapidly absorbed, such as in the case of Lomotil or tricyclics; and (4) patient is suicidal.

Hospital admission is usually required if any of the following criteria are met: (1) patient is symptomatic and has ECG changes after tricyclic ingestion; (2) patient is unresponsive to verbal stimulation, (3) endotracheal intubation was required; and (4) systolic blood pressure is below 80 mm Hg.

Patient Assessment. The examination should include vital signs with a temperature and respiratory rate. Cardiopulmonary stabilization and anticipation of possible deterioration should also occur during initial assessment. Cardiac monitoring, pulse oximetry, and use of a large-bore IV should be considered.

Respiratory Assessment. Respiratory rate and depth can be affected by a number of agents. Check for airway patency. An increased rate and depth can be attributed to sympathomimetics such as cocaine, amphetamines, or caffeine. Noting the rate and pattern may be your first clue to an acid-based disorder. Tachypnea may result in primary alkalosis from salicylates or as a compensation for a dangerous metabolic acidosis that can occur from ethylene glycol, methanol, or other agents.

Assessment of lung sounds is an important part of serial assessments to note the presence of crackles or wheezes in patient's who may have aspirated or are in congestive heart failure. Table 42-5 lists agents associated with tachypnea.

Cardiovascular Assessment. Evidence of cardiac dysrhythmias, hypotension, or hypertension requires advanced cardiac life support as well as intensive care observation. Continuous cardiac monitoring is re-

TABLE 42-5. AGENTS ASSOCIATED WITH TACHYPNEA

Carbon monoxide	Drug-associated metabolic
Salicylates	acidosis
Pentachlorophenol	Drug-associated hepatic failure
Cyanide	

Tables 42-5 to 42-29 are adapted from Bryson PD. (1989) Comprehensive Review of Toxicology. Aspen Publications, 2nd ed.

quired, since life-threatening dysrhythmias can occur rapidly with such agents as tricyclics. Certain agents require cardiac monitoring (Table 42-6); others predispose to hypotension (Table 42-7).

Neurological Assessment. A depressed level of consciousness is a major complication in the overdose patient. Describe the patient's response to stimuli, presence or absence and type of reflexes, as well as vital sign disturbance. Other causes of decreased level of consciousness (trauma, diabetes, anoxia, sepsis, and others) should be investigated. The Glasgow Coma Scale is helpful and commonly used in neurological assessment. A summary of common neurological assessments is provided in Table 42-8. When noting pupillary size and response during your examination of the patient, be aware that certain toxins can cause characteristic eye changes (Table 42-9).

Seizures. Seizures are best managed by treating the underlying cause (e.g., hypoxia, hypoglycemia, or hyponatremia). Diazepam, phenytoin, and phenobarbital can be effective in controlling seizures from nonspecific causes or until underlying causes can be corrected. Physostigmine may be useful in cases of life-threatening anticholenergic poisonings. Halothan or

thiopental can be used for refractory seizures not responsive to the above treatments. The use of general anesthetics is reserved for cardiopulmonary stabilization when conventional methods fail. Although general anesthesia will allow for physiological stabilization, it will not stop the CNS seizures. During generalized seizures, airway protection and maintaining oxygenation are vital. Seizures may be a clue to drug withdrawal; they may be seen after administration of naloxone to a comatose patient who is narcotic dependent. Table 42-10 lists factors that may precipitate seizures. Common treatments for patients with altered mental status are listed in Table 42-11.

Gastrointestinal Assessment. Gastrointestinal disturbances are most frequently associated with the agents listed in Table 42-12. Common symptoms associated with GI poisoning center around the loss of GI fluids and subsequent hypovolemia. Electrolyte imbalances can occur as well. Blood loss can result from irritation of the gastric mucosa or from a Mallory-Weiss tear of the esophagus during protracted vomiting. Gastrointestinal decontamination is of vital importance in treatment of a toxic ingestion. X-ray studies can be diagnostic with agents that may be radiopaque (Table 42-13).

Hepatic and Renal Assessment. Laboratory studies are essential to assess potential damage to hepatic and renal systems. Liver function tests, (e.g., SGPT, SGOT, and alkaline phosphatase) are useful in assessing hepatic functioning. Although jaundice is a latent indicator of liver failure, it is seen with the agents listed in Table 42-14.

When assessing the renal system, urine output, the presence of myoglobinuria or hematuria, as well as

TABLE 42-6. COMMON AGENTS ASSOCIATED WITH HYPERTENSION AND TACHYCARDIA

Anticholinergics	Withdrawal Syndromes	Sympathomimetics
Tricyclics	Alcohol	Amphetamines
Antihistimines	Aldomet	Caffeine
Antipsychotics	Beta blockers	Cocaine
Mushrooms	CNS depressants	Clonidine
Plants	Sedatives/hypnotics	LSD
Over-the-counter		Theophylline
medicines		Phencyclidine
		Monoamine oxidase inhibitors

TABLE 42-7. COMMON AGENTS ASSOCIATED WITH HYPOTENSION

Hypotension and Tachycardia	Hypotension and Bradycardia
Carbon monoxide	Beta blockers
Cyanide	Calcium channel blockers
Narcotics	Clonidine
Nitrites	Digoxin
Phenothiazines	Organophosphates
Sedatives/hypnotics	
Tricyclics	
Iron	
Disulfiram	

laboratories studies (blood urea nitrogen, creatinine) are significant in determining renal failure. Table 42-15 lists agents that are potentially renal toxic.

Skin and Mucous Membrane Assessment. Skin and mucous membrane assessment can provide important clues in determining the causative agent. Observe for burns or erosion of oral mucosa as well as cutaneous bullous lesions. Evidence of unaccounted-for puncture wounds and contusions may be indicative of snake bites, drug abuse, or trauma. Table 42-16 lists some of these agents.

The sense of smell can also provide diagnostic clues when one is dealing with an unknown toxin or can help confirm suspicions. Some agents that have a characteristic odor are listed in Table 42-17.

Treatment of Toxic Emergencies

The goals in treatment of a patient with a known or suspected toxic ingestion are to remove the agent(s),

TABLE 42-8. COMPONENTS OF NEUROLOGICAL EXAMINATION OF THE PATIENT

Focal signs
Gag reflex
Mental status
  Affect
  Behavior and appearance
  Intellectual functioning
  Perceptual disorders
  Thought process and content
Ocular changes
  Nystagmus
  Pupillary size

TABLE 42-9. SUBSTANCES CAUSING CHARACTERISTIC EYE CHANGES

Mydriasis	Substances causing miosis
Anticholenergics	Cholinergics
Glutethimide (Doridan)	Clonidine (Catapres)
Meperidine (Demerol)	Insecticides
Mushrooms (anticholenergics)	Mushrooms (cholinergics)
Withdrawal of abused substances	Narcotics
	Nicotine
Phenothiazines	Sympathomimetics
	Phenylcyclidine (PCP)

Toxins causing nystagmus (acronym: SALEM TIP)

S	Sedatives/hypnotics, solvents	T	Thiamine depletion, tegretol
A	Alcohol	I	Isopropanol
L	Lithium	P	Phenylcyclidine, phenytoin (Dilantin)
E	Ethanol, ethylene glycol		
M	Methanol		

detoxify the patient, and prevent absorption of the suspected agent(s).

Removal of Toxic Agents. Removal can be done with the use of an emetic (ipecac) or through gastric lavage.

Emesis. Syrup of ipecac is the preferred emetic currently used in the United States. It acts locally on the gastric mucosa and centrally on the chemoreceptor trigger zone to stimulate vomiting.

TABLE 42-10. COMMON AGENTS CAUSING SEIZURES (ACRONYM: WITH LA COPS)

W	Withdrawal
I	Isoniazide
T	Theophylline
H	Hypoglycemia agents, hypoxia
L	Lead, lithium, local anesthesia
A	Anticholinergics, amphetamines
C	Camphor, carbon monoxide, carbamazepine, cholinergics, cocaine, chlorinated hydrocarbons, cyanide
O	Organophosphates
P	Phencyclidine, phenothiazines, phenytoin, propoxyphene
S	Salicylates, strychnine, sympathomimetics

TABLE 42-11. SUGGESTED THERAPY FOR PATIENTS WITH ALTERED MENTAL STATUS (ACRONYM: DONT)

	Drug	Dosage
D	Dextrose	Adult: 50 mL of $D_{50}W$
		Child: 1 mL/kg of same solution diluted 1:1
O	Oxygen	As necessary
N	Naloxone	2 mg IV
T	Thiamine	50 to 100 mg IM or IV

TABLE 42-12. AGENTS CAUSING GASTROINTESTINAL DISTURBANCES

Salicylates	Mushrooms
Acetaminophen	Mercury
Lithium	Arsenic
Iron	Phosphorus
Contaminated food	Colchicine

TABLE 42-13. AGENTS THAT MAY BE RADIOPAQUE (ACRONYM: BET A CHIP)

B	Barium
E	Enteric-coated tablets
T	Tricyclic antidepressants
A	Antihistimines
C	Chloral hydrate, cocaine, condoms, calcium
H	Heavy metals
I	Iodides
P	Phenothiazines, potassium

TABLE 42–14. COMMON AGENTS CAUSING HEPATOTOXICITY

Acetaminophen
Arsenic
Carbon tetrachloride
Iron
Toluene (airplane glue)

TABLE 42-15. COMMON AGENTS ASSOCIATED WITH RENAL TOXICITY

Amanita phalloides (mushrooms)
Antibiotics
Ethylene glycol
Methanol

The recommended dose is 30 cc for adults and 15 cc for children 1 to 12 years of age. This dose may be repeated once if emesis has not occurred in 20 to 30 min. Although chronic use of ipecac and large doses can cause neurologic and cardiac complications, ipecac poses little toxicity in the recommended dose.

Ipecac should never be used if a specific oral antidote for the suspected agent is available (*N*-acetylcysteine); if the patient exhibits potential for or history of GI bleeding (salicylates), absent gag reflex (sedatives, narcotics), or impending coma or seizures (sedatives, tricyclics); or if the patient has ingested rapidly absorbed or caustic agents (tricyclics, alkalis, acids). Complications of ipecac include Mallory-Weiss tear of the esophagus, drowsiness, electrolyte imbalance from protracted vomiting, delay in giving activated charcoal or a specific oral antidote, diarrhea, and aspiration. Table 42-18 lists agents for which induced emesis or gastric lavage is not advised. There are certain hydrocarbons that are exceptions for induced emesis or gastric lavage (Table 42-19). Due to the high toxicity of these substances, the risk of aspiration is justified.

Gastric Lavage. Gastric lavage is another method for removal of toxins.

Equipment needed consists of an orogastric tube, 26 to 28 Fr for children or 32 to 40 Fr for adults with large distal and lateral holes. Large-bore orogastric tubes allow pill fragments to be retrieved and decrease the chance of tube occlusion from pills or food particles. Various kits are available for the installation and retrieval of lavage fluid. In adults, warm tap water can be used because it does not alter serum electrolytes or osmolality. In children, warm saline is recommended. Warm lavage fluid is preferred because it decreases gastric peristalsis and increases the rate of pill dissolution, allowing the stomach contents to pass more easily through the tube. Lavage is performed until the fluid is clear, which usually requires 5 to 20 liters of fluid.

The technique for performing lavage requires that the patient be placed in the Trendelenberg, left lateral decubitus position with knees flexed. This position allows for optimum relaxation of the abdominal wall and can reduce the risk of aspiration should vomiting occur. A local anesthetic may be used in the oropharynx to diminish the gag reflex prior to passage of the lavage tube. Warming the lavage tube and treating it with a water-soluble lubricant can ease its passage. As the tube is gently advanced, the patient is instructed to swallow. Coughing, inability to speak, cyanosis, or

TABLE 42-16. AGENTS CAUSING BULLOUS LESIONS

Caustics	Environmental Agents	Sedative/hypnotic Agents
Acids	Carbon monoxide	Barbiturates
Alkalis	Snake venom	Diphenoxylate (Lomotil)
	Insect venom	Glutethimide (Doriden)
		Meprobamate (Equanil, Equagesic)
		Methaqualone (Quaalude)

respiratory distress can indicate unintentional endotracheal intubation. Proper placement should be confirmed prior to instillation of the lavage fluid.

Auscultation of the stomach while air is instilled into the passed tube plus retrieval of stomach contents ensures proper localization of the tube. For patients whose gag reflex is absent, exhibit CNS depression, or are comatose, airway protection is required prior to gastric lavage. For those patients, endotracheal intuba-

TABLE 42-17. AGENTS WITH CHARACTERISTIC ODORS

Odor	Agent
Acetone	Ethyl alcohol
	Isopropyl alcohol
	Lacquer
Bitter almond	Amygdalin
	Apricot pits
	Cyanide
	Laetrile
Burned rope	Marijuana
Carrot	Cicutoxin
Garlic	Arsenic
	Arsine gas
	Organophosphates
	Selenium
	Thallium
	Dimethyl sulfoxide
Mothballs	Naphthalene
	Paradichlorobenzene
Peanuts	Rodenticides
Pear	Chloral hydrate
	Paraldehyde
Pungent aromatic	Ethchlorvynol
Rotten egg	Hydrogen sulfide
	Mercaptans
	Sewer gas
Shoe polish	Nitrobenzene
Violets	Turpentine
Wintergreen	Methyl salicylate

tion is usually required. After passage of the tube and confirmation of its placement, the stomach is initially aspirated of contents.

Larger aliquots 300 to 500 mL of lavage fluid for adults tend to open the rugae of the stomach, thus exposing pill fragments or toxins that may be in the rugal folds. Abdominal massage, (during gastric lavage) at the left upper quadrant is recommended when concretions or bezoars are possible. A concretion or bezoar occurs when numerous pills clump together into a solid mass in the stomach (Table 42-20).

Since gastric lavage is an invasive procedure, it carries certain risks and complications. The risk versus benefit should be determined before this procedure is performed. Complications of gastric lavage are listed in Table 42-21.

Cathartics. Cathartics are used to to decrease the transit time for the nonabsorbed toxin, thereby minimizing absorption in the bowel. Osmotic cathartics, are classified as saline or saccharide. They include sorbitol, magnesium sulfate/citrate, sodium sulfate, disodium phosphate, and are preferred to the stimulant types such as (cascara, castor oil, senna, bisacodyl).

TABLE 42-18. SUBSTANCES FOR WHICH INDUCED EMESIS OR GASTRIC LAVAGE IS CONTRAINDICATED

Caustic agents	Petroleum Distillates
Acids, alkalis, ammonia, coffee pot cleaners, drain cleaners, automatic dishwasher detergent, hair bleaches, lye, metal cleaners, mildew removers, oven cleaners, rust removers, wart removers, toilet bowl cleaners	Furniture polish, gasoline, kerosene, linseed oil, lighter fluid, mineral spirits, naphtha, oils, paint and lacquer thinners, petroleum solvents, pine oil cleaners, turpentine, wood stains

TABLE 42-19. EXCEPTIONS: HYDROCARBONS THAT NEED TO BE EVACUATED FROM THE BOWEL (ACRONYM: CHAMP)

C	Camphor-based hydrocarbons
H	Halogenated hydrocarbons
A	Aromatics
M	Heavy metals
P	Pesticides

Although the use of cathartics is based primarily on empirical and anecdotal evidence, most toxicologists agree with their use as a means of decreasing GI transit time for toxins. Contraindications for cathartics are noted in Table 42-22.

Detoxification and Prevention of Absorption

Activated Charcoal. Activated charcoal is made from the distillation of various types of organic matter, which is then activated by heating to temperatures in excess of 600°C in the absence of air. This cleans and expands the charcoal, increasing its surface area and resulting in enhanced absorption ability. Activated charcoal appears as an inert, fine black powder. It is tasteless and odorless and has a gritty consistency. It is available as a powder, as an aqueous slurry, or in a suspension of 20% activated charcoal in 70% sorbitol. It can be given either orally or through a lavage or nasogastric tube. The charcoal slurry tends to be thick and gritty and is not very palatable when administered orally. It can be difficult to pass through a small-bore nasogastric tube because of its thick consistency. Therefore, whenever lavage is required, it is advantageous to instill the activated charcoal prior to removal of the lavage tube.

Charcoal dosing should provide a 10:1 ratio of charcoal to toxin to provide optimal binding. Because of the inaccuracies of ingested doses of toxins, an arbitrary dose of 1 to 2 g/kg of body weight is recom-

TABLE 42-20. AGENTS CAUSING CONCRETIONS (ACRONYM: BIG MESS)

B	Barbiturates
I	Iron
G	Glutethimide
M	Meprobamate
E	Extended-release theophylline
SS	Salicylates

TABLE 42-21. COMPLICATIONS OF LAVAGE

Aspiration
Respiratory distress
Gastric erosion
Epistaxis
Laryngospasm
Esophageal tear
Mediastinitis
Bolusing of toxins from the stomach into the small bowel

mended. Activated charcoal absorbs not only toxins but other therapeutic drugs as well.

Activated charcoal is thought to be a safe, inert, nontoxic material. No harmful effects have been shown during ingestion or exposure to skin. Although activated charcoal is useful in absorbing many toxins, there are agents that it does not appear to absorb (Table 42-23).

Enhanced Elimination. Enhanced elimination of certain drugs may be assisted by making use of certain pharmokinetic parameters that affect drug excretion. These include forced diuresis (with or without ion trapping), multiple-dose charcoal, dialysis, hemoperfusion, and plasmapheresis.

Forced Diuresis. This method involves enhanced elimination of the agent through urinary excretion. Normally, excretion takes place through glomerular filtration, active tubular secretion, and tubular reabsorption. This method deals with inhibiting tubular reabsorption only by diluting the concentration gradient between the blood and the urine. This will lessen the time of the agent's exposure to the reabsorptive sites in the distal tubules.

TABLE 42-22. CONTRAINDICATIONS FOR USE OF CATHARTICS

Adynamic ileus
Current diarrhea
Intestinal obstruction
No saline cathartics in patient with history of congestive heart failure or salt restrictions
No magnesium sulfate in patient with potential for renal failure
No oil-based cathartics (hazardous if aspirated)
Caution in the very young and very old
In patient with severe fluid and electrolyte imbalance

TABLE 42-23. AGENTS NOT ABSORBED BY ACTIVATED CHARCOAL

Alkali	N-Methyl carbamate	Sorbitol
Boric acid	Potassium hydroxide	Magnesium
DDT	Sodium hydroxide	sulfate
Ferrous sulfate	Sodium metasilicate	Tolbutamide
Mineral acids	N-Acetylcysteine (?)	

Ion-Trapping Methods. Ion-trapping methods cause a solution to become more alkaline or acidic, so that the substance is trapped in the kidney and excretion is enhanced. Weak acids are more ionized in an alkaline solution, and weak bases are more ionized in an acidic solution. If a difference in pH occurs across a membrane, ion trapping will occur. The toxin will collect in the compartment where ionization is greater because the nonionized form crosses the lipid-cell membrane more readily than the ionized form does (Table 42-24).

Alkaline diuresis can be achieved by the administration of sodium bicarbonate in intravenous fluids. Administer fluid amounts to keep urine flow to 3 to 6 mL/kg per hour. Add two to three ampules of sodium bicarbonate to each liter of D_5W. Use enough bicarbonate to achieve a urinary pH of 7.5 or greater. Careful observation of electrolytes is required during diuresis. This is useful for agents that cause metabolic acidosis (Table 42-25).

The risks of acid diuresis currently outweigh the possible benefits. The compounds used to achieve acidification also have the potential to cause acute tubular necrosis secondary to rhabdomyolysis.

Multidose Charcoal. Multiple doses of activated charcoal appear to be effective in enhancing elimina-

tion of certain drugs that undergo enterohepatic or enterogastric circulation. The usual recommended dose for adults is 20 to 100 g every two to eight hours until serum drug levels have been reduced to a subtoxic range (5 to 10 g every four to eight hours is recommended for children). To avoid repeated doses of a cathartic, activated charcoal without the added cathartic is preferred for this method. Also, remember that charcoal will enhance the elimination of therapeutic drugs such as digoxin, theophylline, and carbamazepine (Table 42-26). Careful evaluation of these drug levels is warranted, and the drugs may need to be replaced during this procedure.

Extracorporeal Methods of Elimination Hemodialysis. Hemodialysis can be useful in further clearance of certain substances from the body. It is usually reserved for the patient who has not responded to more conservative and conventional methods.

Patient criteria to determine the need for hemodialysis include the following: stage 3 or 4 coma, hypotension not corrected by adjusting circulating volume, impending renal or hepatic failure, severe acid-base disturbance not responding to therapy, marked hyper- or hypothermia, and severe electrolyte imbalance not responsive to therapy. Certain agents are

TABLE 42-24. DRUGS RESPONSIVE TO ENHANCED DIURESIS OR ION TRAPPING

Neutral Diuresis	Alkaline Diuresis	Acid Diuresis*
Bromides	Phenobarbital	Phencyclidine
Lithium	Salicylates	Amphetamines
(controversial)	Tricyclics	
Isoniazid	Primidone	
(controversial)	Isoniazid	
	(controversial)	
	Lithium	
	(controversial)	

*Not recommended.

TABLE 42-25. AGENTS THAT CAUSE METABOLIC ACIDOSIS (ACRONYM: A MUD PILE CAT)

A	Alcohol
M	Methyl alcohol
U	Uremia
D	Diabetic ketoacidosis
P	Paraldehyde
I	Iron, isoniazid
L	Lactic acidosis
E	Ethylene glycol
C	Carbon monoxide, cyanide
A	Aspirin
T	Toluene

TABLE 42-26. DRUGS RESPONSIVE TO MULTIPLE-DOSE CHARCOAL

Carbamazine (Tegretol)	Meprobamate
Cyclic antidepressants	Nalodol (Corgard)
Dapsone	Phenobarbital
Digitoxin	Phenylbutazone

TABLE 42-27. IMMEDIATE INDICATIONS FOR HEMO-DIALYSIS REGARDLESS OF CLINICAL CONDITION

Amanita phalliodes (mushroom) ingestion
Ethylene glycol
Methanol
Heavy metals in soluble compounds
Heavy metals after chelating

TABLE 42-28. DRUG CRITERIA FOR DIALYSIS

Low molecular weight
Water solubility
Small volume of distribution
Small degree of protein binding
Dialyzable active metabolites

highly toxic, and immediate hemodialysis is needed even if the patient appears stable (Table 42-27).

Various pharmacological properties of the drug(s) or toxin(s) to be eliminated enhance their ability to be dialyzed from the body. These factors are listed in Table 42-28.

Because of their pharmacological properties, the drugs listed in Table 42-29 are responsive to hemodialysis. Keep in mind that although these agents can be dialyzed, hemodialysis and other extracorporeal measures should be used only when conventional and more conservative measures fail.

Hemoperfusion. Hemoperfusion is another method of clearing toxins from the body by passing blood through charcoal columns or resins. Plasma extraction ratios are significantly higher for hemoperfusion than for hemodialysis. The advantage of hemoperfusion is that it is not as restricted by physical drug characteristics, such as molecular weight, water solubility, and protein binding, that limit hemodialysis.

The use of hemoperfusion is controversial but is indicated for a massive ingestion when the extracellular distribution is significant and the plasma level of the toxin is at its maximum. Hemoperfusion is generally successful with the same agents that respond to hemodialysis.

Plasmapheresis. Plasmapheresis is considered a modified exchange transfusion. The method of phlebotomy is used, and then the cellular components of the blood are returned to the patient. The plasma and plasma proteins are then replaced with fresh plasma or a suitable colloid. Plasmapheresis is most effective with drugs that are strongly protein bound, have a long half-life, and are not well dialyzed or hemoperfused.

Antidotes. Certain drugs and toxins have specific antidotes that counteract their harmful effects. It is best to use an antidote if available, although reversal of certain drugs can precipitate withdrawal symptoms and seizures. Table 42-30 provides a list of drugs and antidotes as well as specific precautions needed.

BIBLIOGRAPHY

Advanced Burn Life Support Provider's Manual. (1990). Nebraska Burn Institute.

Bryson, P. *Comprehensive Review of Toxicology, 2nd ed.* Rockville: Aspen Publications, 1989.

Burgess, M. (1991). Initial Management of a Patient with Extensive Burn Injury. *Crit Care Clins of North Am. 3*(2), 165–179.

Cardona, V., Hurn, P., Mason, P., et al. (1988). *Trauma Nursing from Resuscitation Through Rehabilitation.* Philadelphia: W.B. Saunders.

TABLE 42-29. AGENTS RESPONSIVE TO DIALYSIS

Alcohols	Calcium	Meprobamate	Ammonia
Chloral hydrate	Methanol	Amphetamines	Ethylene glycol
Potassium	Antibiotics	Iodides	Quinidine
Barbiturates	Isoniazid	Salicylates	Bromides
Lithium	Strychnine		

TABLE 42-30. AGENTS AND ANTIDOTES

Drug/Toxin	Antidote/Dose	Comment
Acetaminophen	N-Acetylcysteine 140 mg/kg PO (loading) 70 mg/kg PO every 4 hr × 17 doses (maintenance)	No ipecac or charcoal (will delay antidote) Most effective within 12 hr
Anticholinergics	Physostigmine Adult: 0.5–5.0 mg (IV slowly) Child: 0.5 mg or 0.02 mg/kg IV slowly (1–5 mg IV)	Observe for seizures or bradycardia.
Beta-adrenergic blockers	Glucagon: 1–5 mg IV	
Benzodiazepines (Valium, Dalmane, Tranzene)	Flumazenil (Mazicon) Initial: 0.2 mg IV over 15 sec Follow-up: 0.2 mg every 60 sec to 3 mg in 1 hr/1 mg in 5 min	Observe for seizures.
Bromide	Sodium chloride	
Carbamate insecticides	Atropine Adult: up to 5 mg IV every 15 min Child: 0.05 mg/kg IV	Physiological; blocks acetylcholine
Carbon monoxide	Oxygen: 100% reduced half-life of carbon monoxide to 1.5 hr	Hyperbaric chamber at 3 atm reduces half-life to 23 min.
Cardiac glycosides	Fragment, antigen-binding antibody therapy, digibind	Use of severe dysrhythmias, digitoxicity with $K^+ > 5$–6.0 mEq/L. Toxid dose ingestion: Adult: 10 mg Child: 4 mg
Chronic mercury, copper	Penicillamine: 1–4 g	Cuprimine is readily absorbed orally.
Cyanide	Amyl nitrite (pearls) every 2 min Sodium nitrite Adult: 300 mg IV Child: 10 mg/kg Sodium thiosulfate Adult: 12.5 g IV slowly Child: 1.5 mL/kg	Methemoglobin plus cyanide Causes hypotension. Dose assumes normal Hg. Forms harmless sodium thiocyanate.
Ethylene glycol, methanol	Ethyl alcohol (in conjunction with dialysis) 1 cc/kg of 100% ethanol in glucose (loading) 0.1 cc/kg/per hr diluted to maintain level at 100 mg%	Competes for alcohol dehydrogenase; prevents formation of formic acid and oxalates
Gyromitra mushrooms	Pyridoxine: 2–5 mg IV slowly	
Heavy metals 　Lead 　Mercury	Disodium EDTA IV BAL (British antilewisite): 5 mg/kg IM ASAP	Effective chelating agents; form stable, nontoxic, excretable cyclic compounds

(continued)

TABLE 42-30. *(Continued)*

Drug/Toxin	Antidote/Dose	Comment
Gold		
Arsenic		
Iron	Deferoxamine (Desferal) 40–90 mg/kg IM (initial) not to exceed 1 g 10–15 mg/kg/per hr	Deferoxamine mesylate forms excretable ferrioxamine complex.
Isoniazid	Pyridoxine: 2–5 mg IV slowly	
Narcotics/opiates, including Lomotil and propoxyphene (Darvon)	Naloxone: 0.01 mg/kg IV	Frequent repeated doses may be needed; may precipitate acute withdrawal.
Nitrites	Methylene blue: 1–2 mg of 1% solution IV over 5 min	Exchange transfusion may be needed; blocks acetylcholine.
Organophosphates	Atropine Adult: up to 5 mg IV every 15 min Child: 0.05 mg/kg IV Pralidoxime (2-PAM): Initial dose: Adult: 1 g IV Child: 25–50 mg/kg IV	Breaks akyl phosphate-cholinesterase bond
Tricyclic antidepressants	Sodium bicarbonate	Protein binding of drug occurs at alkalotic pH.
Venoms Black widow	Antivenom One vial in 50 cc saline over 30 min	Indicated for patients <12 or >65 years old or with serious medical history
Pit vipers	May require large dose due to lower neutralizing antibody titers in antivenom	For systemic or severe local envenomations Observe for serum sickness, since antivenoms are of equine origin.
Warfarin (Coumadin)	Vitamin K Adult: 5–25 mg IM or IV Child: 1–5 mg IM	Promotes hepatic biosynthesis of prothrombin

Duncan, D. and Driscoll, D. (1991). Burn Wound Management. *Crit Care Clins of North Am. 3*(2), 199–220.

Hartman, G. (1990). Anesthetic Considerations for the Burn Patient. *Welcome Trends in Anesthesiology. 9*(1), 3–11.

Litovitz, T.L., Schmitz, B.F., Bailey, K.M. (1989). Annual Report of the American Association of Poison Control Centers, National Data Collection System.

Metheny, N. (1992). *Fluid and Electrolyte Balance Nursing Considerations.* Philadelphia: J.B. Lippincott.

Mosley, S. (1988). Inhalation Injury: A Review of the Literature. *Heart and Lung.* 17, 1, 3–9.

Tredget, E., Shankowsky, H. Taerum, T., et al. (1990). The Role of Inhalation Injury in Burn Trauma. *Ann Surg. 212,* 720–727.

Trunkey, D. and Lewis, F. (1991). *Current Therapy of Trauma.* Philadelphia: B.C. Decker.

Rue, L. and Cioffi, W. (1991). Resuscitation of Thermally Injured Patients. *Crit Care Clins of North Am. 3*(2), 181–189.

Welch, G. (1991). Anesthesia for the Patient with Thermal Injury. *Current Reviews for Nurse Anesthetists. 14*(12), 94–99.

CHAPTER 43

Sepsis and Multiple Organ Dysfunction Syndrome

Editor's Note

Sepsis and multiple organ dysfunction syndrome (MODS) are a new part of the CCRN exam. This section, along with burns and toxic ingestions, comprises 10% of the CCRN exam (20 questions). This chapter addresses the areas of sepsis and MODS, a section that may have anywhere from 5 to 15 questions on the CCRN exam. Due to the relevance of sepsis and MODS to critical care, it is a valuable area to learn. Understanding these two major concepts involves becoming familiar with relatively complex cellular activities.

In this chapter, a brief summary of these complex activities are given in an attempt to maintain a simplified approach that covers essential CCRN content.

It is unlikely the specific detail in this chapter will be heavily addressed on the CCRN exam. Try to understand the major terms and the general sequence of events that occur in sepsis. If you understand the major therapies and symptoms of sepsis, you will probably be adequately prepared for the exam.

Concepts in sepsis and multisystem organ dysfunction are changing rapidly. Even definitions and terminology are changing in an attempt to keep pace with the improved understanding of concepts involving conditions such as sepsis. In this chapter, definitions and terminology will be employed which are consistent with a recent joint American College of Chest Physicians–Society of Critical Care Medicine committee recommendation. These terms and definitions are listed in Table 43-1. The major reason for these new definitions is the better understanding of the body's response to both infections and inflammation. The key new terms are systemic inflammatory response syndrome and multiple organ dysfunction syndrome (MODS). MODS replaces the term multisystem organ failure (MSOF). MODS is proposed as a more accurate term, since dysfunctions of organs exist along a continuum, rather than being healthy or in failure, as MSOF implies. These definitions are in addition to the slightly revised definition of sepsis.

The rationale for adopting these new terms is

TABLE 43-1. DEFINITIONS USED IN SEPSIS

Infection   Microbial phenomenon characterized by an inflammatory response to the presence of microorganisms or the invasion of normally sterile host tissue by those organisms.

Bacteremia   The presence of viable bacterial in the blood.

Systemic inflammatory response syndrome   The systemic inflammatory response to a variety of severe clinical insults. The response is manifested by two or more of the following conditions:
Temperature >38°C or <36°C
Heart rate >90 bpm
Respiratory rate >20 breaths/min or $Paco_2$ <32 torr
WBC >12,000 cells/mm³ or <4000 cells/mm³, or >10% immature (band) forms

Sepsis   The systemic response to infection. This systemic response is manifested by two or more of the following conditions as a result of infection:
Temperature >38°C or <36°C
Heart rate >90 bpm
Respiratory rate >20 breaths/min or $Paco_2$ <32 torr
WBC >12,000 cells/mm³ or <4000 cells/mm³, or >10% immature (band) forms

Multiple organ dysfunction syndrome   Presence of altered organ function in an acutely ill patient such that homeostasis cannot be maintained without intervention.

based on important diagnostic and therapeutic concepts. To effectively treat any of the above conditions, an understanding of their causative origins is necessary. With the current definitions, the appropriate origin is not always clear. For example, conditions that previously were termed sepsis were frequently associated with an inflammatory process but without any active infection. Sepsis, by definition, must have an active infectious source. Consequently, patients were being diagnosed as having sepsis when they did not meet the definition for sepsis. In this type of patient, the use of antibiotic therapy or even more advanced therapies, such as monoclonal antibodies, may not be effective, since no active infection is present.

Over the next several pages, sepsis and MODS will be briefly explained. From this explanation, an understanding of the appropriate nursing, diagnostic, and therapeutic actions will be possible. This information should prepare you for the CCRN exam in the area of sepsis and MODS.

SEPSIS

Sepsis is one of the leading causes of increased morbidity and mortality in critical care. Sepsis is still a confusing entity for clinicians in that it is a difficult condition to identify, it is difficult to predict who is at risk, and it is even more difficult to treat the condition. Sepsis can present in a mild or severe (septic shock) form, with mortalities ranging anywhere from 20 to 80%, depending on the form of sepsis present. Part of the problem with sepsis is identifying when it is present and why it occurs. In this chapter, potential causes of sepsis and presented along with physical symptoms and responses. Current concepts in treating sepsis will be discussed, as well as controversies in management of the septic patient.

Etiology

Sepsis is defined as the systemic response to infection. It not only is the direct result of an infection but also reflects an inflammatory response produced by the immune system. Sepsis can originate from any antigen, bacterial, viral, or fungal, although by far the most common sources are bacterial. The most significant infections seen in critical care are usually gram-negative bacterial infections (e.g., *Pseudomonas aeruginosa, Klebsiella, Serratia, and Escherichia coli*),

although some gram-positive infections (e.g., *Staphylococcus aureus*) are also responsible for sepsis.

The antigen eventually causing sepsis must take hold in tissues and start to grow in order to produce an infectious process. For example, an antigen can exist on the skin (colonization), or even in the blood, but will not produce an infection until it resides and grows in normal tissue. Normally, most infections are controlled by the immune system, and further progression does not take place. However, in sepsis, the initial infection progresses to a more advanced state.

Septic Cascade

From the initial infection, an extension of the infectious response occurs. The extension involves a series of events, primarily an inflammatory response sequence as well as a direct physiological response to the infection. The extension can be viewed as a cascade of events, which probably becomes self-perpetuating after a certain point. Several events occur that characterize the septic process and subsequent inflammatory response. These events are briefly summarized below. In addition, Table 43-2 shows the primary factors involved in the septic cascade.

The exact sequence of events in sepsis is unclear, although one potential scenario is as follows (Fig. 43-1). The antigen (e.g., bacteria) is attacked by a macrophage (e.g., a segmented neutrophil). The macrophage ingests and destroys most of the antigen. By-products of the damaged antigen, such as endotoxin, are released. The immune system responds to the antigen and the by-products by producing substances designed to control the continued growth of the antigen. For example, the complement system (particularly C3a and C5a) is activated to stimulate neutrophil activity. In addition, platelet activation and aggregation are promoted, perhaps as an attempt to isolate the infection. The neutrophil or other macrophage (e.g., monocytes) will initiate a sequence of events also designed to control the antigen. The major immunologic responses are listed below.

Arachidonic Acid Sequence. In response to the infection, macrophage (neutrophil and monocyte) activity (polymorphonuclear leukocytes [PMN]) in the area increase. PMN attempt to control the infection through a variety of processes, including release of highly destructive molecules such as oxygen free radicals. Another method used by the PMN is through the release of arachidonic acid. As arachidonic acid is gen-

TABLE 43-2. MAJOR IMMUNE SYSTEM MEDIATORS

Arachidonic acid   Phospholipid from cell walls that can produce leukotrienes, thromboxane A_2, and prostaglandins.

Complement   There are two major types, C3 and C5, which have similar actions. Causes mast cells to release vasodilatation mediators, stimulation of arachidonic acid, increased neutrophil and monocyte activity, increased capillary permeability, stimulation of TNF release, and decreased systemic vascular resistance.

Interferons   Increase TNF and interleukin release, activate B-cell activity for antibody formation, and increase neutrophil and monocyte activity.

Leukotrienes   Several different types exist, although the primary actions are to increase platelet aggregation, cause vasoconstriction (reducing capillary blood flow), and increase pulmonary vascular resistance. Stimulate prostacyclin, probably as a feedback control mechanism.

Prostaglandin E_2   Inhibits interleukin-1, causes vasodilation, and can inhibit TNF production.

Prostaglandin I_2   Inhibits platelet aggregation and thrombus formation. Causes vasodilatation and decreased capillary permeability.

Thromboxane A_2   Increases platelet aggregation, leading to capillary obstruction. Increases capillary permeability, vasoconstriction, and broncho-constriction.

Tumor necrosis factor (TNF)   Stimulated from endotoxin or similar substance. Primary action is to increase production

erated, it is further degraded. The degradation of arachidonic acid takes place by one of two pathways, the cyclo-oxygenase or lipo-oxygenase pathway (Fig. 43-2). From the cyclo-oxygenase pathway, two important by-products, thromboxane A_2 and prostacyclin (a prostaglandin), are generated. From the lipo-oxygenase pathway, various leukotrienes (e.g., leukotrienes B_4, C_4, D_4, and E_4) are released.

Both leukotrienes and thromboxane A_2 generate a series of reactions, including an increased tendency for platelet aggregation, increased capillary permeability, and vasoconstriction. Prostacyclin (the precursor to specific prostaglandins) produces essentially the opposite responses, i.e., a decreased tendency for platelet aggregation, decreased capillary permeability, and vasodilatation.

Down Regulation of the Immune/Inflammatory Response. An important aspect of the immune/inflammatory response is the body's ability to neutralize toxic products produced by the immune system. The ability of components of the immune system to control infections is based on the generation of substances that destroy virtually any substance which with they come into contact, including normal cells. For example, oxygen radicals, once released, will damage or destroy any cell with which they come in contact. The body will attempt to produce neutralizing substances, such as peroxidases for oxygen radicals, to avoid injury to normal tissues. One theory of sepsis holds that the down regulation of the immune system malfunctions and allows normal tissue to be damaged by the immune responses.

T-Cell Response. The macrophage also stimulates T-cell activity by altering the T cell to the presence of an ingested antigen through markers on the macrophage cell surface. The T cell senses these markers and promotes the formation of interleukin-2 (IL-2). From IL-2, specific interferons as well as granulocyte-macrophage colony-stimulating factor are released. IL-2 is an active cardiovascular modifier. With release of IL-2, the systemic vascular resistance (SVR) decreases and cardiac output increases.

Tumor Necrosis Factor. Tumor necrosis factor (TNF) is thought to be produced in response to a substance such as endotoxin. TNF produces platelet aggregation, increased capillary permeability, neutrophil activation, and stimulation of the release of IL-1, IL-6, and IL-8. It is thought that TNF may mediate the central response to sepsis, although the exact mechanism for this is unclear. It is also a pyrogenic (fever-producing) substance.

In addition to these responses, the body generates increased quantities of endorphins (endogenous opiate release). The opiate release produces vasodilation (a reduction in SVR) and changes in capillary permeability.

Effect of Immune Response on Endothelial Cells

All of the above activities are designed to help control the growth of antigens. If properly released, the im-

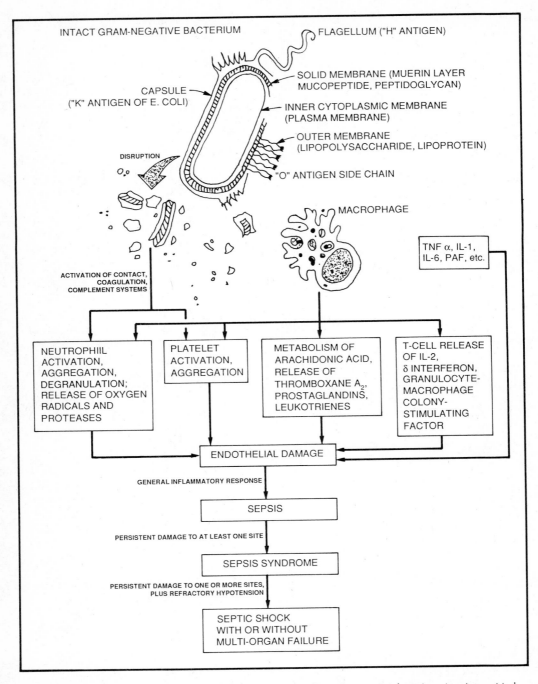

Figure 43-1. The septic cascade. (Modified from Bone, R.C. The pathogenesis of sepsis. Ann Intern Med. 1991;115(6):460.)

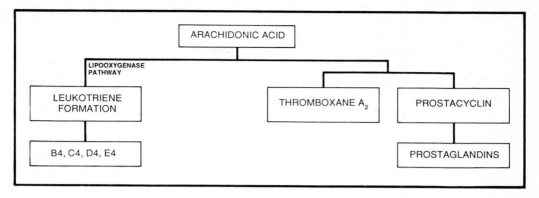

Figure 43-2. Arachidonic acid sequence.

mune/inflammatory response does not injure normal tissue. However, if the response is not controlled, normal cells can be injured. The most likely cells to be at risk of injury in the immune response are the endothelial cells of the blood vessels. If the endothelial layer of blood vessels is damaged, every organ is threatened, since control of vascular fluid and oxygen and nutrient supply may be disrupted.

The immune response is initially a local response. Under normal circumstances, the above responses control antigen growth. Keep in mind, however, that all of these processes, which are designed to control antigen growth, can also damage endothelial cells.

If the immune response spreads beyond a local level, either because the infection is too great to be controlled or because down regulation fails to occur, the immune response may spread systematically. It is the systemic spread that is probably the first major indicator of a septic process.

Extensions of Sepsis. As the septic process manifests, at least one organ will be affected. If the inflammatory response spreads to more than one organ, MODS is likely to occur. In addition, if the systemic spread produces hypotension (see definition in Table 43-1), septic shock is likely to occur. Survival from septic shock is dependent on many factors, with a reduced survival associated with patients who are >65 years old, are immunosuppressed, or are malnourished.

Clinical Presentations

The physical presentation is a combined result of the factors causing sepsis. For example, by-products of arachidonic acid produce systemic vasodilatation, pulmonary hypertension, increased pericapillary shunting, and leakage of fluid from the capillaries (producing third spacing of fluid and edema). The actual physical symptoms produced by these events vary, making clear identification of when the septic process starts difficult.

Several substances, such as TNF, are direct pyrogenic substances. Temperature elevation is common in sepsis, although hypothermia can exist. Temperature elevation is not so much an indicator of sepsis as it is a reflection of the responses of the immune system to the initial infection and the subsequent inflammatory responses.

The patient generally is tachycardiac secondary to an increased cardiac output. The cardiac output increases secondary to a decrease in SVR. The increase in cardiac output is somewhat contradictory, since sepsis has been demonstrated to produce myocardial depressant factors. The increase in cardiac output is probably secondary to an increased end diastolic volume, since ejection fraction is usually reduced.

The patient may have pulmonary symptoms reflective of increased extravascular lung water secondary to increased capillary permeability (such as seen in the adult respiratory distress syndrome). If pulmonary symptoms are present, they may result in refractory hypoxemia (PaO_2 unresponsive to oxygen therapy), generalized crackles heard upon auscultation, shortness of breath, and increased secretion production.

As the septic process continues, any organ system can be affected. For example, a change in level of consciousness may reflect central nervous system involvement, or acute renal or hepatic failure can result. Physical signs of these organ systems failing are the same as if the organ failed for other reasons. Specific signs of individual organ failure can be found in chapters addressing each organ. If the septic process is severe and involves multiple organs, MODS can result.

Treatment

Treatment of sepsis currently is designed to treat the infectious process, control undesirable immune responses, and provide support to any organ system in failure. No curative therapy for sepsis currently exists due to the inability to address the first two objectives. The potential to cure sepsis exists with new therapies designed to control the original infection or immune response, such as monoclonal antibodies. Improved treatment of sepsis is theoretically possible with agents designed to reduce the immune response, such as ibuprofen and naloxone, although research has not verified their role at this time. While great promise exists in eventually controlling sepsis, unfortunately for now most therapy for sepsis is aimed at treating symptoms rather than curing the septic patient.

Therapies that Control the Septic Process

Specific Mediators of the Immune Response
Ibuprofen. Ibuprofen is a thromboxane A_2 inhibitor. Theoretically, it should improve capillary blood flow by blocking capillary vasoconstriction and increased clotting tendencies. Ibuprofen has not been as successful as originally believed in the treatment of sepsis.
Naloxone (Narcan). With the release of endogenous opiates, naloxone should improve the symptoms produced by sepsis by blocking the response of the opiates. While theoretically promising, naloxone has not been effective in clinical trials. At this time, naloxone is unlikely to be useful in the treatment of sepsis.
Prostaglandins. An area of interest in treating septic symptoms is the use of derivatives of prostacyclin. Prostacyclin derivatives (prostaglandins E_1 and E_2) will possibly reduce pulmonary hypertension, reduce coagulopathies, and improve cardiac performance. Studies have indicated conflicting responses to prostaglandins, although clinical results are promising.
Monoclonal Antibodies. The only way to actually cure sepsis is to eliminate the original infection while simultaneously controlling the septic cascade originating from the sepsis. While no drugs are available at this time, within the next few years several drugs that specifically address the infectious agent are likely to be released. Most of these agents are in the category of monoclonal antibodies. Two such antibodies (HA-1A and E5) are examples of monoclonal antibodies for sepsis. These antibodies are specifically designed to neutralize gram-negative bacteria, the most common cause of sepsis. Although the potential of these agents is exciting, their availability is currently limited.

Antibiotic Support. To treat the underlying infectious process that is causing the septic response, specific antibiotic support is required. Cultures are necessary to identify the infectious antigen. If the infectious agent is unknown, broad antibiotic coverage is given. This treatment frequently employs two or three types of antibiotics, e.g., gram-positive coverage (such as a penicillin or cephalosporin), gram-negative coverage (such as an aminoglycoside like gentamicin), and broad gram-negative and gram-positive coverage (imipenem).

Supportive Therapy for Sepsis. General systemic support is usually provided by addressing specific symptoms. While none of these therapies will correct the septic process, they have the potential to improve patient comfort and "buy time" for the other therapies to help control the original problem.

Temperature Changes. Excessive temperature elevation ($>102°F$ or $39°C$) may be treated if the patient is uncomfortable or has excessive oxygen consumption. Oxygenation should be monitored through mixed venous blood gases (Svo_2, Mvo_2) in order to assess the effect of treating temperature elevations.

Fluid Administration. One of the current therapies for sepsis is the administration of potentially large amounts of fluids. Fluid boluses (e.g., normal saline) may be employed in an attempt to maintain capillary blood flow. These therapies may be used even when the cardiac output is normal or elevated, based on the assumption that capillary blood flow is altered and can be maintained only with supranormal blood flow (cardiac outputs).

In sepsis, pulmonary capillary wedge pressures may remain low despite large amounts of fluid administration. This is likely due to the leaking of fluid from the capillaries into the interstitial spaces. Fluid administration may be best controlled by monitoring the critical oxygen delivery point.

Critical Oxygen Delivery Point. In sepsis and particularly septic shock, it has been theorized that a critical oxygen delivery point (Do_2) exists. This point is characterized by the development of a dependence of oxygen consumption on oxygen delivery (Fig. 43-3). This dependence is a result of loss of capillary blood flow.

Under normal circumstances, cells use only the required amount of oxygen for metabolic activities. If more oxygen is provided, such as with an increase in cardiac output with dobutamine, the cells will not use more oxygen just because it is available. Normally then, oxygen consumption should be independent of changes in oxygen delivery.

In pathological states, such as hypoperfusion [from left ventricular failure or hypovolemia] and sepsis, blood flow to cells can be interrupted. The interruption can be due to many factors, such as severely reduced blood flow or microemboli. Whatever the factor, cells will be deprived of oxygen. This point is identified by noting a dependence of oxygen consumption on oxygen delivery. Oxygen consumption dependence on oxygen delivery reflects changes in capillary blood flow. For example, if oxygen delivery falls to abnormally low levels (hypovolemia, left ventricular failure) fewer cells will receive blood flow (and oxygen) with the result of a decrease in oxygen consumption. In sepsis, oxygen delivery is greater than normal secondary to elevated cardiac outputs. However, capillary blood flow is disrupted by local vasoconstriction and microemboli.

If oxygen delivery is increased and oxygen consumption simultaneously increases, it is a reflection of restoration of blood flow to capillary beds. Therapies for treating patients who have a dependence of oxygen consumption or oxygen delivery is focused on increasing oxygen delivery until oxygen consumption once again becomes independent. As long as Vo_2 increases when Do_2 increases, it implies more cells are using oxygen again due to reestablished blood flow. When Vo_2 does not increase when Do_2 increases, the cellular supplies of oxygen are likely to be adequate.

Therapy to treat sepsis and septic shock, used to increase oxygen delivery until Vo_2 is independent of Do_2, has been suggested to improve patient outcome. Studies are still progressing in this area.

To monitor the critical oxygen delivery point, pulmonary artery (Swan-Ganz) catheters are required, preferably fiberoptic catheters to monitor SVo_2 levels at the same time.

Inotropic Support. Normally, when the cardiac output is elevated, as in septic states, one would not expect administration of inotropes. However, some studies have suggested that inotropes (such as dobutamine) be used to help exceed the critical oxygen delivery point. The administration of dobutamine (or other inotropes) is titrated to achieve an optimal balance between oxygen delivery and consumption.

Vasopressors. If the blood pressure falls and is not maintained by fluids and inotropes, vasopressors may be used. The vasopressor generally utilized is either norepinephrine (Levophed), dopamine (Intropin), or phenylephrine (Neosynephrine).

Steroids. Steroid use has been demonstrated to be ineffective in the treatment of sepsis. Despite theoretical advantages, several large studies have indicated that steroids have no major role in the treatment of sepsis.

Nutritional Support. Aggressive support of the septic patient is important to avoid development of malnutrition. Both enteral and parenteral support may be employed to provide adequate calories. Sepsis tends to produce highly catabolic states, requiring adequate protein replacement. Carbohydrates and fats should be administered in adequate levels, with an avoidance of excessive carbohydrates in order to decrease the respiratory work generated by carbohydrate catabolism.

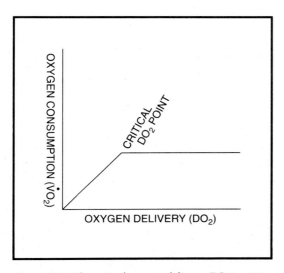

Figure 43-3. The critical oxygen delivery (DO2) point.

General Supportive Measures. Diuretics may be employed if acute renal failure develops. If acute renal failure is present, the cardiac system will be supported by inotropes rather than by fluid therapy.

If hepatic failure exists, therapies designed to reduce hepatic work will be necessary. For example, low-protein diets and lactalose may help reduce symptoms of hepatic failure.

Sepsis is a difficult clinical entity to understand and treat. Symptoms are inconsistent and not clear enough to differentiate sepsis from other conditions. While our understanding of the events that occur in sepsis is improving, treatments are limited in helping improve outcomes for the patient who develops sepsis. While great promise exists for better therapies over the next several years, current therapy is centered on supportive rather than on curative treatment.

SEPTIC SHOCK

Septic shock is a continuation of the septic process. In this situation, however, hypotension develops and is resistant to most therapies. Aggressive fluid resuscitation, inotropic support, and vasopressor application may be required. In septic shock, the likelihood of success in ameliorating these symptoms is limited. Mortality from septic shock is high due to the lack of definitive treatments for the original septic problem.

Septic shock usually presents with hypotension secondary to a markedly reduced SVR. Clinically the patient presents with a reduced blood pressure (<90/60), tachycardia, tachypnea, warm skin (due to peripheral vasodilatation) and reduced urine output. It was originally thought that septic shock may progress to a terminal phase in which the cardiac output falls and the SVR increases, although recent evidence suggests that this stage does not necessarily occur prior to death from septic shock.

MULTIPLE ORGAN DYSFUNCTION SYNDROME

This new category is based upon the understanding that organ dysfunction can take place without actual organ failure. It is probably a precursor to multiple system organ failure, although actual organ failure is likely a preterminal event. MODS may be an extension of the septic process. Widespread organ dysfunction occurs secondary to endothelial injury from the septic cascade. While all organs are affected, the three most common in terms of dysfunction are the lungs, liver, and kidneys. The central nervous system is also commonly affected, as evidenced by a decrease in level of consciousness or change in behavior.

MODS can be classified as either primary or secondary. Primary MODS is the result of direct injury or insult to an organ. The organ failure is the result of the injury or insult, such as acute respiratory failure secondary to aspiration of gastrointestinal contents. The subsequent failure of other organs stems from the primary organ injury. Secondary MODS is a result of organ failure from a distant or unknown site. The organs that fail have not received any direct injury or insult.

Treatment for MODS is supportive of the organs failing, in conjunction with use of any of the therapies described above. It is important to remember that support of an organ is not curative. Consequently, supporting a patient on mechanical ventilation for respiratory failure secondary to sepsis may not improve survival. Perhaps all that is gained is a prolongation of life for several days until the systemic response causes other organs to fail.

BIBLIOGRAPHY

ACCP/SCCM Consensus Conference Committee: American College of Chest Physicians/Society of Critical Care Medicine Consensus Conference. (1992). Definitions for sepsis and organ failure and guidelines for the use of innovative therapies in sepsis. *Crit Care Med 20,* 864–874.

Bernard, G.R., Reines, H.D., Halushka, R.V., et al. (1991). Prostacyclin and thromboxane A2 formation is increased in human sepsis syndrome. Effects of cyclooxygenase inhibition. *Am Rev Respir Dis 144,* 1095–1101.

Bone, R.C. (1991). The pathogenesis of sepsis. *Ann Intern Med 115,* 457–469.

Haupt, M.T., Jastremski, M.S., Clemmer, T.P., et al. (1991). Effect of ibuprofen in patients with severe sepsis: A randomized double blind, multicenter study. The Ibuprofen Study Group. *Crit Care Med 19,* 1339–1347.

Klein, D.M., & Witek-Janusek, L. (1992). Advances in immunotherapy of sepsis. *Dimens Crit Care Nurs 11,* 75–89.

Smith, C.R. Straube, R.C., & Ziegler, E.J. (1992). HA-1A. A human monoclonal antibody for the treatment of gram-negative sepsis. *Infect Dis Clin North Am 6,* 253–266.

Sprung, C.L., Caralis, P.V., Marcial, E.H., et al. (1984). The effects of high-dose glucocorticoid therapy on mortality in patients with clinical signs of systemic sepsis. *N Engl J Med 311,* 1137–1143.

The Veterans Administration Systemic Sepsis Comparative Study Group (1987). Effect of high-dose glucocorticoid therapy on mortality in patients with clinical signs of systemic sepsis. *N Engl J Med 317,* 659–665.

Zimmerman, J.J., & Ringer, T.V. (1992). Inflammatory host responses in sepsis. *Crit Care Clin 8,* 163–189.

Index

Note: Italicized letters following page numbers indicate tables (*t*) and figures (*f*).

Abdomen
blunt or penetrating trauma of, 278, 279
examination of, in head injury, 191
Abdominal aneurysms, 88
Abducens nerve, 192
Aberrant premature contractions (APC), 52, 53*f*, 53*t*
Absences, 207, 208, 210
Absorption, prevention of, in toxic emergencies, 426–482
Accelerated idioventricular rhythm, 50, 51*f*
ACE inhibitors, 15*t*
Acetazolamide, use of, in metabolic acidosis, 123
Acetone, 361
Acetylcholine, 169, 170, 176, 177, 204, 234, 242, 243, 328
Achalsia, 232
Acid
definition of, 120
nonvolatile or fixed, 120
volatile, 120
Acid-base balance, 120
Acid-base disorder, clue to, in toxicologic emergencies, 421
Acid-base disturbances, 120, 122–126
Acidemia, 122
Acidosis
definition of, 107
metabolic, 123, 124, 316
treatment of, 126
respiratory, 123, 126
agents that cause, 427*t*
Acidotic state, 300
Acinar glands, 244
Acini, 359
Acquired immune system, 371, 372
Acquired immunodeficiency syndrome (AIDS)
clinical presentation, 405
etiology of, 402*t*
nursing intervention, 406, 407
treatment, 406
Acromegaly, 338*f*
ACTH. *See* adrenocorticotropic hormone
Actin, 5, 6*f*, 7*f*, 8
Action potential, 8, 9*f*, 175, 176
Activated charcoal, 426, 427*t*
activated partial thromboplastin time (aPTT), 392
Active transport, 238, 295
Acute adrenal insufficiency, 354–356
Acute inflammatory polyradiculoneuropathy. *See* Guillain-Barré syndrome

Acute lymphocytic (lymphoblastic) leukemia (ALL), 407
Acute nonlymphocytic (myelogenous) leukemia (ANLL or AML), 407
Acute renal failure (ARF)
clinical presentation, 315
definition, 313
diagnosis, 315
etiology, 313, 314*t*
management, 316
pathophysiology, 313
phases, 314, 315
uremic signs of, 315*t*
Acute respiratory failure
causes of, 127*t*
clinical presentation, 128
definition of, 127
treatment, 128
Addisonian crisis, 354–356
Addison's disease, 354, 355
Adenohypophysis, 330, 331, 335–337
Adenoids. *See* Pharyngeal tonsils
Adenosine diphosphate (ADP), 6
Adenosine triphosphate (ATP), 6
ADH. *See* Antidiuretic hormone
Adhesions, 273
ADP. *See* Adenosine diphosphate
Adrenal crisis, 354–356
Adrenal gland
anatomy of, 351*f*
cortex of, 351, 352*f*, 353
dysfunction of, 354–357
medulla of, 352*f*
physiology of, 352–354
Adrenaline (epinephrine), 353, 354
Adrenal medulla
anatomy of, 351
hormones of, 330, 353, 354
hyperfunction of, 356
hypofunction of, 356
Adrenergic mechanisms, 19
Adrenergic receptors, and their function, 353*t*
Adrenocorticotropic (ACTH)-releasing factors, 351
Adrenocorticotropic (ACTH)-stimulating factors, 351
Adrenocorticotropin, 329
Adult respiratory distress syndrome (ARDS), 128, 129
associated potential causes and conditions, 128*t*
clinical presentation, 129

Adult respiratory distress syndrome (ARDS) (*cont.*)
    prognosis, 128, 129
    pulmonary surfactant and, 103
    treatment, 129
Afterload, 16–18, 69*t*, 71
Agents and antidotes, 429*t*, 430*t*
AIDS (acquired immunodeficiency syndrome), 405–407
AIDS dementia disorder, 406
Air embolism, 324
Airway
    examination of, in head injury, 191
    lumen, in bronchitis, 138
    pressure release ventilation, 131
    resistance, measurement of, 111
Akinetic seizures (atonic seizures), 208
Albumin, salt-poor, 384
Albuminocytologic dissociation, 203
Aldosterone, 66, 300, 303, 330, 353
Alkalemia, 122
Alkalosis
    definition of, 107
    hemoglobin binding and, 118*f*
    metabolic, 123, 124
        treatment of, 126
    respiratory, 121, 122
        causes of, 123
        identification by blood gases, 125
        treatment of, 126
Alpha 1-antitrypsin deficiencies, chronic obstructive pulmonary disease and, 135
Alpha-amylase, 244
Alpha receptors (alpha 1, alpha 2), 19
Altered mental status, suggested therapy for, 424*t*
Alveolar airways, 103
Alveolar ducts, 102
Alveolar oxygen tensions, 114
Alveolar sacs, 102, 103*f*
Alveolar ventilation, 113, 114, 120, 121, 131, 134
Alveoli, 101, 102
Amine hormones, 328–330
Amino acids, 239
Ammonium chloride, use of, in metabolic acidosis, 123
Ampulla of Vater, 244*f*
Amrinone, 15*t*
Amylase, 244
Amylytic enzyme, 244
Anaerobic glycolysis, 120
Anaphylactic reactions, 375
Anaphylactoid shock, 376–378
Anatomic shunts, 115, 116*f*
Androgens, 353
Anemia, 378, 379
    classification of, 380*t*
    clinical presentation, 378
    definition, 378
    diagnosis, 378
    etiology, 378
    nursing interventions, 378, 379
    sickle-cell, 397, 398
Anergy, 375
Aneurysm graft technique, 89*f*
Aneurysms
    abdominal, 88
    aortic, 88

common postoperative problems with, 89
    diagnosis of, 88
    intracranial, 218–220
    myocardial infarction with, 89
    thoracic, 88, 89
    treatment of, 89
Angelchick prosthesis, 276
Angina pectoris
    coronary artery vasospasm, 64
    Prinz metal's angina, 63, 64
    unstable angina, 63, 64
Angiodysplasia, *See* Arteriovenous malformations
Angioedema, 376
Angiogram studies, in closed head injuries, 198
Angiography, 256
Angioplasty, in myocardial infarction, 67
Angiotensin, 77, 301
Angle of Louis, 101
Anion, 120
Anion gap, 124
Antacids, 256
Anterior cord syndrome, 186*f*
Anterior hemiblock, criteria for, 50*t*
Anterior horns, 183
Anterior pituitary gland, 330
Anterior-septal myocardial infarction, 65
Antibiotics, 436
Antibodies, 373, 374
Anticholinesterase tests, 205
Anticoagulants, for pulmonary embolism, 142
Anticoagulation, 388, 390–392
Anticonvulsants, 209
Antidiuretic hormone (ADH)
    action of, 339
    body water regulation and, 297
    control of, 339
    dysfunctions of
        diabetes insipidus, 339, 340
        syndrome of inappropriate secretion of ADH, 340, 341
    release of, 77
Antidotes, 429*t*, 430*t*
Antigen, in sepsis, 432
Antigen-antibody complex, 399
Antigen-presenting cell (APC), 369
Antimicrobial agents, topical, 419
Antimicrobials, 400
Antithrombin system, 391, 392
Antitrypsin, 135
Antrectomy, 275
Anuria, 315
Aortic aneurysms, 88
Aortic dissection, 88
Aortic pressure, 20*f*
Aortic rupture, 151*f*, 152
    sites of, 151f
Aortic valve, 5*f*, 11*f*
Aortobifemoral bypass, 90*f*
Aortoiliac bypass, 90*f*
Aphasia, 211
Aplastic crisis, 398
Apnea, 105, 107*f*
Appendicitis, 274, 276
Appendix, vermiform, 240
Apneustic breathing, 105, 106*f*

Apraxia, 211
Apresoline, 15*t*
aPTT. *See* Activated partial thromboplastin time
Aqueduct of Sylvius, 164
Arachidonic acid sequence, 432, 433, 435*f*
Arachnoid layer, 158
Arachnoid membrane, 201
Arachnoid villi, 158
Arborization, 167
Argentaffin cells, 234
Arterial blood gases, 122–126, 197
Arterial carbon dioxide pressure, 113, 114
Arterial waveform, normal, 82*f*
Arteriosclerosis, 61
Arteriovenous fistulas
  anastomosis to form shunt, 323*f*
  complications, 321
  for hemodialysis, 320
Arteriovenous malformation, 259
Arteriovenous shunt, 320, 322*f*
Artery, external carotid, 165
Artificial airways, 132–134
Ascites, in cirrhosis, 265
Assisted mandatory ventilation 131, 132
Astereognosis, 211
Asthma, 135, 136*t*, 137*f*
Astrocytes, 167
Ataxic breathing, spirometer patterns of, 106*f*
Atelectasis, 130, 134
Atherectomy, 67, 90
Atherosclerosis
  classification of, 61
  prognosis, 63
  risk factors, 62
Atonic seizures (akinetic seizures), 208
ATP. *See* Adenosine triphosphate
Atria, 19, 28
Atrial contraction, 19
Atrial fibrillation, 38, 39*f*
Atrial flutter, 38*f*
Atrial premature beats. *See* Premature atrial contractions
Atrial pressure, 16, 19, 20*f*
Atrial rate, 29
Atrial tachycardia, 36f
Atrial waveforms, normal, 20*f*
Atrioventricular dissociation, 47*f*
Atrioventricular junctional blocks, 44
Atrioventricular node (AV node), 13
Atrioventricular node and ventricular dysrhythmias, 41–59
Atrioventricular valves, 10*f*, 11*f*, 19
Atrium, 31
Atropine, 19
Auerbach's plexus, 236, 242
Aura, 208
Autonomic dysreflexia (autonomic hyperreflexia), 189, 190
Autonomic nervous system
  heart rate and, 19
  nerve structures of, 169
  parasympathetic nervous system, 169, 170
  sympathetic nervous system, 169, 170
Autonomic regulation, of peripheral vessels, 18
Autopagnosia, 211
"Auto-PEEP," 130
Autoregulation, 180

Autosplenectomy, 398
Axons, 167, 169, 170
Azotemia, 315
AZT (Zidovidine), 406

Bacteroides fragilis, 241
Balloon angioplasties, 90
Balloon tamponade, 258*f*
Banded neutrophils, 399
Band heratopathy, 308
Baroreceptor control, 18
Baroreceptors, 18, 235
Barotrauma, 131
Basal ganglia, 161*f*, 162*t*
Basal rate, 235
Base, definition of, 120
Base excess, 123
Base state, 120
Basilar skull fracture, 194, 195*f*
Basophils, 369
Beta blockers, 15*t*
Beta receptors, (beta 1 and beta 2), 19
Bicarbonate, use of, in metabolic acidosis, 123
Bicarbonate buffer system, 120, 121
Bicarbonate ion, 121, 123, 125
Bilateral myoclonus (myoclonic seizures), 208
Bile, 247
Biliary system, 245–248
Bilirubin, 246–248
Biot's breathing, 105, 107*f*
Biventricular failure, 70
Bleeding time, 392
Blood and component therapy
  clinical presentation, 385
  nursing intervention, 385
  reactions to, 384, 385
  types, 384, 385
Blood-brain barrier, 180
Blood cell, development of, 379*f*
Blood-cerebrospinal fluid barrier, 180
Blood flow
  assessment of, 90
  obstruction to, 89, 90
Blood gases
  arterial 122–126
  normal arterial adult blood gas levels at sea level, 122*t*
  values of, 125
Blood pressure
  effect of aldosterone on, 300
  regulation of, 15, 300, 301
Blood supply, cerebral, 164
Blood urea nitrogen (BUN), 298, 299, 313
B lymphocytes (B cells), 373, 374
Body water, regulation of, 296–298
Bohr equation, 113
Bone marrow transplantation, 408
Bones, long, examination of, in head injury, 191
Bony calvarium, 158
Bowel elimination status, interventions to maintain, 282
Bowel ischemia, following aortic surgery, 89
Bowman's capsule, 288
Brachial plexus, 169

Bradypnea, 105
Brain
  circulatory needs of, 180
  coronal section of, 161f
  functions of specific structures, 162t
  glucose level in, 179
  hypoxia in, 179
  metabolism in, 179
  nutritional needs of, 179
  ventricular system of, 164f
  weight of, 179
Brain herniation
  etiology, 222
  eye movements in, 223–225
  monitoring parameters in, 222
  parameter norms and testing methods, 222, 223
  pathophysiology, 221, 222
  routes of, 221
  stages and parameters, 226t, 227t
  stages of, 222
  through foramen magnum, 225, 228
  types of, 221
Brain scan, in closed head injuries, 198
Brain stem, 179
Brain tissue, 213
Breathing, spontaneous signs of failure of, 132t
Bronchi, 101, 102f
Bronchioles
  anatomy of, 101 102
  respiratory, appearance of, in asthma, 137f
Bronchitis, 135, 137
  airway lumen in, 138
  compared with emphysema, 139t
Bronchodilators, 138, 139
Brown-Sequard's syndrome, 186f
Brudzinski's sign, 202
Brunner's glands, 237
Buffering, 120, 121
Bullous lesions, agents causing, 425t
BUN (blood urea nitrogen), 298, 299
Bundle branch block, 12, 48, 49
Bundle of HIS, 13
BUN-to-creatinine ratio, 299
Burn classifications (American Burn Association), 419
Burn depth, classification of, 416t
Burns
  classification, 414, 419t
    first-degree burns, 414
    second-degree burns (partial thickness), 414
    third-degree (full thickness), 414
  depth of injury, 414f
  fluid remobilization phase, 416, 418
  formulas for fluid replacement/resuscitation, 417t
  inhalation injury, 419, 420
  initial management, 414
  other initial management, 418
  wound management, 418, 419
Burn shock, 414, 415
Bypass techniques, femoral vascular, 90f

Calcitonin, 329, 343–346
Calcium channel blockers, 8, 15t
Calcium gates, 6f

Calcium ions, 7
Calcium
  absorption of, 239
  effect on hydrochloric acid secretion, 234
  factors affecting reabsorption
    corticosteriods, 307
    diuretics, 307
    parathyroid hormone (PTH), 307
    vitamin D, 307
  hypercalcemia, 307, 308
  hypocalcemia, 308, 309
  normal levels of, 307
  regulation of, 307
Caloric needs, 248, 251, 253
cAMP. See Cyclic 31, 51-adenosine monophosphate
Captopril, 15t
Carbohydrates, 236, 238, 239
Carbon dioxide, arterial, 113, 114
Carbon dioxide tension (Pco$_2$), 119
Carbon dioxide transport, 119, 120
Carbonic acid, 119–121
Carbonic anhydrase, 119
Carbon monoxide (CO), 419, 420
Cardia, 234
Cardiac cell, action potential of, 8, 9f
Cardiac contusion, 147, 149
Cardiac cycle
  blood flow and pressure during, 19, 20f
  components of, 25
Cardiac isoenzymes, 65
Cardiac output, 15, 16, 116
Cardiac potential and ion movement, phases of, 9f
Cardiac rupture, 149
Cardiac sphincter, 232, 233
Cardiac tamponade, 149f
Cardiac transplantation
  eligibility criteria for, 87, 88t
  immunosuppression, 88
  postoperative care, 88
  success rate for, 88
Cardiac valves, 11, 19
Cardiac vectors, 23
Cardiogenic shock
  causes, 75t
  compensation mechanisms, 79, 80
  intra-aortic balloon pumps for, 80, 81
  symptoms of, 78t
  treatment of, 80
Cardiomyopathy, 87
Cardiopulmonary bypass, 86
Cardiovascular pressures, normal, 16t
Cardiovascular volumes, normal, 16t
Carina, 101, 102f
Carotid arteries, examination of, in head injury, 191
Cartilages, thyroid-cricoid, 101f
Cascades
  common final pathway, 388
  extrinsic, 388
  intrinsic, 388
Catecholamines, 77, 177, 329, 353
Cathartics, 425, 426t
Catheterization
  cardiac, 16
  pulmonary artery, 16

Cation, 120
CAT scan, use of
    in abdominal trauma, 278
    in head injuries, 198
    in intracranial hematomas, 198
Caustic injury, 279
Cecum, 239, 240
Cell-mediated immunity, 399
Cellular hypoxia, in shock, 75
Cellular immune response, 374
Central cord syndrome, 185
Central herniation, 221, 222, 226t
Central nervous system (CNS), 157
Central neurogenic hyperventilation, 105, 106f
Central venous pressure, 16, 17t, 20, 69t
Cerebellar peduncles, 163f
Cerebellum, 159f, 160f, 162t, 163
Cerebral angiography, in intracranial hematomas, 198
Cerebral blood flow, 180, 213, 214
Cerebral blood supply, internal and external, 164–166
Cerebral cortex, 160f, 162t, 179
Cerebral edema, postoperative, 214
Cerebral perfusion pressure (CPP), 180, 213, 214
Cerebrospinal fluid (CSF)
    circulation and formation of, 163, 164
    in diagnosis of meningitis, 202
    normal amounts and production of, 164
    ph of, 107
    in subarachnoid space, 158
Cerebrovascular accident (CVA)
    clinical presentation, 211
    definition, 211
    diagnosis, 211, 212
    etiology, 211
    nursing intervention, 212
    treatment, 212
Cerebrum, 159, 160f-162t
Cervical plexus, 169
Cervical spine x-rays, 198
Cervical vertebrae, 181
Charcoal
    activated, 426, 427t
    multidose, 427, 428t
Chemical gradient, 8
Chemical synapse, 176f
Chemoreceptors, activation of, 19, 107, 235
Chest trauma
    classification, 143
    closed chest injuries, 143
    flail chest, 143, 144f
    hemothorax, 145
    open chest injuries, 146, 147
    pneumothorax
        open, 145
        simple closed, 144
        tension, 145f
    sternal fracture, 144
    visceral injury, 147, 148
Chest tubes, 144, 145, 146f, 152
Cheyne-Stokes breathing, 105
CHF. See Congestive heart failure
Chief cells, 234
Chloride, role in cardiac cell cycle, 8
Cholecystokinin, 235, 236, 245

Cholinergic crisis, 206
Cholinergic mechanisms, 19
Cholinesterase, 170
Chordae tendineae, 4, 5f
Choroid plexus, 164
Chovstek's sign, 269, 309
Christmas disease, 395
Chromaffin cells, 351
Chronic heart failure, 70
Chronic lymphocytic leukemia (CLL), 408
Chronic myelogeneous leukemia (CML), 407
Chronic obstructive pulmonary disease (COPD)
    causes of, 135, 136
    complications of, 138
    diagnosis of, 135, 136
    nursing intervention and treatment of, 138, 139
Chyme, 235–238
Chymotrypsinogen, 245
Cigarette smoking, chronic obstructive pulmonary disease and 135
Cilia, 103, 104f
Ciliospinal reflex, 223f
Cimetidine (Tagamet), 234, 255–257
Circle of Willis, 164f, 165
Circulatory paths, 13
Circulatory systems of the body
    coronary, 14
    pulmonary, 13
    systemic, 13, 14
Cirrhosis
    advanced signs of, 266f
    clinical presentation, 265, 266
    diagnosis, 266
    esophageal varices in, 257
    etiology, 265
    laboratory tests for, 266t
    nursing intervention, 266, 267
    nutritional intervention, 266, 267
    treatment, 266
    types, 265
Claudication, intermittent, 90
Clotted blood, sequestration of, in the capillaries, 393f
Clotting factors, 387t
CNS. See Central nervous system
CO. See Carbon monoxide
Coagulation process
    normal 387–389f
        common final pathway, 392t
        extrinsic pathway segment, 390f
        intrinsic pathway segment, 391f
Coccyx, 182f
Colloid, 343
Colloidal agents, 15t
Colloidal therapy, 78
Colon
    absorption in, 241
    bacteria in, 241
    carcinoma of, 276, 277
    layers of the colon wall, 240
    mass movements in, 241
    mixing movements in, 240
    motility in, 240
    polyps or tumors of, 259
    propulsive movements in, 240

Coma
  Glascow Scale, 192*t*
  glucose levels and, 179
  hyperosmolars (HHNK), 360, 362, 363
  pathological processes leading to, 221
Complement system, 370
Complete heart block, 46*f*, 47
Complex partial psychomotor
  seizures, 209
Compliance, 110, 111
  causes of decreased compliance, 110*f*, 111*f*
  defined, 110
  intracranial, 213, 214
  types of, 111
Compound injuries, 194
Computerized axial tomography (CAT), 196, 197
Concretions, agents causing, 426*t*
Concussion, 193
Conduction disturbance, 28
Conduction disturbances, dysrhythmias due to, 32*t*
Congestive heart failure (CHF)
  causes of, 70
  clinical presentation, 71*t*
  complications, 71
  definition of, 69
  etiology, 70
    as cause of sinus tachycardia, 33
  left vs. right heart failure, 70, 71
  treatment and nursing intervention, 71
Conn's syndrome, 356
Consciousness, levels of, 191, 192
Consensual right reflex, 222
Continuous positive airway pressure (CPAP), 130, 131
Contracoup force, 193
Contractility, 18, 69*t*
Contusion
  cardiac, 147, 149
  head, 193
  pulmonary, 147, 148*f*
Conus medullaris, 183
COPD. *See* Chronic obstructive pulmonary disease
Coronal suture, 158
Coronary artery bypass grafting, 85
  cardiac tamponade, 87
  criteria for, 86*t*
  determination of need for, 85, 86
  postoperative measures, 86, 87
  surgical procedure, 86
Coronary artery occlusion, four grades of, 62
Coronary artery vasospasm, 64
Corpus callosum, 159, 160*f*
Corticosteroids, 307
Corticosteroids, systemic, 139
Corticosterone, 330
Corticospinal tracts, 163
Corticotropin-releasing hormone, 337
Cortisol, 330, 352, 353
Coughing, 101
Cough reflex, 101
Countercurrent mechanism, in urine concentration, 297*f*, 298
Coup force, 193
Cortex, 287
CPAP. *See* Continuous positive airway pressure
CPP. *See* Cerebral perfusion pressure

Crackles
  cardiac, 108
  pulmonary, 108
Cranial nerves
  component of peripheral nervous system, 168, 169
  dysfunction of, 202
  examination of, in head injury, 192
  origin of, 171*f*
  summary of, 170*t*
Cranial vault, components of, 213
Craniosacral system, 170
Craniotomies
  postop care for, 199
Cranium, 158*f*
Creatinine, 298, 299, 313
Cricoid cartilage, 100*f*, 101*f*
Cricothyroid membrane, 100, 101
Crisis, vaso-occlusive (infarctive), 398
Critical oxygen delivery point, 437*f*
Critical volume, 111
Cryoimmunoglobulins, 383
Cryoprecipitates, 383
Cryptococcal meningitis, 405, 406
Crypts of Lieberkühn, 237*f*
Crystalloid agents, 15*t*
CSF. *See* Cerebrospinal fluid
Cullen's sign, 269
Cushing's syndrome, 356, 357*f*
Cyclic 3',5'-adenosine monophosphate, 329, 336
Cyclo-oxygenase pathway, 433
Cytomegalovirus retinitis, 405, 406
CVP. *See* Central nervous pressure, 16

Dalton's law, 114
Dead space
  anatomic, 13
  physiologic, 14, 113
Decerebrate posture, 225*f*
Decorticate posture, 225*f*
Dehydration, 316
Delta hepatitis. *See* Hepatitis D
Dendrites, 167
Depolarization, of neural cell, 175
Dermatomes, 168*f*, 169
Dermis, 413
Desmopressin acetate (DDAVP), 340
Detoxification, 426–428
Dextran, 384
Diabetes insipidus, 199, 339, 340
Diabetic ketoacidosis, 359–361
Dialysis
  hemodialysis
    complications, 323, 324
    contraindications, 320–322,
    indications, 320, 428*t*
    nursing care, 322, 323
    regional heparinization, 321*f*
  peritoneal
    advantages, 318
    complications, 319, 320
    contraindications, 318
    dialysate, 318, 319

disadvantages, 318
  indications for, 317, 318
  procedure and nursing care, 319
  purpose of, 317
Diamox. *See* Acetazolamide
Diapedesis, of white blood cells, 369
Diaphragm, 95, 96f, 97f
Diaphragma sellae, 159f
Diaphragmatic rupture, 149, 150
Diastolic pressure, 110
Diazepam (Valium), 210, 211
Diencephalon, 159f, 161, 162t
Diffusion, 8, 295, 317
Digestion, accessory organs of, 243–248
  biliary system, 245, 246
  pancreas, 243–245
  salivary glands, 243
Diltiazem, 15t
2,3-Diphosphoglygerate (2,3-DPG), 118, 119
Diploë (diploic space), 158
Disc, slipped, 183
Disequilibrium syndrome, 324
Disseminated intravascular coagulation, 392, 393, 394f, 395–
    397, 408
Distal convoluted apparatus, 289
Diuresis, 416, 418, 426, 427t
Diuretics, 15t, 303, 307
Diverticulosis, 259, 277
Dobutamine, 15t, 18
Doll's eyes, 223, 224t
Dopamine, 15t, 177
Down-regulation, 71
Duct of Wursung, 244
Duodenum, 235, 236
Dura mater, 158, 159f
Dwarfism, 338, 339f
Dynamic compliance, 111
Dysreflexia, autonomic, 189, 190
Dysrhythmias
  atrial fibrillation, 38, 39f
  atrial flutter, 38f
  atrial tachycardia, 36f
  classification of, 32t
  paroxysmal atrial tachycardia, 35f, 36
  premature atrial contraction, 36, 37f
  sinus arrhythmia, 31, 32f
  sinus bradycardia, 31, 32f
  sinus pause/arrest, 34f, 35
  sinus tachycardia, 33, 34f
  wandering atrial pacemaker, 37f, 38

Ears, examination of, in head injury, 191
ECG. *See* Electrocardiogram
Echocardiography, 12
Echoencephalogram, 198
Edrophonium chloride (Tensilon), 205, 206
Effector cells, 373
Ejection fraction, 70
EKG. *See* Electrocardiogram
Elasticity (recoil tendency), 111
Electrical gradient, 8

Electrocardiogram (ECG)
  components of cardiac cycle, 25–27
  interpretation of rhythm strip, 27–29
  normal components of, 23, 24
  paper, 24, 25f
  12-lead, 23, 48t
Electrolyte and fluid balance, interventions to maintain, 280
Electrolytes, 239, 316. *See also specific electrolytes*
Embolectomy, 143
Emboli
  air, 324
  venous, 324
Emergency vs. hospital admissions, criteria for in toxic emergen-
    cies, 421
Emesis, in toxic emergencies, 423–425t
Emphysema
  compared with bronchitis, 139t
  diagnosis, 135, 136
  etiology, 135
  giant bullae of end-stage, 138f
  subcutaneous, 147
Encephalopathies
  brain, 220
  hepatic, 226, 267
End-diastolic volume, 70
Endocardium, 4
End-stage heart disease, 87, 88t
Endocrine glands/hormones
  listing, of, 329t
  negative feedback system of, 330, 331
  pictoral overview, 328f
  stimulus, of gastrointestinal system, 24
Endoscopic therapy, 258
Endoscopy, 256
Endothelial cells, effect of immune response on, 433, 434
Endotracheal tubes, 133, 134
Endovascular therapies, 90
Enteral feedings, 251, 253
Enteral nutrition, 251, 253
Enterogastric reflex, 235
Enzymes, thrombolytic, for pulmonary embolism, 142
Eosinophils, 369
Ependyma, 168
Epicardium, 4
Epidermis, 413
Epidural hematoma, 194, 196f
Epidural monitoring, 214, 215f
Epiglottis, 100f
Epinephrine (Adrenaline), 177, 330, 353, 354
Erosions, gastrointestinal, 255
Erythropoietin, 301
Escape beats, 55
Eschar, 418, 419
Escharotomy incisions, 418f
Escherichia coli, 241
Esophageal carcinoma, surgery for, 275
Esophageal hiatus, 232
Esophageal perforation, 150, 151, 280
Esophageal varices
  clinical presentation, 257
  diagnosis, 257
  nursing intervention, 258
  treatment, 257, 258
Esophagogastrectomy, 275

Esophagus, 232, 233
Eupnea, 105
Eustachian tubes, 98, 100
Exocrine glands, 359
Exocytosis, 336
Exophthalmos, 348
Expiration, 95, 96f
Expiratory reserve volume, 112
Extension response, 225
External carotid artery, 165
Extracellular fluid, maintenance of volume and composition, 300
Extracorporeal membrane oxygenation therapy (ECMO), 129
Extracorporeal methods of elimination, 427
Extradural space (epidural space), 159
Eye changes, (toxins) causing characteristic, 423
Eye movements, in brain herniation, 223–225

Face, examination of, in acute head injury, 191
Facial nerve, 192
Facilitated diffusion, 238
Facilitation, 175
Falx cerebri, 159f
Falx cerebelli, 159f
Famotidine (Pepcid), 256
Fascicles, 13, 48
Fasciculi, 184
Fats
    daily absorption, 239
    digestion of, in stomach, 236
    emulsification of, 239
Fat-soluble vitamins, 239
Femoral-femoral bypass, 90f
Femoral vascular bypass techniques, 90f
Femoropopliteal bypass, 90f
Fenestrae, 294
Fibrinogen (Factor I), 387
Fibrinolytic system, 388
Fibrinolytic therapy, 388, 390
Fibrous pericardium, 4
Filium terminale, 183
Filtration, definition of, 317
First-degree block, 43f, 44
First messenger, 329
Fisher's variant, 203
Fissures, of cerebrum, 160, 161f
Fistulas
    for hemodialysis, 320, 321
    tracheoesophageal, 133, 134
Flail chest, 143, 144f
Flexion response, abnormal, 225
Fluid and electrolyte balance interventions to maintain, 280
Fluid overload, 316
Fluid replacement
    in burns, 415–417t
    crystalloid vs. colloid, 147
Focal motor seizures, 207–209
Follicle-stimulating hormone (FSH), 329
Follicle stimulating hormone-releasing hormone, 337
Follicles, thyroid, 343, 344f
Follicular sacs, 343
Foramen magnum, brain herniation through, 225, 228
Foramina
    Luschka, 164
    Magendie, 164
    Monro, 164
Forced diuresis, 426
Forced vital capacity (FVC), 112
Fossae, 158
FRC. See functional residual capacity
Frontal bones, 158
Frontal lobe dysfunction, central hemisphere, 225
FSH. See Follicle-stimulating hormone
Functional residual capacity (FRC), 112, 130
Fundoplication, Nissen, 275
Fundus, 232, 234
Funiculi, 184, 185f

GABA. See gamma-aminobutyric acid
Gallbladder
    functions of, 247
    location of, 247f
    stimulation of, 248
Gallop sound, 12
Gallstones, 268
Gamma-aminobutyric acid (GABA), 177
Ganglia, of sympathetic nervous system, 172f
Ganglionic fibers, of parasympathetic nervous system, 173f
Gas diffusion principles, 114
Gases, composition of,
    alveolar, 115t
    arterial, 115t
    atmospheric, 115t
    venous, 115t
Gas exchange, pathways of, 103
    lung function of, 109
    pathways of, 103
Gastric digestion, 236
Gastric emptying, 235
Gastric glands, 233, 234
Gastric juice, 233, 235
Gastric lavage, 424, 425t, 426t
Gastric motility, 234, 235
Gastric secretions, control of,
    cephalic phase, 235
    gastric phase, 235
    intestinal phase, 236
Gastrin, 234, 235
Gastroesophageal reflux disease, gastric surgery for, 275
Gastroesophageal sphincter, 232
Gastroilial reflex, 238f
Gastrointestinal and radiologic studies, 253t
Gastrointestinal hemorrhage
    clinical presentation, 255
    complications, 256
    diagnosis, 256
        lower, 256, 259
        upper, 256
    etiology, 255
    nursing intervention, 257
    pathophysiology, 255
    surgery for, 257
    treatment, 256, 257
Gastrointestinal perforation
    clinical presentation, 274
    diagnosis, 274

etiology, 274
nursing intervention, 274
pathophysiology, 274
treatment, 274
Gastrointestinal surgery
for appendicitis, 276
for colonic carcinoma, 276, 277
for diverticulitis, 277
for esophageal carcinoma, 275
nursing intervention for, 277, 278
on small and large intestines, 276
on stomach, 275
Gastrointestinal system
arterial vascularization of, 241, 242*f*
blood supply in, 241
chemical elements in, 249*t*-251*t*
chemical messengers of, 241
disturbances of, nursing interventions for, 280–283
innervation of, 242
intrinsic nervous system of, 242
venous circulation of, 241, 242, 243*f*
Gastrointestinal trauma
blunt/penetrating abdominal trauma
clinical manifestations, 278, 279
diagnosis, 278
nursing intervention, 279
esophageal perforation, 280
other GI trauma, 279, 280
General hormones, listing of, 329*t*
GFR. *See* Glomerular filtration rate
GH. *See* Growth hormone
Giant V waves in a PCWP
tracing, 21*f*
Gigantism, 337, 338
Glands, endocrine, 327, 328*f*, 329*t*
Glands. *See also* specific gland
Glasgow Coma Scale, 192*t*
Glial cells, types of, 166*f*, 167, 168
Glomerular filtration, 293, 294
Glomerular filtration rate
average GFR, 294
equation for calculating, 295
factors affecting, 295
Glomerular membrane, layers of, 295*f*
Glomerular ultrafiltrate, composition of, 294
Glomerulus, 288, 289*f*
Glottis, 100
Glucagon, 329, 359, 360
Glucocorticoids, 199, 330, 352, 353
Gluconeogenesis, 360
Glucose, metabolic dysfunctions, 360–363
Glycogenolysis, 360
Glycolysis, anaerobic, 120
Goblet cells, 103, 104*f*, 237
Gonads, 327
Graft, for hemodialysis, 323*f*
Graft-versus-host-disease (GVHD), 407
Graham's law, 115
Gram-negative bacteria, 375, 432
Grand mal seizures (tonic-clonic), 207, 208, 210
Granulocyte-macrophage colony-stimulating factor, 401
Granulocytes, 368, 384
Graves' disease, 346
Gray matter, 159, 163, 179, 183, 184

Greater curvature, 232
Greater omentum, 234*f*
Grey-Turner's sign, 269
Growth-hormone releasing hormone, 337, 338
Growth hormone (GH), 329, 337–339
Guillain-Barré syndrome, 202–204
clinical presentation, 203
complications, 203
definition, 203, 204
diagnosis, 203
etiology, 203
plasmapheresis in, 204
prognosis for, 204
treatment and nursing intervention, 203, 204
Gyri, cerebral, 160, 161*f*

Haemophilus influenzae, 136, 138, 201
Harris-Benedict equation, 251
Haustra, 239, 240
HCG. *See* Human chorionic gonadotropin
Head injuries
acute, examination of patient with, 191–193
classification of, 193–195
complications of, 196
diagnostic test and findings, 196–198
ICP monitoring of, 214
nursing intervention for, 196
Heart
action potential of cardiac cell, 8, 9*f*
anatomy of, 3
chambers of, 9, 10*f*
electrical activity in, 23
frontal view of the, 9*f*
location and size, 3, 4*f*
muscle cells of, 4–7
normal conduction system of, 12, 13*f*
wall, structure of, 4
Heart block
first degree, 43*f*, 44
second degree, 44*f*, 45*f*, 46
third degree (complete), 44, 45, 46*f*, 47
Heart rate
elevations in, 19
parameters of, 16*t*
in regulation of cardiac output, 19
Heart sounds
abnormal
electrical conduction defects, 12
valve regurgitation, 11
valvular stenosis, 11
ventricular and atrial failure, 12
usefulness of, 12
Heart transplantation. *See* Cardiac transplantation
Heart valves, 10*f*, 11*f*
Hematemesis, 255
Hematochezia, 255
Hematomas, subdural, 159, 194, 195
Hematopoiesis, 378
Hemianopsia, 198, 199
Hemiblocks, 48
Hemodialysis, 320–324, 427, 428*t*
Hemodynamic assessment and intervention, 15–17*t*

Hemoglobin
  binding, 117–119
  oxygen transportation and, 378
  saturation, normal valve, 117
Hemolytic crisis, 398
Hemoperfusion, 428
Hemophilia, 395
Hemorrhage
  intracerebral, 195
  subarachnoid, 195
Hemorrhagic shock, 75–79. *See also* Hypovolemic shock
Hemostatic screening tests, 392
Hemothorax, 145, 146*f*
Henderson-Hasselbalch equation, 121
Henry's law, 114–116, 119
Heparin, for pulmonary embolism, 142
Hepatic encephalopathy, 266, 267
Hepatic failure
  clinical presentation, 267
  diagnosis, 267, 268
  etiology, 267
  nursing intervention, 268
  treatment, 268
Hepatitis A (HAV), 261, 265
Hepatitis B, 262, 265, 266
Hepatitis C, 262, 263
Hepatitis D, 262
Hepatotoxicity, common agents causing, 424*t*
Hering-Breuer stretch reflex, 107
Herniation, brain. *See* Brain herniation
Herniation, in abdominal trauma, 149, 150
Hespan (hetastarch), 15*t*, 384
Hetastarch (Hespan), 15*t*, 384
Heterozygous inheritance, 398
Hiatal hernia, 232
Hilum, 97*f*, 287
Hippocampus, 179
Histamine, 234, 376
HIV, 405
HIV wasting syndrome, 406
Hodgkin's disease, 408, 409
Homeostasis, ion, 175
Homozygous inheritance, 398
Hormone factors, 336
Hormones. *See also* specific hormones
  action of, 329, 330
  classification (local vs. general), 327, 328
  important, general, 328, 329*t*
  negative feedback system of, 330, 331
  tropic, 330
  types of, 328
Human chorionic gonadotropin (HCG), 337
Human placental lactogen, 337
Humoral immune response, 374, 375
Humoral immunity, 399
Hyaline membrane disease (neonatal), 103
Hydrocarbons, evacuation from bowel, 426*t*
Hydrochloric acid
  functions of, 234
  use of, in metabolic alkalosis, 123
Hydrochloric acid, use of, in metabolic alkalosis, 123
Hydrogen ion
  concentration, 120
  increased elimination of, 122

Hydrolysis, 238
Hypercalcemia, 307, 308
Hypercapnia, 180
Hypercarbia, 118*f*
Hypercorticism (Cushing's syndrome), 356
Hyperextension, of spinal cord, 183*f*
Hyperflexion, of spinal cord, 183*f*
Hyperglycemia, 179
Hyperkalemia, 306, 316
Hypermagnesemia, 310, 311
Hypernatremia, 303, 304
Hyperosmolality, 297*f*
Hyperosmolar coma (HHNK), 360, 362, 363
Hyperphosphatemia, 309
Hyperpnea, 105
Hyperreflexia, autonomic, 189, 190
Hypersensitivity reactions
  Type I (allergic/anaphylactic), 375
  Type II, 375, 376
  Type III (immune-complex mediated reactions), 376
  Type IV (delayed type), 376
Hypertension, 82, 141, 422
Hypertensive crisis
  characteristics of emergency hypertension, 82*t*
  medications to treat, 83*t*
Hyperthermia, 118*f*
Hyperthyroidism
  clinical presentation, 348, 349*f*
  complications, 348
  diagnosis, 348
  etiology, 348
  treatment, 348
Hyperventilation
  in cardiogenic shock, 80
  of central neurogenic, 105, 106*f*
Hypocalcemia, 308, 309
Hypocarbia, 118*f*
Hypoglossal nerve, 192
Hypoglycemia, 179
Hypoglycemia reaction, 363
Hypokalemia, 306, 307
Hypomagnesemia, 311
Hyponatremia, 304, 305, 340
Hypo-osmolality, 340
Hypopharyngeal sphincter, 232
Hypophosphatemia, 310
Hypophysis, 335*f*, 336*f*
Hypotension, 134, 256, 423*t*
Hypothalamic-hypophysial portal vessels, 337
Hypothalamic releasing hormone (factor), 343
Hypothalamus, 161, 162*t*, 329, 330*t*, 331*f*
Hypothermia, 118*f*
Hypothyroidism (myxedema), 346
  clinical presentation, 346, 347*f*
  complications, 346
  etiology, 346
  treatment, 346, 347
Hypoventilation, 115, 123
Hypovolemia, 16, 17*t*, 77, 79
Hypovolemic shock, 75*t*, 76, 77, 78*t*, 79
Hypoxemia, 115, 117, 128, 136
Hypoxia, 117, 179, 180

Ibuprofen, 436
Iced saline lavage, use in GI bleeding, 256
Ice water caloric test, 223, 224*f*
ICP. *See* Intracranial pressure
Idioventricular rhythm, 50, 51*f*
Ileocecal sphincter, 238
Ileocecal valve, 236, 238
Ileum, 236
Immune response, 399, 433, 434
Immune serum globulin, 261
Immune system, 367, 399, 400. *See also* Innate immune
    system
Immune system mediators, 433*t*
Immunity, comparison of B- and T-cell immunity, 401*t*
Immunocompromise and infection, in the critically
    ill, 375
Immunoglobulins, 373, 400*t*
Immunosuppression
  definition of, 375
  etiology, 400
  infection, 400
  nursing care, 401, 403–405
  treatment, 400, 401, 402*t*, 404*t*
Immunotherapy, 401
Inderal (propranolol), 15*t*, 349
Industrial exposure, chronic obstructive pulmonary disease (COPD)
    and, 135
Infarction, intestinal, 271, 272
Infarctive crisis, 398
Infection
  interventions to prevent, 283
  opportunistic, 375
Infectious polyneuritis. *See* Guillain-Barré syndrome
Inferior myocardial infarctions, 65, 66*f*
Inflammation, 369–371
Inflammatory response, 399
Inhalation injury, 419, 420
Inherent automaticity, 12
Innate immune system defenses
  anatomic defenses, 368
  chemical defenses, 368
  natural defenses, 367, 368
Inotropes, 15, 16, 437
Inspiration, 96*f*
Inspiratory capacity, 112
Inspiratory center, 105
Inspiratory reserve volume, 112
Insulin, 329, 359, 360
Insulin shock, 360, 363
Intercalated discs, 5
Intercostal muscles, 96
Interferon, 401
Intermittent claudication, 90
Intermittent mandatory ventilation, 132
Interneurons, 178
Internodal tracts, 12
Interleukin-1, 369
Interleukin-2, 369
Intervertebral discs, 182, 183
Intestinal infarction
  clinical presentation 271, 272
  diagnosis, 272
  etiology, 271
  nursing intervention, 272

pathophysiology, 271
  treatment, 272
Intestinal obstruction
  clinical presentation, 273
  diagnosis, 273
  etiology, 273
  nursing intervention, 273
  pathophysiology, 272, 273
  treatment, 273
Intra-aortic balloon pump, 80, 81*f*, 82, 87
Intracerebral hemorrhage, 195, 196, 197*f*
Intracranial aneurysms
  classification, 219*t*
  clinical presentation, 219
  definition, 218
  diagnosis, 219
  etiology, 219
  incidence, 218, 219
  location, 218
  nursing intervention, 219, 220
  pathophysiology, 218
  prognosis, 219
  surgical intervention, 220, 221*f*
Intracranial compliance, 213
Intracranial mass lesions, 194
Intracranial pressure (ICP)
  compensatory mechanisms for, 180, 213
  monitoring, 213–217
    disadvantages, 215*t*
    implications, 217
    indicators for, 214
    measurement sites, 214
    systems, 214*f*
    techniques, 214, 215, 216*f*, 217*f*
    waveforms, 215, 217
  normal values, 213
  nursing interventions, 217
Intrapleural pressure, 109, 110
Intrapulmonary shunt, 114, 115
Intravascular fluid, 213
Intraventricular conduction defects. *See* bundle
    branch block
Intraventricular hemorrhage, complications of,
    196
Intraventricular monitoring, 215
Intrinsic factor, 234
Intubation, nasotracheal, 133, 134
Intubation, orotracheal, 133
Inverse ratio ventilation, 129, 131
Iodide trapping, 344
Iodine, 344
Ion, 120
Ion homeostasis, 175
Ion trapping, 427*t*
Ipecac, syrup of, 423, 424, 425*t*, 426*t*
Iron, 239
Ischemia
  bowel and spinal cord, 89
  cardiac, 26
  mesenteric, 271
Islets of Langerhans, 359
Isoelectric waves, 24
Isometric contraction phase, 20
Isoproterenol, 19

Jacksonian seizures, 207
Jaundice, 265
Jejunum, 236
Junctional ischemia, 42
Junctional rhythm, 41, 42*f*
Juxtaglomerular apparatus, 289, 290*f*
Juxtaglomerular nephron, 289*f*

Kallikrein, 388
Kaposi's sarcoma, 406
Kernig's signs, 202
Ketoacidosis, diabetic, 359–361
Kidney(s)
    anatomy, 287, 288*f*
    disturbances of, 121, 122
    function of, in acid-base regulation, 120
    infection of, 316
    nerve supply of, 290*f*
    physiological processes of, 293–295
    vascular supply of, 290*f*
Krebs cycle, 179
Kupffer cells, 246
Kussmaul breathing, 105

Laceration, pulmonary, 147
Lactate levels, in shock, 77
Lacteal, 237
Lactic acidosis, treatment of in cardiogenic shock, 80
Lamboidal suture, 158
Lamina, 181
Laminar air flow, ·112*f*
Landry-Guillain-Barré disease. *See* Guillain-Barré syndrome
Laplace's law, 234
Large intestine, 239, 240*f*, 241, 276
Laryngeal pharynx, 232
Laryngopharynx, 98, 100
Larynx, 100*f*
Laser angioplasties, 90
Lateral myocardial infarction, 67*f*
Lavage, gastric
    complications of, 426*t*
    contraindicated with, 425*t*
Lead II normal sinus rhythm, 28
Lead placement, 24*f*
Left atrial pressure, 110
Left atrium, 9, 10*f*
Left axis deviation, 48
Left bundle branch block, 13, 48, 50*t*
Left-heart failure, 70, 71
Left ventricle, 9, 10*f*, 19
Left ventricular end diastolic pressure (LVEDP), 16, 17
Left ventricular failure, 17, 70, 71*t*
Left ventricular hypertrophy (LVH), 48, 49*t*
Left ventricular performance, methods to assess, 69*t*
Left ventricular pressure, 16
Left ventricular pump failure, 70
Leiberkühn, crypts of, 237*f*
Lesions, of the eye, 198
Lesser curvature, 232

Leukemias
    categories of, 407
    complications, 407, 408
    manifestations of, 407*t*
    nursing intervention, 408
    treatment, 408
Leukocytes, 368
Leukostasis, 408
Levophed. *See* norepinephrine
Lidocaine, 211
Light reflexed, 222*f*, 223
Limbic system, 161, 162*t*
Linton tube, 258
Lipolytic enzymes, 244
Lipo-oxygenase pathway, 433
Liver, 245, 246*f*
    anatomy of, 245
    blood supply to, 245, 246
    functions of, 246, 247
    lobule of, 246*f*
    tests to measure biosynthetic function of, 252*t*
Liver function tests, in hepatitis A, 261
Liver rupture, 279
Liver tests, 251*t*, 252*t*
Lobes
    cerebral, 160, 161
    lung, 981*f*
LOC. *See* note p. 220
Loop diuretics, 303
Loop of Henle, 290*f*, 296, 298, 299
Lower airway, 101
    lung parenchyma, 102–104
    tracheobronchial tree, 101, 102
Lower gastrointestinal bleeding, 259
L-tubules, 5
Lugol's solution, 349
Lumbar cistein, 183
Lumbar puncture, 197, 225, 228
Lumbar vertebra, 182*f*
Lumbosacral plexus, 169
Lung function tests, 112
Lung(s)
    air flow in, 11, 12*f*
    anatomy, 97*f*
    contusion, 147, 148*f*
    diseases, 123, 139
    function of, 112
    in acid-base disturbances, 121, 122
    lobes of, 98*f*
Lung sounds, 107, 108
Lung parenchyma, 97, 102, 103, 104*f*
Lung parenchyma, pulmonary circulation of, 104
    lung parenchyma, entrance of freshly oxygenated blood of, 104*f*
    (and oxygenated blood)
Lung pressures, 110
Lung volumes, 111, 112, 113*f*
Luteinizing hormone, 329
Luteinizing hormone-releasing hormone, 337
LVEDP. *See* left ventricular end diastolic pressure
Lymph nodes, 371*f*, 372*f*
Lymphatic system, 371
Lymphocytes, 372–374, 399
Lymphoid tissue, primary and secondary, 371, 372
Lymphokines, 373

Lymphomas, 408, 409
Lymphopoiesis, 371
Lymphoresis, 204

Macrophages, 399
Macula densa, 289
Magnesium
    hypermagnesemia, 310, 311
    hypomagnesemia, 311
    normal level of, 310
    regulation of, 310
Malabsorption, tests useful in the diagnosis of, 252*t*
Maltose, 244
Maxillary arteries, 165
Mean arterial pressure (MAP), 18*t*
Mean pulmonary arterial pressure (MPAP), 18*t*
Mechanical ventilation, 131, 132
Mediastinum, 97*f*
Medulla oblongata, 18, 159*f*, 162*t*, 163
Medullary center (respiratory center), 105
Megaloblastic crisis, 398
Meissner's plexus, 236, 242
Melanin, oversecretion of, in Addison's disease, 355*f*
Memory T cells, 373
Meninges, 158*f*
Meningismus, 219
Meningitis
    clinical presentation, 202
    complications, 202
    definition, 201
    diagnosis, 202
    etiology, 201
    nursing intervention in, 202
    pathophysiology, 201
Mental status, altered, suggested therapy for, 424*t*
Mentation, examination of, in acute head injury, 191, 192
Mesencephalon (midbrain), 159*f*, 161, 162*t*, 163
Mesenteric ischemia
    nonocclusive, 271, 272
    occlusive, 271, 272
Messengers, first and second, 329
Mestinon (pyridostigmine bromide), 205, 206
Metabolic acidosis
    agents that cause, 427*t*
    causes of, 124
    classification of, 124
    treatment of, 126
Metabolic alkalosis
    causes of, 124
    treatment of, 126
Metabolic disturbances, 123
Metabolic waste products, excretion of, 298, 299
Metamyelocytes, 368, 369
MI. See Myocardial infarction
Microcirculation, 76*f*
Microcirculatory system, regulation of, 76*t*
Microglia, 167
Micronodular cirrhosis, 265
Microvilli, 236, 237
Midbrain (mesencephalon), 159*f*, 160*f*, 161, 162*t*
Mineralocorticoids, 330, 353
Mitochondria, 6*f*
Mitral regurgitation, 10

Mitral valve, 5*f*, 10*f*, 11*f*
Mobitz I block, 44
Monoamines, 177
Monoclonal antibodies, 436
Monocytes, 368, 369, 399
Monosynaptic reflex arc, 177, 178*f*
Monro, foramen of, 164
"Moon face," 356
Motor function, examination of, in acute head injury, 193
Mouth, 265
Mucociliary escalator, 101, 103
Mucosa, 236
Mucous blanket, 103, 104*f*
Mucus, 233
Multiple myeloma, 409*t*
Multiple organ dysfunction syndrome, 431, 435, 438
Multisystem organ failure, 431
Munro-Kellie hypothesis, 213
Murmurs, 11, 12
Muscle spindle, 177, 178*f*
Muscularis mucosa, 236
Myasthenia gravis (and crisis), 204–206
    associated conditions, 205
    clinical presentation, 205
    complications, 206
    definition, 204
    diagnosis, 205
    etiology, 205
    nursing intervention, 206
    pathophysiology, 206
    postthymectomy, 206
    treatment, 205, 206
Myelin, 167, 179
Myelin sheath, 175, 176
Myenteric plexus, 236, 242
Myenteric reflex, 238
Myocardial failure, assessment of, 69
Myocardial infarction (MI)
    acute, 64*f*
    anterior-septal, 65*f*
    atherectomy for, 67
    inferior, 65, 67*f*
    lateral, 67*f*
    medical therapy for, 67, 68
    recovery from, 68
    thrombolytic therapy for, 66
Myocardial injury, 26
Myocardial oxygen consumption (MVO$_2$), 18
Myocardium, 4
Myoclonic seizures (bilateral myoclonus), 207, 208
Myofibrals, 5, 6*f*
Myosin, 5, 6*f*, 7*f*, 8
Myxedema, 346, 347*f*
Myxedema coma, 347, 348

Naloxone (Narcan), 436
Nasal cannula, 129
Nasopharynx, 98, 232
Nasotracheal intubation, 133
Negative base excess, 123, 124
Negatively deflected waves, 25
Negative-pressure ventilators, 131
Neoplastic disease, gastric surgery for, 275

Neostigmine (Prostigmin), 206
Nephron, 288–290
  anatomy, 288, 289
  capillary beds of, 294f
  cortical, 288f
  juxtamedullary, 289f
Nerves, cranial, 169
Nervous tissue, components of, 166–168
Neural cell
  depolarization of, 175
  repolarization of, 175
Neuroendocrine messenger, 241
Neurofibrils, 167
Neurogenic hyperventilation, spirometer pattern of central, 106f
Neuroglia, 165, 166f, 167
Neurohypophysial hormone-releasing and -inhibiting factors, 331
Neurohypophysis, 330, 331, 335, 336
Neurohypophysis, hormones of, 336, 339
Neurologic examination
  components of 423t
  in head injury, 191, 192
Neurological dysfunction, residual, 202
Neuromuscular junction, 176f
Neurons
  diagram of structures of, 166f
  shapes of, 165f
  types of, 167
Neurotransmitters, 176, 177, 241
Neutrophils, 368, 399
Nicardipine, 15t
Nicotinic acid, 179
Nissen fundoplication, 275
Nissl bodies, 167
Nitrates, 15t
Nitroglycerin, 15t
Nitroprusside, 15t, 18
Nizatidime, 234
Nodes of Ranvier, 167, 176f
Non-Hodgkin's lymphoma, 406, 408, 409
Nonionic movement, 238
Nonvolatile fixed acids, 120
  sources of, 120
Norepinephrine, 15t, 169, 177, 243, 330, 354
Normal saline, 15t
Normal sinus rhythm, 29
Nose, 97
Nosocomial infection, 375
Nuchal rigidity, 202
Nucleosus pulposis, 183
Nutrient digestion and absorption, 238
Nutritional support methods, 251
Nutritional status, interventions to maintain, 280–282

Obstruction, intestinal, 272, 273
  arterial and venous flow, 89, 90
Occipital arteries, 165
Occipital bones, 158
Occlusions, 88
Occlusive disorders, 89, 90
Oculocephalic response (doll's eyes), 223, 224f
Oculomotor nerve, 192
Oculovestibular reflex, 223, 224f
Odors, characteristic, agents with, 425t

Oligodendroglia, 167, 168
Oliguria, 313
Open pneumothorax, 145
Open tension pneumothorax, 146f
Opisthotonus, 225
Opportunistic infection, 375
Optic nerve, 192
Optic nerve fibers, 198
Optic radiation, 199
Oral cavity, 265
Oropharynx, 98, 100, 232
Orotracheal intubation, 133
Osmolarity, 296
Osmoreceptors, 235
Osmosis, 8, 295, 317
Otorrhea, 194
Ovaries, 327
Overhydration, 316
Oximetry, 119
Oxygen capacity, 117
Oxygen consumption, 117
Oxygen content, 116, 117
Oxygen extraction rate, 117
Oxygen saturation, 117
Oxygen tension, normal value, 117
Oxygen therapy, 129t, 130
Oxygen toxicity, 130
Oxygen transport, 115–117
Oxygenation, assessment of, 119
Oxygenation failure, 128
Oxygen-hemoglobin binding, 117
Oxyhemoglobin dissociation curve, 117, 118
Oxytocin, 339

PAC. *See* Premature atrial contraction
Pacemakers
  definition, 55
  electrical patterns of, 58f
  five-position pacemaker code, 57t
  indications for, 56
  modes of pacing, 55, 56
  type of pacing modes, 56
Pancreas
  anatomy, 244f, 359f
  cells, 359, 360f
  physiology, 359, 360
  secretions of, 244, 245
Pancreatectomy, 277
Pancreatic cancer, 277
Pancreaticoduodenectomy, 277
Pancreatitis, acute, 268–270
Pancreatitis, traumatic, 279
Papillac, 231
Papillary muscles, 4, 5f, 10
Paraldehyde, 211
Parasympathetic nervous system, ganglionic fibers of, 170, 173f
Parathormone, 345, 346
Parathyroid dysfunction
  clinical presentation, 350
  complications, 350
  diagnosis, 350
  etiology, 350

nursing interventions, 350
treatment, 350
Parathyroid glands
anatomy, 345*f*
chief cells and oxphil cells, 345*f*
physiology, 345, 346
Parathyroid hormone, 307, 329, 345
Parenteral nutrition, 253
Parietal cell vagotomy, 275
Parietal bones, 158
Parietal (oxyntic) cells, 234
Parkland formula, 415
Parotid gland, 243
Paroxysmal atrial tachycardia, 35*f*, 36
Paroxysmal junctional tachycardia, 43*f*
Paroxysmal supraventricular tachycardia. *See* Paroxysmal atrial
tachycardia
Passive diffusion, 238
Passive transport, 295
PCWP. *See* Pulmonary capillary wedge pressure
PEEP. *See* Positive end expiratory pressure
Pepcid (Famotidine), 256
Pepsin, 239
Peptic disease, 255
Peptide hormones, 329, 330
Peptides, 328
Peptones, 239
Perforation
esophageal, 149, 150, 280
gastrointestinal, 274
Pericardiocentesis, 149, 150*f*
Pericarditis, 72, 73
Pericardium, 4
Pericranium, 158
Perikaryon, 167
Peripheral nervous system, 157, 168
Peristaltic contractions, 238
Peristaltic waves, 232
Peritoneal dialysis, 317*f*-320
Peritoneum, 317
Peritonitis, 240, 270, 318
Pernicious anemia, 179
Pesticides, chronic obstructive pulmonary disease and, 135
Petit mal seizures, 207, 208, 210
Peyer's patches, 237
pH
defined, 120
interventions to correct, 123
of cerebrospinal fluid, 107
Phagocytosis, 368, 369, 370*f*, 399
Pharyngeal tonsils (adenoids), 100
Pharynx, 98, 99*f*, 232
Phenobarbital, 211
Phenylephrine, 15*t*
Phenytoin, 211
Pheochromocytoma, 357
Phosphate
hyperphosphatemia, 309
hypophasphatemia, 310
normal level of, 309
regulation of, 309
Phosphate buffer system, 120, 121
Phospholipase A, 244
Phosphorylation, 6

Physical assessment, 3
Physiologic shunting, causes of, 115, 116*f*
Pia mater, 158
Pitressin. *See* Antidiuretic hormone
Pituicytes, 336
Pituitary gland
anatomy of, 335, 336
anterior (master gland), 330
lobes of, 335
location, 335
physiology, 327, 330, 337
size, 335
Plasmapheresis, 204, 428
Plasmin, 388
Plateau phase. *See* Action potential, phases of
Platelet count, 380, 392
Platelet production, 379, 380
Platelet transfusions, 380
Platelets, 384
Pleura, 97, 97*f*
Pleural drainage
chest tubes, 152
system design, 152
water seal chamber, 152
Plexuses, spinal nerve
brachial, 169
cervical, 169
lumbosacral, 169
Pneumocystis carinni pneumonia, 406
Pneumotaxic breathing, 106*f*
Pneumotaxic center, 105
Pneumothorax, 133, 144, 145*f*
Poikilothermism, 188
Poisoning mortality, agents responsible for highest, 421
Poisons, 420
Pollution, COPD and, 135
Polycythemia, 136
Polymorphonuclear granulocytes, 368
Polymorphonuclear leukocytes, 399
Polysynaptic reflex arc, 177, 178, 179*f*
Pons, 159*f*, 160*f*, 162*t*, 163
Portal-hypophysial system, 331
Portal vein system, 241, 242
Portosystemic shunt surgery, 258
Positive base excess, 124
Positive end expiratory pressure (PEEP), 129–131
Positive pressure ventilators, 131, 134
Posterior hemiblock, criteria for, 50*t*
Posterior horns, 184
Postganglionic fibers, 170
Postsplenectomy sepsis syndrome, 372
Postthymectomy nursing interventions, 206
Potassium
hyperkalemia, 306
hypokalemia, 306, 307
normal levels, 305
regulation of, 305
Potassium chloride (KCl), use of, in metabolic alkalosis, 123
Potassium ions
involvement in cardiac cell cycle, 8
PR interval, 26*f*, 28
Prazosin, 15*t*
Preganglionic fibers, 169, 170
Preload, 16, 69*t*, 71, 77

Premature atrial contraction (PAC), 36, 37f
Premature junctional contraction, 42f
Premature ventricular contractions (PVC), 51, 52f, 53t
Pressoreceptors. *See* Baroreceptors
Pressure, average diastolic, 110
Pressure, average pulmonary artery systolic, 110
Pressure-controlled inverse
    ratio ventilation, 131
Pressure support ventilation, 132
Prinz metals' angina, 63, 64
Procarboxypeptidase, 245
Proenzymes, 245
Prolactin, 329
Prolactin-inhibiting hormone, 337
Propranolol hydrochloride, 349
Propranolol (Inderal), 15t
Prostacyclin, 433
Prostaglandins, 301, 328, 436
Prosthesis, Angelchick, 276
Prostigmin (Neostigmine), 206
Protein buffer system, 120, 121
Protein catabolism, 316
Protein hormones, 329, 330
Proteins, 236, 239, 328
Prothrombin (Factor II), 387
Prothrombin time (PT), 392
Proteases, 239
Proteolytic enzymes, 244
Proximal gastric vagotomy, 275
Proximal convoluted tubule, 288
PR segment, 26, 27f
Psychomotor seizures, 207, 209
PT. *See* Prothrombin time
Pulmonary air flow, 111
Pulmonary anatomy, components of, 95
Pulmonary artery systolic pressure, 110
Pulmonary blood circulation, volume and rate, 104
Pulmonary capillary wedge pressure (PCWP)
    atrial pressure and, 20
    hemodynamic assessment, use in, 17t
    in hypovolemia, 77
    LVEDP estimate, use in, 16
    normal values, 110
    use of, 69t
Pulmonary contusion, 147, 148f
Pulmonary edema, 71, 72, 103
Pulmonary embolism, 141f
    clinical presentation, 142
    complications, 142
    diagnosis, 142
    etiology, 141, 142
    massive, 142
    predisposing factors, 141, 142
    submassive, 142
    symptoms of, 90
    treatment, 142
Pulmonary fibrosis, 139
Pulmonary function, physiologic basis of, 109
Pulmonary hypertension, 141
Pulmonary laceration, 147
Pulmonary surfactant, 103
Pulmonary valve, 5f, 11f
Pulmonary vascular resistance (PVR), 17, 18t, 69t
Pulmonary veins, 19

Pulmonary ventilation, 109, 110
Pulse oximetry, 119
Pulsus paradoxus, 12, 87
(Pupil) light reflex, 222f, 223
Purkinje fibers, 13, 27
PVC. *See* Premature ventricular contraction
Pyloric sphincter, 233, 236
Pyloroplasty, 275
Pylorus, 232
Pyridostigmine bromide (Mestinon), 205, 206
Pyrixdoxine, 179
Pyrogens, 370
P wave, 25, 28, 29

QRS complex, 25, 26f, 28, 29
QRS measurement, 29
QRS, ST, and QT intervals, 27f

Radiopaque agents, 424t
Rales. *See* Crackles
Ranitidine (Zantac), 234, 255–257
Rapid ejection phase, 20
Ravier, nodes of, 167
Reabsorption atelectasis, 130
Rebreathing masks, 129
Rectum, 239, 240f
Red blood cells
    formation of, 378, 379f
    synthesis and maturation, 301
Reduced-ejection phase, 21
Reed-Sternberg cells, 408
Reflexes
    Hering-Breur (stretch), 107
    monosynaptic, 177, 178f
    polysynaptic, 177, 178
Reflux, 232
Regulatory cells, 373
Renal artery, 290
Renal erythropoietic factor, 301
Renal failure, acute, 313–316
Renal function, useful definitions for understanding, 295
Renal toxicity, common agents associated with, 424t
Renin-angiotensin-aldosterone cascade, 77
Renin-angiotensin mechanism, 300, 301
Repolarization, of neural cell, 175, 176
Residual volume, 112
Respiratory acidosis, 123, 126, 127
Respiratory alkalosis, 123, 126
    treatment of, 126
Respiratory bronchioles, appearance of in asthma, 137f
Respiratory center (medullary center), 105
Respiratory disturbances, 123
Respiratory failure, oxygenation-induced, 129t
Respiratory membrane, 114
Resting interval, 8, 9f
Resting membrane potential, 175
Resting potential, 8
Restrictive lung disease, 139
Reticular activating system (RAS), 161, 163f
Retinal fibers, 198
Retrovir (zidovidine), 406
Reye-Johnson syndrome, 214

Rhonchi. *See* Wheeze
Rhythm strip, 26, 27
Rib, 97*f*
Rib, fractures of, 143
Right atrial pressure, 16
Right atrium, 9, 10*f*
Right axis deviation, 48
Right bundle branch block, 48, 50*t*
Right bundle branches, 13
Right precordial leads, 49*f*
Right ventricle, 9, 10*f*, 19
Right ventricular end diastolic pressure, 16
Right ventricular failure, 70, 71*t*
Right ventricular performance, methods to assess, 69*t*
Right ventricular preload assessments, 17
Right ventricular pressure, 16
Right ventricular hypertrophy, criteria for, 49*t*
Right ventricular hypertrophy (RVH), 48
Rolando, fissure of, 160
R-on-T phenomenon, 52
Roto-bed, 188*f*
R-to-R intervals, 28
Rule of nines, 415*f*
Rupture
    aortic, 151*f*, 152
    diaphragmatic, 149, 150
RVEDP. *See* Right ventricular end diastolic pressure
R wave, 26–29

Sagittal suture, 158
Sacral vertebrae, 182*f*
Saline, normal, 15*t*
Saliva, 231
Salivary glands, 231, 243, 244*f*
Salivary secretions, 243
Saltatory conduction, 176*f*
SA node. *See* Sinoatrial node
Sarcolemma, 5, 6*f*
Sarcomere, 5, 6*f*, 8
Sarcoplasmic reticulum, 5, 6*f*
Scalp, 157*f*, 158, 191
Sciatic nerve, 168
Second-degree block, 44*f*, 45*f*, 46
Second messenger, 329
Secretin, 235, 245
Secretory IgA, 368
Segmental demyelination, 203
Seizures, 207–210
    classification of, 207*t*
    clinical presentation, 208, 209
    common agents causing, 423*t*
    complications, 209, 210
    definition, 207
    etiology, 208
    nursing intervention, 209, 210
    treatment, 209
Semilunar valves, 11*f*
Sengstaken-Blakemore tube, 258*f*
Sensation, examination of, in acute head injury, 193
Septa, 102
Septic shock, 438
Serotonin, 177
Shaldon catheters, 320, 323*f*

Shock, examination for, in head injury, 191
Silastic catheters, 320
Serum sickness, 376
Sex hormones, 330
Shock
    cardiogenic
        causes of, 75*t*
        symptoms of, 78*t*
    cellular hypoxia in, 75
    complications of, 77, 78
    hemorrhagic, 75
    hypovolemic
        causes of, 75*t*
        symptoms of, 78*t*
    low-SVR, 75
Shunts, for hemodialysis, 320
SIADH. *See* Syndrome of inappropriate antidiuretic hormone
Sickle-cell disease, 397, 398
Simple closed pneumothorax, 144
Sinoatrial arrest or block, 34*f*, 35
Sinoatrial node (SA node), 12, 31
Sinus arrhythmia, 31, 32*f*
Sinus bradycardia, 31, 33*f*
Sinus dysrhythmia, 31
Sinus pause/arrest, 34
Sinus tachycardia, 19, 33*f*, 34
Skin, anatomy of, 414*f*
Skull
    anatomy of, 158
    x-ray of, in head injuries, 198
Skull fractures, 193, 194*f*
Slipped disc, 183
Slit pore, 294
Small intestine
    absorption mechanisms in, 238, 239
    anatomy of, 236, 237
    glands of, 237
    movements of, 237, 238
    nutrient digestion and absorption, 238, 239
    surgery for, 276
Sneezing, 101
Sodium
    effect of aldosterone on, 303
    hypernatremia, 303, 304
        clinical presentation of, 304
        etiology, 304
    involvement in cardiac cell cycle, 8
    normal levels, 303
    regulation of, 303
Sodium bicarbonate, 245
Sodium pump, 175
Sodium threshold, 8
Soma (perikaryon), 167
Somatostatin, 359
Somatotropin. *See* Growth hormone
Somogyi effect, 363
Sounds, lung, 107
Sphenoid bones, 158
Sphincter of Oddi, 244*f*, 248
Spinal accessory nerve, 192
Spinal cord
    hyperextension of, 183*f*
    hyperflexion of, 183*f*
    location, 183

significant ascending and descending tracts, 185*f*
structure, 183, 184*f*
Spinal cord injuries
classification of, 184–186
complications, 187
metabolic needs, 189
nursing intervention, 189
Spinal ganglia, 168
Spinal ischemia, following aortic surgery, 89
Spinal nerve fibers, types of, 168
Spinal nerve plexuses, 169*f*
Spinal nerve roots, their attachment to the spinal cord, 167*f*
Spinal shock, definition of, 186
complications, 187, 189
cardiovascular system, 187
gastrointestinal system, 188
metabolic needs, 189
musculoskeletal system, 188
renal system, 187, 188
respiratory system, 187
Spirometer patterns of ventilation, 105–107
Spleen, 372
Spontaneous depolarization, 12
ST segment, 26, 27*f*
Staphylococcus aureus, 201
Staphylococcus epidermidis, 201
Starling's law, 16, 17*f*, 295
Static compliance, 111
Status asthmaticus, 136, 137
Status epilepticus
clinical presentation, 210
definition, 210
etiology, 210
incidence, 210
nursing intervention, 211
pathophysiology, 210
prognosis, 210
treatment, 210, 211
Steal syndrome, 321, 322
Stem cells, 378
Sternal fracture, 144
Sternomanibrial junction, 101
Sternum, 95, 96*f*
Steroid hormones, involvement of liver in metabolism of, 246
Steroids, 328, 329, 437
Stomach, 232–235
anatomy of, 232
capacity of, 232
divisions and curvatures, 232*f*
layers of stomach wall, 232*f*
openings of, 233
size, 232
Streptococcus pneumoniae, 136
Streptokinase, 390
Stretch receptors, 18, 235
Stroke volume, 10, 19, 16*t*, 69*t*, 70
Subarachnoid cisterns, 159
Subarachnoid hemmorhage, 195, 197
Subarachnoid monitoring, 214
Subarachnoid space, 159
Subcutaneous emphysema, 147

Subdural hematomas, 159, 194, 196*f*
Subdural space, 159
Sublingual gland, 243
Submandibular gland, 243
Sucking chest wound, 146*f*
Sucral fate (Carafate), 256
Suctioning, with artificial airways, 133
Sulci, cerebral, 160, 161*f*
Summation, 175
Supraventricular tachycardia (SVT), 43
Surfactant, pulmonary, 103
Surgery, for pulmonary embolism, 142, 143
SVR. *See* Systemic vascular resistance
Swallowing, 231, 232
S wave, 26, 29
Sylvius, Aqueduct of, 164
Sylvius, fissure of, 160
Sympathetic nervous system ganglia, 172*f*
Sympathetic regulation, 19
Sympathetic stimulation, in cardiogenic shock, 79
Syndrome of inappropriate antidiuretic hormone (SIADH), 304, 340, 341
Syneresis, 388
Syrup of ipecac, 423, 424
Systemic inflammatory response syndrome, 431
Systemic vascular resistance (SVR), 15, 17, 18*t*, 69*t*, 75
Systemic vascular response, 433

Tachycardia
atrial tachycardia, 36*f*, 37
paroxysmal atrial tachycardia, 35*f*, 36
sinus, 33*f*, 34
Tachypnea, 105, 422*t*
T-cell response, 433
Telencephalon, 159*f*, 161*f*
Temporal arteries, 165
Temporal bones, 158
Tensilon. *See* Edrophonium chloride
Tension pneumothorax, 144, 145*f*
Tentorium cerebelli, 159*f*, 163
Testes, 327
Thalamus (diencephalon), 161, 162*t*
Thiamine (Vitamin B1), 179
Third-degree block, 44, 45, 46*f*, 47
Thirst, 296, 297
Thoracic aneurysms, 88, 89
Thoracic cage, 95*f*
Thoracic vertebra, 182*f*
Thoracolumbar system. *See* sympathetic nervous system
Thrombocytopenia
causes of, 381*t*
clinical presentation, 380
treatment, 380
Thrombolytic enzymes, for pulmonary embolism, 142
Thrombopoietin, 379
Thymectomy, 206
Thymus, 372
Thyroglobulin, organification of, 344
Thyroid, 327
Thyroid gland
anatomy, 343*f*
dysfunction, 346

Thyroid hormone replacement, 347
Thyroid-stimulating hormone, 329, 343, 344
Thyroid storm, 346, 348–350
Thromlytic therapy, for myocardial infarction, 66
Thrombus, 141
Thyrotoxic crisis
  clinical presentation, 348
  complications, 348
  etiology, 348
  pathophysiology, 348
  treatment, 348, 349
Thyrotoxicosis, 348
Thyrotropin-releasing hormone, 337
Thyrotropin-releasing hormone factors, 344
Thyroxine, 328, 329, 343, 344
Tidal volume, 112
Tissue plasminogen activator, 390
Todd's paralysis, 208
Tongue, 231, 232
Tonic-clonic (grand mal) seizures, 208
Total lung capacity, 111, 112
Toxic goiter, 348
Toxicologic emergencies
  cardiovascular assessment, 421, 422*t*, 423*t*
  GI assessment, 422, 424*t*
  hepatic and renal assessment, 422, 423, 424*t*
  neurological assessment, 422, 423*t*
  patient assessment, 421
  respiratory assessment, 421, 422*t*
  seizures in, 422, 423*t*, 424*t*
  skin and mucous membrane assessment, 423, 425*t*
  treatment, 423–428
    activated charcoal, 426
    cathartics, 425, 426*t*
    emesis (syrup of ipecac), 423–425
    gastric lavage, 424, 425*t*, 426*t*
Trabeculae, 372
Trachea, 98*f*, 101, 102*f*
Tracheobronchial injuries, 151
Tracheobronchial tree, 101, 102
Tracheoesophageal fistula, 133, 134
Tracheostomy, 133
Transfusion
  cryoprecipitates, 383
  fresh frozen plasma, 383
  reactions to, 384, 385
  red blood cells (RBCs), 383
  whole blood, 383, 384
Tricuspid valve, 5*f*, 10, 11*f*
Trifascicular blocks, 48
Trigeminal nerve, 192
Triiodothyronine, 343, 344
Trochlear nerve, 192
Tropic hormones, 330
Tropomyosin, 5, 7
Troponin, 5, 7
Trousseau's sign, 269, 309
Trypsin, 135, 239, 245
Trypsinogen, 245
Tubes, endotracheal, 133
Tubular absorption and secretion, 295–298
Tubular necrosis, acute, 313

Tumor necrosis factor, 433
T wave, 26*f*
Type I and type II heart blocks, 46
Tyrosine, 344

Ulcers, 255, 275
Uncal herniation, 221, 222, 227*t*
Unstable angina, 63, 64
Upper airway, 97, 99*f*, 101
Urea, 298
Uremic signs of acute renal failure, 315*t*
Urinary output, normal, 315
Urine formation, 296*t*
Urine output, normal, 295
Ureter, 291*f*
Urethra, 291*f*
Urinary bladder, 291*f*
Urokinase, 390
U wave, 27*f*

Vagotomy, 275
Vagus nerve, 192
Valium, 210, 211
Valvular injury, 149
Vascular surgery
  aneurysm graft technique, 89*f*
  assessment of need for, 90
  indications for, 88
  postoperative considerations, 89
Vasoconstriction, 18, 19
Vasoconstrictor, 15
Vasodilation, 18, 19
Vasopressin. *See* Antidiuretic hormone
Vasopressors, 437
Venae cavae, 19
Venous emboli, 324
Venous oximetry, 119
Venous sinuses, 166
Ventilation
  alveolar, 113
  controlling factors of, 105
  factors that alter, 107
  failure, 127, 128
  physiology, 120–127
  protection of, 80
  spirometer pattern of normal, 105
Ventilation/perfusion ratios, 115
Ventilator support, complications of, 134
Ventricles, 28
Ventricular conduction defects, criteria for, 50*t*
Ventricular failure, assessment of, 69
Ventricular fibrillation, 53, 54, 55*f*
Ventricular pressure, 20*f*
Ventricular rate, 29
Ventricular tachycardia, 53, 54*f*
Vertebrae, C-1 and C-2, articulation of, 182*f*
Vertebral column, 181–183
  divisions of, 181
  typical vertebra, 181*f*
Villi, 236, 237*f*

Viral hepatitis
  hepatitis A, 261
  hepatitis B, 262
  hepatitis C, 262, 263
  hepatitis D, 262
  nursing intervention, 263
Virchow's triad, 141
Visceral injuries, 143, 147–149
Visual field defects, 198f
Visual pathway defects, 198, 199
Vital capacity, 112
Vitamin B1, (Thiamine), 179
Vitamin B12, 179
Vitamin D, 307
Vitamins
  fat-soluble, 239
  water-soluble, 239
Volatile acids, 120
Volume expanders, 384
Von Willebrand's disease, 395

Wandering atrial pacemaker, 37f
Waste products, 298, 299
Water, distribution of, through the body, 297f
Water-soluble vitamins, 239, 240
Waveform, normal arterial, 82f
Wave of depolarization, 175
Wenckebach block, 44f
Wernicke-Korsakoff syndrome, 179
Wheezes, 108, 137
Whipple's procedure, 277
White matter, 163, 179, 183, 184
Willis, circle of, 164f
Withdrawal reflex, 177
Wursung, duct of, 244, 245

Zidovidine (AZT), 406
Zona fasciculata, 351, 352f
Zona glomerulosa, 351, 352f
Zona reticularis, 351, 352f
Zymogenic (chief) cells, 234